REHABILITATION TECHNIQUES
in Sports Medicine

REHABILITATION TECHNIQUES
in Sports Medicine

Second Edition

WILLIAM E. PRENTICE, Ph.D., P.T., A.T.,C.
Professor, Coordinator of the Sports Medicine Program
Department of Physical Education, Exercise and Sport Science
Clinical Professor, Division of Physical Therapy
Department of Medical Allied Professions
Associate Professor of Orthopedics
School of Medicine
The University of North Carolina,
Chapel Hill, North Carolina

Director of Sports Medicine Education and Fellowship Programs
HEALTHSOUTH Rehabilitation Corporation,
Birmingham, Alabama

with 661 *illustrations*

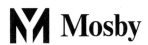 Mosby

St. Louis Baltimore Boston Chicago London Madrid Philadelphia Sydney Toronto

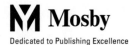

Mosby

Dedicated to Publishing Excellence

Editor-in-Chief: James M. Smith
Acquisitions Editor: Vicki Malinee
Developmental Editor: Wendy Schiff
Project Manager: Carol Sullivan Wiseman
Production Editor: Shannon Canty
Designer: Betty Schulz
Cover Design: GW Graphics & Publishing

SECOND EDITION

Printed in the United States of America
Composition by Graphic World, Inc.
Printing/binding by R.R. Donnelley & Sons Company

Mosby–Year Book, Inc.
11830 Westline Industrial Drive
St. Louis, Missouri 63146

Library of Congress Cataloging-in-Publication Data
Rehabilitation techniques in sports medicine   /   [edited by] William E.
    Prentice.—2nd ed.
        p.   cm.
    Includes bibliographical references and index.
    ISBN 0-8016-7675-4
    1. Sports—Accidents and injuries—Patients—Rehabilitation.
    2. Sports physical therapy.   I. Prentice, William E.
RD97.R44 1993
617.1´027—dc20   93-35546
                                                                    CIP

93 94 95 96 97 / 9 8 7 6 5 4 3 2 1

Preface

One of the primary goals of every sports medicine professional is to create a playing environment for the athlete that is as safe as it can possibly be. Regardless of that effort, the nature of athletic participation dictates that injuries will eventually occur. Fortunately, few of the injuries that occur in an athletic setting are life-threatening. The majority of the injuries are not serious and lend themselves to rapid rehabilitation. When injuries do occur the focus of the sports therapist shifts from injury prevention to injury treatment and rehabilitation.

The process of rehabilitation begins immediately after injury. Initial first aid and management techniques can have substantial impact on the course and ultimate outcome of the rehabilitative process. In a sports medicine setting, the athletic trainer and/or physical therapist generally assumes the primary responsibility for design, implementation, and supervision of the rehabilitation program for the injured athlete. Thus, in addition to possessing sound understanding of how injuries can be prevented, the sports therapist must also be competent in providing correct and appropriate initial care when injury does occur.

Designing programs for rehabilitation is relatively simple and involves several basic short-term goals: 1) controlling pain, 2) maintaining or improving flexibility, 3) returning or increasing strength, 4) reestablishing neuromuscular control, and 5) maintaining levels of cardiorespiratory fitness. The long-term goal is to return the injured athlete to practice or competition as quickly and safely as possible. This is the easy part of supervising a rehabilitation program. The difficult part comes in knowing exactly when and how to change or alter the rehabilitation protocols to most effectively accomplish both long- and short-term goals.

The approach to rehabilitation in a sports medicine environment is considerably different than in most other rehabilitation settings. The competitive nature of athletics necessitates an aggressive approach to rehabilitation. Since the competitive season in most sports is relatively short, the athlete does not have the luxury of being able to simply sit around and do nothing until the injury heals. Their goal is to return to activity as soon as safely possible. Thus the sports therapist who is supervising the rehabilitation program must perform a balancing act walking along a thin line between not pushing the athlete hard enough or fast enough and being overly aggressive. In either case, a mistake in judgment on the part of the sports therapist may hinder the athlete's return to activity.

Decisions as to when and how to alter and progress a rehabilitation program should be based within the framework of the healing process. The sports therapist must possess a sound understanding of both the sequence and time frames for the various phases of healing, realizing that certain physiological events must occur during each of the phases. Anything that is done during a rehabilitation program that interferes with this healing process will likely increase the length of time required for rehabilitation and slow return to full activity. The healing process must have an opportunity to accomplish what it is supposed to. At best the sports therapist can only try to create an environment that is conducive to the healing process. There is little that can be done to speed up the process physiologically, but there are many things that may be done during rehabilitation to impede healing.

The sports therapist has many tools at his/her disposal that can facilitate the rehabilitative process. How they choose to utilize those tools is often a matter of individual preference and experience. Additionally, each individual patient is a little different, and their response to various treatment protocols is somewhat variable. Thus it is impossible to "cookbook" specific protocols that can be followed like a recipe. In fact, use of rehabilitation "recipes" should be strongly discouraged. Instead the sports therapist must develop a broad theoretical knowledge base from which specific techniques of rehabilitation may be selected and practically applied to each individual case.

EXPERT CONTRIBUTORS

As the art and science of sports medicine becomes more sophisticated and specialized, the need arises for textbooks that deal with specific aspects of sports injury management. Rehabilitation is certainly one of the major areas of responsibility for the sports therapist. For the classroom instructor there are a number of texts available that present a general overview of the various aspects of sports medicine. However, in the past many instructors have relied on a collection of handout materials that deal with information specific to rehabilitation techniques to be used in advanced courses. The contributing authors have attempted to combine their expertise and knowledge to produce a single text that encompasses all aspects of rehabilitation in a sports medicine setting.

This second edition of *Rehabilitation Techniques in Sports Medicine* is for the student of sports medicine who is interested in gaining more in-depth exposure to the theory and practical application of rehabilitation techniques in a sports medicine environment.

The purpose of this text is to provide the sports therapist with a comprehensive guide to the design, implementation and supervision of rehabilitation programs for sport-related injuries. It is intended for use in advanced courses in sports medicine that deal with practical application of theory in a clinical setting.

ORGANIZATION

The text is essentially divided into two sections. The first seventeen chapters describe the healing process and discuss the various techniques and theories on which rehabilitation protocols should be based. New chapters on the use of isokinetic exercise, plyometric exercise, closed-kinetic chain exercise, cardiorespiratory fitness, and one on proprioception, kinesthesia, joint position sense, and neuromuscular control have been added. Separate chapters devoted to proprioceptive neuromuscular facilitation techniques (PNF) and to aquatic therapy have been added.

Chapters 18 through 26 discuss the practical application of the theoretical basis for rehabilitation relative to specific regional anatomical areas. Included are chapters concerning the rehabilitation of injuries to the spine, the shoulder, the elbow, the wrist and hand, the hip and thigh, the knee, the lower leg, the ankle, and finally the foot. Each chapter briefly identifies the pathophysiology of the various injuries fol-

lowed by a discussion of potential techniques of rehabilitation that may be applied relative to different phases of the healing process.

Thus, the second edition of *Rehabilitation Techniques in Sports Medicine* has been significantly expanded and updated to offer a comprehensive reference and guide on sports injury rehabilitation to the sports therapist overseeing programs of rehabilitation.

COMPREHENSIVE COVERAGE OF RESEARCH BASED MATERIAL

Relative to some of the other health-care specializations, sports medicine is still in its infancy. Growth dictates the necessity for expanding our research efforts to identify new and more effective methods and techniques for dealing with sport-related injury. Any sports therapist charged with the responsibility of supervising a rehabilitation program knows that the most currently accepted and up-to-date rehabilitation protocols tend to change rapidly. A sincere effort has been made by the contributing authors to present the most recent information on the various aspects of injury rehabilitation currently available from the literature.

Additionally, this manuscript has been critically reviewed by selected athletic trainers and physical therapists who are well respected clinicians, educators, and researchers in this field to further ensure that the material presented is accurate and current.

PERTINENT TO SPORTS MEDICINE

There are many texts currently available that deal with the subject of rehabilitation of injury in various patient populations. However, the second edition of this text concentrates exclusively on the application of rehabilitation techniques in a sport-related setting. The emphasis on sports medicine makes this text somewhat unique.

PEDAGOGICAL AIDS

The aids provided in this text to assist the student in its use include the following:

Objectives. These are listed at the beginning of each individual chapter to identify the concepts to be presented.

Figures and Tables. The number of figures and tables included throughout the text has been significantly increased in an effort to provide as much visual and graphic demonstration of specific rehabilitation techniques and exercises as possible.

Summary. Each chapter has a summary that outlines the major points presented.

References. A comprehensive list of up-to-date references is provided at the end of each chapter to provide additional information relative to chapter content.

ACKNOWLEDGEMENTS

The preparation of the manuscript for a textbook is long term and extremely demanding of effort that requires input and cooperation on the part of many different individuals.

I would like to personally thank each of the contributing authors. They were asked to contribute to this text because I have tremendous respect for them both personally and professionally. These individuals have distinguished themselves as educators and clinicians dedicated to the field of sports medicine. I am exceedingly grateful for their input.

Wendy Schiff, my developmental editor at Mosby, has been persistent and diligent in the completion of this text. She has patiently encouraged me along, and I certainly have appreciated her support.

Shannon Canty, my production editor, has been diligent in her attention to essential details in the production process. I rely heavily on, and appreciate, her expertise.

The following individuals have invested a significant amount of time and energy as reviewers for this manuscript, and I appreciate their efforts.

William D. Bandy, Ph.D., P.T., SCS, A.T., C.
University of Central Arkansas

Neil Curtis, M.S., A.T., C.
William Patterson College

Steve Dickoff-Hoffman, M.S., P.T., SCS, A.T., C.
North Hills Orthopedic and Sports Physical Therapy

Magie Lacambra, M.Ed., A.T., C.
Arizona State University

Christine Stopka, Ph.D., A.T., C.
University of Florida

Steve Tippett, M.D., P.T., SCS, A.T., C.
Great Plains Sports Medicine and Rehabilitation Center

Lori A. Thein, M.S., P.T., SCS, A.T., C.
University of Wisconsin

Finally, and most importantly this is for Tena, Brian, and Zachary, who make it all worth it.

William E. Prentice

Contributors

John Marc Davis, P.T., A.T., C.
Physical Therapist/Athletic Trainer
Division of Sports Medicine
The University of North Carolina
Chapel Hill, North Carolina

Bernard DePalma, M.Ed., P.T., A.T., C.
Head Athletic Trainer
Cornell University
Ithaca, New York

Danny T. Foster, M.A., A.T., C.
Associate Director of Athletic Training Services
Curriculum Director of Athletic Training Education
The University of Iowa
Iowa City, Iowa

Joe Gieck, Ed.D, P.T., A.T., C.
Associate Professor, Department of Human Services,
    Curry School of Education
Assistant Clinical Professor, Department of
    Orthopaedics and Rehabilitation
Head Athletic Trainer
The University of Virginia
Charlottesville, Virginia

Steven A. Dickoff-Hoffman, M.S., P.T., A.T., C., SCS
Director
North Hills Orthopedic and Sports Physical
    Therapy
Sewickley, Pennsylvania

Daniel N. Hooker, Ph.D., P.T., SCS, A.T., C.
Coordinator of Athletic Training
The University of North Carolina
Chapel Hill, North Carolina

Patsy Huff, B.S. Pharm.
Director of the Pharmacy, Student Health Service
Clinical Assistant Professor, School of Pharmacy
The University of North Carolina
Chapel Hill, North Carolina

Stuart L. (Skip) Hunter, P.T., A.T., C.
Director, Clemson Physical Therapy
Clemson, South Carolina

Scott M. Lephart, Ph.D., A.T., C.
Director, Athletic Training/Sports Medicine
    Program
Assistant Professor, Education
Assistant Professor of Orthopaedic Surgery
University of Pittsburgh
Pittsburgh, Pennsylvania

Gina Lorence-Konin, P.T., A.T., C.
Physical Therapist/Athletic Trainer, Pike Creek
    Sports Medicine Center Physical Therapy,
    Wilmington, Delaware
Adjunct Professor, Delaware Technical and
    Community College, Wilmington, Delaware
Clinical Supervisor, University of Delaware,
    Newark, Delaware

Michael McGee, M.A., A.T., C.
Director of Sports Medicine
Instructor, Department of Physical Education,
    Lenoir Rhyne
Hickory, North Carolina

Julie Ann Moyer, Ed.D., P.T., A.T., C.
Clinical Assistant Professor, Thomas Jefferson
    University, Philadelphia, Pennsylvania
Adjunct Professor, University of Delaware, Newark,
    Delaware
Adjunct Professor, Delaware Technical and
    Community College, Wilmington, Delaware
Director, Pike Creek Sports Medicine Center
    Physical Therapy, Wilmington, Delaware

Janine Oman, M.S., P.T., A.T., C.
Athletic Trainer/Physical Therapist
The University of North Carolina
Chapel Hill, North Carolina

David H. Perrin, Ph.D., A.T., C.

Director, Graduate Athletic Training Program
Associate Professor, Curry School of Education
The University of Virginia
Charlottesville, Virginia

William E. Prentice, Ph.D., P.T., A.T., C.

Professor, Coordinator of the Sports Medicine
    Program, Department of Physical Education,
    Exercise, and Sport Science
Clinical Professor, Division of Physical Therapy
Department of Medical Allied Professions
Associate Professor, Department of Orthopedics
School of Medicine
The University of North Carolina
Chapel Hill, North Carolina

Director, Sports Medicine Education and
    Fellowship Programs
HEALTHSOUTH Rehabilitation Corporation
Birmingham, Alabama

Rich Reihl, M.A., A.T., C.

Head Athletic Trainer
Adjunct Faculty, Department of Sports Medicine
Pepperdine University
Malibu, California

Gina Selepak, M.A., A.T., C.

Athletic Trainer
Deerfield Academy
Deerfield, Massachusetts

Lori A. Thein, M.S., P.T., SCS, A.T., C.

University of Wisconsin Sports Medicine Center
Madison, Wisconsin

Steve Tippett, M.S., P.T., SCS, A.T., C.

Director, Great Plains Sports Medicine and
    Rehabilitation Center
Peoria, Illinois

Michael L. Voight, M.Ed, P.T., A.T., C., SCS

Director, Berkshire Institute of Orthopedic and
    Sports Physical Therapy
Wyomissing, Pennsylvania
Instructor, Department of Orthopaedics, Division of
    Physical Therapy
University of Miami
Coral Gables, Florida

Contents

The Healing Process and the Pathophysiology of Musculoskeletal Injuries

1

William E. Prentice

OBJECTIVES

After completion of this chapter, the student should be able to do the following:

- Describe the pathophysiology of the healing process.

- Identify those factors that may impede the healing process.

- Identify the four types of tissue in the human body.

- Discuss the etiology and pathology of various musculoskeletal injuries associated with various types of tissue.

- Discuss the healing process relative to specific musculoskeletal structures.

- Explain the importance of initial first aid and injury management of these injuries and their impact on the rehabilitation process.

Rehabilitation of sports-related injuries requires some knowledge and understanding of the etiology and pathology involved in various musculoskeletal injuries that may occur.[4,31,53] When injury occurs, the sports therapist is charged with designing, implementing, and supervising the rehabilitation program. Rehabilitation protocols and progressions must be based primarily on the physiological responses of the tissues to injury and on an understanding of how various tissues heal. Thus the sports therapist must understand the healing process to effectively supervise the rehabilitative process. This chapter discusses the healing process relative to the various musculoskeletal injuries that may be encountered in a sports medicine setting.

UNDERSTANDING THE HEALING PROCESS

Rehabilitation programs must be based on the framework of the healing process. The sports therapist must have a sound understanding of that process in terms of the sequence of the various phases of healing that take place. Decisions on how and when to alter and progress a rehabilitation program should be primarily based on recognition of signs and symptoms, as well as some awareness of the time frames associated with the various phases of healing.[1,38]

Basically the healing process consists of the inflammatory response phase, the fibroblastic-repair phase, and the maturation-remodeling phase. It must be stressed that although the phases of healing are presented as three separate entities, the healing process is a continuum. Phases of the healing process overlap one another and have no definitive beginning or end points.[17]

Inflammatory Response Phase

Once a tissue is injured, the process of healing begins immediately[5] (Figure 1-1, *A*). The destruction of tissue produces direct injury to the cells of the various soft tissues. Cellular injury results in altered metab-

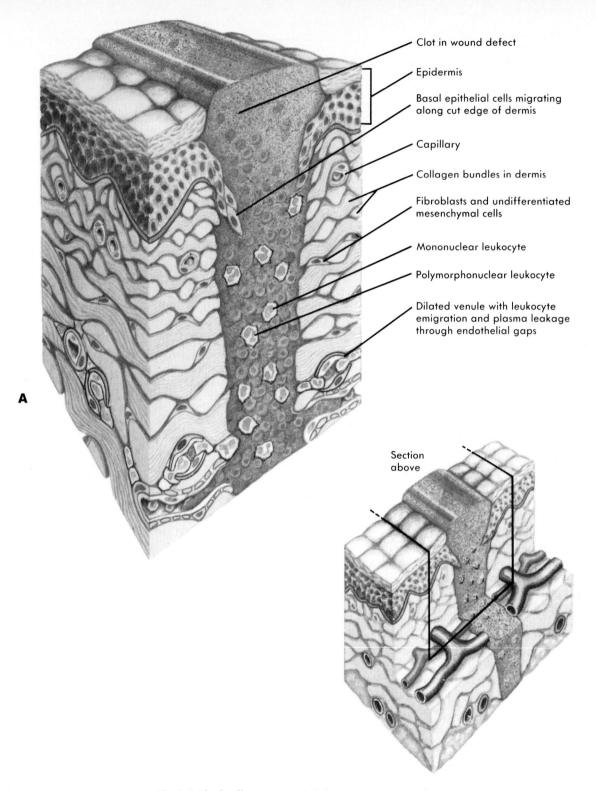

Clot in wound defect

Epidermis

Basal epithelial cells migrating along cut edge of dermis

Capillary

Collagen bundles in dermis

Fibroblasts and undifferentiated mesenchymal cells

Mononuclear leukocyte

Polymorphonuclear leukocyte

Dilated venule with leukocyte emigration and plasma leakage through endothelial gaps

A

Section above

Fig. 1-1. The healing process. A, Inflammatory response phase.

olism and the liberation of materials that initiate the inflammatory response. It is characterized symptomatically by redness, swelling, tenderness, and increased temperature.[8,35]

Inflammation is a process through which **leukocytes** and other **phagocytic cells** and exudate are delivered to the injured tissue. This cellular reaction is generally protective, tending to localize or dispose of injury by-products (for example, blood and damaged cells) through phagocytosis and thus setting the stage for repair. Locally vascular effects, disturbances of fluid exchange, and migration of leukocytes from the blood to the tissues occur.

The vascular reaction involves vascular spasm, formation of a platelet plug, blood coagulation, and growth of fibrous tissue.[51] The immediate response to damage is a vasoconstriction of the vascular walls that lasts for approximately 5 to 10 minutes. This spasm presses the opposing endothelial linings together to produce a local anemia that is rapidly replaced by hyperemia of the area due to dilation. This increase in blood flow is transitory and gives way to slowing of the flow in the dilated vessels, which then progresses to stagnation and stasis. The initial effusion of blood and plasma lasts for 24 to 36 hours.

Three chemical mediators, **histamine, leukotaxin,** and **necrosin,** are important in limiting the amount of exudate and thus swelling after injury. Histamine released from the injured mast cells causes vasodilation and increased cell permeability, owing to swelling of endothelial cells and then separation between the cells. Leucotaxin is responsible for margination in which leukocytes line up along the cell walls. It also increases cell permeability locally, thus affecting passage of the fluid and white blood cells through cell walls via diapedesis to form exudate. Therefore vasodilation and active hyperemia are important in exudate (plasma) formation and supplying leukocytes to the injured area. Necrosin is responsible for phagocytic activity. The amount of swelling that occurs is directly related to the extent of vessel damage.

Platelets do not normally adhere to the vascular wall. However, injury to a vessel disrupts the endothelium and exposes the collagen fibers. Platelets adhere to the collagen fibers to create a sticky matrix on the vascular wall, to which additional platelets and leukocytes adhere and eventually form a plug. These plugs obstruct local lymphatic fluid drainage and thus localize the injury response.

The initial event that precipitates clot formation is the conversion of **fibrinogen** to **fibrin.** This transformation occurs because of a cascading effect beginning with the release of a protein molecule called **thromboplastin** from the damaged cell. Thromboplastin causes **prothrombin** to be changed into **thrombin,** which in turn causes the conversion of fibrinogen into a very sticky fibrin clot that shuts off blood supply to the injured area. Clot formation begins around 12 hours after injury and is completed within 48 hours.

As a result of a combination of these factors, the injured area becomes walled off during the inflammatory stage of healing. The leukocytes phagocytize most of the foreign debris toward the end of the inflammatory phase, setting the stage for the fibroblastic phase. This initial inflammatory response lasts for approximately 2 to 4 days after initial injury.

CHRONIC INFLAMMATION. A distinction must be made between the acute inflammatory response as described previously and chronic inflammation. Chronic inflammation occurs when the acute inflammatory response does not eliminate the injuring agent and restore tissue to its normal physiological state. Chronic inflammation involves the replacement of leukocytes with **macrophages, lymphocytes,** and **plasma cells.** These cells accumulate in a highly vascularized and innervated loose connective tissue matrix in the area of injury.[34]

The specific mechanisms that convert an acute inflammatory response to a chronic inflammatory response are to date unknown, however, they seem to be associated with situations that involve overuse or overload with cumulative microtrauma to a particular structure.[16,34] Likewise there is no specific time frame in which the classification of acute is changed to chronic inflammation.

Fibroblastic-Repair Phase

During the fibroblastic phase of healing, proliferative and regenerative activity leading to scar formation and repair of the injured tissue follows the vascular and exudative phenomena of inflammation[27] (Figure 1-1, *B*). The period of scar formation referred to as *fibroplasia* begins within the first few hours after injury and may last for as long as 4 to 6 weeks. During this period, many of the signs and symptoms associated with the inflammatory response subside. The athlete may still indicate some tenderness to touch and will usually complain of pain when particular movements stress the injured structure. As scar for-

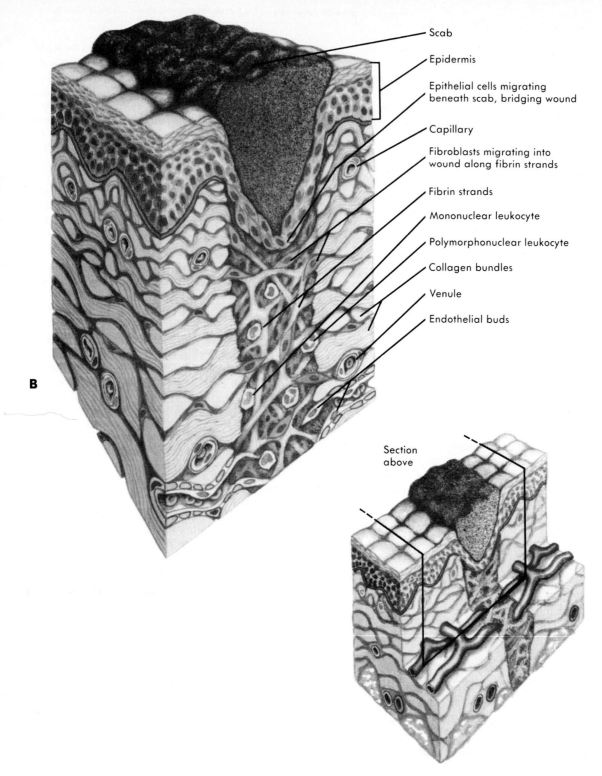

Scab

Epidermis

Epithelial cells migrating beneath scab, bridging wound

Capillary

Fibroblasts migrating into wound along fibrin strands

Fibrin strands

Mononuclear leukocyte

Polymorphonuclear leukocyte

Collagen bundles

Venule

Endothelial buds

B

Section above

Fig. 1-1, cont'd. B, Fibroblastic-repair phase.

mation progresses, complaints of tenderness or pain gradually disappear.[48]

During this phase, growth of endothelial capillary buds into the wound is stimulated by a lack of oxygen, after which the wound is capable of healing aerobically. Along with increased oxygen delivery comes an increase in blood flow, which delivers nutrients essential for tissue regeneration in the area.[9]

The formation of a delicate connective tissue called *granulation tissue* occurs with the breakdown of the fibrin clot. Granulation tissue consists of **fibroblasts,** collagen, and capillaries. It appears as a reddish granular mass of connective tissue that fills in the gaps during the healing process.

As the capillaries continue to grow into the area, fibroblasts accumulate at the wound site, arranging themselves parallel to the capillaries. Fibroblastic cells begin to synthesize an **extracellular matrix** that contains protein fibers of **collagen** and **elastin,** a **ground substance** that consists of nonfibrous proteins called *proteoglycans,* **glycosaminoglycans,** and fluid. On about day 6 or 7, fibroblasts also begin producing collagen fibers that are deposited in a random fashion throughout the forming scar. As the collagen continues to proliferate, the tensile strength of the wound rapidly increases in proportion to the rate of collagen synthesis. As the tensile strength increases, the number of fibroblasts diminishes to signal the beginning of the maturation phase.

This normal sequence of events in the repair phase leads to the formation of minimal scar tissue. Occasionally, a persistent inflammatory response and continued release of inflammatory products can promote extended fibroplasia and excessive fibrogenesis that can lead to irreversible tissue damage.[58] Fibrosis can occur in synovial structures as with adhesive capsulitis in the shoulder, in extraarticular tissues including tendons and ligaments, in bursa, or in muscle.

Maturation-Remodeling Phase

The maturation-remodeling phase of healing is a long-term process (Figure 1-1,*C*). This phase features a realignment or remodeling of the collagen fibers that make up scar tissue according to the tensile forces to which that scar is subjected. Ongoing breakdown and synthesis of collagen occur with a steady increase in the tensile strength of the scar matrix. With increased stress and strain the collagen fibers realign in a position of maximum efficiency parallel to the lines of tension. The tissue gradually assumes normal appearance and function, although a scar is rarely as strong as the normal injured tissue. Usually by the end of approximately 3 weeks, a firm, strong, contracted, nonvascular scar exists. The maturation phase of healing may require several years to be totally complete.

THE ROLE OF PROGRESSIVE CONTROLLED MOBILITY IN THE MATURATION PHASE. Wolff's law states that bone and soft tissue will respond to the physical demands placed on them, causing them to remodel or realign along lines of tensile force.[61] Therefore it is critical that injured structures be exposed to progressively increasing loads, particularly during the remodeling phase. Controlled mobilization is superior to immobilization for scar formation, revascularization, muscle regeneration, and reorientation of muscle fibers and tensile properties in animal models.[64] However, immobilization of the injured tissue during the inflammatory response phase will likely facilitate the process of healing by controlling inflammation, thus reducing clinical symptoms. As healing progresses to the repair phase, controlled activity directed toward return to normal flexibility and strength should be combined with protective support or bracing.[30] Generally, clinical signs and symptoms disappear at the end of this phase.

As the remodeling phase begins, aggressive active range-of-motion and strengthening exercises should be incorporated to facilitate tissue remodeling and realignment. To a great extent, pain will dictate rate of progression. With initial injury, pain is intense and tends to decrease and eventually subside altogether as healing progresses. Any exacerbation of pain, swelling, or other clinical symptoms during or after a particular exercise or activity indicates that the load is too great for the level of tissue repair or remodeling. The sports therapist must be aware of the time required for the healing process and realize that being overly aggressive can interfere with that process.

Factors That Impede Healing

EXTENT OF INJURY. The nature or amount of the inflammatory response is determined by the extent of the tissue injury. **Microtears** of soft tissue involve only minor damage and are most often associated with overuse. **Macrotears** involve significantly greater destruction of soft tissue and result in clinical symptoms and functional alterations. Macrotears are generally caused by acute trauma.[30]

EDEMA. The increased pressure caused by swelling

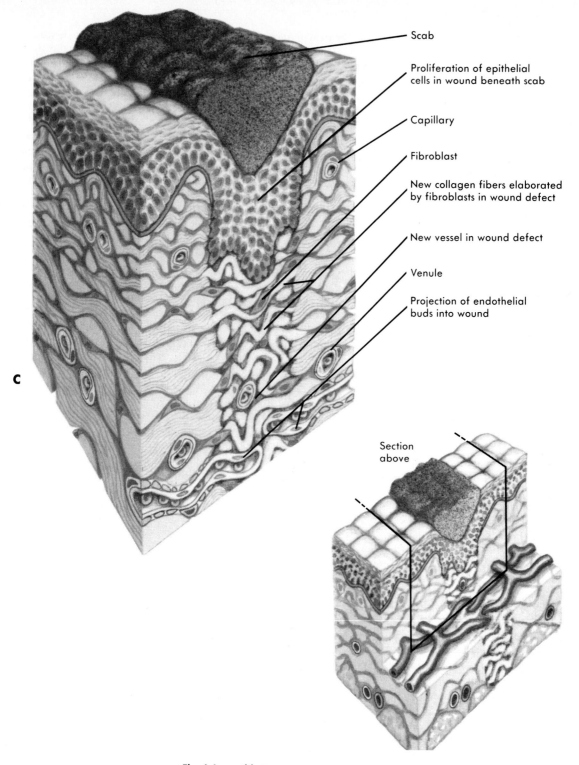

Scab

Proliferation of epithelial cells in wound beneath scab

Capillary

Fibroblast

New collagen fibers elaborated by fibroblasts in wound defect

New vessel in wound defect

Venule

Projection of endothelial buds into wound

Section above

Fig. 1-1, cont'd. C, Maturation-remodeling phase.

retards the healing process, causes separation of tissues, inhibits neuromuscular control, produces reflexive neurological changes, and impedes nutrition in the injured part. Edema is best controlled and managed during the initial first-aid management period as described previously.[7]

HEMORRHAGE. Bleeding occurs with even the smallest amount of damage to the capillaries. Bleeding produces the same negative effects on healing as does the accumulation of edema, and its presence produces additional tissue damage and thus exacerbation of the injury.

POOR VASCULAR SUPPLY. Injuries to tissues with a poor vascular supply heal poorly and at a slow rate. This response is likely related to a failure in the initial delivery of phagocytic cells and fibroblasts necessary for scar formation.

SEPARATION OF TISSUE. Mechanical separation of tissue can significantly impact the course of healing. A wound that has smooth edges that are in good apposition will tend to heal by primary intention with minimal scarring. Conversely, a wound that has jagged, separated edges must heal by secondary intention, with granulation tissue filling the defect and excessive scarring.[49]

MUSCLE SPASM. Muscle spasm causes traction on the torn tissue, separates the two ends, and prevents approximation. Local and generalized ischemia may result from spasm.

ATROPHY. Wasting away of muscle tissue begins immediately with injury. Strengthening and early mobilization of the injured structure retard atrophy.

CORTICOSTEROIDS. Use of corticosteroids in the treatment of inflammation is controversial. Steroid use in the early stages of healing has been demonstrated to inhibit fibroplasia, capillary proliferation, collagen synthesis, and increases in tensile strength of the healing scar. Their use in the later stages of healing and with chronic inflammation is debatable.

KELOIDS AND HYPERTROPHIC SCARS. Keloids occur when the rate of collagen production exceeds the rate of collagen breakdown during the maturation phase of healing. This process leads to hypertrophy of scar tissue, particularly around the periphery of the wound.

INFECTION. The presence of bacteria in the wound can delay healing, causes excessive granulation tissue, and frequently causes large, deformed scars.[24]

HUMIDITY, CLIMATE, AND OXYGEN TENSION. Humidity significantly influences the process of epithelization. Occlusive dressings stimulate the epithelium to migrate twice as fast without crust or scab formation. The formation of a scab occurs with dehydration of the wound and traps wound drainage, which promotes infection. Keeping the wound moist provides an advantage for the necrotic debris to go to the surface and be shed.

Oxygen tension relates to the neovascularization of the wound, which translates into optimal saturation and maximal tensile strength development. Circulation to the wound can be affected by ischemia, venous stasis, hematomas, and vessel trauma.

HEALTH, AGE, AND NUTRITION. The elastic qualities of the skin decrease with aging. Degenerative diseases, such as diabetes and arteriosclerosis, also become a concern of the older athlete and may affect wound healing. Nutrition is important for wound healing. In particular, vitamins C (collagen synthesis and immune system), K (clotting), and A (immune system); zinc for the enzyme systems; and amino acids play critical roles in the healing process.

PATHOPHYSIOLOGY OF HEALING RELATIVE TO VARIOUS BODY TISSUES

There are four types of fundamental tissues in the human body: epithelial, connective, muscular, and nervous[56] (Table 1-1). According to Guyton, all tissues of the body can be defined as soft tissue except bone.[25] Cailliet, however, more technically defines **soft tissue** as the matrix of the human body comprised of cellular elements within a ground substance. Furthermore, Cailliet believes that soft tissue is the most common site of functional impairment of the musculoskeletal system.[6] Therefore most sports-related injuries occur to the soft tissues. With this in mind, soft tissue structure is explained and bone structure is briefly described in this chapter.[36]

Epithelial Tissue

The first fundamental tissue is epithelial tissue (Figure 1-2). This specific tissue covers all internal and external body surfaces and therefore encompasses structures such as the skin, the outer layer of the internal organs, and the inner lining of the blood vessels and glands. A basic purpose of epithelial tissue, as presented by Fahey, is to protect and form structure for other tissues and organs.[15] In addition, this tissue functions in absorption (for example, in the digestive tract) and secretion (as in glands). A principal physiological characteristic of epithelial tissue

TABLE 1-1
Tissues

Tissue	Location	Function
EPITHELIAL		
Simple squamous	Alveoli of lungs	Absorption by diffusion of respiratory gases between alveolar air and blood
	Lining of blood and lymphatic vessels	Absorption by diffusion, filtration, and osmosis
Stratified squamous	Surface of lining of mouth and esophagus	Protection
	Surface of skin (epidermis)	
Simple columnar	Surface layer of lining of stomach, intestines, and parts of respiratory tract	Protection; secretion; absorption
Stratified transitional	Urinary bladder	Protection
CONNECTIVE (most widely distributed of all tissues)		
Areolar	Between other tissues and organs	Connection
Adipose (fat)	Under skin	Protection
	Padding at various points	Insulation; support; reserve food
Dense fibrous	Tendons; ligaments	Flexible but strong connection
Bone	Skeleton	Support; protection
Cartilage	Part of nasal septum; covering articular surfaces of bones; larynx; rings in trachea and bronchi	Firm but flexible support
	Disks between vertebrae	
	External ear	
Blood	Blood vessels	Transportation
MUSCLE		
Skeletal (striated voluntary)	Muscles that attach to bones	Movement of bones
	Eyeball muscles	Eye movements
	Upper third of esophagus	First part of swallowing
Cardiac (striated involuntary)	Wall of heart	Contraction of heart
Visceral (nonstriated involuntary or smooth)	In walls of tubular viscera of digestive, respiratory, and genitourinary tracts	Movement of substances along respective tracts
	In walls of blood vessels and large lymphatic vessels	Changing of diameter of blood vessels
	In ducts of glands	Movement of substances along ducts
	Intrinsic eye muscles (iris and ciliary body)	Changing of diameter of pupils and shape of lens
	Arrector muscles of hairs	Erection of hairs (gooseflesh)
NERVOUS		
	Brain; spinal cord; nerves	Irritability; conduction

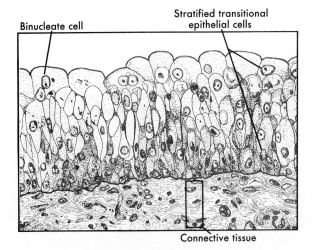

Binucleate cell

Stratified transitional epithelial cells

Connective tissue

Fig. 1-2. Epithelial cells exist in several layers.

is that it contains no blood supply per se, so it must depend on the process of diffusion for nutrition, oxygenation, and elimination of waste products. Most sports-related injuries to this type of tissue are traumatic, including abrasions, lacerations, punctures, and avulsions. Other injuries to this tissue may include infection, inflammation, or disease.

Connective Tissue

The functions of connective tissue in the body are to support, provide a framework, fill space, store fat, help repair tissues, produce blood cells, and protect against infection. It consists of various types of cells separated from one another by some type of extracellular matrix. This matrix consists of fibers and ground substance and may be solid, semisolid, or fluid. The primary types of connective tissue cells are **macrophages,** which function as phagocytes to clean up debris; **mast cells,** which release chemicals (histamine and heparin) associated with inflammation; and the **fibroblasts,** which are the principal cells of the connective tissue.

Fibroblasts produce collagen and elastin found in varying proportions in different connective tissues. Collagen is a major structural protein that forms strong, flexible, inelastic structures that hold connective tissue together. Collagen enables a tissue to resist mechanical forces and deformation. Elastin, however, produces highly elastic tissues that assist in recovery from deformation. Collagen fibrils are the

load-bearing elements of connective tissue. They are arranged to accommodate tensile stress but are not as capable of resisting shear or compressive stress. Consequently the direction of orientation of collagen fibers is along lines of tensile stress.

Collagen has several mechanical and physical properties that allow it to respond to loading and deformation, permitting it to withstand high tensile stress. The mechanical properties of collagen include elasticity, which is the capability to recover normal length after elongation; viscoelasticity, which allows for slow return to normal length and shape after deformation; and plasticity, which allows for permanent change or deformation. The physical properties include force-relaxation, which indicates the decrease in the amount of force needed to maintain a tissue at a set amount of displacement or deformation over time; the creep response, which is the ability of a tissue to deform over time while a constant load is imposed; and hysteresis, which is the amount of relaxation a tissue has undergone during deformation and displacement. If the mechanical and physical limitations of connective tissue are exceeded, injury results.

There are several different types of connective tissue.[3,28,52] **Fibrous connective tissue** is composed of strong collagenous fibers that bind tissues together. There are two types of fibrous connective tissue. **Dense connective tissue** is composed primarily of collagen and is found in tendons, fascia, aponeurosis, ligaments, and joint capsule. **Tendons** connect muscles to bone. An **aponeurosis** is a thin, sheetlike tendon. A **fascia** is a thin membrane of connective tissue that surrounds individual muscles and tendons or muscle groups. **Ligaments** connect bone to bone. All synovial joints are surrounded by a **joint capsule,** which is a type of connective tissue similar to a ligament. The orientations of collagen fibers in ligaments and joint capsules are less parallel than in tendons. **Loose connective tissue** forms many types of thin membranes found beneath the skin, between muscles, and between organs. **Adipose tissue** is a specialized form of loose connective tissue that stores fat, insulates, and acts as a shock absorber. The blood supply to fibrous connective tissue is relatively poor, so healing and repair are slow processes.

Cartilage is a type of rigid connective tissue that provides support and acts as a framework in many structures. It is composed of chondrocyte cells contained in small chambers called *lacunae* surrounded completely by an intracellular matrix. The matrix consists of varying ratios of collagen and elastin and a ground substance made of proteoglycans and glycosaminoglycans, which are nonfibrous protein molecules. These proteoglycans act as sponges and trap large quantities of water, which allows cartilage to spring back after being compressed. Cartilage has a poor blood supply, thus healing after injury is very slow. There are three types of cartilage. **Hyaline cartilage** is found on the articulating surfaces of bone and in the soft part of the nose. It contains large quantities of collagen and proteoglycan. **Fibrocartilage** forms the intervertebral disks and menisci located in several joint spaces. It has greater amounts of collagen than proteoglycan and is capable of withstanding a great deal of pressure. **Elastic cartilage** is found in the auricle of the ear and the larynx. It is more flexible than the other types of cartilage and consists of collagen, proteoglycan, and elastin.

Reticular connective tissue is also composed primarily of collagen. It provides the support structure of the walls of various internal organs including the liver and kidneys.

Elastic connective tissue is composed primarily of elastic fibers. It is found primarily in the walls of blood vessels, airways, and hollow internal organs.

Bone is a type of connective tissue consisting of both living cells and minerals deposited in a matrix (Figure 1-3). Each bone consists of three major components. The **epiphysis** is an expanded portion at each end of the bone that articulates with another bone. Each articulating surface is covered by an articular or **hyaline** cartilage. The **diaphysis** is the shaft of the bone. The **epiphyseal** or **growth plate** is the major site of bone growth and elongation. Once bone growth ceases, the plate ossifies and forms the epiphyseal line. With the exception of the articulating surfaces, the bone is completely enclosed by the **periosteum,** a tough, highly vascularized and innervated fibrous tissue.

The two types of bone material are **cancellous,** or spongy, bone and **cortical,** or compact, bone. Cancellous bone contains a series of air spaces referred to as *trabeculae,* whereas cortical bone is relatively solid. Cortical bone in the diaphysis forms a hollow **medullary canal** in long bone, which is lined with **endosteum** and filled with bone **marrow.** Bone has a rich blood supply that certainly facilitates the healing process after injury. Bone has the functions of support, movement, and protection. Furthermore, bone stores and releases calcium into the bloodstream and manufactures red blood cells.

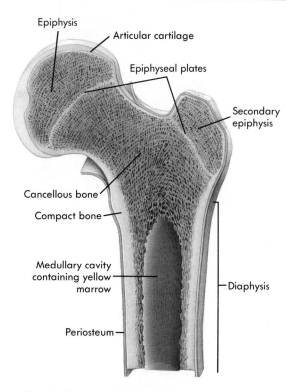

Fig. 1-3. Structure of bone shown in cross-section.

One other type of connective tissue in the body is **blood.** Blood is composed of various cells suspended in a fluid intracellular matrix referred to as *plasma.* Plasma contains red blood cells, white blood cells, and platelets. Although this component does not function in structure, it is essential for the nutrition, cleansing, and physiology of the body.

Injuries to Connective Tissue

With connective tissue playing such a major role throughout the human body, it is not surprising that many sports-related injuries involve structures composed of connective tissue. Although tendons are classified as connective tissue, injuries to tendons and tendon healing will be incorporated into the discussion of the musculotendinous unit.

LIGAMENT SPRAINS. A sprain involves damage to a ligament that provides support to a joint. A ligament is a tough, relatively inelastic band of tissue that connects one bone to another.

Before discussing injuries to ligaments, a review of joint structure is in order[43] (Figure 1-4). All **synovial**

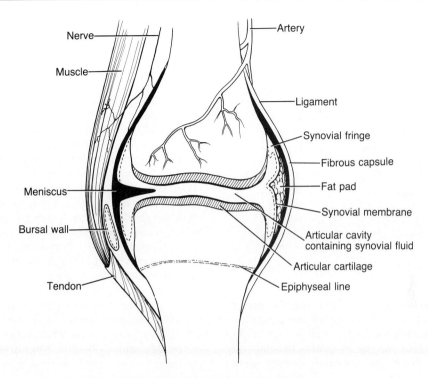

Fig. 1-4. Structure of a synovial joint.

joints are composed of two or more bones that artic-ulate with one another to allow motion in one or more places. The articulating surfaces of the bone are lined with a very thin, smooth, cartilaginous covering called a *hyaline cartilage*. All joints are entirely surrounded by a thick, ligamentous **joint capsule.** The inner sur-face of this joint capsule is lined by a very thin **syno-vial membrane** that is highly vascularized and inner-vated. The synovial membrane produces **synovial fluid,** the functions of which include lubrication, shock absorption, and nutrition of the joint.

Some joints contain a thick fibrocartilage called a *meniscus.* The knee joint, for example, contains two wedge-shaped menisci that deepen the articulation and provide shock absorption in that joint. Finally, the main structural support and joint stability is pro-vided by the ligaments, which may be either thick-ened portions of a joint capsule or totally separate bands. Ligaments are composed of dense connective tissue arranged in parallel bundles of collagen com-posed of rows of fibroblasts. Although bundles are arranged in parallel, not all collagen fibers are ar-ranged in parallel.

Ligaments and tendons are very similar in struc-ture. However, ligaments are usually more flattened than tendons, and collagen fibers in ligaments are more compact. The anatomical positioning of the lig-aments determines in part what motions a joint can make.

If stress is applied to a joint that forces motion beyond its normal limits or planes of movement, in-jury to the ligament is likely[12] (Figure 1-5). The se-verity of damage to the ligament is classified in many different ways; however, the most commonly used system involves three degrees of ligamentous sprain.

- First-degree sprain: There is some stretching or perhaps tearing of the ligamentous fibers with little or no joint instability. Mild pain, little swell-ing, and joint stiffness may be apparent.
- Second-degree sprain: There is some tearing and separation of the ligamentous fibers and mod-erate instability of the joint. Moderate-to-severe pain, swelling, and joint stiffness should be ex-pected.
- Third-degree sprain: There is total rupture of the ligament, manifested primarily by gross insta-

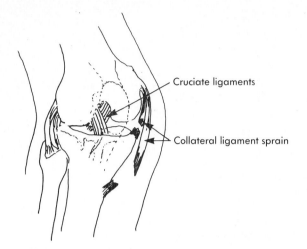

Cruciate ligaments

Collateral ligament sprain

Fig. 1-5. Example of a ligament sprain in the knee joint.

bility of the joint. Severe pain may be present initially, followed by little or no pain due to total disruption of nerve fibers. Swelling may be profuse, and thus the joint tends to become very stiff some hours after the injury. A third-degree sprain with marked instability usually requires some form of immobilization lasting several weeks. Frequently the force producing the ligament injury is so great that other ligaments or structures surrounding the joint may also be injured. With cases in which there is injury to multiple joint structures, surgical repair or reconstruction may be necessary to correct an instability.

Ligament healing. The healing process in the sprained ligament follows the same course of repair as with other vascular tissues. Immediately after injury and for approximately 72 hours there is a loss of blood from damaged vessels and attraction of inflammatory cells into the injured area.

During the next 6 weeks, vascular proliferation with new capillary growth begins to occur along with fibroblastic activity, resulting in the formation of a fibrin clot. Synthesis of collagen and ground substance of proteoglycan as constituents of an intracellular matrix contributes to the proliferation of the scar. Collagen fibers are initially arranged in a random woven pattern with little organization. Gradually there is a decrease in fibroblastic activity, a decrease in vascularity, and an increase to a maximum in collagen density of the scar.[2]

Over the next several months the scar continues to mature with the realignment of collagen occurring in response to progressive stresses and strains. The maturation of the scar may require as long as 12 months to complete.[2] The exact length of time required for maturation depends on mechanical factors such as apposition of torn ends and length of immobilization.

Surgically repaired extraarticular ligaments have healed with decreased scar formation and are generally stronger than unrepaired ligaments initially, although this strength advantage may not be maintained as time progresses. Nonrepaired ligaments heal by fibrous scarring effectively lengthening the ligament and producing some degree of joint instability. With intraarticular ligament tears the presence of synovial fluid dilutes the hematoma, thus preventing formation of a fibrin clot and spontaneous healing.[28]

Several studies have shown that actively exercised ligaments are stronger than those that are immobilized. Ligaments that are immobilized for periods of several weeks after injury tend to decrease in tensile strength and also exhibit weakening of the insertion of the ligament to bone.[44] Thus it is important to minimize periods of immobilization and progressively stress the injured ligaments while exercising caution relative to biomechanical considerations for specific ligaments.[2,42]

It is not likely that the inherent stability of the joint provided by the ligament before injury will be regained. Thus to restore stability to the joint, the other structures that surround that joint, primarily muscles and their tendons, must be strengthened. The increased muscle tension provided by strength training can improve stability of the injured joint.[54,55]

BONE FRACTURES. Fractures are extremely common injuries among the athletic population. They can be generally classified as being either **open** or **closed.** A closed fracture involves little or no displacement of bones and thus little or no soft tissue disruption. An open fracture involves enough displacement of the fractured ends that the bone actually disrupts the cutaneous layers and breaks through the skin. Both fractures can be relatively serious if not managed properly, but an increased possibility of infection exists in an open fracture. Fractures may also be considered complete, in which the bone is broken into at least two fragments, or incomplete, where the fracture does not extend completely across the bone.

The varieties of fractures that can occur include greenstick, transverse, oblique, spiral, comminuted, impacted, avulsive, and stress. A **greenstick** fracture

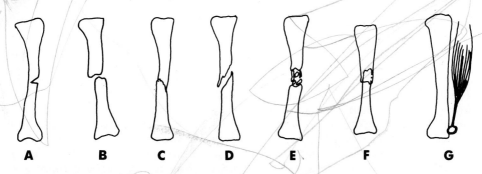

Fig. 1-6. Fractures of bone. **A,** Greenstick; **B,** transverse; **C,** oblique; **D,** spiral; **E,** comminuted; **F,** impacted; **G,** avulsion.

(Figure 1-6, *A*) occurs most often in children whose bones are still growing and have not yet had a chance to calcify and harden. It is called a *green-stick fracture* because of the resemblance to the splintering that occurs to a tree twig that is bent to the point of breaking. Because the twig is green, it splinters but can be bent without causing an actual break.

A **transverse** fracture (Figure 1-6, *B*) involves a crack perpendicular to the longitudinal axis of the bone that goes all the way through the bone. Displacement may occur; however, because of the shape of the fractured ends, the soft tissue (for example, muscles, tendons, and fat) that surrounds it sustains relatively little damage. A **linear** fracture runs parallel to the long axis of a bone and is similar in severity to a transverse fracture.

An **oblique** fracture (Figure 1-6, *C*) results in a diagonal crack across the bone and two very jagged, pointed ends that, if displaced, can potentially cause a good bit of soft tissue damage. Oblique and spiral fractures are the two types most likely to result in compound fractures.

A **spiral** fracture (Figure 1-6, *D*) is similar to an oblique fracture in that the angle of the fracture is diagonal across the bone. In addition, an element of twisting or rotation causes the fracture to spiral along the longitudinal axis of the bone. Spiral fractures used to be fairly common in ski injuries occurring just above the top of the boot when the bindings on the ski failed to release when the foot was rotated. These injuries are now less common due to improvements in equipment design.

A **comminuted** fracture (Figure 1-6, *E*) is a serious problem that may require an extremely long time for rehabilitation. In the comminuted fracture, multiple fragments of bone must be surgically repaired and fixed with screws and wires. If a fracture of this type

occurs to a weight-bearing bone, as in the leg, a permanent discrepancy in leg length may develop.

In an **impacted** fracture (Figure 1-6, *F*), one end of the fractured bone is driven up into the other end. As with the comminuted fracture, correcting discrepancies in the length of the extremity may require long periods of intensive rehabilitation.

An **avulsion** fracture (Figure 1-6, *G*) occurs when a fragment of bone is pulled away at the bony attachment of a muscle, tendon, or ligament. Avulsion fractures are common in the fingers and some of the smaller bones but can also occur in larger bones whose tendinous or ligamentous attachments are subjected to a large amount of force.

Perhaps the most common fracture resulting from physical activity is the **stress fracture.** Unlike the other types of fractures that have been discussed, the stress fracture results from overuse or fatigue rather than acute trauma.[33,40] Common sites for stress fractures include the weight-bearing bones of the leg and foot. In either case, repetitive forces transmitted through the bones produce irritations and microfractures at a specific area in the bone. The pain usually begins as a dull ache that becomes progressively more painful day after day. Initially, pain is most severe during activity. However, when a stress fracture actually develops, pain tends to become worse after the activity is stopped.

The biggest problem with a stress fracture is that often it does not show up on an x-ray film until the osteoblasts begin laying down subperiosteal callus or bone, at which point a small white line, or a callus, appears. However, a bone scan may reveal a potential stress fracture in as little as 2 days after onset of symptoms. If a stress fracture is suspected, the athlete should stop any activity that produces added stress or fatigue to the area for a minimum of 14 days. Stress fractures do not usually require casting but may become normal fractures that must be immobilized if handled incorrectly. If a fracture occurs, it should be managed and rehabilitated by a qualified orthopedist and sports therapist.

Bone healing. Healing of injured bone tissue is similar to soft tissue healing in that all phases of the healing process may be identified, although bone regeneration capabilities are somewhat limited. However, the functional elements of healing differ significantly from those of soft tissue. Tensile strength of the scar is the single most critical factor in soft tissue healing, whereas bone has to contend with a number of additional forces including torsion, bending, and compression.[18] Trauma to bone may vary from contusions of the periosteum to closed, nondisplaced fractures to severely displaced open fractures that also involve significant soft tissue damage. When a fracture occurs, blood vessels in the bone and the periosteum are damaged, resulting in bleeding and subsequent clot formation. Hemorrhaging from the marrow is contained by the periosteum and the surrounding soft tissue in the region of the fracture. In about 1 week, fibroblasts have begun laying down a fibrous collagen network. The fibrin strands within the clot serve as the framework for proliferating vessels. **Chondroblast** cells begin producing fibrocartilage, creating a **callus** between the broken bones. At first, the callus is soft and firm because it is composed primarily of collagenous fibrin. The callus becomes firm and more rubbery as cartilage begins to predominate. Bone producing cells called ***osteoblasts*** begin to proliferate and enter the callus, forming cancellous bone trabeculae, which eventually replace the cartilage. Finally the callus crystalizes into bone, at which point remodeling of the bone begins. The callus can be divided into two portions, the external callus located around the periosteum on the outside of the fracture and the internal callus found between the bone fragments. The size of the callus is proportional both to the damage and to the amount of irritation to the fracture site during the healing process. Also during this time, **osteoclasts** begin to appear in the area to resorb bone fragments and clean up debris.[28,52]

The remodeling process is similar to the growth process of bone in that the fibrous cartilage is gradually replaced by fibrous bone and then by more structurally efficient lamellar bone. Remodeling involves an ongoing process during which osteoblasts lay down new bone and osteoclasts remove and break down bone according to the forces placed upon the healing bone.[60] Wolff's law maintains that a bone will adapt to mechanical stresses and strains by changing size, shape, and structure. Therefore, once the cast is removed, the bone must be subjected to normal stresses and strains so that tensile strength may be regained before the healing process is complete.[23,57]

The time required for bone healing is variable and based on a number of factors such as severity of the fracture, site of the fracture, extensiveness of the trauma, and age of the patient. Normal periods of immobilization range from as short as 3 weeks for the small bones in the hands and feet to as long as 8 weeks for the long bones of the upper and lower extremities. In some instances, for example, the four small toes, immobilization may not be required for healing. The healing process is certainly not complete when the splint or cast is removed. Osteoblastic and osteoclastic activity may continue for 2 to 3 years after severe fractures.

OSTEOARTHROSIS. Osteoarthrosis needs to be mentioned because it is a degenerative condition of bone and cartilage in and about the joint. **Arthritis** should be defined as primarily an inflammatory condition with possible secondary destruction. **Arthrosis** is primarily a degenerative process with destruction of cartilage, remodeling of bone, and possible secondary inflammatory components.

Cartilage fibrillates, that is, releases fibers or groups of fibers and ground substance into the joint. Peripheral cartilage that is not exposed to weight-bearing or compression-decompression mechanisms is particularly likely to fibrillate. Fibrillation is typically found in the degenerative process associated with poor nutrition or disuse. This process can then extend even to weight-bearing areas with progressive destruction of cartilage proportional to stresses applied on it. When forces are increased, thus increasing stress, osteochondral or subchondral fractures can occur. Concentration of stress on small areas may produce pressures that overwhelm the tissue's capabilities. Typically, lower limb joints have to handle greater stresses, but their surface area is usually larger than the surface area of upper limbs. The articular cartilage is protected to some extent by the synovial fluid, which acts as a lubricant. It is also protected by the subchondral bone, which responds to stresses in an elastic fashion. It is more compliant than compact bone, and microfractures may be a means of force absorption. Trabeculae may fracture or may be displaced due to pressures applied on the subchondral bone. In compact bone, fracture may be a means of defense to dissipate force. In the joint also, forces may be absorbed by joint movement and eccentric contraction of muscles.

In the majority of joints where the surfaces are not congruent, the applied forces tend to concentrate in certain areas, which favors joint degeneration. Osteophytosis is a response of bone to increase its surface area. Typically people describe this growth as "bone spurs." Chondromalacia is the nonprogressive transformation of cartilage with irregular surfaces and areas of softening. Typically it occurs in nonweight–bearing areas at first and may progress to areas of excessive stress.

In athletes, certain joints may be more susceptible to a response resembling osteoarthrosis.[46] The proportion of body weight resting on the joint, the pull of musculotendinous tissue, and any significant external force applied to the joint are predisposing factors. Altered joint mechanics caused by laxity or previous trauma are also factors that come into play. The intensity of forces may be great, as in the hip, where the above-mentioned factors can produce pressures or forces that may be four times that of body weight and up to ten times that of body weight on the knee.

Typically, muscle forces generate more stress than body weight itself. Particular injuries are conducive to osteoarthritic changes such as subluxation and dislocation of the patella, osteochondritis dissecans, recurrent synovial effusion, and hemarthrosis. Also, ligamentous injuries may bring about a disruption of proprioceptive mechanisms, loss of adequate joint alignment, and meniscal damage in the knees with removal of the injured meniscus.[26] Other factors that have an impact are loss of full range of motion, poor muscular power and strength, and altered biomechanics on the joint. Different joints are affected in different sports: the knee and ankle in European football, the hand in boxing, the shoulder and elbow in baseball, and the patella in cycling. This list is not exhaustive. In sports participation, however, spurring and spiking of bone are not synonymous with osteoarthrosis if the joint space is maintained and the cartilage lining is intact. It may simply be an adaptation to the increased stress of physical activity.

Cartilage healing. Cartilage has a relatively limited healing capacity. When chondrocytes are destroyed and the matrix is disrupted, the course of healing is variable, depending on whether damage is to cartilage alone or also to subchondral bone. Injuries to articular cartilage alone fail to elicit clot formation or a cellular response. For the most part the chondrocytes adjacent to the injury are the only cells that show any signs of proliferation and synthesis of matrix. Thus the defect fails to heal, although the extent of the damage tends to remain the same.[20,39]

If subchondral bone is also affected, inflammatory cells enter the damaged area and formulate granulation tissue. In this case, the healing process proceeds normally with differentiation of granulation tissue cells into chondrocytes occurring in about 2 weeks. At approximately 2 months normal collagen has been formed.

Muscle Tissue

Muscle tissue is often considered to be a type of connective tissue, but here it is treated as the third of the fundamental tissues. Muscle tissue is designed to contract and thus provide movement of other tissues and organs. The three types of muscles are smooth (involuntary), cardiac, and skeletal (voluntary). **Smooth muscle** is found within the viscera, where it forms the walls of the internal organs, and within many hollow chambers. **Cardiac muscle** is found only in the heart and is responsible for its contraction. A significant characteristic of the cardiac muscle is that it contracts as a single fiber, unlike smooth and skeletal muscles, which contract as separate units. This characteristic forces the heart to work as a single unit continuously; therefore if one portion of the muscle should die (as in myocardial infarction), the entire contraction of the heart does not cease.

Skeletal muscle is the striated muscle within the body responsible for the movement of bony levers (Figure 1-7). Skeletal muscle consists of two portions: (1) the muscle belly and (2) its tendons, which are collectively referred to as a *musculotendinous unit*. The muscle belly is composed of separate, parallel elastic fibers called *myofibrils*. Myofibrils are composed of thousands of small **sarcomeres,** which are the functional units of the muscle. Sarcomeres contain the contractile elements of the muscle, as well as a substantial amount of connective tissue that holds the fibers together. **Myofilaments** are small contractile elements of protein within the sarcomere. There are two distinct types of myofilaments: thin **actin** myofilaments and thicker **myosin** myofilaments. Fingerlike projections, or **crossbridges,** connect the actin and myosin myofilaments. When a muscle is stimulated to contract, the crossbridges pull the myofilaments closer together, thus shortening the muscle

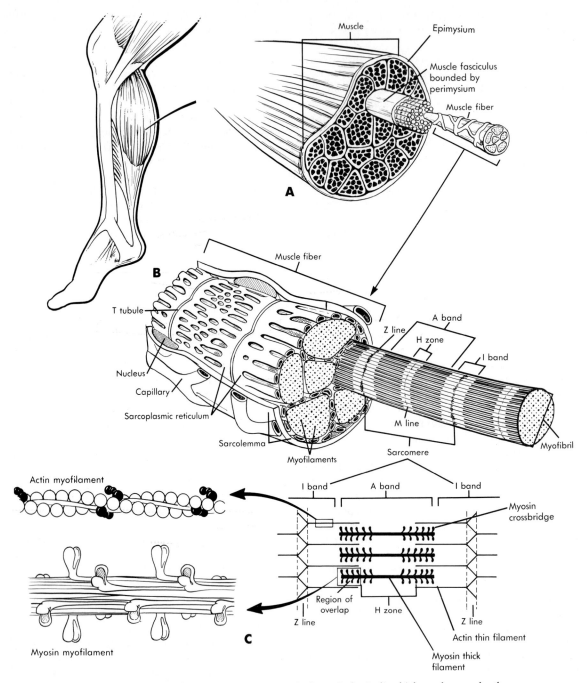

Fig. 1-7. Parts of a muscle. A, Muscle is composed of muscle fasciculi, which can be seen by the unaided eye as striations in the muscle. The fasciculi are composed of bundles of individual muscle fibers (muscle cells). **B,** Each muscle fiber contains myofibrils in which the banding patterns of the sarcomeres are seen. **C,** The myofibrils are composed of actin myofilament and myosin myofilaments, which are formed from thousands of individual actin and myosin molecules.

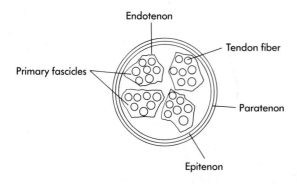

Fig. 1-8. Structure of a tendon.

and producing movement at the joint that the muscle crosses.[16]

The **muscle tendon** attaches muscle directly to bone. The muscle tendon is composed primarily of collagen fibers and a matrix of proteoglycan, which is produced by the **tenocyte** cell. The collagen fibers are grouped together into **primary bundles.** Groups of primary bundles join together to form hexagonal shaped **secondary bundles.** Secondary bundles are held together by intertwined loose connective tissue containing elastin called the *endotenon.* The entire tendon is surrounded by a connective tissue layer called the *epitenon.* The outermost layer of the tendon is the **paratenon,** which is a double layer connective tissue sheath lined on the inside with synovial membrane (Figure 1-8).

All skeletal muscles exhibit four characteristics: (1) the ability to change in length or stretch, elasticity; (2) the ability to shorten and return to normal length, extensibility; (3) the ability to respond to stimulation from the nervous system, excitability; and (4) the ability to shorten and contract in response to some neural command, contractility.

Skeletal muscles show considerable variation in size and shape. Large muscles generally produce gross motor movements at large joints, such as knee flexion produced by contraction of the large, bulky hamstring muscles. Smaller skeletal muscles, such as the long flexors of the fingers, produce fine motor movements. Muscles producing movements that are powerful in nature are usually thicker and longer, whereas those producing finer movements requiring coordination are thin and relatively shorter. Other muscles may be flat, round, or fan-shaped.[28,52]

Muscles may be connected to bone by a single tendon or by two or three separate tendons at either end. Those muscles that have two separate muscle and tendon attachments are called *biceps,* and those muscles with three separate muscle and tendon attachments are called *triceps.*

Muscles contract in response to stimulation by the central nervous system. An electrical impulse transmitted from the central nervous system through a single motor nerve to a group of muscle fibers causes a depolarization of those fibers. The motor nerve and the group of muscle fibers that it innervates are referred to collectively as a ***motor unit.*** An impulse coming from the central nervous system and traveling to a group of fibers through a particular motor nerve causes all the muscle fibers in that motor unit to depolarize and contract. This is referred to as the ***all-or-none*** response and applies to all skeletal muscles in the body.[28]

Injuries to Musculotendinous Structures

STRAINS. If a musculotendinous unit is overstretched or forced to contract against too much resistance exceeding the extensibility limits or the tensile capabilities of the weakest component within the unit, damage may occur to the muscle fibers, at the musculotendinous juncture, in the tendon, or at the tendinous attachment to the bone.[21,29] Any of these injuries may be referred to as a ***strain*** (Figure 1-9). Muscles strains, like ligament sprains, are subject to various classification systems. The following is a simple system of classification of muscle strains:

- First-degree strain: Some muscle or tendon fibers have been stretched or actually torn. Active motion produces some tenderness and pain. Movement is painful, but full range of motion is usually possible.
- Second-degree strain: Some muscle or tendon fibers have been torn, and active contraction of the muscle is extremely painful. Usually a palpable depression or divot exists somewhere in the muscle belly at the spot where the muscle fibers have been torn. Some swelling may occur because of capillary bleeding.
- Third-degree strain: There is a complete rupture of muscle fibers in the muscle belly, in the area where the muscle becomes tendon, or at the tendinous attachment to the bone. The athlete has significant impairment to or perhaps total loss of movement. Pain is intense initially but diminishes quickly because of complete separation of the nerve fibers. Musculotendinous

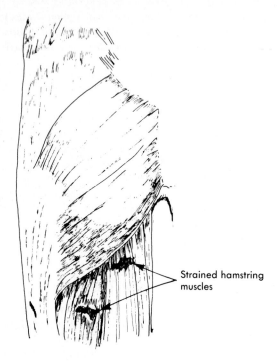

Fig. 1-9. A muscle strain results in tearing or separation of fibers.

Strained hamstring muscles

ruptures are most common in the biceps tendon of the upper arm or in the Achilles heelcord in the back of the calf. When either of these tendons rupture, the muscle tends to bunch toward its proximal attachment. With the exception of an Achilles rupture, which is frequently surgically repaired, the majority of third-degree strains are treated conservatively with some period of immobilization.

Muscle healing. Injuries to muscle tissue involve similar processes of healing and repair as discussed with other tissues. Initially there will be hemorrhage and edema followed almost immediately by phagocytosis to clear debris. Within a few days there is a proliferation of ground substance, and fibroblasts begin producing a gel-type matrix that surrounds the connective tissue, leading to fibrosis and scarring. At the same time, myoblastic cells form in the area of injury, which will eventually lead to regeneration of new myofibrils. Thus regeneration of both connective tissue and muscle tissue has begun.[62]

Collagen fibers undergo maturation and orient themselves along lines of tensile force according to

Wolff's law. Active contraction of the muscle is critical in regaining normal tensile strength.

Regardless of the severity of the strain, the time required for rehabilitation is fairly lengthy. In many instances, rehabilitation time for a muscle strain is longer than for a ligament sprain. These incapacitating muscle strains occur most frequently in the large, force-producing hamstring and quadriceps muscles of the lower extremity. The treatment of hamstring strains requires a healing period of at least 6 to 8 weeks and a considerable amount of patience. Trying to return to activity too soon frequently causes reinjury to the area of the musculotendinous unit that has been strained, and the healing process must begin again.

TENDINITIS. Of all the overuse problems associated with physical activity, tendinitis is among the most common. **Tendinitis** is a catch-all term that can describe many different pathological conditions of a tendon. It essentially describes any inflammatory response within the tendon without inflammation of the paratenon. The term *paratenonitis* describes inflammation of the outer layer of the tendon only and usually occurs when the tendon rubs over a bony prominence. **Tendinosis** describes a tendon that has significant degenerative changes with no clinical or histological signs of an inflammatory response.[11]

In cases of what is most often called *chronic tendinitis,* there is evidence of significant tendon degeneration, loss of normal collagen structure, loss of cellularity in the area, but absolutely no inflammatory cellular response in the tendon. The inflammatory process is an essential part of healing. Inflammation is supposed to be a brief process with an end point after its function in the healing process has been fulfilled. The point or the cause in the pathological process where the acute inflammatory cellular response terminates and the chronic degeneration begins has not been determined. As mentioned previously, with chronic tendinitis the cellular response involves a replacement of leukocytes with macrophages and plasma cells.

During muscle activity a tendon must move or slide on other structures around it whenever the muscle contracts. If a particular movement is performed repeatedly, the tendon becomes irritated and inflamed. This inflammation is manifested by pain on movement, swelling, possibly some warmth, and usually crepitus. Crepitus is a crackling sound similar to the sound produced by rolling hair between the fingers by the ear. Crepitus is usually caused by the adherance of the paratenon to the surrounding structures while it slides back and forth. This adhesion is caused primarily by the chemical products of inflammation that accumulate on the irritated tendon.[11]

The key to treating tendinitis is rest. If the repetitive motion causing irritation to the tendon is eliminated, chances are the inflammatory process will allow the tendon to heal. Unfortunately, an athlete who is seriously involved with some physical activity may have difficulty in resting for 2 weeks or more while the tendinitis subsides. Antiinflammatory medications and therapeutic modalities are also helpful in reducing the inflammatory response. An alternative activity, such as bicycling or swimming, is necessary to maintain fitness levels to a certain degree while allowing the tendon a chance to heal.

Tendinitis most commonly occurs in the Achilles tendon in the back of the lower leg in runners or in the rotator cuff tendons of the shoulder joint in swimmers or throwers, although it can certainly flare up in any tendon in which overuse and repetitive movements occur.

TENOSYNOVITIS. Tenosynovitis is very similar to tendinitis in that the muscle tendons are involved in inflammation. However, many tendons are subject to an increased amount of friction due to the tightness of the space through which they must move. In these areas of high friction, tendons are usually surrounded by synovial sheaths that reduce friction on movement. If the tendon sliding through a synovial sheath is subjected to overuse, inflammation is likely to occur. The inflammatory process produces by-products that are "sticky" and tend to cause the sliding tendon to adhere to the synovial sheath surrounding it.

Symptomatically, tenosynovitis is very similar to tendinitis, with pain on movement, tenderness, swelling, and crepitus. Movement may be more limited with tenosynovitis because the space provided for the tendon and its synovial covering is more limited. Tenosynovitis occurs most commonly in the long flexor tendons of the fingers as they cross over the wrist joint and in the biceps tendon around the shoulder joint. Treatment for tenosynovitis is the same as for tendinitis. Because both conditions involve inflammation, mild antiinflammatory drugs, such as aspirin, may be helpful in chronic cases.

Tendon healing. Unlike most soft tissue healing, tendon injuries pose a particular problem in rehabilitation. The injured tendon requires dense fibrous union of the separated ends and extensibility and flexibility at the site of attachment. Thus an abundance of collagen is required to achieve good tensile strength. Unfortunately, collagen synthesis can become excessive, resulting in fibrosis, in which adhesions form in surrounding tissues and interfere with the gliding that is essential for smooth motion. Fortunately, over a period of time the scar tissue of the surrounding tissues becomes elongated in its structure because of a breakdown in the cross-links between fibrin units and thus allows the necessary gliding motion. A tendon injury that occurs where the tendon is surrounded by a synovial sheath can be potentially devastating.

A typical time frame for tendon healing would be that during the second week the healing tendon adheres to the surrounding tissue to form a single mass. During the third week, the tendon separates to varying degrees from the surrounding tissues. However, the tensile strength is not sufficient to permit a strong pull on the tendon for at least 4 to 5 weeks, the danger being that a strong contraction can pull the tendon ends apart.

Nerve Tissue

The final fundamental tissue is nerve tissue (Figure 1-10). This tissue provides sensitivity and communication from the central nervous system (brain and spinal cord) to the muscles, sensory organs, various systems, and the periphery. The basic nerve cell is the neuron. The neuron cell body contains a large **nucleus** and branched extensions called *dendrites,* which respond to neurotransmitter substances released from other nerve cells. From each nerve cell arises a single **axon,** which conducts the nerve impulses. Large axons found in peripheral nerves are enclosed in sheaths composed of **Schwann cells,** which are tightly wound around the axon. A nerve is a bundle of nerve cells held together by some connective tissue, usually a lipid-protein layer called the *myelin sheath* on the outside of the axon. Neurology is an extremely complex science, and only a brief presentation of its relevance to sports-related injuries is covered here.

INJURIES TO NERVES. In a sports medicine setting, nerve injuries usually involve either contusions or inflammations. More serious injuries involve the crushing of a nerve or complete division (severing). This type of injury may produce a life-long physical disability, such as paraplegia or quadriplegia, and should therefore not be overlooked in any circumstance.

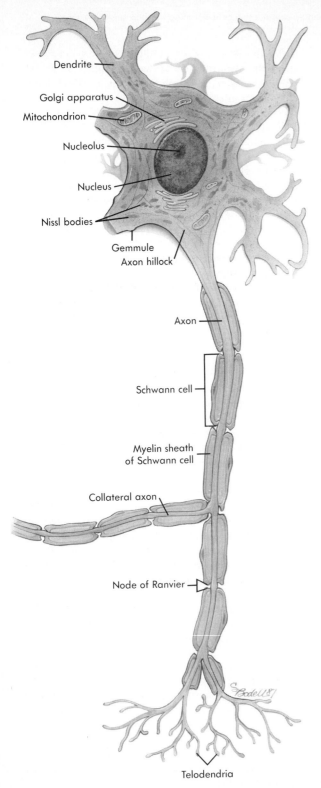

Dendrite

Golgi apparatus

Mitochondrion

Nucleolus

Nucleus

Nissl bodies

Gemmule
Axon hillock

Axon

Schwann cell

Myelin sheath
of Schwann cell

Collateral axon

Node of Ranvier

Telodendria

Fig. 1-10. Structural features of a nerve cell.

Of critical concern to the sports therapist is the importance of the nervous system in proprioception and neuromuscular control of movement as an integral part of a rehabilitation program. This will be discussed in great detail in Chapter 9.

Nerve healing. Specialized tissue, such as nerve cells, cannot regenerate once the nerve cell dies. In an injured peripheral nerve, however, the nerve fiber can regenerate significantly if the injury does not affect the cell body. The proximity of the axonal injury to the cell body can significantly affect the time required for healing. The closer an injury is to the cell body, the more difficult the regenerative process. In the case of a severed nerve, surgical intervention can markedly enhance regeneration.

For regeneration to occur, an optimal environment for healing must exist. When a nerve is cut, several degenerative changes occur that interfere with the neural pathways. Within the first 3 to 5 days the portion of the axon distal to the cut begins to degenerate and breaks into irregular segments. There is also a concomitant increase in metabolism and protein production by the nerve cell body to facilitate the regenerative process. The neuron in the cell body contains the genetic material and produces chemicals necessary for maintenance of the axon. These substances cannot be transmitted to the distal part of the axon, and eventually there will be complete degeneration.

In addition, the myelin portion of the Schwann cells around the degenerating axon also degenterates, and the myelin is phagocytized. the Schwann cells divide, forming a column of cells in place of the axon. If the cut ends of the axon contact this column of Schwann cells, the chances are good that an axon may eventually reinnervate distal structures. If the proximal end of the axon does not make contact with the column of Schwann cells, reinnervation will not occur.

The axon proximal to the cut has minimal degeneration initially and then begins the regenerative process with growth from the proximal axon. Bulbous enlargements and several axon sprouts form at the end of the proximal axon. Within about 2 weeks, these sprouts grow across the scar that has developed in the area of the cut and enter the column of Schwann cells. Only one of these sprouts will form the new axon while the others will degenerate. Once the axon grows through the Schwann cell columns, remaining Schwann cells proliferate along the length of the degenerating fiber and form new myelin around the growing axon, which will eventually reinnervate distal structures.

Regeneration is slow, at a rate of only 3 to 4 millimeters per day. Axon regeneration can be obstructed by scar formation due to excessive fibroplasia. Damaged nerves within the central nervous system regenerate very poorly compared to nerves in the peripheral nervous system. Central nervous system axons lack connective tissue sheaths, and the myelin-producing Schwann cells fail to proliferate.[28,52]

OTHER MUSCULOSKELETAL PROBLEMS
Dislocations and Subluxations

A dislocation occurs when at least one bone in an articulation is forced out of its normal and proper alignment and stays out until it is either manually or surgically put back into place or reduced.[41] Dislocations most commonly occur in the shoulder joint, elbow, and fingers, but they can occur wherever two bones articulate.

A subluxation is like a dislocation except that in this situation a bone pops out of its normal articulation but then goes right back into place. Subluxations most commonly occur in the shoulder joint, as well as in the knee cap in females.

Dislocations should never be reduced immediately, regardless of where they occur. The sports therapist should take the athlete to an x-ray facility and rule out fractures or other problems before reduction. Inappropriate techniques of reduction may only exacerbate the problem. Return to activity after dislocation or subluxation is largely dependent on the degree of soft tissue damage.

Bursitis

In many areas, particularly around joints, friction occurs between tendons and bones, skin and bone, or two muscles. Without some mechanism of protection in these high-friction areas, chronic irritation would be likely.

Bursae are essentially pieces of synovial membrane that contain small amounts of synovial fluid. This presence of synovium permits motion of surrounding structures without friction.

If excessive movement or perhaps some acute trauma occurs around these bursae, they become irritated and inflamed and begin producing large amounts of synovial fluid. The longer the irritation continues or the more severe the acute trauma, the more fluid is produced. As the fluid continues to accumulate in a limited space, pressure tends to increase and causes irritation of the pain receptors in the area.

Bursitis can be extremely painful and can severely restrict movement, especially if it occurs around a joint. Synovial fluid continues to be produced until the movement or trauma producing the irritation is eliminated.

A bursa that occasionally completely surrounds a tendon to allow more freedom of movement in a tight area is referred to as a *synovial sheath.* Irritation of this synovial sheath may restrict tendon motion.

All joints have many bursae surrounding them. The three bursae most commonly irritated as a result of various types of physical activity are the subacromial bursa in the shoulder joint, the olecranon bursa on the tip of the elbow, and the prepatellar bursa on the front surface of the patella. All three of these bursae have produced large amounts of synovial fluid, affecting motion at their respective joints.

Muscle Soreness

Overexertion in strenuous muscular exercise often results in muscular pain. At one time or another most everyone has experienced **muscle soreness,** usually resulting from some physical activity to which we are unaccustomed.

There are two types of muscle soreness. The first type of muscle pain is acute and accompanies fatigue. It is transient and occurs during and immediately after exercise. The second type of soreness involves delayed muscle pain that appears approximately 12 hours after injury. It becomes most intense after 24 to 48 hours and then gradually subsides so that the muscle becomes symptom free after 3 or 4 days. This second type of pain may best be described as a syndrome of delayed muscle pain, leading to increased muscle tension, edema formation, increased stiffness, and resistance to stretching.[22]

The cause of delayed-onset muscle soreness (DOMS) has been debated. Initially it was hypothesized that soreness was due to an excessive buildup of lactic acid in exercised muscles. However, recent evidence has essentially ruled out this theory.[14]

It has also been hypothesized that DOMS is caused by the tonic, localized spasm of motor units, varying in number with the severity of pain. This theory maintains that exercise causes varying degrees of ischemia in the working muscles. This ischemia causes pain, which results in reflex tonic muscle contraction that increases and prolongs the ischemia. Consequently a cycle of increasing severity is begun.[13] As with the lactic acid theory, the spasm theory has also been discounted.

Currently there are two schools of thought relative to the cause of DOMS. DOMS seems to occur from very small tears in the muscle tissue, which seem to be more likely with eccentric or isometric contractions.[14] It is generally believed that the initial damage caused by eccentric exercise is mechanical damage to either the muscular or connective tissue. Edema accumulation and delays in the rate of glycogen repletion are secondary reactions to mechanical damage.[45]

DOMS may be caused by structural damage to the elastic components of connective tissue at the musculotendinous junction. This damage results in the presence of hydroxyproline, a protein by-product of collagen breakdown, in blood and urine.[10]

It has also been documented that structural damage to the muscle fibers results in an increase in blood serum levels of various protein/enzymes, including creatine kinase. This increase indicates that there is likely some damage to the muscle fiber as a result of strenuous exercise.[14]

Muscle soreness may best be prevented by beginning at a moderate level of activity and gradually progressing the intensity of the exercise over time. Treatment of muscle soreness usually also involves some type of stretching activity. As for other conditions discussed in this chapter, ice is important as a treatment for muscle soreness, particularly within the first 48 to 72 hours.

Contusions

A **contusion** is synonymous with the term *bruise*. The mechanism that produces it is a blow from some external object that causes soft tissues (for example, skin, fat, muscle, ligaments, joint capsule) to be compressed against the hard bone underneath. If the blow is hard enough, capillaries rupture and allow bleeding into the tissues. The bleeding, if superficial enough, causes a bluish-purple discoloration to the skin that persists for several days. The contusion may be very sore to the touch. If damage has occurred to muscle, pain may be elicited on active movement. In most cases the pain ceases within a few days, and discoloration disappears in usually 2 to 3 weeks.

The major problem with contusions occurs where an area is subjected to repeated blows. If the same area, or more specifically a muscle, is bruised over and over again, small calcium deposits may begin to accumulate in the injured area. These pieces of calcium may be found between several fibers in the muscle belly, or calcium may form a spur that projects from the underlying bone. These calcium formations, which may significantly impair movement, are referred to as *myositis ossificans.* In some cases myositis ossificans may develop from a single trauma.

The key to preventing myositis ossificans from occurring from repeated contusion is protection of the injured area by padding. If the area is properly protected after the first contusion, myositis ossificans may never develop. Protection, along with rest, may frequently allow the calcium to be reabsorbed and eliminate any need for surgical intervention.

The two areas that seem to be the most vulnerable to repeated contusions during physical activity are the quadriceps muscle group on the front of the thigh and the biceps muscle on the front of the upper arm. The formation of myositis ossificans in either of these or any other areas may be detected on x-ray films.

INITIAL MANAGEMENT OF INJURIES

Initial first aid and management techniques are perhaps the most critical part of any rehabilitation program. The initial management unquestionably has a significant impact on the course of the rehabilitative process.[37] Regardless of the type of injury, the one problem they all have in common is swelling. Swelling may be caused by any number of factors, including bleeding, production of synovial fluid, an accumulation of inflammatory by-products, edema, or a combination of several factors. No matter which mechanism is involved, swelling produces an increased pressure in the injured area, and increased pressure causes pain.[59] Swelling can also cause neuromuscular inhibition, which results in weak muscle contraction. Swelling is most likely during the first 72 hours after an injury. Once swelling has occurred, the healing process is significantly retarded. The injured area cannot return to normal until all the swelling is gone.

Therefore everything that is done in first aid management of any of these conditions should be directed toward controlling the swelling.[1] If the swelling can be controlled initially in the acute stage of injury, the time required for rehabilitation is likely to be significantly reduced. To control and severely limit the

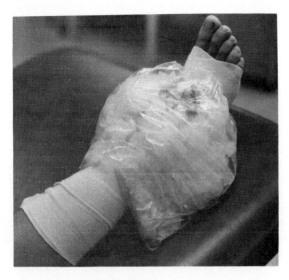

Fig. 1-11. Musculoskeletal injuries should be treated initially with protection, restricted activity, ice, compression, and elevation.

amount of swelling, the PRICE principle—protection, restricted activity, ice, compression, and elevation—can be applied (Figure 1-11). Each factor plays a critical role in limiting swelling, and all factors should be used simultaneously.

Protection

The injured area should be protected from additional injury by applying appropriate splints, braces, pads, or other immobilization devices. If the injury involves the lower extremity, it is recommended that the athlete go nonweight bearing on crutches at least until the acute inflammatory response has subsided.

Restricted Activity (Rest)

Rest after any type of injury is an extremely important component of any treatment program. Once an anatomical structure is injured, it immediately begins the healing process. If the injured structure is not rested and is subjected to external stress and strains, the healing process never really gets a chance to begin. Consequently, the injury does not get well, and the time required for rehabilitation is markedly increased. The number of days necessary for resting varies with the severity of the injury, but most minor injuries should rest for approximately 48 to 72 hours before an active rehabilitation program is begun.

It must be emphasized that rest does not mean that the athlete does nothing. The term *rest* applies only to the injured body part. During this period, the athlete should continue to work on cardiovascular fitness and strengthening and flexibility exercises for the other parts of the body not affected by the injury.[63]

Ice

The use of cold is the initial treatment of choice for virtually all conditions involving injuries to the musculoskeletal system.[50] It is most commonly used immediately after injury to decrease pain and promote local vasoconstriction, thus controlling hemorrhage and edema. It is also used in the acute phase of inflammatory conditions, such as bursitis, tenosynovitis, and tendinitis, in which heat may cause additional pain and swelling. Cold is also used to reduce the reflex muscle spasm and spastic conditions that accompany pain. Its analgesic effect is probably one of its greatest benefits. One explanation of the analgesic effect is that cold decreases the velocity of nerve conduction, although it does not entirely eliminate it. Cold may also bombard cutaneous sensory nerve receptor areas with so many cold impulses that pain impulses are lost. With ice treatments, the athlete reports an uncomfortable sensation of cold, followed by burning, an aching sensation, and finally complete numbness.[32,47]

Because of the low thermal conductivity of underlying subcutaneous fat tissues, applications of cold for short periods are ineffective in cooling deeper tissues. For this reason longer treatments of 20 to 30 minutes are recommended. Cold treatments are generally believed to be more effective in reaching deeper tissues than most forms of heat. Cold applied to the skin is capable of significantly lowering the temperature of tissues at a considerable depth. The extent of this lowered tissue temperature depends on the type of cold applied to the skin, the duration of its application, the thickness of the subcutaneous fat, and the region of the body to which it is applied. Ice should be applied to the injured area until the signs and symptoms of inflammation have disappeared and there is little or no chance that swelling will be increased by using some form of heat. Ice should be used for at least 72 hours after an acute injury.[32,47]

Compression

Compression is likely the single most important technique for controlling initial swelling. The purpose of compression is to mechanically reduce the amount of space available for swelling by applying pressure around an injured area. The best way of applying pressure is to use an elastic wrap, such as an Ace bandage, to apply firm but even pressure around the injury.

Because of the pressure build up in the tissues, having a compression wrap in place for a long time may become painful. However, the wrap must be kept in place despite significant pain because it is so important in the control of swelling. The compression wrap should be left in place continuously for at least 72 hours after an acute injury. In many overuse problems, such as tendinitis, tenosynovitis, and particularly bursitis, which involve ongoing inflammation, the compression wrap should be worn until the swelling is almost entirely gone.

Elevation

The fourth factor that assists in controlling swelling is elevation. The injured part, particularly an extremity, should be elevated to eliminate the effects of gravity on blood pooling in the extremities. Elevation assists venous drainage of blood and other fluids from the injured area back to the central circulatory system. The greater the degree of elevation, the more effective the reduction in swelling. For example, in an ankle sprain, the leg should be placed in such a position that the ankle is virtually straight up in the air. The injured part should be elevated as much as possible during the first 72 hours.

The appropriate technique for initial management of the acute injuries discussed in this chapter, regardless of where they occur, would be the following:

1. Apply a compression wrap directly over the injury. Wrapping should be from distal to proximal. Tension should be firm and consistent. Wetting the elastic wrap to facilitate the passage of cold from ice packs may be helpful.
2. Surround the injured area entirely with ice bags, and secure them in place. Ice bags should be left on for 45 minutes initially and then 1 hour off and 30 minutes on as much as possible over the next 24 hours. During the following 48-hour period, ice should be applied as often as possible.
3. The injured part should be elevated as much

as possible during the initial 72-hour period after injury. Keeping the injured part elevated while sleeping is particularly important.
4. Allow the injured part to rest for approximately 72 hours after the injury.

MANAGING THE HEALING PROCESS THROUGH REHABILITATION

In sports medicine, the rehabilitation philosophy relative to inflammation and healing after injury is to assist the natural processes of the body while doing no harm.[34] The course of rehabilitation chosen by the sports therapist must focus on their knowledge of the healing process and its therapeutic modifiers to guide, direct, and stimulate the structural function and integrity of the injured part. The primary goal should be to have a positive influence on the inflammation and repair process to expedite recovery of function in terms of range of motion, muscular strength and endurance, neuromuscular control, and cardiorespiratory endurance.[18] The sports therapist must try and minimize the early effects of excessive inflammatory processes including pain modulation, edema control, and reduction of associated muscle spasm, which can produce loss of joint motion and contracture. Finally, the sports therapist should concentrate on preventing the recurrence of injury by influencing the structural ability of the injured tissue to resist future overloads by incorporating various training techniques.[34] The subsequent chapters throughout this text can serve as a guide for the sports therapist in using the many different rehabilitation tools available.

SUMMARY

1. The three phases of the healing process are the inflammatory response phase, the fibroblastic-repair phase, and maturation-remodeling phase, which occur in sequence but overlap one another in a continuum.
2. Factors that may impede the healing process include edema, hemorrhage, lack of vascular supply, separation of tissue, muscle spasm, atrophy, corticosteroids, hypertrophic scars, infection, climate and humidity, age, health, and nutrition.
3. The four fundamental types of tissue in the human body are epithelial, connective, muscle, and nerve.
4. Ligament sprains involve stretching or tearing the fibers that provide stability at the joint.
5. Fractures may be classified as either greenstick,

transverse, oblique, spiral, comminuted, impacted, avulsive, or stress.

6. Osteoarthritis involves degeneration of the articular cartilage or subchondral bone.

7. Muscle strains involve a stretching or tearing of muscle fibers and their tendons and cause impairment to active movement.

8. Tendinitis, an inflammation of a muscle tendon that causes pain on movement, usually occurs because of overuse.

9. Tenosynovitis is an inflammation of the synovial sheath through which a tendon must slide during motion.

10. Dislocations and subluxations involve disruption of the joint capsule and ligamentous structures surrounding the joint.

11. Bursitis is an inflammation of the synovial membranes located in areas where friction occurs between various anatomical structures.

12. Muscle soreness may be caused by spasm, connective tissue damage, muscle tissue damage, or some combination of each of these factors.

13. Repeated contusions may lead to the development of myositis ossificans.

14. All injuries should be initially managed with rest, ice, compression, and elevation to control swelling and thus reduce the time required for rehabilitation.

REFERENCES

1 Arnheim D, Prentice W: *Principles of athletic training,* ed 8, St Louis, 1993, Mosby.

2 Arnoczky SP: Physiologic principles of ligament injuries and healing. In Scott WN, editor: *Ligament and extensor mechanism injuries of the knee,* St Louis, 1991, Mosby.

3 Beck EW: *Mosby's atlas of functional human anatomy,* St Louis, 1982, Mosby.

4 Booher JM, Thibodeau GA: *Athletic injury assessment,* ed 2, St Louis, 1989, Mosby.

5 Bryant MW: Wound healing, *CIBA Clinical Symposia* 29(3):2-36, 1977.

6 Cailliet R: *Soft tissue pain and disability,* ed 2, Philadelphia, 1988, FA Davis.

7 Carley PJ, Wainapel SF: Electrotherapy for acceleration of sound healing: low intensity direct current, *Arch Phys Med Rehabil* 66:443-446, 1985.

8 Carrico TJ, Mehrhof AI, Cohen IK: Biology and wound healing, *Surg Clin North Am* 64(4):721-734, 1984.

9 Cheng N: The effects of electrocurrents on A.T.P. generation, protein synthesis and membrane transport, *J Orth Res* 171:264-272, 1982.

10 Clancy W: Tendon trauma and overuse injuries. In Leadbetter W, Buckwalter J, Gordon S, editors: *Sports-induced inflammation,* Park Ridge, Ill, 1990, American Academy of Orthopaedic Surgeons.

11 Clarkson PM, Tremblay I: Exercise-induced muscledamage, repair and adaptation in humans, *J Appl Physiol* 65:1-6, 1988.

12 Derscheid GL, Garrick JG: Medial collateral ligament injuries in football: nonoperative management of grade I and grade II sprains, *Am J Sports Med* 9(6):365-368, 1981.

13 deVries HA: Quantitative EMG investigation of spasm theory of muscle pain, *Am J Phys Med* 45:119-134, 1966.

14 Evans WJ: Exercise induced skeletal muscle damage, *Phys Sports Med* 15:189-200, 1987.

15 Fahey TD: *Athletic training: principles and practice,* Palo Alto, Calif, 1986, Mayfield Publishing.

16 Fantone J: Basic concepts in inflammation. In Leadbetter W, Buckwalter J, Gordon S, editors: *Sports-induced inflammation,* Park Ridge, Ill, 1990, American Academy of Orthopaedic Surgeons.

17 Fernandez A, Finlew JM: Wound healing: helping a natural process, *Postgrad Med J* 74(4):311-318, 1983.

18 Flynn M, Rovee D: Influencing repair and recovery, *Am J Nurs* 82:1550-1558, 1982.

19 Frankel VH, Nordin M: *Basic biomechanics of the skeletal system,* Philadelphia, 1980, Lea & Febiger.

20 Gelberman R, Goldberg V, An K-N, et al. *Soft tissue healing.* In Woo SL-Y, Buckwalter J, editors: *Injury and repair of musculoskeletal soft tissues,* Park Ridge, Ill, 1988, American Academy of Orthopaedic Surgeons.

21 Glick JM: Muscle strains: prevention and treatment, *Phys Sports Med* 8(11):73-77, 1980.

22 Gould JA, Davies GJ, editors: *Orthopaedic and sports physical therapy,* St Louis, 1990, Mosby.

23 Gradisar IA: Fracture stabilization and healing. In Gould JA, Davies GJ, editors: *Orthopaedic and sports physical medicine,* St Louis, 1985, Mosby.

24 Gross A, Cutright D, Bhaskar S, et al.: Effectiveness of pulsating water jet lavage in treatment of contaminated crush wounds, *Am J Surg* 124:373-375, 1972.

25 Guyton AC: *Textbook of medical physiology,* Philadelphia, 1986, WB Saunders.

26 Henning CE: Semilunar cartilage of the knee: function and pathology. In Pandolf KB, editor: *Exercise and sport science review,* New York, 1988, Macmillan Publishing.

27 Hettinga DL: Inflammatory response of synovial joint structures. In Gould JA, Davies GJ, editors: *Orthopaedic and sports physical therapy,* St Louis, 1985, Mosby.

28 Hole J: *Human anatomy and physiology,* Dubuque, Iowa, 1984, William C. Brown.

29 Keene JS: Ligament and muscle tendon unit injuries. In Gould JA, Davies GJ, editors: *Orthopaedic and sports physical therapy,* St Louis, 1985, Mosby.

30 Kibler WB: Concepts in exercise rehabilitation of athletic injury. In Leadbetter W, Buckwalter J, Gordon S, editors: *Sports-induced inflammation,* Park Ridge, Ill, 1990, American Academy of Orthopaedic Surgeons.

31 Kissane JM: *Anderson's pathology,* ed 8, St Louis, 1985, Mosby.

32 Knight KL: *Cryotherapy: theory, technique and physiology,* Chattanooga, Tenn, 1985, Chattanooga Corporation.

33 Lane NE, Bloch D, Wood P, et al.: Aging, long-distance running, and the development of musculoskeletal disability, *Am J Med* 82:772-780, 1987.

34 Leadbetter W: Introduction to sports-induced soft-tissue inflammation. In Leadbetter W, Buckwalter J, Gordon S, editors: *Sports-induced inflammation*, Park Ridge, Ill, 1990, American Academy of Orthopaedic Surgeons.

35 Leadbetter W, Buckwalter J, Gordon S: *Sports-induced inflammation*, Park Ridge, Ill, 1990, American Academy of Orthopaedic Surgeons.

36 Leonard PC: *Building a medical vocabulary*, ed 2, Philadelphia, 1988, WB Saunders.

37 MacMaster JH: *The ABC's of sports medicine*, Melbourne, Fla, 1982, RE Kreiger Publishing.

38 Marchesi VT: Inflammation and healing. In Kissane JM, editor: *Anderson's pathology*, ed 8, St Louis, 1985, Mosby.

39 Martinez-Hernandez A, Amenta P: Basic concepts in wound healing. In Leadbetter W, Buckwalter J, Gordon S, editors: *Sports-induced inflammation*, Park Ridge, Ill, 1990, American Academy of Orthopaedic Surgeons.

40 Messier SP, Pittala KA: Etiologic factors associated with selected running injuries, *Med Sci Sports Exerc* 20(5):501-505, 1988.

41 Muckle DS: *Outline of fractures and dislocations*, Bristol, England, 1985, Wright Publishing.

42 Musacchia XJ: Disuse atrophy of skeletal muscle: animal models. In Pandolf KB, editor: *Exercise and sport sciences review*, New York, 1988, Macmillan Publishing.

43 Norkin C, Levangie P: *Joint structure and function: a comprehensive analysis*, Philadelphia, 1983, FA Davis.

44 Noyes FR: Functional properties of knee ligaments and alterations induced by immobilization, *Clin Orthop* 123:210-242, 1977.

45 O'Reilly K, Warhol M, Fielding R, et al.: Eccentric exercise induced muscle damage impairs muscle glycogen depletion, *J Appl Physiol* 63:252-256,1987.

46 Panush RS, Brown DG: Exercise and arthritis, *Sports Med* 4:54-64, 1987.

47 Prentice WE, editor: *Therapeutic modalities in sports medicine*, St Louis, 1990, Mosby.

48 Riley WB: Wound healing, *Am Fam Physician* 24:5, 1981.

49 Robbins SL, Cotran RS, Kumar V: *Pathologic basis of disease*, ed 3, Philadelphia, 1984, WB Saunders.

50 Roy S, Irvin R: *Sports medicine, prevention, evaluation, management and rehabilitation*, Englewood Cliffs, NJ, 1983, Prentice Hall.

51 Rywlin AM: Hemopoietic system. In Kissane JM, editor: *Anderson's pathology*, ed 8, St Louis, 1985, Mosby.

52 Seeley R, Stephens T, Tate P: *Anatomy and physiology*, St Louis, 1989, Mosby.

53 Seller RH: *Differential diagnosis of common complaints*, Philadelphia, 1986, WB Saunders.

54 Stanish WD, Gunnlaugson B: Electrical energy and soft tissue injury healing, *Sportcare and Fitness* 9:12, 1988.

55 Stanish WD, Rubinovich M, Kozey J, et al.: The use of electricity in ligament and tendon repair, *Phys Sports Med* 13:8, 1985.

56 Stewart J: *Clinical anatomy and physiology*, Miami, 1986, Medmaster.

57 Stone MH: Implications for connective tissue and bone alterations resulting from rest and exercise training, *Med Sci Sports Exerc* 20(5):S162-168, 1988.

58 Wahl S, Renstrom P: *Fibrosis in soft-tissue injuries*. In Leadbetter W, Buckwalter J, Gordon S, editors: *Sports-induced inflammation*, Park Ridge, Ill, 1990, American Academy of Orthopaedic Surgeons.

59 Wells PE, Frampton V, Bowsher D: *Pain management in physical therapy*, Norwalk, Conn, 1988, Appleton and Lange.

60 Whiteside JA, Fleagle SB, Kalenak A: Fractures and refractures in intercollegiate athletes: an eleven year experience, *Am J Sports Med* 9(6):369-377, 1981.

61 Wolff J: *Gesetz der transformation der knochen*, Berlin, 1892, Aug. Hirschwald.

62 Woo SL-Y, Buckwalter J, editors: *Injury and repair of musculoskeletal soft tissues*, Park Ridge, Ill, 1988, American Academy of Orthopaedic Surgeons.

63 Woodman R, Pare L: Evaluation and treatment of soft tissue lesions of the ankle and foot using the Cyriax approach, *Phys Ther* 62:1144-1147, 1982.

64 Zachezewski J: Flexibility for sports. In Sanders B, editor: *Sports physical therapy*, Norwalk, Conn, 1990, Appleton and Lange.

Rehabilitation Goals in Sports Medicine

2

Julie Moyer and Gina Lorence-Konin

OBJECTIVES

After completion of this chapter, the student should be able to do the following:

- Describe the two primary rehabilitation goals of sports medicine.

- Discuss factors involved in the prevention of athletic injuries.

- Describe short- and long-term rehabilitation goals and general treatment management programs.

A rehabilitative goal is an end that one tries to achieve via therapeutic intervention. These goals are used to direct the treatment management programs and are established after a thorough initial evaluation and subsequent reevaluations. The two primary rehabilitative goals in sports medicine are: (1) the prevention of injuries to athletes and (2) the safe return of an injured athlete to the previous level of competition as quickly as possible.

INJURY PREVENTION
Physical Conditioning

The primary goal in rehabilitation, injury prevention, can be aided by proper physical conditioning. Off-season conditioning is essential for an athlete seeking maximal in-season performance.[11,12] Off-season conditioning (1) decreases the athlete's risk of injury, (2) decreases the rehabilitation time once an injury has occurred, (3) promotes excellence, (4) maintains an athlete's previous education of task performance, and (5) provides a close, positive bond between the athlete and the sport, thus aiding in the athlete's mental well-being and sport enjoyment.[7]

The first 4 weeks of a season are the most dangerous because the participants are generally out of condition.[2] Therefore the major goal of off-season conditioning is to achieve the highest level of fitness possible and thus enter the season in a conditioned rather than an unconditioned state. This goal is best accomplished by structuring a well-balanced conditioning program that can be performed as effectively yet efficiently as possible. This program should include seven major phases: (1) the warm-up, primarily performed to prepare the cardiovascular system for stress, (2) stretching, to promote proper range of motion, (3) strengthening exercises, (4) endurance activities, (5) sport-specific or functional activities, to meet the special demands and skills a particular sport requires, (6) cool-down, and (7) relaxation techniques, to aid in the recovery from fatigue and promote stress reduction (Figures 2-1, *A* and *B* and 2-2). The off-season gives the sports therapist an opportunity to rehabilitate injuries incurred during in-season participation.

Preparticipation Physical

A physical examination should be mandatory before and specific to participation at all levels and ages of sports participation (Figure 2-3). The examination determines if the athlete is physically capable of withstanding the stresses of the sport and helps to reveal imbalances and weaknesses that may be corrected through rehabilitation.

Ideally the examination should be performed 4 to

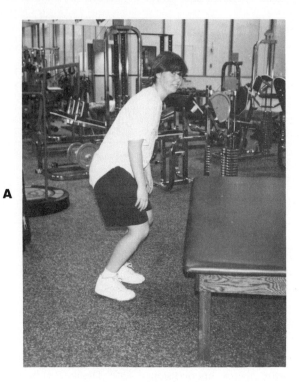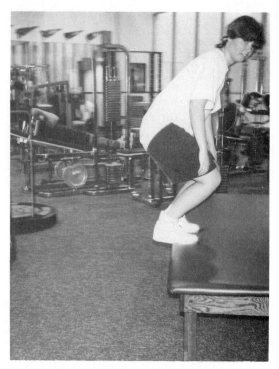

Fig. 2-1. Functional activities. Functional activities are used to meet the special demands and skills a particular sport requires. **A,** Starting position. **B,** Terminal position.

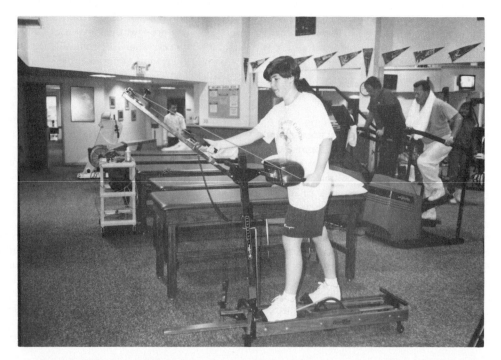

Fig. 2-2. Endurance activities. Endurance activities are one phase of a seven-step conditioning program.

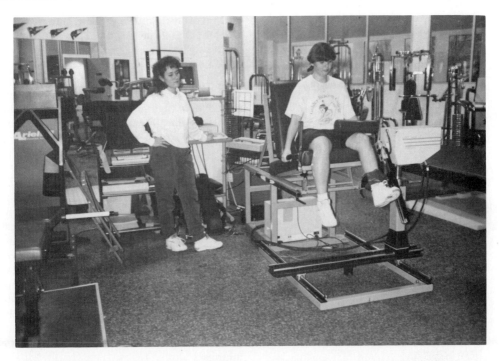

Fig. 2-3. Isokinetic testing. Isokinetic testing may be performed for preparticipation data collection.

6 weeks before the start of the season to give the physician a good indication of the athlete's level of health and, if necessary, give the sports therapist adequate time to adopt goals and develop a rehabilitation program before the season begins.

The seven major parts of a sports examination are (1) past medical history and current medical information; (2) measurements including range of motion, body type, strength, percentage body fat, girth, posture, level of maturation, and cardiovascular fitness; (3) orthopedic examination; (4) eye examination; (5) dental screening; (6) laboratory tests; (7) and review of the examination by a physician to allow, disallow, or restrict athletic participation.[15]

Preinjury Data Collection

Preinjury data collection can help identify possible problem areas and set goals in rehabilitation.[10]

Testing, including muscle strength, power, and endurance, in various muscle groups provides objective data. This data may be used to devise short- and long-term goals after an injury is sustained. The sports therapist or physician may now set goals such as "in-

crease strength to 80% of preinjury level" or "return to full preinjury status." Subsequent testing may be performed, and the athlete's progress or status is objectively identified.

Nutrition and Diet

Nutrition is an important component of in-season and off-season conditioning. A good nutritional program should consist of low-fat, high-fiber, nutritious foods from the major food groups including dairy products, fruits and vegetables, breads and cereals, meats and meat alternatives such as nuts. The recommended ratio of these foods is about 55% carbohydrates, 30% fat, and 15% protein.[18] Nutritional supplements, such as protein, vitamins, and minerals, are expensive and are often not necessary if the athlete's diet is nutritionally well balanced.

The major difference between in-season and off-season nutritional conditioning is caloric intake. The caloric intake of individuals is very dependent upon activity level. The average sedentary person may require about 1500 Calories per day, whereas moderately training athletes average 3000 Calories per day

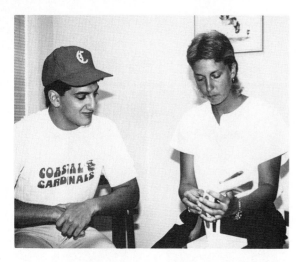

Fig. 2-4. Education prevents injury. Education of athletes assists in the prevention and treatment of injuries.

and intensely training endurance athletes may require over 5000 Calories per day.

During a lowered training level, such as off-season conditioning, the athlete's basal metabolic rate (BMR) lowers. The BMR is the lowest amount of energy needed to keep the body running during waking hours. When the BMR lowers, fewer Calories are burned by the athlete, thus the potential of increased body fat exists. Therefore most off-season conditioning programs should include caloric restrictions.

Education

Education is the best form of preventive medicine. The educated athlete studies off-season conditioning programs, biomechanics, diet and nutrition, equipment fitting, sports psychology, injury prevention techniques, and injury treatment procedures (Figure 2-4). The educated athlete also becomes familiar with the rules and regulations of the sport, especially as they relate to drug control and banned substances. Knowledge and understanding of these concepts aid the athlete in the prevention and treatment of injuries.

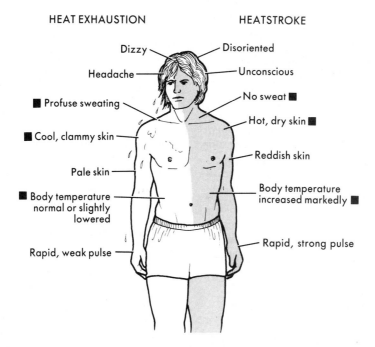

Fig. 2-5. Signs and symptoms—heat exhaustion and heatstroke. Main signs and symptoms with heat exhaustion and heatstroke.
(From Booher JM, Thibodeau GA: *Athletic injury assessment,* St Louis, 1985, Mosby.)

Safe Playing Environment and Equipment

The sports medicine practitioner carefully inspects all playing facilities to ensure that they are safe for play. Weather conditions should also be monitored with recommendations made to the coach or athletic director. Such weather conditions include heat, cold, rain, and lightning.

The most common types of disorders associated with heat are heat cramps, heat exhaustion, and heatstroke. These serious heat-related problems primarily occur when the temperature and humidity are high; the body begins to absorb heat at a faster rate than heat is expelled by means such as perspiration and evaporation. When this heat absorption occurs, the athlete is at risk of overheating, (Figure 2-5) which may be monitored using a sling psychrometer.[4]

Several authors have previously found a relationship between dehydration and decreased muscle strength.[1,6,14,17] In addition, dehydration causes a loss of plasma volume, which leads to a decreased stroke volume and an increased heart rate during submaximal aerobic exercise.[3,9,16]

Lightning is another serious weather occurrence that must be treated with respect. As with all potential injuries, the best treatment is prevention. The rule of thumb when playing during lightning is if you can count 15 seconds or less between the time you see lightning and the time you hear thunder, the athletic competition should be postponed (1 mile = 5 seconds; lightning can strike up to 3 miles away).[13]

Injuries can be prevented with appropriate clothing and equipment (Figure 2-6). Also, the correct fitting of the equipment is essential. Protective clothing and equipment not only are used to protect the athlete from acquiring an injury but also can be used to further protect an injury already sustained.

INITIAL EVALUATION, TREATMENT, AND REHABILITATION
Rehabilitation

The second primary goal of rehabilitation is the safe return of injured athletes to their prior level of competition as quickly as possible. This goal is best achieved by a thorough initial evaluation, proper immediate treatment, and a comprehensive rehabilitation program (Figure 2-7). Rehabilitation in sports medicine should involve a multidisciplinary team approach including athletic trainers, physical therapists, physicians, coaches, and athletes.

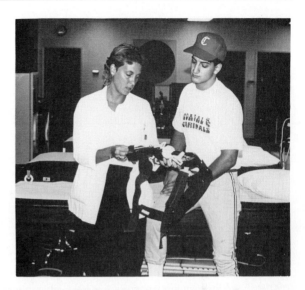

Fig. 2-6. Protective equipment. Proper instruction for wear and care is essential when using protective equipment.

The most efficient and effective form of rehabilitation is therapeutic exercise (see Chapter 3). Appropriate therapeutic exercise helps the athlete achieve increased strength, increased power, improved proprioception and kinesthesia, increased range of motion, improved cardiovascular and muscular endurance, and relaxation. Increased coordination, decreased biomechanical and anatomical deficits, improved balance, maximized function, and minimized swelling can also be assisted through exercise. Exercise also helps minimize damage that results from osteoporosis.

For these goals to be achieved, four principles must be observed. First, therapeutic exercises must be adapted based upon the individualized needs of the athlete. Second, the initial exercise program should not aggravate the disorder. Third, the exercises should be performed in orderly, progressive steps (Tables 2-1 and 2-2). Last, the exercise program should be well rounded: (1) use a wide variety of exercise techniques, (2) constantly change the exercise program to avoid boredom, (3) make sure the uninvolved areas of the body remain conditioned so that the risk of incurring other injuries is reduced when the athlete returns to competition, (4) set realistic goals for and with the athlete, with constant reevaluation and modification of the goals and treatment program, and (5) have the athlete actively en-

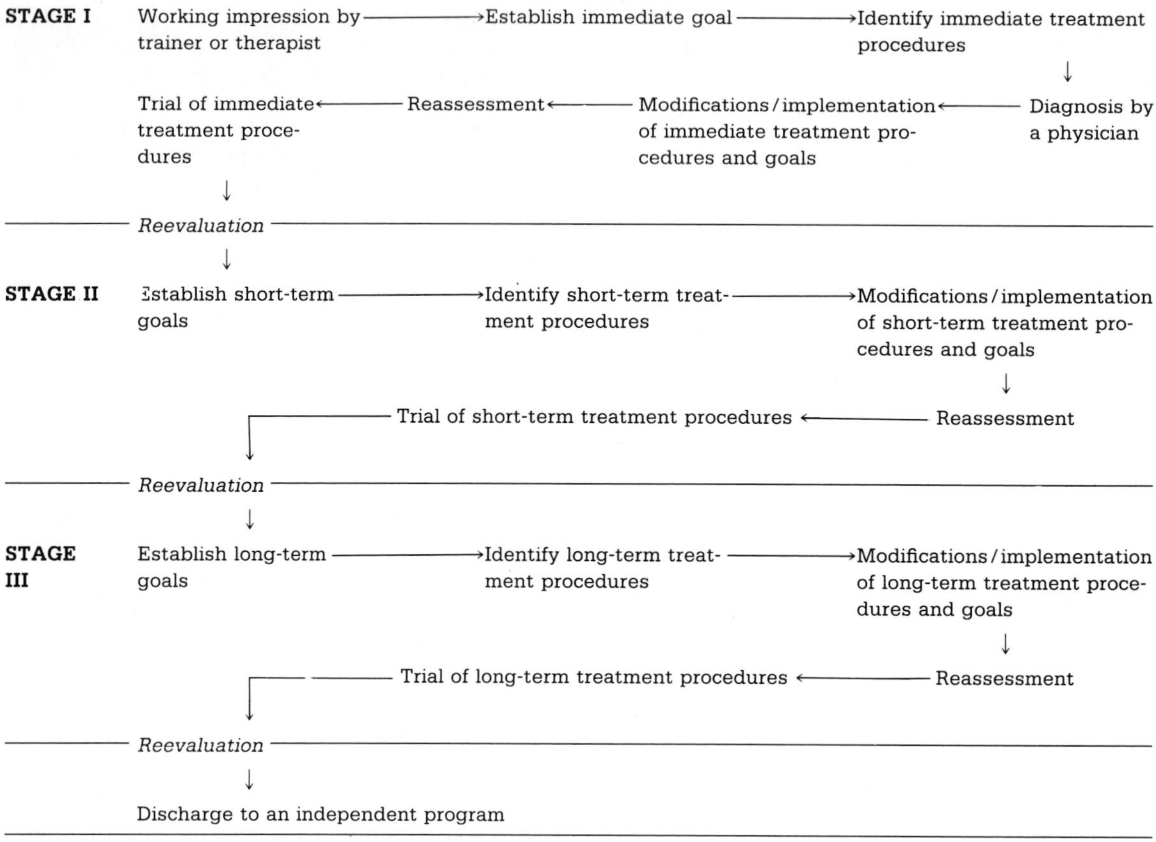

STAGE I Working impression by ⟶ Establish immediate goal ⟶ Identify immediate treatment
trainer or therapist   procedures
                                                                                          ↓
Trial of immediate ⟵ Reassessment ⟵ Modifications/implementation ⟵ Diagnosis by
treatment proce-   of immediate treatment pro-   a physician
dures   cedures and goals
         ↓
──────── *Reevaluation* ──
         ↓

STAGE II Establish short-term ⟶ Identify short-term treat- ⟶ Modifications/implementation
goals   ment procedures   of short-term treatment pro-
                                                                                          cedures and goals
                                                                                                       ↓
         ┌──────── Trial of short-term treatment procedures ⟵──────── Reassessment
         ↓
──────── *Reevaluation* ──
         ↓

STAGE III Establish long-term ⟶ Identify long-term treat- ⟶ Modifications/implementation
goals   ment procedures   of long-term treatment proce-
                                                                                          dures and goals
                                                                                                       ↓
         ┌──────── Trial of long-term treatment procedures ⟵──────── Reassessment
         ↓
──────── *Reevaluation* ──
         ↓
Discharge to an independent program

Fig. 2-7. Goal setting and treatment sequencing.

TABLE 2-1
Sample of Progressive, Resistive Knee Exercise Stages by Davies[5]

Stage	Exercise	Specifics
I	Submaximal, multiple-angle isometrics	10 sets of 10 repetitions, a 10-sec contraction, performed at 10 angles
II	Maximal, multiple-angle isometrics	
III	Submaximal, short-arc isokinetics	Primarily intermediate contractile velocity speeds at 60–180 deg/sec, using a velocity spectrum rehabilitation program (10 repetitions at every 30 deg/sec)
IV	Short-arc isotonics	Used with or in place of maximal, short-arc isokinetics
V	Maximal, short-arc isokinetics	
VI	Submaximal, full-range isokinetics	Primarily fast contractile velocity speeds at 180–300 deg/sec, using a velocity spectrum rehabilitation program
VII	Maximal, full-range isokinetics	

TABLE 2-2
Nonspecific Progression of Resistive Therapeutic Exercise

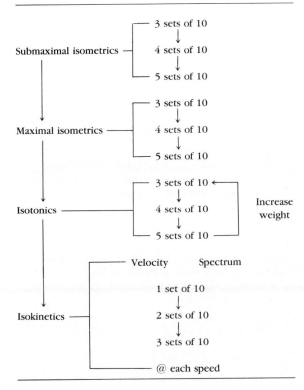

rolled in a home therapy program, as well as outpatient physical therapy and the athletic training room program.

Goals

In *Webster's Ninth New Collegiate Dictionary,* goal is defined as the end toward which effort is directed.[19] In sports medicine, goals are established to identify the outcome of rehabilitation and treatment. Goals should be measurable; for example, increase passive shoulder flexion by 20% or increase range of motion to 90 degrees of shoulder flexion in 2 weeks; decrease effusion by 2 cm displayed with girth measurement at the joint line in 4 weeks, increase isokinetic strength to 90% of contralateral side before discharge, etc.[10]

SHORT- AND LONG-TERM GOALS. Rehabilitation goals (after insult) may be divided into two main categories, short- and long-term goals (Table 2-3).

Collectively, these rehabilitation goals provide a guideline to get the athlete back to the highest level of function in the shortest amount of time that is safely feasible. Establishing appropriate rehabilitation goals is often the most difficult aspect of the rehabilitative program.

Short-term goals. Stage I of postinjury goal setting begins at the time of injury insult. The immediate rehabilitative goal is established at the time of injury and is based upon a quick but relatively thorough on-the-field evaluation and working impression by the sports therapist along with an immediate diagnosis by the sports physician if available and indicated (Figure 2-8).

When an athlete is evaluated, measurements should be taken initially, then periodically as the athlete progresses toward attaining the goals. As stated previously, the goals of rehabilitation would be to attain the preinjury status identified in the preparticipation examination. If preparticipation examinations are not performed, then an injured extremity may be compared to measurements from the uninjured extremity. These measurements should include: 1) strength of each muscle group, 2) power of each muscle group, 3) endurance of each muscle group, 4) balance between antagonistic muscle groups, 5) flexibility of muscles around the joint rehabilitated, 6) proprioception of the affected limb, 7) effusion remaining, and 8) functional use of that limb in the required sport.[19]

After the evaluation, a conservative short-term goal must be established along with the treatment management to accomplish this goal. This immediate goal setting and treatment implementation may range from protective padding for reentry into competition to emergency care and transportation to a hospital with appropriate referrals to a physician specialist such as a neurologist or orthopedic surgeon.

One of the most frequently used immediate treatment management acronyms is PRICE: Protection, Restricted activity, Ice, Compression, and Elevation (Figure 2-9). Protection means protecting the injured area from further insult, which may be performed in a variety of ways, including padding and strapping. With more serious injuries or when there is doubt as to the severity of an injury, protection may also include slings, splints, and assistive ambulatory devices.

Restricted activity is probably the most controversial aspect of the PRICE treatment program. It protects an injury from further damage. Restricted activity in the form of rest may be indicated for some

TABLE 2-3
Rehabilitation Stages, Goals, and General Treatment Methods

Stage	Goal	General Treatment Methods
I		
Short-Term Goals	Protection from further damage	Protective padding and strapping
	Resistive activity	Splints, braces, and immobilizers
	Control/minimize pain and swelling	Ice
	Assist the healing process and enable the symptoms and level of dysfunction to subside	Compression wrap tape and other devices Elevate the injured area Therapeutic modalities: cold agents, heat/diathermy, electric stimulation, intermittent compression devices, massage, taping/padding/immobilization as indicated
	Maintain normal function	Therapeutic exercise: isometric-PROM-AAROM-AROM of injured area, general vigorous exercise regime to uninvolved body parts, psychological exercises, education of the athlete
II		
Long-Term Goals	Achieve normal strength, power, muscular and cardiovascular endurance, agility, anatomical alignment, sensory feedback (proprioception, stereognosis), balance, timing, coordination, biomechanical motions, psychological conditioning	Therapeutic modalities: to a lesser extent than stage I. Therapeutic exercise: PROM-AAROM-AROM, hydro-aquatherapy, psychological training, isometrics, isotonics (concentric and eccentric), isokinetics, PNF techniques, cardiovascular and muscular endurance activities, progressive sport-specific activities
	Discharge to an independent program	Education of the athlete

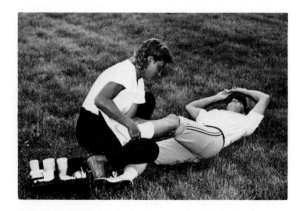

Fig. 2-8. Certified athletic trainer. The NATA–certified athletic trainer provides immediate on-the-field care of injured athletes.

serious injuries; however, prolonged immobilization may lead to a decreased functional length of musculotendinous tissue and decreased sport performance. Therefore the term *restricted activity* is preferred to rest. Restricted activity allows the athlete to participate at the maximally safe level.

Ice application produces a decrease in metabolic production and therefore lowers the cell's oxygen and nutrient requirements. In turn, these reduced requirements decrease blood flow, edema, and muscular fatigue. Decreased pain is also noted. Cold application may be provided in many ways, including ice packs, ice massage, cold whirlpool (approximately 55° F), inflatable splints with refrigerant gas, and ice towels.

Compression may be performed with tape, wraps, compression sleeves, exercise, massage, or intermit-

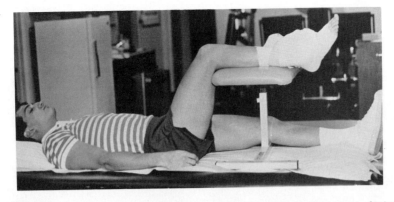

Fig. 2-9. PRICE. PRICE is a commonly used acronym in the immediate treatment of injuries.

tent compression devices. The purpose of compression is to enhance lymphatic and venous return, normalize osmotic pressure, minimize fluid accumulation in the intercellular space, and hence minimize swelling and edema at the injury site. Elevation of the injured part also assists in this process and is accomplished via gravity by raising the injured part higher than the heart.

After the immediate treatment program has been implemented and when the environment allows (return to the outpatient clinic or training room), the athlete must be reevaluated so that short-term treatment goals and procedures may be revised and long-term goals developed. These treatment procedures and short-term goals are primarily concerned with assisting the healing process and enabling the subsidence of the symptoms associated with the injury, such as pain, swelling, and decreased function. Short-term goals are therefore goals that may be achieved in 2 to 4 weeks after injury.[8] Symptoms may be minimized with the assistance of therapeutic modalities, therapeutic exercises, and education of the athlete.

Hot and cold applications, shortwave and microwave diathermy, phonophoresis and iontophoresis, radiation, ultrasound, electrical stimulation, and intermittent compression devices are all examples of physical modalities that may be used to achieve these short-term goals (Figure 2-10). Other physical measures that are helpful are massage, joint mobilization, constant passive motion devices, and traction.

Exercise is the most critical part of a rehabilitation program. The primary goals of therapeutic exercise during this stage of recovery are as follows: (1) to maintain or promote normal function without aggravation to the injury and (2) to decrease swelling and

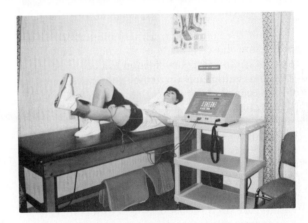

Fig. 2-10. Therapeutic modalities. Therapeutic modalities, such as functional electrical stimulation, are an integral part of injury rehabilitation.

edema via rhythmic isometric or active muscular contractions, thus assisting lymphatic return.

Long-term goals. Long-term goals require more than 4 weeks until an optimal level of function is achieved.[8] Therapeutic exercise plays an important part in the achievement of long-term goals. Therapeutic exercise is used to increase strength, agility, speed, power, range of motion, sensory feedback, posture, endurance, coordination, balance, relaxation, and other psychological training skills (Figure 2-11).

The SAID principle (specific adaptations to imposed demands) must be reemphasized during the development of the long-term goals and treatment programs. Rehabilitation must be adapted to the specific demands placed upon the athlete's body and on the injured part by the specific requirements of the sport and playing position.

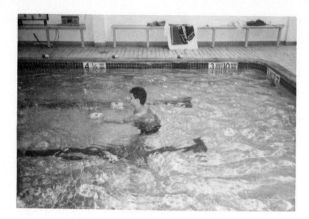

Fig. 2-11. Hydrotherapy. Hydrotherapy may be a beneficial form of exercise.

While the long-term treatment program advances, a decision must be made as to whether or when a safe return to sport participation can take place. This decision is ultimately up to the sports physician, with the assistance of the sports therapist, coach, and athlete. Results of reevaluation, along with understanding the specific physical demands of the athlete's individual sport and position, must be reviewed to determine whether the healing and functional level of the athlete are adequate for safe reentry in sports (Figure 2-12). Whenever in doubt concerning the degree of healing and safe return of the athlete, the health-care professional must be conservative.

FACTORS THAT INFLUENCE REHABILITATION GOALS. Adherence to the SAID principle is necessary for rehabilitation goals. Many athlete-specific factors can cause a practitioner to modify the rehabilitation goals. Such factors include type of sport, time remaining in the season, other sports of participation, game rules, outside sporting influences, psyche of the athlete, type and severity of the injury, stage of healing, and treatment techniques (see box).[15]

Different sports place different demands on an injury. For example, a shoulder injury to a soccer player does not produce as great a playing deficit as a shoulder injury to a baseball player. Likewise, the position played within the same sport is also influential; for example, a shoulder injury to a first baseman vs. to a pitcher.

Time remaining in the season and other sport participations can produce modifications in the rehabilitation goals. If an injury occurs at the end of the season and there is no postseason championship play, the athlete may choose to be conservative and not strive for active participation in the last game. This

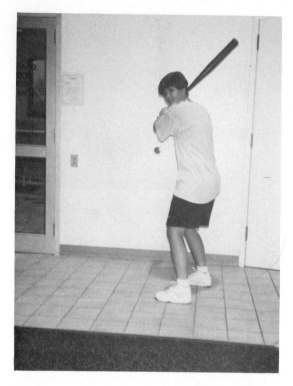

Fig. 2-12. Functional testing. Functional testing may be performed to determine the athlete's functional level for safe reentry in sports.

choice may especially be the case if the athlete will soon be involved with another sport season.

Game rules also cause modifications in goals through protective padding or bracing restrictions regarding substitutions. Although outside sporting influences, such as scholarship possibilities and coach or parental influence, should not sway a health-care practitioner's decision on the resumption of activity, those pressures exist and should be weighed with extreme caution.

Sports psychology is an interesting but often overlooked aspect of athletic rehabilitation. Injury and illness produce a wide range of emotional reactions; therefore the health-care practitioner needs to understand and develop the individual psyche of each athlete. Athletes vary in terms of pain threshold, cooperation and compliance, competitiveness, denial of disability, depression, intrinsic and extrinsic motivation, anger, fear, guilt, and the ability to adjust to injury. Besides dealing with the mental aspect of the injury, sports psychology may also be used to improve total athletic performance through the use of visu-

---

OUTLINE OF FACTORS THAT INFLUENCE REHABILITATION GOALS

1. Type of sport
   a. Demands that particular sport will make upon the injury
   b. Position played
2. Time remaining in the season
   a. Beginning vs. end of season
   b. Postseason play and championships
3. Other sports
   a. Other sports in which the athlete participates
   b. Priorities of these sports
4. Sport rules
   a. As they relate to injuries and substitutions
   b. Protective equipment
5. Outside sporting influence
   a. Possibility of scholarships
   b. Parents' or coach's involvement with the injury
6. Psyche of the athlete
   a. Intrinsic and extrinsic motivation
   b. Cooperation and compliance
   c. Competitiveness
   d. Pain threshold
7. Type of injury
   a. Sprain vs. contusion vs. fracture
   b. Secondary injuries
8. Severity of the injury
   a. Amount and degree of dysfunction
9. Type of treatment and rehabilitation
   a. The requirement of surgical intervention including precautions, contraindications, and complications
   b. Speed in controlling initial pain and swelling
   c. Type of surgical procedure (for example, meniscal repair vs. meniscectomy)

---

alization, self-hypnosis, and relaxation techniques.

The severity of the injury, along with the type of treatment and rehabilitation that is instituted, will influence short- and long-term goals. The amount of pain, swelling, and dysfunction; whether surgery (and the type of surgery) is required; and the existence of precautions, complications, or contraindications of treatment can all produce modifications in goal setting. Last, the stage of healing is a strong factor influencing rehabilitation goals and treatment management.

SUMMARY

1. The best way to treat a sports injury is to prevent the injury from occurring.
2. After an athlete has acquired an injury, a speedy but thorough initial evaluation must be performed so that appropriate, immediate rehabilitation goals and a treatment management program may be established.
3. Goals include specific data.
4. The most efficient and effective form of rehabilitation is therapeutic exercise.
5. The rehabilitation goals after injury are based upon the safe return of an injured athlete to the previous level of competition as quickly as possible.

REFERENCES

1. Armstrong LE: The impact of hyperthermia and hypohydration on circulation, strength, endurance, and health, *J Appl Sport Sci Res* 2(4):60-65, 1988.
2. Arnheim DD, Prentice W: *Principles of athletic training* ed 8, St Louis, 1993, Mosby.
3. Åstrand PO, Rodahl K: *Textbook of work physiology,* New York, 1977, McGraw Hill.
4. Booher JM, Thibodeau GA: *Athletic injury assessment,* St Louis, 1985, Mosby.
5. Davies GJ: *A compendium of isokinetics in clinical usage,* ed 3, LaCrosse, WI, 1987, S & S Publishers.
6. Houston ME, Green HJ, Thomas JA: The effects of rapid weight loss on physiological functions in wrestlers, *Phys Sports Med* 9:173, 1981.
7. Hunter LY, Funk FJ: *Rehabilitation of the injured knee,* St Louis, 1984, Mosby.
8. Kettenbach G: *Writing S.O.A.P. notes,* Philadelphia 1990, FA Davis.
9. Klinzing JE, Kapowicz W: The effects of rapid weight loss and rehydration on a wrestling performance test, *J Sports Med* 16:82, 1986.
10. Konin JG: *Pre-injury data collection,* presented at Injuries in Baseball Course, Birmingham, AL, 1992 American Sports Medicine Institute.
11. Mellion MB: Sports injuries and athletic problems, St Louis, 1988, Mosby.
12. Moffroid MT, Kusiak ET: The power struggle, *Phys Ther* 55:1098-1104, 1975.
13. Moyer JA: Playing in lightning is risky business, *Softball News* 6(7):2, 1988.
14. Neilsen B, Sjogaard G, Ugeluig J, et al.: Fluid balance in exercise dehydration and rehydration with different glucose-electrolyte drinks, *Eur J Appl Physiol* 55:318-325, 1986.
15. Roy S, Irvin R: *Sports medicine: prevention, evaluation, management, and rehabilitation,* Englewood Cliffs, NJ, 1983, Prentice-Hall.
16. Saltin B: Circulatory response to submaximal and maximal exercise after thermal dehydration. *J Appl Physiol* 19:1114, 1964.
17. Torranin C, Smith DP, Byrd R: The effect of acute thermal dehydration and rapid rehydration on isometric and isotonic endurance, *J Sports Med Phys Fit* 19:1-9, 1979.
18. Wardlaw G, Insel P: *Perspectives in nutrition,* St Louis, 1993, Mosby.
19. *Webster's Ninth New Collegiate Dictionary,* Springfield, Mass, 1984, Merriam-Webster.

Maintaining and Improving Flexibility

3

William E. Prentice

OBJECTIVES

After completion of this chapter, the student should be able to do the following:

- Define flexibility, and describe its importance in injury rehabilitation.

- Identify factors that limit flexibility.

- Differentiate between active and passive range of motion.

- Explain the difference between ballistic, static, and PNF stretching.

- Discuss the neurophysiological principles of stretching.

- Describe stretching exercises that may be used to improve flexibility at specific joints throughout the body.

The sports therapist is responsible for designing, monitoring, and progressing programs of rehabilitation for injured athletes. The goals for a sports medicine rehabilitation program differ from goals for other patient populations. The athlete must return to competitive fitness levels, and the intensity of the rehabilitation must be adjusted appropriately during the course of the program. The sports therapist has to understand the principles and techniques involved in reconditioning the injured athlete. The term *therapeutic exercise* is commonly used to refer to techniques of reconditioning.

FLEXIBILITY

Flexibility has been defined as the ability to move a joint or series of joints through a full, nonrestricted, pain-free range of motion.[1,2,14,22,32] For the sports therapist, a return to or improvement on this preinjury range is an important goal of any rehabilitation program. Most sports activities require relatively "normal" amounts of flexibility. However, some activities, such as gymnastics, ballet, diving, or karate, require

increased flexibility for superior performance (Figure 3-1). An athlete who has a restricted range of motion will probably realize a decrease in performance capabilities. For example, a sprinter with tight, inelastic hamstring muscles probably loses some speed because the hamstring muscles restrict the ability to flex the hip joint and thus shorten stride length. Lack of flexibility may also result in uncoordinated or awkward movement patterns.

Most sports therapists would agree that good flexibility is essential to successful physical performance, although their ideas are based primarily on observation rather than scientific research. Likewise, they also believe that maintaining good flexibility is important in prevention of injury to the musculotendinous unit, and they will generally insist that stretching exercises be included as part of the warm-up before engaging in strenuous activity,[13,27,34] although little or no research evidence is available to support this practice.

Flexibility can be discussed in relation to movement involving only one joint, such as the knees, or movement involving a whole series of joints, such as

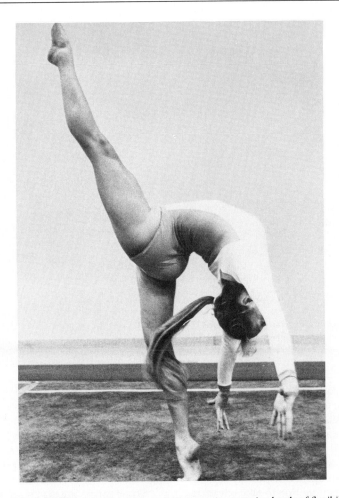

Fig. 3-1. Flexibility. Certain sports activities require superior levels of flexibility.

the spinal vertebral joints, which must all move together to allow smooth bending or rotation of the trunk. Flexibility is specific to a given joint or movement. A person may have good range of motion in the ankles, knees, hips, back, and one shoulder joint. If the other shoulder joint lacks normal movement, however, then a problem exists that needs to be corrected before the person can function normally.[7]

FACTORS THAT LIMIT FLEXIBILITY

A number of anatomical factors may limit the ability of a joint to move through a full, unrestricted range of motion. The **bony structure** may restrict the endpoint in the range. An elbow that has been fractured through the joint may lay down excess calcium in the joint space, causing the joint to lose its ability to fully extend. However in many instances we rely on bony prominences to stop movements at normal endpoints in the range.

Fat may also limit the ability to move through a full range of motion. A person who has a large amount of fat on the abdomen may have severely restricted trunk flexion when asked to bend forward and touch the toes. The fat may act as a wedge between two lever arms, restricting movement wherever it is found.

Skin might also be responsible for limiting movement. For example, a person who has had some type of injury or surgery involving a tearing incision or

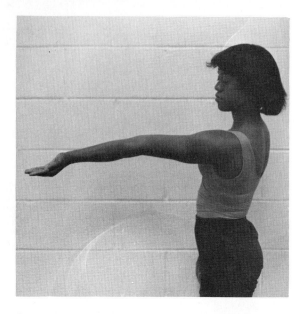

Fig. 3-2. Excessive joint motion. Excessive joint motion, such as the hyperextended elbow, can predispose a joint to injury.

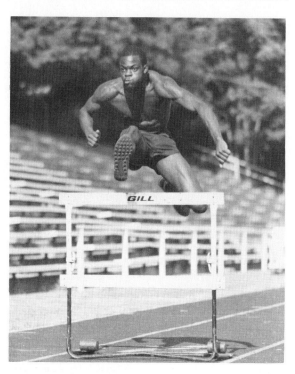

Fig. 3-3. Flexibility. Flexibility is an essential component of many sports-related activities.

laceration of the skin, particularly over a joint, will have inelastic scar tissue formed at that site. This scar tissue is incapable of stretching with joint movement.

Muscles and their tendons, along with their surrounding fascial sheaths, are most often responsible for limiting range of motion. When performing stretching exercises to improve flexibility about a particular joint, you are attempting to take advantage of the highly elastic properties of a muscle. Over time it is possible to increase the elasticity, or the length that a given muscle can be stretched. Persons who have a good deal of movement at a particular joint tend to have highly elastic and flexible muscles. **Connective tissue** surrounding the joint, such as ligaments on the joint capsule, may be subject to **contractures.** Ligaments and joint capsules have some elasticity; however, if a joint is immobilized for a period of time, these structures tend to lose some elasticity and actually shorten. This condition is most commonly seen after surgical repair of an unstable joint, but it can also result from long periods of inactivity.

It is also possible for a person to have relatively slack ligaments and joint capsules. These people are generally referred to as being *loose-jointed.* Examples of this trait would be an elbow or knee that hyper-

extends beyond 180 degrees (Figure 3-2). Frequently there is instability associated with loose-jointedness that may present as great a problem in movement as ligamentous or capsular contractures.

Skin contractures caused by scarring of ligaments, joint capsules, and musculotendinous units are each capable of improving elasticity to varying degrees through stretching over time. With the exception of bony structure, age, and gender, all the other factors that limit flexibility may be altered to increase range of joint motion.

ACTIVE AND PASSIVE RANGE OF MOTION

Active range of motion, also called *dynamic flexibility,* refers to the degree to which a joint can be moved by a muscle contraction, usually through the midrange of movement. Dynamic flexibility is not necessarily a good indicator of the stiffness or looseness of a joint because it applies to the ability to move a joint efficiently, with little resistance to motion.[17]

Passive range of motion, sometimes called *static flexibility,* refers to the degree to which a joint may

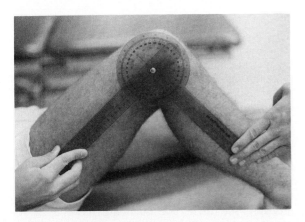

Fig. 3-4. Goniometric measurement. Measurement of active knee joint flexion using a goniometer.

be passively moved to the endpoints in the range of motion. No muscle contraction is involved to move a joint through a passive range.

When a muscle actively contracts, it produces a joint movement through a specific range of motion.[32,35] However, if passive pressure is applied to an extremity, it is capable of moving farther in the range of motion. It is essential in sports activities that an extremity be capable of moving through a nonrestricted range of motion.[33] For example, a hurdler who cannot fully extend the knee joint in a normal stride is at considerable disadvantage because stride length and thus speed will be reduced significantly (Figure 3-3).

Passive range of motion is important for injury prevention. There are many situations in sports in which a muscle is forced to stretch beyond its normal active limits. If the muscle does not have enough elasticity to compensate for this additional stretch, it is likely that the musculotendinous unit will be injured.

Assessment of Active and Passive Range of Motion

Accurate measurement of active and passive range of joint motion is difficult.[19] Various devices have been designed to accommodate variations in the size of the joints, as well as the complexity of movements in articulations that involve more than one joint.[21] Of these devices, the simplest and most widely used is the **goniometer** (Figure 3-4).

A goniometer is a large protractor with measure-

TABLE 3-1
Active Ranges of Joint Motions

Joint	Action	Degrees of Motion
Shoulder	Flexion	0-180 degrees
	Extension	0-50 degrees
	Abduction	0-180 degrees
	Medial rotation	0-90 degrees
	Lateral rotation	0-90 degrees
Elbow	Flexion	0-160 degrees
Forearm	Pronation	0-90 degrees
	Supination	0-90 degrees
Wrist	Flexion	0-90 degrees
	Extension	0-70 degrees
	Abduction	0-25 degrees
	Adduction	0-65 degrees
Hip	Flexion	0-125 degrees
	Extension	0-15 degrees
	Abduction	0-45 degrees
	Adduction	0-15 degrees
	Medial rotation	0-45 degrees
	Lateral rotation	0-45 degrees
Knee	Flexion	0-140 degrees
Ankle	Plantarflexion	0-45 degrees
	Dorsiflexion	0-20 degrees
Foot	Inversion	0-30 degrees
	Eversion	0-10 degrees

ments in degrees. By aligning the individual arms of the goniometer parallel to the longitudinal axis of the two segments involved in motion about a specific joint, it is possible to obtain reasonably accurate measurement of range of movement. To enhance reliability, standardization of measurement techniques and methods of recording active and passive ranges of motion are critical in individual clinics where successive measurements may be taken by different sports therapists to assess progress. Table 3-1 provides a list of what would be considered normal active ranges for movements at various joints.

The goniometer has an important place in a rehabilitation setting, where it is essential to assess improvement in joint flexibility to modify injury rehabilitation programs.

STRETCHING TECHNIQUES

Flexibility has been defined as the range of motion possible about a single joint or through a series of articulations. The maintenance of a full, nonrestricted range of motion has long been recognized as an essential component of athletic fitness.[8,9,10] Flexibility is important not only for successful physical performance but also for the prevention of injury.[5]

The goal of any effective flexibility program should be to improve the range of motion at a given articulation by altering the extensibility of the musculotendinous units that produce movement at that joint. It is well documented that exercises that stretch these musculotendinous units over time will increase the range of movement possible about a given joint.[29]

Stretching techniques for improving flexibility have evolved over the years.[24] The oldest technique for stretching is called *ballistic stretching,* which makes use of repetitive bouncing motions. A second technique, known as *static stretching,* involves stretching a muscle to the point of discomfort and then holding it at that point for an extended time. This technique has been used for many years. Recently another group of stretching techniques known collectively as *proprioceptive neuromuscular facilitation (PNF),* involving alternating contractions and stretches, has also been recommended.[25] Researchers have had considerable discussion about which of these techniques is most effective for improving range of motion.

Agonist vs. Antagonist Muscles

Before discussing the three different stretching techniques, it is essential to define the terms *agonist* and *antagonist muscles.* Most joints in the body are capable of more than one movement. The knee joint, for example, is capable of flexion and extension. Contraction of the quadriceps group of muscles on the front of the thigh causes knee extension, whereas contraction of the hamstring muscles on the back of the thigh produces knee flexion.

To achieve knee extension, the quadriceps group contracts while the hamstring muscles relax and stretch. Muscles that work in concert with one another in this manner are called *synergistic muscle groups.*[4] The muscle that contracts to produce a movement, in this case the quadriceps, is referred to as the *agonist muscle.* Conversely, the muscle being stretched in response to contraction of the agonist muscle is called the *antagonist muscle.* In this example of knee extension, the antagonist muscle would be the hamstring group. Some degree of balance in strength must exist between agonist and an-

tagonist muscle groups. This balance is necessary for normal, smooth, coordinated movement, as well as for reducing the likelihood of muscle strain caused by muscular imbalance.

Comprehension of this synergistic muscle action is essential to understanding the three techniques of stretching.

Ballistic Stretching

If you were to walk out to the track on any spring or fall afternoon and watch people who are warming up with stretching exercises before they run, you would probably see them use bouncing movements to stretch a particular muscle. This bouncing technique is more appropriately known as *ballistic stretching,* in which repetitive contractions of the agonist muscle are used to produce quick stretches of the antagonist muscle.

Over the years, many fitness experts have questioned the safety of the ballistic stretching technique.[3,23] Their concerns have been primarily based on the idea that ballistic stretching creates somewhat uncontrolled forces within the muscle that may exceed the extensibility limits of the muscle fiber, thus producing small microtears within the musculotendinous unit. Certainly this may be true in sedentary individuals or perhaps in athletes who have sustained muscle injuries.

Most sports activities are dynamic and require ballistic-type movements. For example, forcefully kicking a soccer ball 50 times involves a repeated dynamic contraction of the agonist quadriceps muscle. The antagonist hamstrings are contracting eccentrically to decelerate the lower leg. Ballistic stretching of the hamstring muscle before engaging in this type of activity should allow the muscle to gradually adapt to the imposed demands and reduce the likelihood of injury. Since ballistic stretching is functional, it should be integrated into training and reconditioning programs when appropriate.

Static Stretching

The static stretching technique is another extremely effective and popular technique of stretching. This technique involves passively stretching a given antagonist muscle by placing it in a maximal position of stretch and holding it there for an extended time. Recommendations for the optimal time for holding this stretched position vary, ranging from as short as

3 seconds to as long as 60 seconds.[25] One study has indicated that holding a stretch for 15 seconds is as effective as 2 minutes for increasing muscle flexibility. Stretches lasting for longer than 30 seconds seem to be uncomfortable for the athlete. A static stretch of each muscle should be repeated 3 or 4 times. A static stretch may be accomplished by using a contraction of the agonist muscle to place the antagonist muscle in a position of stretch. A passive static stretch requires the use of *body* weight, assistance from the sports therapist or partner, or use of a T-bar, primarily for stretching the upper extremity.

Much research has been done comparing ballistic and static stretching techniques for the improvement of flexibility. Static and ballistic stretching appear to be equally effective in increasing flexibility, and there is no significant difference between the two. However, much of the literature states that with static stretching there is less danger of exceeding the extensibility limits of the involved joints because the stretch is more controlled. Most of the literature indicates that ballistic stretching is apt to cause muscular soreness, especially in sedentary individuals, whereas static stretching generally does not cause soreness and is commonly used in injury rehabilitation of sore or strained muscles.[15]

Static stretching is likely a much safer stretching technique, especially for sedentary or untrained individuals. However, since many physical activities involve dynamic movement, stretching in a warm-up should begin with static stretching followed by ballistic stretching, which more closely resembles the dynamic activity.

PNF Stretching Techniques

PNF techniques were first used by physical therapists for treating patients who had various neuromuscular disorders.[25] Only recently have PNF stretching exercises been used as a stretching technique for increasing flexibility.[28,31]

There are a number of different PNF techniques currently being used for stretching, including slow-reversal-hold-relax, contract-relax, and hold-relax techniques.[36] All techniques involve some combination of alternating isometric or isotonic contractions and relaxation of both agonist and antagonist muscles (a 10-second pushing phase followed by a 10-second relaxing phase). PNF stretching techniques are described in detail in Chapter 11.

PNF stretching techniques can be used to stretch any muscle in the body.[11,12] PNF stretching techniques are perhaps best performed with a partner, although they may also be done using a wall as resistance.

NEUROPHYSIOLOGICAL BASIS OF STRETCHING

All three stretching techniques are based on a neurophysiological phenomenon involving the **stretch reflex** (see Figure 11-1).[30] Every muscle in the body contains various types of mechanoreceptors that when stimulated inform the central nervous system of what is happening with that muscle. Two of these mechanoreceptors are important in the stretch reflex: the **muscle spindle** and the **Golgi tendon organ.** Both types of receptors are sensitive to changes in muscle length. The Golgi tendon organs are also affected by changes in muscle tension. When a muscle is stretched, the muscle spindles are also stretched, sending a volley of sensory impulses to the spinal cord that inform the central nervous system that the muscle is being stretched. Impulses return to the muscle from the spinal cord, which causes the muscle to reflexively contract, thus resisting the stretch.[30] If the stretch of the muscle continues for an extended period of time (at least 6 seconds), the Golgi tendon organs respond to the change in length and the increase in tension by firing off sensory impulses of their own to the spinal cord. The impulses from the Golgi tendon organs, unlike the signals from the muscle spindle, cause a reflex relaxation of the antagonist muscle. This reflex relaxation serves as a protective mechanism that will allow the muscle to stretch through relaxation before the extensibility limits are exceeded, causing damage to the muscle fibers.[37]

With the jerking, bouncing motion of ballistic stretching, the muscle spindles are being repetitively stretched, thus there is continuous resistance by the muscle to further stretch. The ballistic stretch is not continued long enough to allow the Golgi tendon organs to have a relaxing effect.

The static stretch involves a continuous sustained stretch lasting anywhere from 6 to 60 seconds, which is sufficient time for the Golgi tendon organs to begin responding to the increase in tension. The impulses from the Golgi tendon organs can override the impulses coming from the muscle spindles, allowing the muscle to reflexively relax after the initial reflex resistance to the change in length. Thus lengthening the muscle and allowing it to remain in a stretched position for an extended period of time is unlikely to produce any injury to the muscle.

The effectiveness of the PNF techniques may be attributed in part to these same neurophysiological principles. The slow-reversal-hold technique discussed previously takes advantage of two additional neurophysiological phenomena.[29]

The maximal isometric contraction of the muscle that will be stretched during the 10-second "push" phase again causes an increase in tension that stimulates the Golgi tendon organs to affect a reflex relaxation of the antagonist even before the muscle is placed in a position of stretch. This relaxation of the antagonist muscle during contractions is referred to as *autogenic inhibition.*

During the relaxing phase the antagonist is relaxed and passively stretched while there is a maximal isotonic contraction of the agonist muscle pulling the extremity further into the agonist pattern. In any synergistic muscle group, a contraction of the agonist causes a reflex relaxation in the antagonist muscle, allowing it to stretch and protecting it from injury. This phenomenon is referred to as *reciprocal inhibition* (see Figure 11-2).

Thus with the PNF techniques the additive effects of autogenic and reciprocal inhibition should theoretically allow the muscle to be stretched to a greater degree than is possible with static or ballistic stretching.[30]

PRACTICAL APPLICATION

Although all three stretching techniques have been demonstrated to effectively improve flexibility, there is still considerable debate as to which technique produces the greatest increases in range of movement. The ballistic technique is recommended for any athlete who is involved in dynamic activity despite its potential for causing muscle soreness in the sedentary or untrained individual. In highly trained individuals, it is unlikely that ballistic stretching will result in muscle soreness.

Static stretching is perhaps the most widely used technique. It is a simple technique and does not require a partner. A fully nonrestricted range of motion can be attained through static stretching over time. PNF stretching techniques are capable of producing dramatic increases in range of motion during one stretching session. Studies comparing static and PNF stretching suggest that PNF stretching is capable of producing greater improvement in flexibility over an extended training period.[16,29] The major disadvantage of PNF stretching is that a partner is usually required to assist with the stretch, although stretching with a partner may have some motivational advantages. More and more athletic teams seem to be adopting the PNF technique as the method of choice for improving flexibility.

THE RELATIONSHIP OF STRENGTH AND FLEXIBILITY

We often hear about the negative effects that strength training has on flexibility. For example, someone who develops large bulk through strength training is often referred to as *muscle bound.* The expression muscle bound has negative connotations in terms of the ability of that person to move. We tend to think of people who have highly developed muscles as having lost much of their ability to move freely through a full range of motion.[26]

Occasionally a person develops so much bulk that the physical size of the muscle prevents a normal range of motion. Strength training that is not properly done can impair movement, however, there is no reason to believe that weight training, if done properly through a full range of motion, will impair flexibility. Proper strength training probably improves dynamic flexibility and, if combined with a rigorous stretching program, can greatly enhance powerful and coordinated movements that are essential for success in many athletic activities. In all cases a heavy-weight training program should be accompanied by a strong flexibility program (Figure 3-5).

GUIDELINES AND PRECAUTIONS FOR STRETCHING

The following guidelines and precautions should be incorporated into a sound stretching program:

- Warm up using a slow jog or fast walk before stretching vigorously.
- To increase flexibility, the muscle must be overloaded or stretched beyond its normal range but not to the point of pain.
- Stretch only to the point where you feel tightness or resistance to stretch or perhaps some discomfort. Stretching should not be painful.[6]
- Increases in range of motion will be specific to whatever muscle or joint is being stretched.
- Exercise caution when stretching muscles that surround painful joints. Pain is an indication that

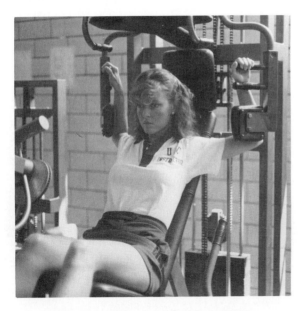

Fig. 3-5. Strength training can improve flexibility.
Strength training through a full range of motion will not impair flexibility.

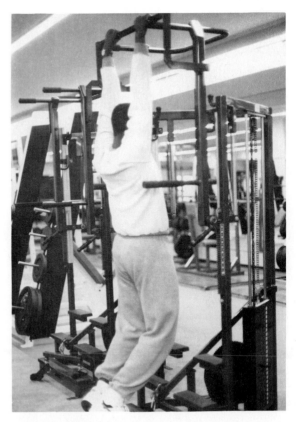

Fig. 3-6. Hanging stretch. Muscles: General stretch for shoulder girdle muscles.

something is wrong and should not be ignored.

- Avoid overstretching the ligaments and capsules that surround joints.
- Exercise caution when stretching the low back and neck. Exercises that compress the vertebrae and their discs may cause damage.
- Stretching from a seated rather than a standing position takes stress off the low back and decreases the chances of back injury.
- Stretch those muscles that are tight and inflexible.
- Strengthen those muscles that are weak and loose.
- Always stretch slowly and with control.
- Be sure to continue normal breathing during a stretch. Do not hold your breath.
- Static and PNF techniques are most often recommended for individuals who want to improve their range of motion.
- Ballistic stretching should be done only by those who are already flexible or accustomed to stretching and done only after static stretching.
- Stretching should be done at least three times per week to see minimal improvement. It is recommended that you stretch between five and six times per week to see maximum results.

STRETCHING EXERCISES

Figure 3-6 to 3-26 illustrate stretching exercises that may be used to improve flexibility at specific joints throughout the body. The exercises described may be done statically or with slight modification; they may also be done with a partner using a PNF technique.

There are many possible variations to each of these exercises.[20] The exercises selected are those that seem to be the most effective for stretching of various muscle groups.

SUMMARY

1. Flexibility is the ability to move a joint or a series of joints smoothly through a full range of motion.
2. Flexibility is specific to a given joint, and the term

Text continued on page 50.

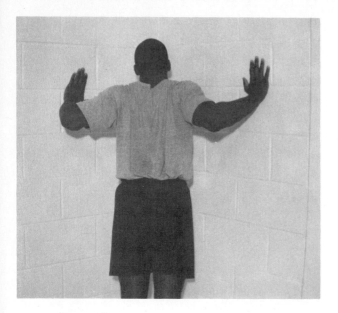

Fig. 3-7. Wall corner stretch. Muscles: Greater and smaller pectoral, anterior deltoid, coracobrachial.

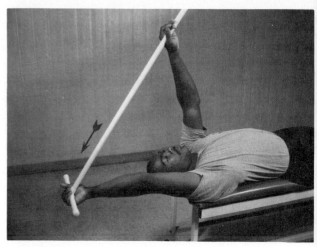

Fig. 3-8. Shoulder extensors stretch using T-Bar. Muscles: Latissimus dorsi, teres major and minor, posterior deltoid, triceps.

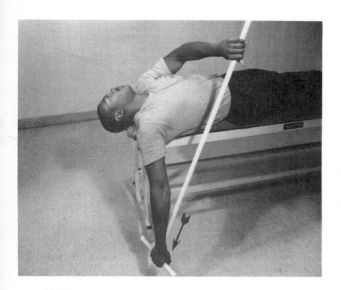

Fig. 3-9. Shoulder flexors stretch using T-Bar. Muscles: Anterior deltoid, coracobrachialis, pectoralis major, biceps.

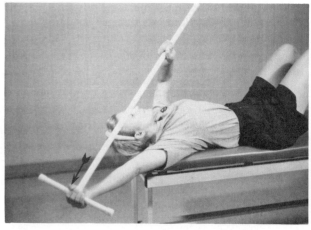

Fig. 3-10. Shoulder adductors stretch using T-Bar. Muscles: Latissimus dorsi, teres major and minor, pectoralis major; pectoralis minor, posterior deltoid, triceps.

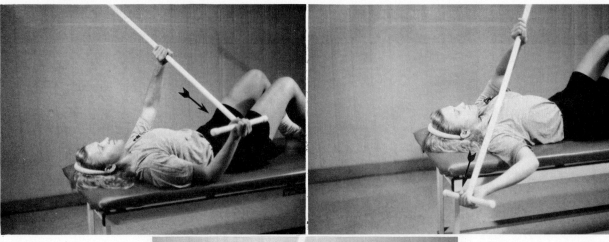

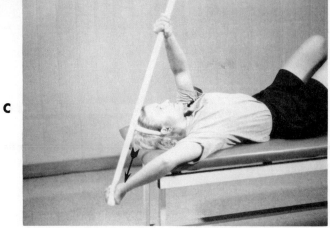

B

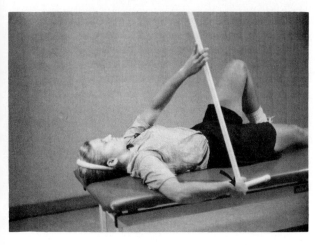

C

Fig. 3-11. Shoulder internal rotators stretch using T-Bar. Muscles: Subscapularis, pectoralis major, latissimus dorsi, teres major, anterior deltoid. NOTE: Stretch should be done with arm at **A,** 0 degrees, **B,** 90 degrees, and **C,** 135 degrees.

Fig. 3-12. Shoulder external rotators stretch using T-Bar.
Muscles: Infraspinatus, teres minor, posterior deltoid.

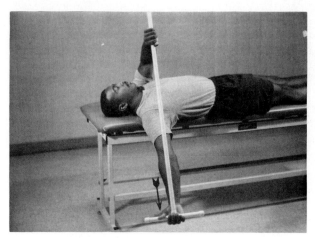

Fig. 3-13. Horizontal adductors stretch using T-Bar.
Muscles: Pectoralis major, anterior deltoid, biceps.

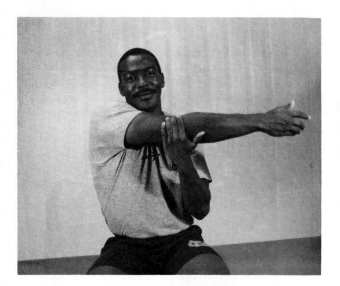

Fig. 3-14. Horizontal abductors stretch. Muscles: Posterior deltoid, infraspinatus, teres minor, rhomboids, middle trapezius.

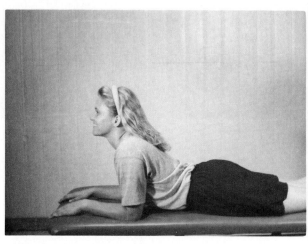

Fig. 3-15. Trunk and low back flexors stretch. Muscles: Rectus abdominis, internal and external obliques.

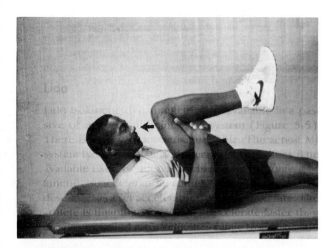

Fig. 3-16. Trunk and low back extensors stretch. Muscles: Erector spinae, iliocostalis thoracis, longissimus thoracis, spinalis thoracis, iliocostalis lumborum, quadratus lumborum.

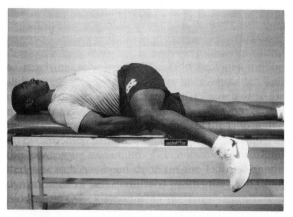

Fig. 3-17. Trunk and low back rotators stretch. Muscles: Internal oblique on side toward rotation, external oblique on side opposite rotation, rectus abdominis, latissimus dorsi on side opposite rotation, semispinalis, multifidus, rotator.

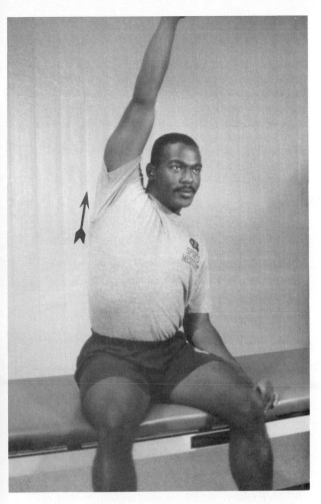

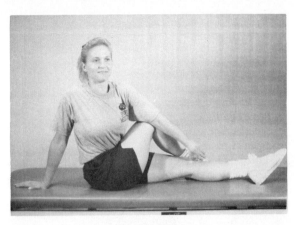

Fig. 3-19. Figure 4. Muscles: Piriformis, internal and external obturator, quadriceps gluteus maximus.

Fig. 3-18. Trunk lateral flexors stretch. Muscles: Latissimus dorsi, internal and external obliques, rectus abdominis.

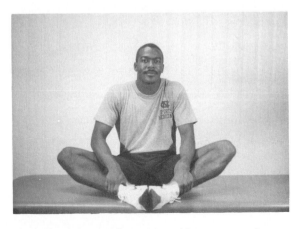

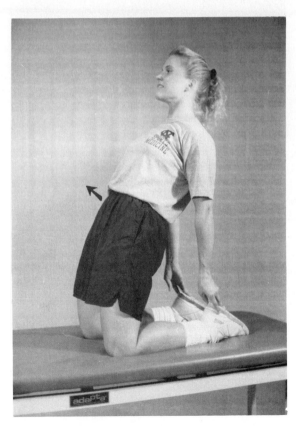

Fig. 3-20. Groin stretch. Muscles: Adductor magnus, longus, and brevis; pectineus; gracilis.

Fig. 3-21. Kneeling thrusts. Muscles: Rectus femoris.

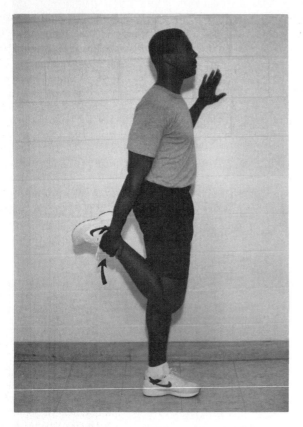

Fig. 3-22. Knee extensors stretch. Muscles: Quadriceps.

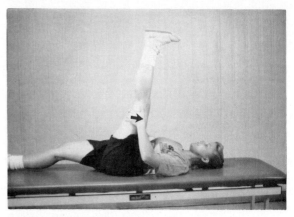

Fig. 3-23. Knee flexors stretch. Muscles: Hamstrings. NOTE: Externally rotated tibia stretches semimembranous and semitendinous; internally rotated tibia stretches biceps femoris.

good flexibility implies that there are no joint abnormalities restricting movement.

3. Flexibility may be limited by fat, bone structure, skin, connective tissue, ligaments, or muscles and tendons.

4. Passive range of motion refers to the degree to which a joint may be passively moved to the endpoints in the range of motion, whereas active range of motion refers to movement through the midrange of motion resulting from active contraction.

5. Measurement of joint flexibility is accomplished through the use of a goniometer.

6. An agonist muscle is one that contracts to produce joint motion; the antagonist muscle is stretched with contraction of the agonist.

7. Ballistic, static, and proprioceptive neuromuscular facilitation (PNF) techniques have all been used as stretching techniques for improving flexibility.

8. Each of these stretching techniques is based on the neurophysiological phenomena involving the muscle spindles and Golgi tendon organs. PNF techniques appear to be the most effective in producing increases in flexibility.

9. Stretching should be included as part of the warm-up period to prepare the muscles for what they are going to be asked to do and to prevent injury, as well as in the cool-down period to help reduce injury. Stretching after an activity may prevent muscle soreness and will help increase flexibility by stretching a loose, warmed up muscle.

10. Strength training, if done correctly through a full range of motion, will probably improve flexibility.

REFERENCES

1 Alter MJ: *The science of stretching,* Champaign, Ill, 1988, Human Kinetics Publishers.

2 Arnheim DD, Prentice WE: *Principles of athletic training,* St Louis, 1993, Mosby.

3 Åstrand PO, Rodahl K: *Textbook of work physiology,* New York, 1986, McGraw-Hill.

4 Basmajian J: *Therapeutic exercise,* ed 4, Baltimore, 1984, Williams & Wilkins.

5 Bealieu JE: *Stretching for all sports,* Pasadena, Calif, 1980, Athletic Press.

6 Bealieu JE: Developing a stretching program, *Phys Sports Med* 9(11):59, 1981.

7 Chapman EA, deVries HA, Swezey R: Joint stiffness: effect of exercise on young and old men, *J Gerontol* 27:218, 1972.

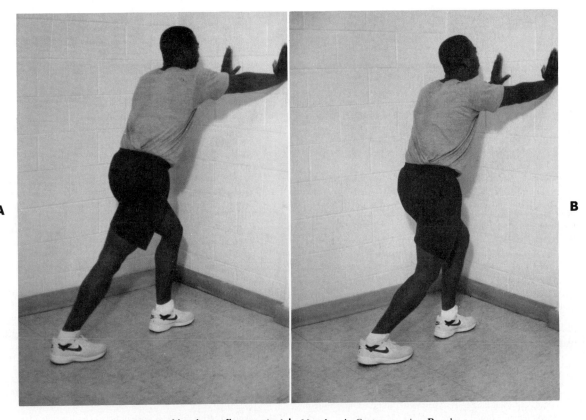

Fig. 3-24. Ankle plantarflexors stretch. Muscles: **A,** Gastrocnemius, **B,** soleus.

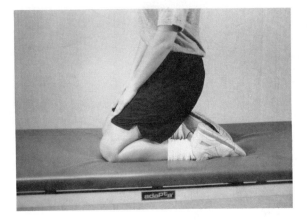

Fig. 3-25. Ankle dorsiflexors stretch. Muscles: Anterior tibialis.

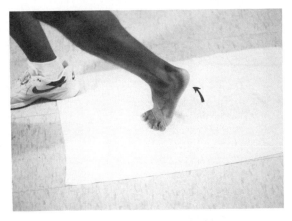

Fig. 3-26. Plantar fascia stretch. Structure: Plantar fascia.

8 Corbin C, Fox K: Flexibility: the forgotten part of fitness, *J Phys Educ* 16(6):191, 1985.

9 Corbin C, Noble L: Flexibility, *J Phys Educ Rec Dance* 51:23, 1980.

10 Corbin C, Noble L: Flexibility: a major component of physical fitness. In Cundiff DE, editor: *Implementation of health fitness exercise programs,* Reston, Va, 1985, American Alliance for Health, Physical Education, Recreation, and Dance.

11 Cornelius WL: Two effective flexibility methods, *Athletic Training* 16(1):23, 1981.

12 Cornelius WL: *PNF and other flexibility techniques,* Arlington, Va, 1986, Computer Microfilm International (microfiche; 20 fr).

13 Cornelius WL, Hagemann RW Jr, Jackson AW: A study on placement of stretching within a workout, *J Sports Med Phys Fitness* 28(3):234, 1988.

14 Couch J: *Runners world yoga book,* Mountain View, Calif, 1982, World Publications.

15 deVries H: *Physiology of exercise for physical education and athletics,* Dubuque, Iowa, 1986, WC Brown.

16 Godges JJ, MacRae H, Longdon C, et al.: The effects of two stretching procedures on hip range of motion and joint economy, *J Ortho Sports Phys Ther* 11:350-357, 1989.

17 Herling J: It's time to add strength training to our fitness programs, *J Phys Educ Program* 79:17, 1981.

18 Humphrey LD: Flexibility, *J Phys Educ Rec Dance* 52:41, 1981.

19 Hutinger P: How flexible are you? *Aquatic World Magazine,* Jan 1974.

20 Ishii DK: Flexibility strexercises for co-ed groups, *Scholastic Coach* 45:31, 1976.

21 Jackson AW, Baker AA: The relationship of the sit-and-reach test to criterion measures of hamstring and back flexibility in young females, *Res Q Exerc Sport* 57(3):183, 1986.

22 Jensen C, Fisher G: *Scientific basis of athletic conditioning,* Philadelphia, 1979, Lea & Febiger.

23 Johnson P: *Sport, exercise and you,* New York, 1975, Holt, Rinehart, & Winston.

24 Knortz K, Ringel C: Flexibility techniques, *National Strength and Conditioning Association Journal* 7(2):50, 1985.

25 Knott M, Voss P: *Proprioceptive neuromuscular facilitation,* ed 3, New York, 1985, Harper & Row.

26 Liemohn W: Flexibility and muscular strength, *J Phys Educ Rec Dance* 59(7):37, 1988.

27 Murphy P: Warming up before stretching advised, *Phys Sports Med* 14(3):45, 1986.

28 Prentice WE: An electromyographic analysis of heat or cold and stretching for inducing muscular relaxation, *J Orthop Sports Phys Ther* 3:133-140, 1982.

29 Prentice WE: A comparison of static and PNF stretching for improvement of hip joint flexibility, *Athletic Training* 18(1):56, 1983.

30 Prentice WE: A review of PNF techniques—implications for athletic rehabilitation and performance, *Forum Medicum* (51):1-13, 1989.

31 Prentice WE, Kooima E: The use of PNF techniques in rehabilitation of sport-related injury, *Athletic Training* 21(1):26-31, 1986.

32 Rasch P: *Kinesiology and applied anatomy,* Philadelphia, 1989, Lea & Febiger.

33 Sapega AA, Quedenfeld T, Moyer R, et al.: Biophysical factors in range-of-motion exercise, *Phys Sports Med* 9(12):57, 1981.

34 Shellock F, Prentice WE: Warm-up and stretching for improved physical performance and prevention of sport related injury, *Sports Med:* 2:267-278, 1985.

35 *Staying flexible: the full range of motion,* Alexandria, Va, 1987, Time Life Books.

36 Tanigawa MC: Comparison of the hold relax procedure and passive mobilization on increasing muscle length, *Phys Ther* 52:725, 1972.

37 Verrill D, Pate R: Relationship between duration of static stretch in the sit and reach position and biceps femoris electromyographic activity, *Med Sci Sports Exerc* 14:124, 1982.

Muscular Strength and Endurance

4

William E. Prentice

OBJECTIVES

After completion of this chapter, the student should be able to do the following:

- Define strength, and indicate its significance to health and skill of performance.

- Discuss the anatomy and physiology of skeletal muscle.

- Discuss the physiology of strength development and factors that determine strength.

- Describe specific methods for improving muscular strength.

- Differentiate between muscle strength and muscle endurance.

- Discuss differences between males and females in terms of strength development.

- Identify strength-training exercises for developing specific muscle groups.

- Demonstrate proper techniques for using weights to develop strength and muscular endurance.

THE IMPORTANCE OF MUSCULAR STRENGTH

One of the primary rehabilitation program goals of any sports therapist is to return muscular strength and endurance to preinjury levels. The development of muscular strength is an essential component of any reconditioning program. By definition, **strength** is the ability of a muscle to generate force against some resistance. Maintenance of at least a normal level of strength in a given muscle or muscle group is important for normal healthy living. Muscle weakness or imbalance can result in abnormal movement or gait and can impair normal functional movement. Muscle weakness can also produce poor posture.

THE IMPORTANCE OF MUSCULAR ENDURANCE

Muscular strength is closely associated with muscular endurance. **Muscular endurance** is the ability to perform repetitive muscular contractions against some resistance for an extended period of time. As we will

see later, as muscular strength increases, there tends to be a corresponding increase in endurance. For example, a person can lift a weight 25 times. If muscular strength is increased by 10% through weight training, it is very likely that the maximal number of repetitions would be increased because it is easier for the person to lift the weight.

For most people, developing muscular endurance is more important than developing muscular strength, since muscular endurance is probably more critical in carrying out the everyday activities of living. This statement becomes increasingly true with age. However, a tremendous amount of strength is necessary for anyone involved in competition.

THE IMPORTANCE OF POWER

Most movements in sports are explosive and must include elements of strength and speed if they are to be effective. If a large amount of force is generated quickly, the movement can be referred to as a **power** movement. Without the ability to generate power, an athlete will be limited in his or her performance capabilities.[34] Strength training plays a critical role in achieving competitive fitness levels and also in injury rehabilitation.

TYPES OF SKELETAL MUSCLE CONTRACTION

Skeletal muscle is capable of three different types of contraction: (1) an **isometric contraction,** (2) a **concentric contraction,** and (3) an **eccentric contraction.** An isometric contraction occurs when the muscle contracts to produce tension, but there is no change in muscle length. Considerable force can be generated against some immovable resistance even though no movement occurs. In a concentric contraction the muscle shortens in length while tension develops to overcome or move some resistance. In an eccentric contraction, the resistance is greater than the muscular force being produced, and the muscle lengthens while producing tension. Concentric and eccentric contractions are considered dynamic movements.[37]

FACTORS THAT DETERMINE THE ABILITY TO GENERATE FORCE AGAINST RESISTANCE

Muscular strength is proportional to the cross-sectional diameter of the muscle fibers. The greater the cross-sectional diameter or the bigger a particular muscle, the stronger it is, and thus the more force it is capable of generating. The size of a muscle tends to increase in cross-sectional diameter with weight training. This increase in muscle size is referred to as **hypertrophy.**[23] Conversely a decrease in the size of a muscle is referred to as **atrophy.** Strength is a function of the number and diameter of muscle fibers composing a given muscle. The number of fibers is an inherited characteristic, thus a person with a large number of muscle fibers to begin with has the potential to hypertrophy to a much greater degree than does someone with relatively few fibers.[19]

Strength is also directly related to the efficiency of the neuromuscular system and the function of the motor unit in producing muscular force. As will be indicated later in this chapter, initial increases in strength during the first 8 to 10 weeks of a weight-training program can be attributed primarily to increased neuromuscular efficiency. Strength training will increase neuromuscular efficiency in three ways: there is an increase in the number of motor units

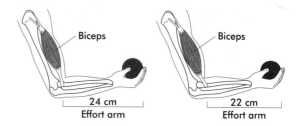

Fig. 4-1. Muscle attachments. The position of attachment of the muscle tendon on the lever arm can affect the ability of that muscle to generate force. **B** should be able to generate greater force than **A** because the tendon attachment on the lever arm is closer to the resistance.

being recruited, there is an increase in the firing rate of each motor unit, and there is increased synchronization of motor unit firing.[5] Strength in a given muscle is determined not only by the physical properties of the muscle but also by biomechanical factors that dictate how much force can be generated through a system of levers to an external object.[40]

If we think of the elbow joint as one of these lever systems, we would have the biceps muscle producing flexion of this joint (Figure 4-1). The position of attachment of the biceps muscle on the forearm will largely determine how much force this muscle is capable of generating. If there are two athletes, A and B, and A has a biceps attachment that is closer to the fulcrum (the elbow joint) than B, then A must produce a greater effort with the biceps muscle to hold the weight at a right angle because the length of the effort arm will be greater than with B.

The length of a muscle determines the tension that can be generated. By varying the length of a muscle, different tensions may be produced. This length-tension relationship is illustrated in Figure 4-2. At position B in the curve, the interaction of the crossbridges between the actin and myosin myofilaments within the sarcomere is at maximum. Setting a muscle at this particular length will produce the greatest amount of tension. At position A, the muscle is shortened, and at position C the muscle is lengthened. In either case the interaction between the actin and myosin myofilaments through the crossbridges is greatly reduced,

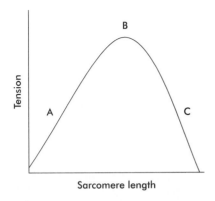

Fig. 4-2. The length-tension relation of the muscle.
Greatest tension is developed at point *B* with less tension developed at points *A* and *C*.

thus the muscle is not capable of generating significant tension.

The ability to generate muscular force is also related to age.[4] Both men and women seem to be able to increase strength throughout puberty and adolescence, reaching a peak around 20 to 25 years of age, at which time this ability begins to level off and in some cases decline. After about age 25 a person generally loses an average of 1% of his or her maximal remaining strength each year. Thus at age 65 a person would have only about 60% of the strength he or she had at age 25.[27] This loss in muscle strength is definitely related to individual levels of physical activity. Those people who are more active or perhaps those who continue to strength train considerably decrease this tendency toward declining muscle strength. In addition to retarding this decrease in muscular strength, exercise may also have an effect in slowing the decrease in cardiorespiratory endurance and flexibility, as well as slowing increases in body fat. Thus strength maintenance is important for all athletes regardless of age or the level of competition for achieving total wellness and good health and in rehabilitation after injury.

Gains in muscular strength resulting from resistance training are reversible. Individuals who interrupt or stop resistance because of injury will see rapid decreases in strength gains. "If you don't use it you'll lose it."

Overtraining can have a negative effect on the development of muscular strength. The statement "if you abuse it you will lose it" is very applicable. Overtraining can result in psychological breakdown

(staleness) or physiological breakdown, which may involve musculoskeletal injury, fatigue, or sickness. Engaging is proper and efficient resistance training, eating a proper diet, and getting appropriate rest can all minimize the potential negative effects of overtraining.

Fast-Twitch vs. Slow-Twitch Fibers

All fibers in a particular motor unit are either **slow-twitch or fast-twitch fibers,** each of which has distinctive metabolic and contractile capabilities. Slow-twitch fibers are also referred to as *type I fibers.* They are more resistant to fatigue than are fast-twitch fibers; however, the time required to generate force is much greater in slow-twitch fibers.[20] Because they are relatively fatigue resistant, slow-twitch fibers are associated primarily with long-duration, aerobic-type activities.

Fast-twitch fibers (type II) are capable of producing quick, forceful contractions but have a tendency to fatigue more rapidly than do slow-twitch fibers. Fast-twitch fibers are useful in short-term, high-intensity activities, which mainly involve the anaerobic system. Fast-twitch fibers are capable of producing powerful contractions, whereas slow-twitch fibers produce a long-endurance force. There are two subdivisions of fast-twitch fibers. While both types of fast-twitch fibers are capable of rapid contraction, type IIa fibers are moderately resistant to fatigue, while type IIb fibers fatigue rapidly and are considered the "true" fast-twitch fibers.

Within a particular muscle are both types of fibers, and the ratio in an individual muscle varies with each person.[18] Those muscles whose primary function is to maintain posture against gravity require more endurance and have a higher percentage of slow-twitch fibers. Muscles that produce powerful, rapid, explosive strength movements tend to have a much greater percentage of fast-twitch fibers.

Because this ratio is genetically determined, it may play a large role in determining ability for a given sports activity. Sprinters and weight lifters for example have a large percentage of fast-twitch fibers in relation to slow-twitch fibers.[8] Conversely, marathon runners generally have a higher percentage of slow-twitch fibers. The question of whether fiber types can change as a result of training has to date not been conclusively resolved. However, both types of fibers can improve their metabolic capabilities through specific strength and endurance training.[25]

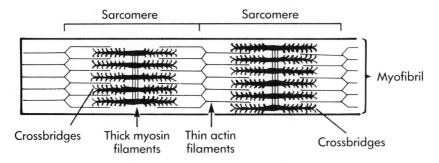

Fig. 4-3. Muscle contraction. Muscles contract when an electrical impulse from the central nervous system causes the myofilaments in a muscle fiber to move closer together.

PHYSIOLOGY OF STRENGTH DEVELOPMENT

There is no question that weight training to improve muscular strength results in an increased size, or hypertrophy, of a muscle. What causes a muscle to hypertrophy? A number of theories have been proposed to explain this increase in muscle size.[14]

Some evidence exists that there is an **increase in the number of muscle fibers** due to fibers splitting in response to training.[19] However, this research has been conducted in animals and should not be generalized to humans. It is generally accepted that the number of fibers is genetically determined and does not seem to increase with training.

It has been hypothesized that because the muscle is working harder in weight training, more blood is required to supply that muscle with oxygen and other nutrients. Thus it is thought that the **number of capillaries is increased.** This hypothesis is only partially correct; no new capillaries are formed during strength training; however, a number of dormant capillaries may well become filled with blood to meet this increased demand for blood supply.

A third theory to explain this increase in muscle size seems the most credible. Muscle fibers are composed primarily of small protein filaments, called *myofilaments,* which are contractile elements in muscle. **Myofilaments** are small contractile elements of protein within the sarcomere. There are two distinct types of myofilaments: thin **actin** myofilaments and thicker **myosin** myofilaments. Fingerlike projections or **crossbridges** connect the actin and myosin myofilaments. When a muscle is stimulated to contract, the crossbridges pull the myofilaments closer together, thus shortening the muscle and producing movement at the joint that the muscle crosses (Figure 4-3).[16]

These **myofilaments increase in size and number** as a result of strength training, causing the individual muscle fibers to increase in cross-sectional diameter.[28] This increase is particularly true in men, although women will also see some increase in muscle size. More research is needed to further clarify and determine the specific reasons for muscle hypertrophy.

Other Physiological Adaptations to Resistance Exercise

In addition to muscle hypertrophy, there are a number of other physiological adaptations to resistance training. The strength of non-contractile structures, including tendons and ligaments, is increased. The mineral content of bone is increased, thus making the bone stronger and more resistant to fracture. Maximal oxygen uptake is improved when resistance training is of sufficient intensity to elicit heart rates at or above training levels. There is also an increase in several enzymes important in aerobic and anaerobic metabolism.[1,15,16]

TECHNIQUES OF RESISTANCE TRAINING

There are a number of different techniques of resistance training for strength improvement including isometric exercise, progressive resistive exercise, isokinetic training, circuit training, and plyometric exercise. Regardless of which of these techniques is used, one basic principle of reconditioning is extremely important. For a muscle to improve in strength, it must be forced to work at a higher level than that to which it is accustomed. In other words, the muscle must be *overloaded.* Without overload the muscle will be able to maintain strength as long as training is continued against a resistance to which the muscle is accustomed. However, no additional strength gains will be realized. This maintenance of existing levels of muscular strength may be more important in weight-training programs that emphasize muscular endurance rather than strength gains. Many individuals can benefit more in terms of overall health by concentrating on improving muscular endurance. However, to most effectively build muscular strength, weight training requires a consistent, increasing effort against progressively increasing resistance.[39]

Resistive exercise is based primarily on the principles of overload and progression. If these principles are applied, all of the following training techniques will produce improvement of muscular strength over time.

In a rehabilitation setting, progressive overload is limited to some degree by the healing process. Since the sports therapist takes an aggressive approach to rehabilitation, the rate of progression is perhaps best determined by the injured athlete's response to a specific exercise. Exacerbation of pain or increased swelling should signal the sports therapist that their rate of progression is too aggressive.

Isometric Exercise

An **isometric exercise** involves a muscle contraction in which the length of the muscle remains constant, while tension develops toward a maximal force against an immovable resistance[30] (Figure 4-4). Isometric exercises are capable of increasing muscular strength.[35] However, strength gains are relatively specific with as much as a 20% overflow to the joint angle at which training is performed. At other angles, the strength curve drops off dramatically because of a lack of motor activity at that angle. Thus strength is increased at the specific angle of exertion, but there is no corresponding increase in strength at other positions in the range of motion.

Another major disadvantage of these isometric exercises is that they tend to produce a spike in systolic blood pressure that can result in potentially life-threatening cardiovascular accidents.[20] This sharp increase in systolic blood pressure results from a Valsalva maneuver, which increases intrathoracic pressure. To avoid or minimize this effect, it is recommended that breathing be done during the maximal contraction to prevent this increase in pressure.

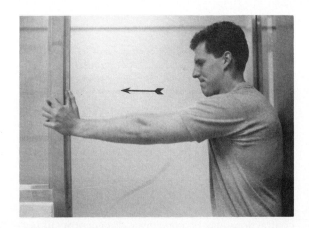

Fig. 4-4. Isometric exercises. Isometric exercises involve contraction against some immovable resistance.

The use of isometric exercises in injury rehabilitation or reconditioning is widely practiced. There are a number of conditions or ailments resulting from trauma or overuse that must be treated with strengthening exercises. Unfortunately, these problems may be exacerbated with full range-of-motion strengthening exercises. It may be more desirable to make use of positional isometric exercises until the healing process has progressed to the point that full-range activities can be performed. During rehabilitation, it is often recommended that a muscle be contracted isometrically for 10 seconds at a time at a frequency of 10 or more contractions per hour. Isometric exercises may also offer significant benefit in a strengthening program.[41] There are certain instances in which an isometric contraction can greatly enhance a particular movement. For example, one of the exercises in power weight lifting is a squat. A squat is an exercise in which the weight is supported on the shoulder in a standing position. The knees are then flexed, and the weight is lowered to a three-quarter squat position, from which the lifter must stand completely straight once again.

It is not uncommon for there to be one particular angle in the range of motion at which smooth movement is difficult because of insufficient strength. This joint angle is referred to as a *sticking point.* A power lifter will typically use an isometric contraction against some immovable resistance to increase strength at this sticking point. If strength can be improved at this joint angle, then a smooth, coordinated power lift can be performed through a full range of movement.

Progressive Resistive Exercise

A second technique of resistance training is perhaps the most commonly used and most popular technique among sports therapists for improving muscular strength in a reconditioning program. **Progressive resistive exercise** training uses exercises that strengthen muscles through a contraction that overcomes some fixed resistance such as with dumbells, barbells, or various weight machines. Progressive resistive exercise uses isotonic contractions in which force is generated while the muscle is changing in length.

CONCENTRIC VS. ECCENTRIC CONTRACTIONS. Isotonic contractions may be concentric or eccentric. In performing a bicep curl, to lift the weight from the starting position the biceps muscle must contract and shorten in length. This shortening contraction is referred to as a **concentric** or **positive** contraction. If the biceps muscle does not remain contracted when the weight is being lowered, gravity would cause this weight to simply fall back to the starting position. Thus to control the weight as it is being lowered, the biceps muscle must continue to contract while at the same time gradually lengthening. A contraction in which the muscle is lengthening while still applying force is called an **eccentric** or **negative** contraction.

It is possible to generate greater amounts of force against resistance with an eccentric contraction than with a concentric contraction because eccentric contractions require a much lower level of motor unit activity to achieve a certain force than do concentric contractions. Since fewer motor units are firing to produce a specific force, additional motor units may be recruited to generate increased force. In addition, oxygen use is much lower during eccentric exercise than in comparable concentric exercise. Thus eccentric contractions are less resistant to fatigue than are concentric contractions. The mechanical efficiency of eccentric exercise may be several times higher than that of concentric exercise.[37]

Traditionally, progressive resistive exercise has concentrated primarily on the concentric component without paying much attention to the importance of the eccentric component.[23] The use of eccentric contractions, particularly in rehabilitation of various sports-related injuries, has received considerable emphasis in recent years. Eccentric contractions are critical for deceleration of limb motion, especially during high-velocity dynamic activities. For example, a baseball pitcher relies on an eccentric contraction of the external rotators of the glenohumeral joint to decelerate the humerus, which may be internally rotating at speeds as high as 8000 degrees/second. Certainly, strength deficits or an inability of a muscle to tolerate these eccentric forces can predispose an injury. Thus in a rehabilitation program the sports therapist should incorporate eccentric strengthening exercises. Eccentric contractions are possible with all free weights, with the majority of isotonic exercise machines, and with most isokinetic devices. Eccentric contractions are used with plyometric exercise discussed in Chapter 6 and may also be incorporated with functional PNF strengthening patterns discussed in Chapter 11.

ISOTONIC EXERCISE EQUIPMENT. There are various types of exercise equipment that can be used with progressive resistive exercise including free weights (barbells and dumbells) or exercise machines such as Universal, Nautilus, Eagle, Body Master, Keiser, Paramount, Continental, Pyramid, Sprint, Hydrafitness, Dynatrac, Future, and Bull. Dumbells and barbells require the use of iron plates of varying weights that can be easily changed by adding or subtracting equal amounts of weight to both sides of the bar. The exercise machines for the most part have stacks of weights that are lifted through a series of levers or pulleys. The stack of weights slides up and down on a pair of bars that restrict the movement to only one plane. Weight can be increased or decreased simply by changing the position of a weight key (Figure 4-5).

There are advantages and disadvantages to free-weights and machines. The machines are relatively safe to use in comparison with free weights. For example, a bench press with free weights requires a partner to help lift the weight back onto the support racks if the lifter does not have enough strength to complete the lift; otherwise the weight may be dropped on the chest. With the machines the weight may be easily and safely dropped without fear of injury.

It is also a simple process to increase or decrease the weight by moving a single weight key with the exercise machines, although changes can generally be made only in increments of 10 or 15 pounds. With free weights, iron plates must be added or removed from each side of the barbell.

Surgical tubing, as a means of providing resistance, has been widely used in sports medicine (Figure 4-6). The advantage of exercising with surgical tubing is that the direction of movement is less restricted

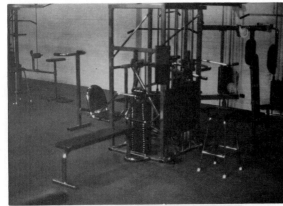

A

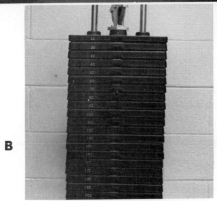

B

Fig. 4-5. Isotonic equipment. A, Universal equipment is isotonic. **B,** Resistance may be easily changed by changing the key in the stack of weights.

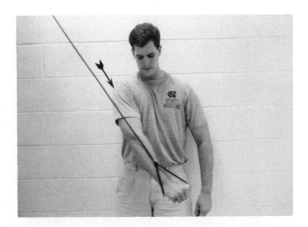

Fig. 4-6. Strengthening exercises. Strengthening exercises using surgical tubing are widely used in sports injury rehabilitation.

onstrated that the muscle should be overloaded and fatigued both concentrically and eccentrically for the greatest strength improvement to occur.[2,14,27] When training specifically for the development of muscular strength, the concentric portion of the exercise should require 1 to 2 seconds, while the eccentric portion of the lift should require 2 to 4 seconds. The ratio of the concentric component to the eccentric component should be approximately 1 to 2. Physiologically the muscle will fatigue much more rapidly concentrically than eccentrically.

Athletes who have strength trained using free weights and exercise machines realize the difference in the amount of weight that can be lifted. Unlike the machines, free weights have no restricted motion and can thus move in many different directions, depending on the forces applied. With free weights, an element of muscular control on the part of the lifter to prevent the weight from moving in any other direction other than vertical will usually decrease the amount of weight that can be lifted.[42]

One problem often mentioned in relation to progressive resistive exercise reconditioning is that the amount of force necessary to move a weight through a range of motion changes according to the angle of pull of the contracting muscle. It is greatest when the angle of pull is approximately 90 degrees. In addition, once the inertia of the weight has been overcome and momentum has been established, the force required to move the resistance varies according to the force that muscle can produce through the range of

than with free weights or exercise machines. Thus exercise can be done against resistance in more functional movement planes. The use of surgical tubing exercise in plyometrics and PNF strengthening techniques will be discussed in Chapters 6 and 11. Surgical tubing may be used to provide resistance with the majority of the exercises shown in Figures 4-9 through 4-44. Regardless of which type of equipment is used, the same principles of progressive resistive exercise may be applied. In progressive resistive exercise it is essential to incorporate concentric and eccentric contractions. Research has clearly dem-

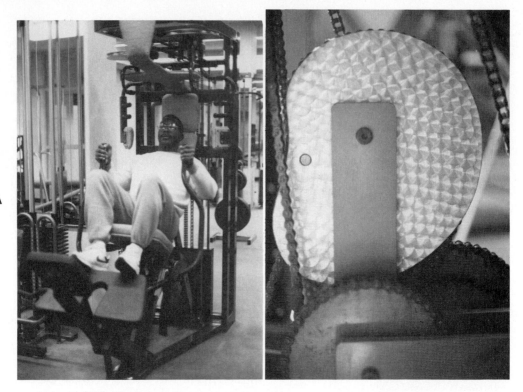

Fig. 4-7. Nautilus equipment. A, Nautilus bench press machine. **B,** The cam on Nautilus is designed to equalize resistance throughout the full range of motion.

motion. Thus it has been argued that a disadvantage of any type of isotonic exercise is that force required to move the resistance is constantly changing throughout the range of movement.

Nautilus has attempted to alleviate this problem of changing force capabilities by using a cam in its pulley system (Figure 4-7). The cam is individually designed for each piece of equipment so that the resistance is variable throughout the movement. It attempts to alter resistance so that the muscle can handle a greater load, but at the points where the joint angle or muscle length is mechanically disadvantageous, it reduces the resistance to muscle movement. Whether this design does what it claims is debatable. This change in resistance at different points in the range of motion has been labeled *accommodating resistance* or *variable resistance.*

PROGRESSIVE RESISTIVE EXERCISE TECHNIQUES. Perhaps the single most confusing aspect of progressive resistive exercise is the terminology used to describe specific programs.[21] The following list of terms with their operational definitions may help clarify the confusion:

Repetitions = Number of times you repeat a specific movement.

Repetition Maximum (RM) = Maximum number of repetitions at a given weight.

Set = A particular number of repetitions.

Intensity = The amount of weight or resistance lifted.

Recovery Period = The rest interval between sets.

Frequency = The number of times an exercise is done in a week's period.

SPECIFIC TECHNIQUES OF STRENGTH TRAINING. Specific recommendations for techniques of improving muscular strength are controversial among sports therapists. A considerable amount of research has been done in the area of resistance training relative to (1) the amount of weight to be used, (2) the number of repetitions, (3) the number of sets, and (4) the frequency of training.

A variety of specific programs have been proposed that recommend the optimal amount of weight,

TABLE 4-1
DeLorme's Program

Set	Amount of Weight	Repetitions
1	50% of 10 RM	10
2	75% of 10 RM	10
3	100% of 10 RM	10

TABLE 4-2
The Oxford Technique

Set	Amount of Weight	Repetitions
1	100% of 10 RM	10
2	75% of 10 RM	10
3	50% of 10 RM	10

TABLE 4-3
MacQueen's Technique

Sets	Amount of Weight	Repetitions
3 (Beginning/intermediate)	100% of 10 RM	10
4–5 (Advanced)	100% of 2–3 RM	2–3

TABLE 4-4
The Sanders' Program

Sets	Amount of Weight	Repetitions
Total of 4 sets (3 times per week)	100% of 5 RM	5
Day 1–4 sets	100% of 5 RM	5
Day 2–4 sets	100% of 3 RM	5
Day 3–1 set	100% of 5 RM	5
2 sets	100% of 3 RM	5
2 sets	100% of 2 RM	5

TABLE 4-5
Knight's DAPRE Program

Set	Amount of Weight	Repetitions
1	50% of RM	10
2	75% of RM	6
3	100% of RM	Maximum
4	Adjusted working weight*	Maximum

*See Table 4-6.

number of sets, number of repetitions, and frequency for producing maximal gains in levels of muscular strength. However, regardless of the techniques used, the healing process must dictate the specifics of any strength-training program. Certainly to improve strength the muscle must be overloaded. The amount of weight used and the number of repetitions must be sufficient to make the muscle work at higher intensity than it is used to working. This factor is the most critical in any strength-training program. The strength-training program must also be designed to ultimately meet the specific competitive needs of the athlete.

One of the first widely accepted strength-development programs to be used in a rehabilitation program was developed by DeLorme and was based on a repetition maximum of 10 (10 RM).[11] The amount of weight used is what can be lifted exactly 10 times (Table 4-1).

Zinovieff proposed the Oxford technique, which, like DeLorme's program, was designed to be used in beginning, intermediate, and advanced levels of rehabilitation.[44] The only difference is that the percent of maximum was reversed in the three sets (Table 4-2). MacQueen's technique[26] differentiates between beginning to intermediate and advanced levels as is shown in Table 4-3.

Sanders' program (Table 4-4) was designed to be used in the advanced stages of rehabilitation and was based on a formula that used a percentage of body weight to determine starting weights.[37] The percent-

ages below represent median starting points for different exercises:

Barbell squat—45% of body weight
Barbell bench press—30% of body weight
Leg extension—20% of body weight
Universal bench press—30% of body weight
Universal leg extension—20% of body weight
Universal leg curl—10 to 15% of body weight
Universal leg press—50% of body weight
Upright rowing—20% of body weight

Knight applied the concept of progressive resistive exercise in rehabilitation. His DAPRE (daily adjusted progressive resistive exercise) program (Tables 4-5

TABLE 4-6
DAPRE Adjusted Working Weight

Number of Repetitions Performed During Third Set	Adjusted Working Weight During Fourth Set	Next Exercise Session
0–2	−5–10 lb	−5–10 lb
3–4	−0–5 lb	Same weight
5–6	Same weight	+5–10 lb
7–10	+5–10 lb	+5–15 lb
11	+10–15 lb	+10–20 lb

TABLE 4-7
Berger's Adjustment Technique

Sets	Amount of Weight	Repetitions
3	100% of RM	6–8

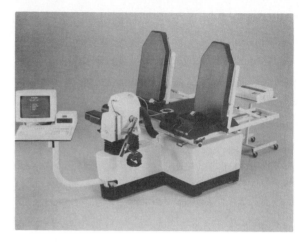

Fig. 4-8. KinCom. The KinCom is an isokinetic device that provides resistance at a constant velocity.

and 4-6) allows for individual differences in the rates at which patients progress in their rehabilitation programs.[24]

Berger has proposed a technique that is adjustable within individual limitations (Table 4-7). For any given exercise, the amount of weight selected should be sufficient to allow 6 to 8 RM in each of the three sets with a recovery period of 60 to 90 seconds between sets. Initial selection of a starting weight may require some trial and error to achieve this 6 to 8 RM range. If at least three sets of 6 RM cannot be completed, the weight is too heavy and should be reduced. If it is possible to do more than three sets of 8 RM, the weight is too light and should be increased.[7] Progression to heavier weights then is determined by the ability to perform at least 8 RM in each of three sets. When progressing weight, an increase of about 10% of the current weight being lifted should still allow at least 6 RM in each of three sets.

For rehabilitation purposes, strengthening exercises should be performed on a daily basis initially, with the amount of weight, number of sets, and number of repetitions governed by the injured athlete's response to the exercise. As the healing process progresses and pain or swelling is no longer an issue, a particular muscle or muscle group should be exercised consistently every other day. At that point the frequency of weight training should be at least three times per week but no more than four times per week. It is common for serious weight lifters to lift every day; however, they exercise different muscle groups on successive days. For example, Monday, Wednesday, and Friday may be used for upper body muscles, whereas Tuesday, Thursday, and Saturday are used for lower body muscles.

Arthur Jones, inventor of the Nautilus machine, has suggested that if training is done properly with the Nautilus equipment, that is, using both concentric and eccentric contractions, strength training is necessary only twice each week, although this schedule has not been sufficiently documented.

Isokinetic Exercise

An **isokinetic exercise** involves a muscle contraction in which the length of the muscle is changing while the contraction is performed at a constant velocity. In theory, maximal resistance is provided throughout the range of motion by the machine. The resistance provided by the machine will move only at some preset speed, regardless of the torque applied to it by the individual. Thus the key to isokinetic exercise is not the resistance but the speed at which resistance can be moved.

Several isokinetic devices are available commercially; the Ariel Computerized Exercise System, Cybex, Orthotron, Biodex, KinCom, Lido, MERAC, and Mini-gym are among the more common isokinetic devices (Figure 4-8). In general, they rely on hydraulic, pneumatic, and mechanical pressure systems to produce this constant velocity of motion. The majority of isokinetic devices are capable of resisting concentric and eccentric contractions at a fixed speed to exercise a muscle.

ISOKINETICS AS A CONDITIONING TOOL. Isokinetic devices are designed so that regardless of the amount of force applied against a resistance, it can only be moved at a certain speed. That speed will be the same whether maximal force or only half the maximal force is applied. Consequently, when training isokinetically, it is absolutely necessary to exert as much force against the resistance as possible (maximal effort) for maximal strength gains to occur. Maximal effort is one of the major problems with an isokinetic strength-training program.

Anyone who has been involved in a weight-training program knows that on some days it is difficult to find the motivation to work out. Because isokinetic training requires a maximal effort, it is very easy to "cheat" and not go through the workout at a high level of intensity. In a progressive resistive exercise program, the athlete knows how much weight has to be lifted with how many repetitions. Thus isokinetic training is often more effective if a partner system is used primarily as a means of motivation toward a maximal effort. When isokinetic training is done properly with a maximal effort, it is theoretically possible that maximal strength gains are best achieved through the isokinetic training method in which the velocity and force of the resistance are equal throughout the range of motion. However there is no conclusive research to support this theory.

Whether this changing force capability is a deterrent to improving the ability to generate force against some resistance is debatable. In real life it does not matter whether the resistance is changing; what is important is that an individual develops enough strength to move objects from one place to another. The amount of strength necessary for athletes is largely dependent on their level of competition.

Another major disadvantage of using isokinetic devices as a conditioning tool is their cost. With initial purchase costs ranging between $40,000 and $60,000 and the necessity of regular maintenance and software upgrades, the use of an isokinetic device for general conditioning or resistance training is for the most part unrealistic. Thus isokinetic exercises are primarily used as a diagnostic and rehabilitative tool.

ISOKINETICS IN REHABILITATION. Isokinetic strength testing gained a great deal of popularity throughout the 1980s in rehabilitation settings. This trend stems from it providing an objective means of quantifying existing levels of muscular strength and thus becoming useful as a diagnostic tool.

Because the capability exists for training at specific speeds, comparisons have been made regarding the relative advantages of training at fast or slow speeds in a rehabilitation program. The research literature seems to indicate that strength increases from slow-speed training are relatively specific to the velocity used in training. Conversely, training at faster speeds seems to produce a more generalized increase in torque values at all velocities. Minimal hypertrophy was observed only while training at fast speeds, affecting only type II or fast-twitch fibers.[10,33] An increase in neuromuscular efficiency caused by more effective motor unit firing patterns has been demonstrated with slow-speed training.[27]

During the early 1990s, the value of isokinetic devices for quantifying torque values at functional speeds has been questioned. This issue, in addition to the theory and use of isokinetic exercise in a rehabilitation setting, will be discussed in detail in Chapter 5.

Circuit Training

Circuit training is a technique that may be useful to the sports therapist to maintain or perhaps improve levels of muscular strength or endurance in other parts of the body while the athlete allows for healing and reconditioning of an injured body part. Circuit training uses a series of exercise stations that consist of various combinations of weight training, flexibility, calisthenics, and brief aerobic exercises. Circuits may be designed to accomplish many different training goals. With circuit training the athlete moves rapidly from one station to the next, performing whatever exercise is to be done at that station within a specified time period. A typical circuit would consist of 8 to 12 stations, and the entire circuit would be repeated three times.

Circuit training is most definitely an effective technique for improving strength and flexibility. Certainly if the pace or time interval between stations is rapid and if work load is maintained at a high level of intensity with heart rates at or above target training levels, the cardiorespiratory system may benefit from this circuit. However, there is little research evidence that shows that circuit training is very effective in improving cardiorespiratory endurance. It should be and is most often used as a technique for developing and improving muscular strength and endurance.[17]

Plyometric Exercise

Plyometric exercise is a technique that is being increasingly incorporated into later stages of the reconditioning program by the sports therapist. Plyometric training includes specific exercises that encompass a rapid stretch of a muscle eccentrically, followed immediately by a rapid concentric contraction of that muscle to facilitate and develop a forceful explosive movement over a short period of time.[12] The greater the stretch put on the muscle from its resting length immediately before the concentric contraction, the greater the resistance the muscle can overcome. Plyometrics emphasize the speed of the eccentric phase. The rate of stretch is more critical than the magnitude of the stretch. An advantage to using plyometric exercises is that they can help to develop eccentric control in dynamic movements.

Plyometric exercises involve hops, bounds, and depth jumping for the lower extremity and the use of medicine balls and other types of weighted equipment for the upper extremity. Depth jumping is an example of a plyometric exercise in which an individual jumps to the ground from a specified height and then quickly jumps again as soon as ground contact is made.[3]

Plyometrics tend to place a great deal of stress on the musculoskeletal system. The learning and perfection of specific jumping skills and other plyometric exercises must be technically correct and specific to one's age, activity, physical, and skill development. Plyometric exercise will be discussed in detail in Chapter 6.

OPEN VS. CLOSED KINETIC CHAIN EXERCISES

The concept of the kinetic chain deals with the anatomical functional relationships that exist in the upper and lower extremities. In a weight-bearing position, the lower extremity kinetic chain involves the transmission of forces between the foot, ankle, lower leg, knee, thigh, and hip. In the upper extremity, when the hand is a weight-bearing surface, forces are transmitted to the wrist, forearm, elbow, upper arm, and shoulder girdle.

An **open kinetic chain** exists when the foot or hand is not in contact with the ground or some other surface. In a **closed kinetic chain,** the foot or hand

is weight bearing. Movements of the more proximal anatomical segments are affected by these open vs. closed kinetic chain positions. For example, the rotational components of the ankle, knee, and hip reverse direction when changing from an open to closed kinetic chain activity. In a closed kinetic chain the forces begin at the ground and work their way up through each joint. Also, in a closed kinetic chain, forces must be absorbed by various tissues and anatomical structures rather than simply dissipating as would occur in an open chain.

In rehabilitation, the use of closed chain strengthening techniques has become the treatment of choice for many sports therapists. Since most sports activities involve some aspect of weight bearing with the foot in contact with the ground or the hand in a weight-bearing position, closed kinetic chain strengthening activities are more functional than are open chain activities. Therefore rehabilitative exercises should be incorporated that emphasize strengthening of the entire kinetic chain rather than an isolated body segment. Chapter 7 will discuss closed kinetic chain activities in detail.

TRAINING FOR MUSCULAR STRENGTH VS. MUSCULAR ENDURANCE

Muscular endurance was defined as the ability to perform repeated muscle contractions against resistance for an extended period of time. Most weight-training experts believe that muscular strength and muscular endurance are closely related.[13,31,38] As one improves, there is a tendency for the other to improve also.

It is generally accepted that when weight training for strength, heavier weights with a lower number of repetitions should be used. Conversely, endurance training uses relatively lighter weights with a greater number of repetitions.

It has been suggested that endurance training should consist of three sets of 10 to 15 repetitions[6] using the same criteria for weight selection progression and frequency as recommended for progressive resistive exercise. Thus suggested training regimens for muscular strength and endurance are similar in terms of sets and numbers of repetitions.[43] Persons who possess great levels of strength tend to also exhibit greater muscular endurance when asked to perform repeated contractions against resistance.[29]

STRENGTH TRAINING DIFFERENCES BETWEEN MALES AND FEMALES. Strength training is absolutely essential for an athlete. The approach to strength training is

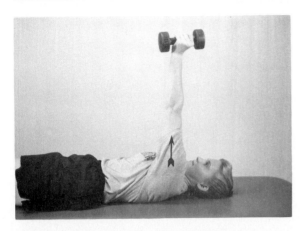

Fig. 4-9. Scapular abduction and upward rotation.
Primary muscle: Serratus anterior.

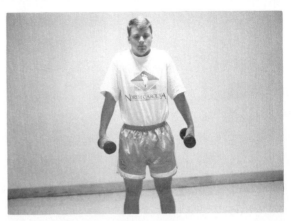

Fig. 4-10. Scapular elevation (shoulder shrugs). Primary muscles: Upper trapezius, levator scapula.

no different for female than for male athletes. However, some obvious physiological differences exist between the sexes.

The average woman does not build significant muscle bulk through weight training. Significant muscle hypertrophy is dependent on the presence of a steroidal hormone known as **testosterone.** Testosterone is considered a male hormone, although some women possess some testosterone in their systems. Women with higher testosterone levels tend to have more masculine characteristics, such as increased facial and body hair, a deeper voice, and the potential to develop a little more muscle bulk.[32] For the average female athlete, developing large, bulky muscles through strength training is unlikely, although muscle tone may be improved. Muscle tone basically refers to the firmness of tension of the muscle during a resting state. The initial stages of a strength-training program are likely to produce dramatic increases in levels of strength very rapidly. For a muscle to contract, an impulse must be transmitted from the nervous system to the muscle. Each muscle fiber is innervated by a specific motor unit. By overloading a particular muscle, as in weight training, the muscle is forced to work more efficiently. Efficiency is achieved by getting more motor units to fire, thus causing more muscle fibers to contract, which results in a stronger contraction of the muscle. Consequently, women and men often see extremely rapid gains in strength when a weight-training program is first begun. In the female, these tremendous initial strength gains, which can be attributed to improved neuromuscular system efficiency, tend to plateau, and

minimal improvement in muscular strength is realized during a continuing strength-training program. These initial neuromuscular strength gains are also seen in men, although their strength continues to increase with appropriate training. Again, women who possess higher testosterone levels have the potential to increase their strength further because of the development of greater muscle bulk.

Differences in strength levels between males and females are best illustrated when strength is expressed in relation to body weight minus fat. The reduced strength/body weight ratio in women is the result of their percentage of body fat. The strength/body weight ratio may be significantly improved through weight training by decreasing the body fat percentage while increasing lean weight.

The absolute strength differences are considerably reduced when body size and composition are considered. Leg strength may actually be stronger in the female than in the male, although upper extremity strength is much greater in the male.[32]

SPECIFIC STRENGTHENING EXERCISES IN REHABILITATION

Because muscle contractions result in joint movement, the goal of resistance training in a rehabilitation program should be to regain and perhaps increase the strength of either a specific muscle that has been injured or to increase the efficiency of movement about a given joint.[36]

Figures 4-9 through 4-44 are organized to show exercises for all motions about a particular joint
Text continued on page 73.

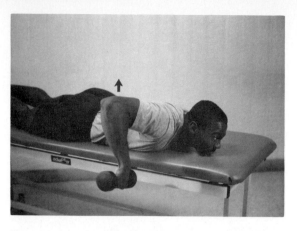

Fig. 4-11. Scapular adduction (Bent arm reverse flys). Primary muscles: Middle trapezius.

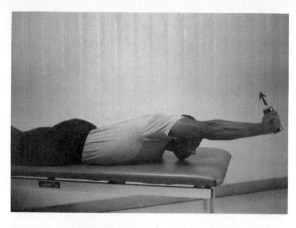

Fig. 4-12. Scapular depression and adduction. Primary muscles: Inferior trapezius.

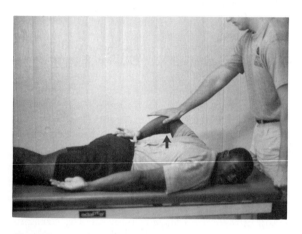

Fig. 4-13. Scapular adduction and downward rotation. Primary muscles: Rhomboids. Secondary muscles: Inferior trapezius.

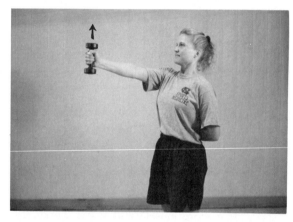

Fig. 4-14. Shoulder flexion to 90 degrees. Primary muscles: Anterior deltoid, coracobrachialis. Secondary muscles: Middle deltoid, pectoralis major, biceps.

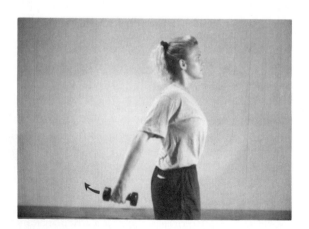

Fig. 4-15. Shoulder extension. Primary muscles: Latissimus dorsi, teres major, posterior deltoid. Secondary muscles: Teres minor, triceps.

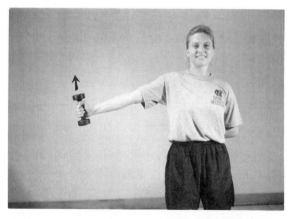

Fig. 4-16. Shoulder abduction to 90 degrees. Primary muscles: Middle deltoid, supraspinatus. Secondary muscles: Anterior deltoid.

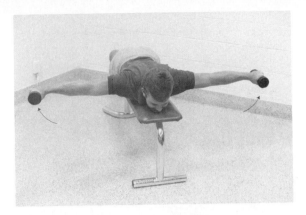

Fig. 4-17. Shoulder horizontal abduction. Primary muscles: Posterior deltoid. Secondary muscles: Infraspinatus, teres minor.

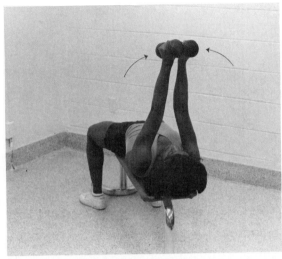

Fig. 4-18. Shoulder horizontal adduction. Primary muscles: Pectoralis major. Secondary muscles: Anterior deltoid.

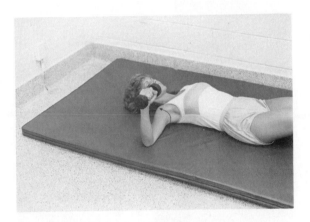

Fig. 4-19. Shoulder external rotation. Primary muscles: Infraspinatus, teres minor. Secondary muscles: Posterior deltoid. NOTE: Should be done at both 0 and 90 degrees.

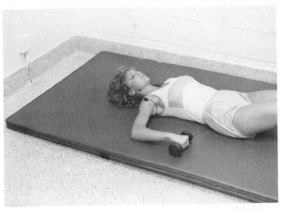

Fig. 4-20. Shoulder internal rotation. Primary muscles: Subscapularis, pectoralis major, latissimus dorsi, teres minor. Secondary muscles: Anterior deltoid. NOTE: Should be done at 0, 90, and 135 degrees.

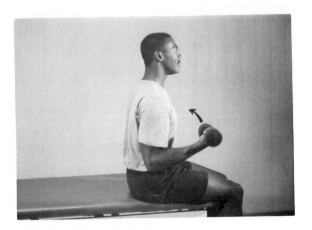

Fig. 4-21. Elbow flexion. Primary muscles: Biceps, brachialis, brachioradialis. NOTE: Palm up more biceps, thumb up more brachioradialis, palm down more brachialis.

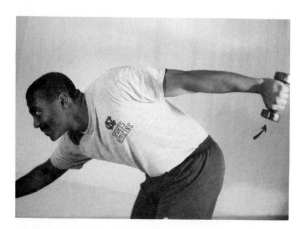

Fig. 4-22. Elbow extension. Primary muscles: Triceps. Secondary muscles: Forearm extensors.

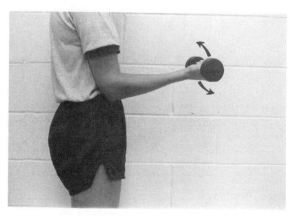

Fig. 4-23. Forearm pronation-supination. Primary muscles: Supination—Biceps, supinator. Pronation—Pronator peres, pronator quadratus.

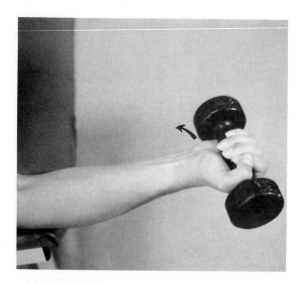

Fig. 4-24. Wrist flexion. Primary muscles: Flexor carpi radialis, flexor carpi ulnaris, palmaris longus.

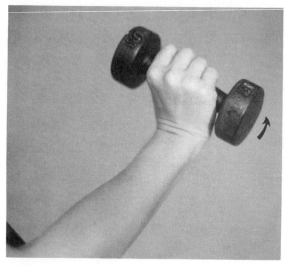

Fig. 4-25. Wrist extension. Primary muscles: Extensor carpi radialis longus and brevis, extensor carpi ulnaris.

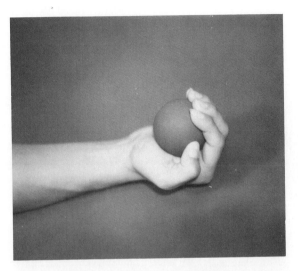

Fig. 4-26. Flexion of hand and fingers. Primary muscles: Intrinsic muscles of the hand, long flexors in the forearm.

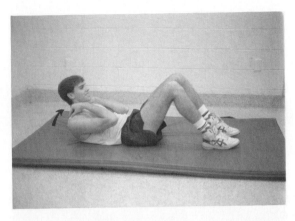

Fig. 4-27. Trunk flexion. Primary muscles: Rectus abdominis. Secondary muscles: Internal oblique, external oblique.

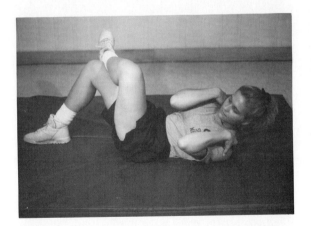

Fig. 4-28. Trunk rotation. Primary muscles: Internal oblique on the side of the direction of rotation, external oblique on the opposite side. Secondary muscles: Rectus abdominis, latissimus dorsi, multifidus.

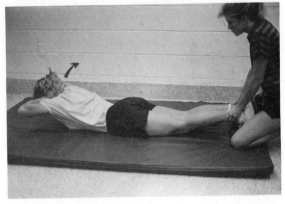

Fig. 4-29. Trunk extension. Primary muscles: Erector spinae, longissimus thoracis, iliocostalis thoracis, spinalis thoracis, iliocostalis lumborum, quadratus lumborum.

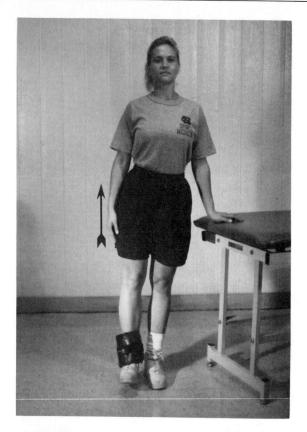

Fig. 4-30. Elevation of pelvis. Primary muscles: Quadratus lumborum, iliocostalis lumborum. Secondary muscles: Internal and external oblique abdominals, hip adductors.

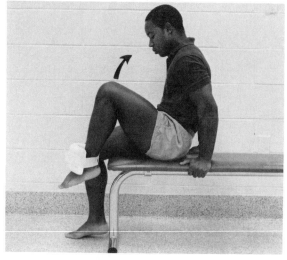

Fig. 4-31. Hip flexion. Primary muscles: Psoas major, iliacus. Secondary muscles: Rectus femoris, sartorius, pectineus, tensor fascia lata, adductor longus and brevis.

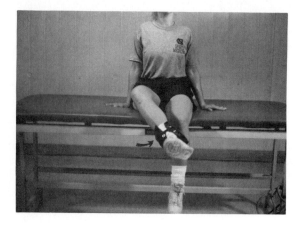

Fig. 4-32. Hip flexion, abduction, lateral rotation. Primary muscles: Sartorius. Secondary muscles: Hip external rotators, hip flexors, hip abductors.

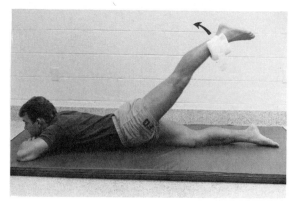

Fig. 4-33. Hip extension. Primary muscles: Gluteus maximus, hamstrings. NOTE: Flexing knee isolates gluteus maximus.

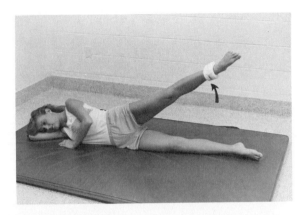

Fig. 4-34. Hip abduction. Primary muscles: Gluteus medius. Secondary muscles: Tensor fascia lata, gluteus medius and maximus. NOTE: Bringing the hip into flexion exercises the tensor fascia lata.

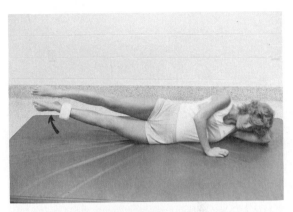

Fig. 4-35. Hip adduction. Primary muscles: Adductor magnus, longus, and brevis; pectineus, gracilis.

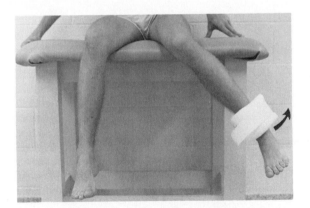

Fig. 4-36. Hip medial rotation. Primary muscles: Gluteus minimus, tensor fascia lata. Secondary muscles: Gluteus medius, semitendinous, semimembranous.

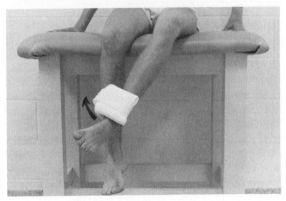

Fig. 4-37. Hip lateral rotation. Primary muscles: Internal and external obturator, quadriceps, piriform, superior and inferior gemelli, gluteus maximus.

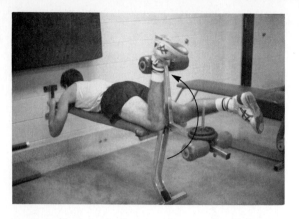

Fig. 4-38. Knee flexion. Primary muscles: Biceps femoris, semimembranous, semitendinous. Secondary muscles: Gracilis, gastrocnemius, sartorius, popliteus. NOTE: Biceps femoris is best strengthened with tibia rotated externally, semimembranous and semitendinous muscles are best strengthened with tibia rotated internally.

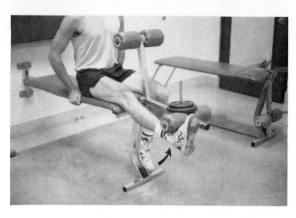

Fig. 4-39. Knee extension. Primary muscles: Rectus femoris, vastus lateralis, intermedialis, medialis.

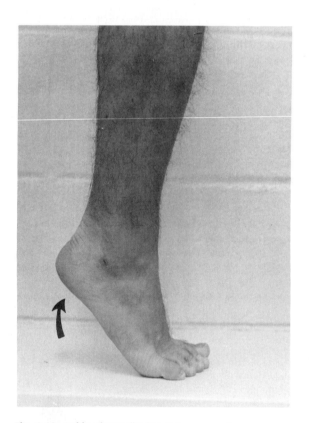

Fig. 4-40. Ankle plantarflexion. Primary muscles: Gastrocnemius, soleus. Secondary muscles: Posterior tibialis, peroneus longus and brevis, flexor hallicus longus, flexor digitorum longus, plantaris. NOTE: Extended knee strengthens the gastrocnemius, flexed knee strengthens soleus.

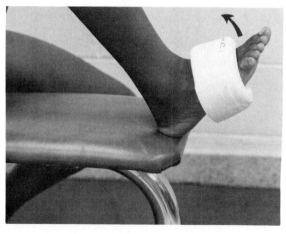

Fig. 4-41. Foot dorsiflexion and inversion. Primary muscles: anterior tibialis.

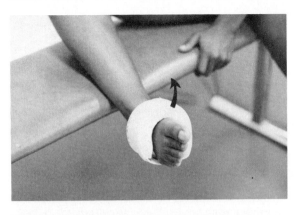

Fig. 4-42. Foot inversion. Primary muscles: Posterior tibialis. Secondary muscles: Flexor digitorum longus, flexor hallicus longus.

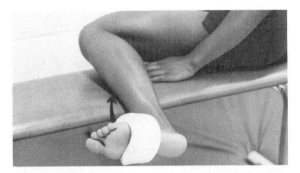

Fig. 4-43. Foot eversion. Primary muscles: Peroneus longus and brevis. Secondary muscles: Extensor digitorum longus, peroneus tertius.

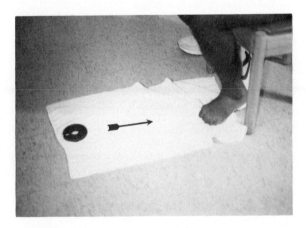

Fig. 4-44. Flexion of toes. Primary muscles: Flexor digitorum longus and brevis, lumbricales, flexor hallicus longus.

rather than for each specific muscle. These exercises are demonstrated using free weights (dumbells or bar weights) and some exercise machines. Other strengthening techniques widely used for injury rehabilitation involving isokinetic exercise, plyometrics, closed kinetic chain exercises, and PNF strengthening techniques will be discussed in subsequent chapters.

SUMMARY

1. Muscular strength may be defined as the maximal force that can be generated against resistance by a muscle during a single maximal contraction.

2. Muscular endurance is the ability to perform repeated isotonic or isokinetic muscle contractions or to sustain an isometric contraction without undue fatigue.

3. Muscular endurance tends to improve with muscular strength thus training techniques for these two components are similar.

4. Muscular strength and endurance are essential components of any rehabilitation program.

5. Muscular power involves the speed with which a forceful muscle contraction is performed.

6. The ability to generate force is dependent on the physical properties of the muscle, neuromuscular efficiency, as well as the mechanical factors that dictate how much force can be generated through the lever system to an external object.

7. Hypertrophy of a muscle is caused by increases in the size and perhaps the number of actin and myosin protein myofilaments, which result in an increased cross-sectional diameter of the muscle.

8. The key to improving strength through resistance training is using the principle of overload within the constraints of the healing process.

9. Five resistance training techniques that can improve muscular strength are isometric exercise, progressive resistive exercise, isokinetic training, circuit training, and plyometric training.

10. Improvements in strength with isometric exercise occur at specific joint angles.

11. Progressive resistive exercise is the most common strengthening technique used by the sports therapist for reconditioning after injury.

12. Circuit training involves a series of exercise stations consisting of weight training, flexibility, and calisthenic exercises that can be designed to maintain fitness while reconditioning an injured body part.

13. Isokinetic training provides resistance to a muscle at a fixed speed.

14. Plyometric exercise uses a quick eccentric stretch to facilitate a concentric contraction.

15. Closed kinetic chain exercises may provide a more functional technique for strengthening of injured muscles and joints in the athletic population.

16. Women can significantly increase strength levels but generally will not build muscle bulk as a result of strength training because of a relative lack of the hormone testosterone.

REFERENCES

1 Alway SE, MacDougall D, Sale G, et al: Functional and structural adaptations in skeletal muscle of trained athletes, *J Appl Physiol* 64:1114, 1988.

2 American College of Sports Medicine: *Position statement on the use and abuse of arabolic-androgenic steroids in sports,* 1977.

3 Arnheim D, Prentice WE: *Principles of athletic training,* St Louis, 1993, Mosby.

4 Åstrand PO, Rodahl K: *Textbook of work physiology,* New York, 1986, McGraw-Hill.

5 Bandy W, Lovelace-Chandler V, Bandy B, et al: Adaptation of skeletal muscle to resistance training, *J Ortho Sports Phys Ther* 12(6):248–255, 1990.

6 Berger R: Effect of varied weight training programs on strength, *Res Q Exerc Sport* 33:168, 1962.

7 Berger R: *Conditioning for men,* Boston, 1973, Allyn & Bacon.

8 Costill D, Daniels J, Evan W, et al.: Skeletal muscle enzymes and fiber compositions in male and female track athletes, *J Appl Physiol* 40:149, 1976.

9 Cowart V: If youngsters overdose with anabolic steroids what is the cost anatomically and otherwise, *JAMA* 261:1856, 1989.

10 Coyle E, Feiring D, Rotkis T, et al: Specificity of power improvements through slow and fast speed isokinetic training, *J Appl Physiol* 51:1437, 1981.

11 DeLorme T, Wilkins A: *Progressive resistance exercise,* New York, 1951, Appleton-Century-Crofts.

12 Duda M: Plyometrics: a legitimate form of power training, *Phys Sports Med* 16:213, 1988.

13 Dudley GA, Fleck SJ: Strength and endurance training: are they mutually exclusive? *Sports Med* 4(2):79, 1987 (review).

14 Etheridge G, Thomas T: Physiological and biomedical changes of human skeletal muscle induced by different strength training programs, *Med Sci Sports Exerc* 14:141, 1982.

15 Fleck SJ, Kramer WJ: Resistance training: physiological responses and adaptations, *Phys Sports Med* 16:108, 1988.

16 Gettman L: Circuit weight training: a critical review of its physiological benefits, *Phys Sports Med* 9(1):44, 1981.

17 Gettman L, Ward P, Hagan R: A comparison of combined running and weight training with circuit weight training, *Med Sci Sports Exerc* 14:229, 1982.

18 Gollnick P, Sembrowich W: Adaptations in human skeletal muscle as a result of training. In Amsterdam EA, editor: *Exercise in cardiovascular health and disease,* New York, 1977, York Medical Books.

19 Gonyea W: Role of exercise in inducing increases in skeletal muscle fiber number, *J Appl Physiol* 48:421, 1980.

20 Graves JE, Pollack M, Jones A, et al: Specificity of limited range of motion variable resistance training, *Med Sci Sports Exerc* 21:84, 1989.

21 Hickson J, Rosenkaffer M: Characterization of standardized weight training exercise, *Med Sci Sports Exerc* 14:169, 1982.

22 Hortobagyi T, Katch FI: Role of concentric force in limiting improvement in muscular strength, *J Appl Physiol* 68:650, 1990.

23 Jensen C, Fisher G: *Scientific basis of athletic conditioning,* Philadelphia, 1979, Lea & Febiger.

24 Knight K: Knee rehabilitation by the DAPRE technique, *Am J Sports Med Phys Fitness* 7:336, 1979.

25 Lamb DR: Anabolic steroids. In Williams MH, editor: *Ergogenic aids in sport,* Champaign, Ill, 1983, Human Kinetics Publishers.

26 MacQueen I: Recent advances in the technique of progressive resistance, *Br Med J* 11:11993, 1954.

27 McArdle W, Katch F, Katch V: *Exercise physiology, energy, nutrition, and human performance,* Philadelphia, 1991, Lea & Febiger.

28 McGlynn GH: A reevaluation of isometric training, *J Sports Med Phys Fitness* 12:258, 1972.

29 Meredith CN, Frontera W, Fisher E, et al.: Peripheral effects of endurance training in young and old subjects, *J Appl Physiol* 66(6):2844, 1989.

30 Nicholas JJ: Isokinetic testing in young nonathletic able-bodied subjects, *Arch Phys Med Rehabil* 70(3):210, 1989 (review).

31 Nygard CH, Luophaarui T, Suurnakki T, et al.: Muscle strength and muscle endurance of middle-aged women and men associated to type, duration and intensity of muscular load at work, *Int Arch Occup Environ Health* 60(4):291, 1988.

32 O'Shea JP: Power weight training and the female athlete, *Phys Sports Med* 9(6):109, 1981.

33 Pipes T, Wilmore J: Isokinetic vs. isotonic strength training in adult men, *Med Sci Sports Exerc* 7:262, 1975.

34 President's Council on Physical Fitness and Sports: *Weight training for strength and power,* Washington, DC, 1980, US Government Printing Office.

35 Rehfeldt H, Caffiber G, Kramer H, et al.: Force, endurance time, and cardiovascular responses in voluntary isometric contractions of different muscle groups, *Biomed Biochim Acta* 48(5–6):S509, 1989.

36 Sale D, MacDougall D: Specificity in strength training: a review for the coach and athlete, *Can J Appl Sports Sci* 6:87, 1981.

37 Sanders M: Weight training and conditioning. In Sanders B, editor: *Sports physical therapy,* Norwalk, Conn, 1990, Appleton & Lange.

38 Smith TK: Developing local and general muscular endurance, *Athletic J* 62:42, 1981.

39 Stone M: Physiological effects of a short-term resistive training program on middle-aged untrained men, *National Strength Coaches Association Journal* 4:16, 1982.

40 Strauss RH, editor: *Sportsmedicine,* Philadelphia, 1984, WB Saunders.

41 Ulmer H, Knierman W, Warlow T, et al.: Interindividual variability of isometric endurance with regard to the endurance performance limit for static work, *Biomed Biochim Acta* 48(5-6):S504, 1989.

42 Weltman A, Stamford B: Strength training: free weights vs. machines, *Phys Sports Med* 10:197, 1982.

43 Yates JW: Recovery of dynamic muscular endurance, *Eur Appl Physiol* 56(6):662, 1987.

44 Zinovieff A: Heavy resistance exercise, the Oxford technique, *Br J Physiol Med* 14:129, 1951.

Isokinetics in Rehabilitation

5

Janine Oman

OBJECTIVES

After completion of this chapter, the student should be able to do the following:

- Describe isokinetic exercise.

- Identify the advantages and disadvantages of isokinetic exercise.

- List the various computerized isokinetic systems.

- Describe the use of isokinetic evaluation in the athletic population.

- Discuss the use of isokinetic exercise as a rehabilitation tool in the athletic population.

ISOKINETIC EXERCISE

The concept of isokinetic exercise was described in 1967 by Hislop and Perrine.[20] Isokinetic exercise can best be described as movement that occurs at a constant angular velocity with accommodating resistance. Maximum muscle tension can be generated throughout the range of motion because the resistance is variable to match the muscle tension produced at the various points in the range of motion. Isokinetic machines allow the angular velocity to be preset. Once the specified angular velocity is achieved, the machine provides accommodating resistance throughout the specified range of motion.[16]

Isokinetic evaluation and rehabilitation is limited by the technological advances of isokinetic dynamometers. Isokinetic dynamometers now provide concentric and eccentric resistance. Velocities are variable depending on the machine, although the average range is from zero to 300 degrees/second. Some machines allow velocities greater than 400 degrees/second.

Historically, the two primary advantages associated with isokinetic exercise are the ability to work maximally throughout the range of motion and the ability to work at various velocities to simulate functional activity.[37] Care should be taken, however, when inferring functional capacity based on results of dynamic isokinetic testing.[28] Velocities achieved during functional activity greatly exceed the velocity capacities of isokinetic dynamometers. Velocities measured at the hip and knee during a soccer kick exceeded 400 degrees/second and 1200 degrees/second, respectively.[27] The majority of isokinetic testing is done in a nonweight-bearing position that is not representative of functional activities. However, given these limitations, isokinetic exercise can be a very powerful tool for the sports therapist in evaluation and rehabilitation of sports-related injuries.

ISOKINETIC DYNAMOMETERS

Various isokinetic dynamometers are commercially available to the sports therapist. The different systems all offer variable types of resistance and velocities. This section is not meant to endorse a particular isokinetic system but is provided to give the sports therapist information on the specifications of some of the more common commercially available isokinetic dynamometers. Table 5-1 provides a comparison of the different dynamometers with information related to the manufacturer's address, exercise modes available, velocities, and torque maximums.

TABLE 5-1
Isokinetic Equipment Information

Isokinetic Equipment and Manufacturer	Exercise Modes Available	Speeds	Torque Maximum*
Ariel Computerized Exercise System Ariel Life Systems, Inc. PO Box 1169 La Jolla, CA 92038	Isometric Isokinetic (concentric only) Isotonic	1-1000/sec	1000 ft lbs

BIODEX
Biodex Corporation
PO Box S
Shirley, NY 11967
	Isokinetic (concentric and eccentric)
	Isometric
	Continuous Passive Motion (CPM)
		Isokinetic:
		  Concentric: 30-450/sec
		  Eccentric: 10-120/sec
		CPM: 2-120/sec
			Concentric: 650 ft lbs
			Eccentric: 300 ft lbs

CYBEX
Cybex Corporation
2100 Smithtown Ave.
PO Box 9003
Ronkonkoma, NY 11779-0903
	Isokinetic
	Concentric: powered and non-powered mode
	Eccentric: powered mode
	CPM
		Powered Concentric: 15-120/sec
		Non-powered Concentric: 15-500/sec
		Powered Eccentric: 30-120/sec
		CPM: 5-120/sec
			Powered Concentric:
			  500 ft lbs
			Powered Eccentric:
			  30-55/sec: 250 ft lbs
			  60-120/sec: 300 ft lbs

KIN-COM
Chattex Corporation
4717 Adams Road
PO Box 489
Hixson, TN 37343
	Isometric
	Isokinetic (concentric and eccentric)
	Isotonic
	CPM
		Isokinetic:
		  Concentric: 1-250/sec
		  Eccentric: 1-250/sec
		Isotonic: 1-250/sec
		CPM: 1-250/sec
			Isometric: 450 ft lbs
			Isokinetic:
			  Concentric: 450 ft lbs
			  Eccentric: 450 ft lbs
			Isotonic: 2-450 ft lbs

LIDO ACTIVE
Loredan Biomedical
3650 Industrial Blvd.
West Sacramento, CA 95691
	Isometric
	Isokinetic (concentric and eccentric)
	Isotonic
	Isoacceleration
	CPM
		Isokinetic:
		  Concentric: 1-400/sec
		  Eccentric: 1-250/sec
		CPM: 1-120/sec
			Isometric: 400 ft lbs
			Isokinetic:
			  Concentric: 400 ft lbs
			  Eccentric: 250 ft lbs
			Isotonic: 400 ft lbs

MERAC Universal Gym Equipment PO Box 1270 930 27th Ave. Cedar Rapids, IA 52406	Isometric Isokinetic (concentric only) Isotonic	Isokinetic: 15-500/sec Isotonic: 1000/sec	Isokinetic: 500 ft lbs Isotonic: 500 ft lbs

*To convert foot-pounds to Newton-meters multiply by 4.45

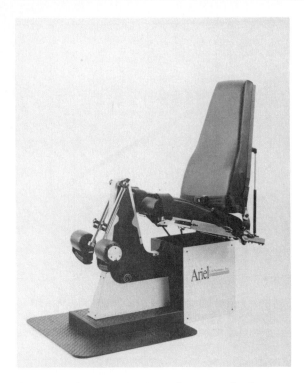

Fig. 5-1. Ariel computerized exercise system (CES) 500 multifunction.

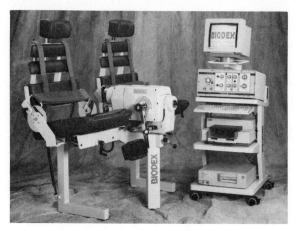

Fig. 5-2. Biodex isokinetic dynamometer.

Ariel Computerized Exercise System (CES)

Three different machines designated as CES are available by Ariel. The CES 500 multifunction allows closed kinetic chain testing and rehabilitation (Figure 5-1). The multifunction machine tests more functional exercise, such as the squat or bench press, instead of isolated joint motions. The CES Back is designed to rest and rehabilitate lumbar flexion and extension. The CES 5000 Arm-Leg is designed for isolated motions of the knee, ankle, shoulder, or elbow. The CES dynamometers provide only concentric resistance but allow velocities up to 1000 degrees/second. The CES allows for isometric and isotonic modes. All dynamometers are computer controlled. The primary limitation of this machine is that it does not operate in an eccentric mode. Also, there is limited research available on the reliability and validity of the CES machines, as well as normative comparison data performed on these dynamometers.[2]

Biodex

The Biodex isokinetic dynamometer allows concentric and eccentric motion (Figure 5-2). This system has isometric, CPM, and isokinetic exercise modes. Concentric velocities range from 30 to 450 degrees/second. Eccentric velocities range from 10 to 120 degrees/second. Maximum torque values allowed for safety purposes are 650 ft lb concentrically and 300 ft lb eccentrically.[4]

One advantage of the Biodex is that it allows for high-speed concentric activity while being fairly user friendly. The Biodex also can be set up easily for strengthening in diagonal planes. The Biodex generates a very comprehensive report after isokinetic evaluation. However, the low eccentric torque maximum and low eccentric velocities are a limitation of this machine when used in the athletic population.

Cybex 6000

The Cybex 6000 is the newest dynamometer manufactured by Cybex that allows concentric and eccentric motion (Figure 5-3). All other Cybex dynamometers allow only concentric activity. The 6000 has a powered and nonpowered mode. The nonpowered mode allows free limb acceleration with concentric/concentric activity that is similar to previous Cybex dynamometers. The powered mode provides both concentric and eccentric activity and CPM. The Cybex 6000 has 18 exercise/test patterns available.

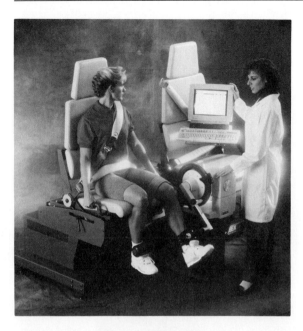

Fig. 5-3. Cybex 6000.

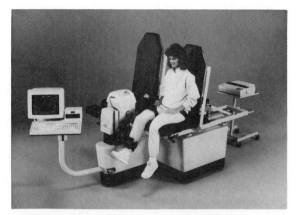

Fig. 5-4. Kin-Com 500H isokinetic dynamometer.

Nonpowered concentric velocities range between 15 to 500 degrees/second. The torque maximum for nonpowered concentric activity is 500 ft lb. Powered concentric velocities range from 15 to 120 degrees/ second. The torque maximum for this mode is also 500 ft lb. Powered eccentric velocities range from 30 to 120 degrees/second. The torque maximums vary depending on the velocity in this mode. The torque maximum for velocities between 30 and 55 degrees/second is 250 ft lb. The torque maximum in the eccentric powered mode for velocities between 60 and 120 degrees/second is 300 ft lb. The velocities in the continuous passive motion mode vary between 5 and 120 degrees/second.[8]

One of the primary advantages of this dynamometer is that it is a Cybex product. The nonpowered mode of this dynamometer is the same as previous Cybex dynamometers, so the normative and research data can be used as comparison data with this machine. This machine also is very versatile in that it can be used for many exercise patterns for the upper and lower extremity. The disadvantage of the Cybex is similar to the Biodex, with low eccentric torque maximums and low eccentric velocities when used in the athletic population.

Kin-Com

The Kin-Com isokinetic dynamometer was the first active system available that allowed concentric and eccentric activity (Figure 5-4). This system is available with either a two seat (500H) or one seat (125E) testing apparatus. The Kin-Com 500H can simultaneously measure internal muscular activity with integrated electromyographic (EMG) capabilities as an option on this machine. A back attachment is available with the 500H. The Kin-Com dynamometers offer isometric, isotonic, continuous passive motion (CPM), and isokinetic modes. The velocities for isotonic, CPM, and isokinetic (concentric and eccentric) modes range between 1 and 250 degrees/second. The force maximums are 450 ft lb (2000 Newtons) for all of the exercise modes. All of the Kin-Com dynamometers are computer controlled.[21]

The Kin-Com dynamometers offer one of the highest force maximums, as well as the highest velocities for eccentric testing and rehabilitation, a distinct advantage in the athletic setting. The Kin-Com is also extremely user friendly. The Kin-Com, however, only provides torque/force comparison data after isokinetic testing. The Kin-Com does not provide any work or power data in the results comparison after testing. The Kin-Com is limited to 250 degrees/second in the concentric mode, which is considerably slower than other available isokinetic dynamometers.

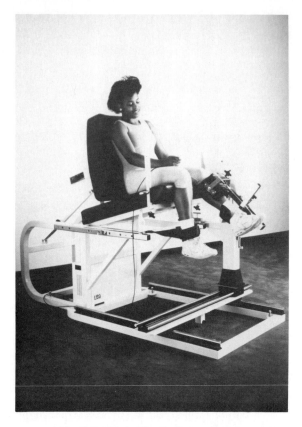

Fig. 5-5. Lido isokinetic dynamometer.

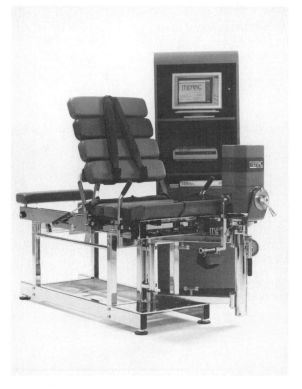

Fig. 5-6. MERAC system.

Lido

Lido isokinetic dynamometers are available in a passive or active multijoint (MJ) system (Figure 5-5). There is also a back system available. The active MJ system has concentric and eccentric capabilities. The available exercise modes are isometric, isotonic, isokinetic, isoacceleration, and CPM. Isoacceleration is described as a set acceleration/deceleration rate. The athlete is unable to accelerate/decelerate faster than the programmed rate. Velocities range from 1 to 400 degrees/second for concentric exercise and 1 to 250 degrees/second for eccentric exercise. CPM has an upper velocity limit of 120 degrees/second. The torque maximum for isometric, isotonic, and concentric isokinetic modes is 400 ft lb. The eccentric isokinetic maximum is 250 ft lb. The Lido isokinetic dynamometers are computer controlled.[24]

The Lido active MJ dynamometer is like the Kin-Com in that it allows higher velocity eccentric training and evaluation. The Lido has a Challenge software program that gives the athlete gamelike biofeedback displays during training to provide extra motivation to reach exercise goals. The Lido provides unique sliding cuff attachments for hip, knee, shoulder, and elbow exercise. The sliding cuff compensates for movement of the axis of rotation during reciprocal exercise. The primary disadvantage of the Lido active MJ dynamometer in the athletic population relates to the low torque maximum of eccentric exercise. Limited research has been done on the Lido isokinetic dynamometers as compared with the Kin-Com, Biodex, or Cybex systems.

Merac

The Musculoskeletal Evaluation, Rehabilitation, and Conditioning (MERAC) system was designed and developed by Universal Gym Equipment (Figure 5-6). The MERAC offers isokinetic, isometric, isotonic, and individualized dynamic variable resistance (IDVR) exercise modes. The MERAC is limited to concentric isokinetic activity. The IDVR mode measures the limb's strength isokinetically to establish a motor performance curve (MPC). IDVR provides variable isotonic resistance to match a selected percentage of the MPC throughout the range of motion. Exercise velocities in the isokinetic mode range from 15 to 500 degrees/second. Isotonic velocities range from 15 to 1000 degrees/second. The torque maximum for all exercise modes is 500 ft lb. The MERAC is computer controlled.[25]

The advantages of the MERAC system are the increased velocities and high torque maximum offered in the isokinetic and isotonic modes. The primary disadvantage is that the MERAC provides only concentric resistance. Also, limited research has been performed on the MERAC isokinetic dynamometer.

Noncomputerized Isokinetic Equipment

Several manufacturers have isokinetic equipment available on the market that is not interfaced with computer-driven software. The Orthotron, manufactured by Cybex, and Hydrafitness equipment are the two most widely used types of noncomputerized isokinetic exercise equipment. The major advantage of this type of equipment is that the cost is substantially lower, yet they may still be used for training and strengthening. The disadvantage is that they do not afford the sports therapist the capacity to produce quantifiable, objective evaluation data for an individual athlete.

ISOKINETIC EVALUATION
Parameters

Various parameters of force and torque are used to compare extremities during isokinetic evaluation. One of the limitations of the isokinetic literature is that an abundance of parameters is used in describing isokinetic strength characteristics of muscle. The sports therapist is faced with evaluating the results of specific isokinetic tests and correctly applying the results with normative data that is available in the literature.

Primarily, force or torque data are used in isokinetic literature. Force can best be described as the push or pull produced by the action of one object on another. Force is measured in pounds or Newtons. Torque is the moment of force applied during rotational motion. Torque is measured in foot-pounds or

Newton-meters.[23] Either parameter can be used in isokinetic testing, but force and torque are not interchangeable terms. Most of the isokinetic dynamometers use torque as the measured parameter.

The force and torque parameters in the literature relate to either peak or average force/torque production. Peak force/torque is the point of highest force/torque production.[14] Average force/torque is the force/torque produced across the whole range of motion.[19] Peak and average force/torque can also be compared to body weight for a weight-adjusted force/torque.

Work and power parameters are also identified in isokinetic literature. Work is defined as force multiplied by displacement.[23] Work is best represented as the area under the torque or force curve. Power is defined as the rate of performing work. Data relating to power characteristics are best evaluated by identifying the amount of work performed in a specific time period. This information is not readily available on all isokinetic dynamometers.

Testing

Isokinetic evaluation is dependent on many different variables to produce a reliable test. Two of the variables are speed of testing and the position of the athlete during testing. These variables need to be controlled and should be consistent from test session to test session. The sports therapist needs to test the athlete at specific speeds if comparison to normative data is desired.

The literature provides a vast array of testing speeds for upper and lower extremity isokinetic evaluations.[13,19,22,33] Some researchers state that testing at different speeds allows the sports therapist to test different characteristics of muscular strength and power.[9] There is limited research evidence, however, to support this view.[28]

Generally, 60 degrees/second has been used as the primary test speed for concentric isokinetic testing. Eccentric testing speeds tend to be more variable. Hageman and Sorenson[14] recommend 120 degrees/second as the upper limit for eccentric testing in the general population and 180 degrees/second as the upper limit in the athletic population. Coactivation of the antagonistic musculature occurs with faster speed testing.[15] This coactivation happens because the antagonistic musculature produces force to slow down the lever arm in preparation for the endpoint of the range of motion with open kinetic testing. Reciprocal testing of antagonistic musculature may not be accurate at faster speeds because of the increased force produced by the antagonistic musculature.

Recommended positioning of the athlete during an isokinetic evaluation varies depending on the specific literature reviewed. Positioning of the joint should account for the gravity effect and the healing phase of the injured structures. The gravity effect torque must be calculated if the sports therapist is analyzing reciprocal group ratios such as the quadriceps and hamstrings. Failure to account for this torque skews the agonist/antagonist ratio if the sports therapist tests the two muscles in the same position. An easy way to control this effect is to test the different muscles in different positions so that each muscle is in an antigravity position during testing. Many of the new dynamometers correct for the gravity effect torque if desired. The sports therapist may need to modify the testing position to protect healing structures. For example, early testing of the shoulder musculature after an episode of subluxation/dislocation should be performed with the arm at the side and not in the abducted position.

Positioning the tested joint so that it reproduces functional activity may be beneficial for the sports therapist. The effect of hip position on the torque values of the quadriceps and hamstrings has been studied by Worrell et al.[36] Their results indicated that peak torque was greater in the seated position and less in the supine position. However, the authors state that evaluation of peak torque may be more appropriate from the supine position to mimic hip position during functional activity.

The length of the lever arm of the dynamometer affects the ability to produce torque. Torque production is significantly affected when the lever arm is changed in length greater than 25%. As the lever is shortened, the ability to produce torque is decreased.[30] The sports therapist can limit torque production early in the healing phase of injury by decreasing the length of the lever arm. However, the length of the lever arm needs to be consistent between testing sessions if the sports therapist is comparing previous testing sessions to the current test.

Reliability

It is important to the sports therapist to have reliable and reproducible test results. Test reliability is dependent on many factors but is probably the most overlooked aspect of isokinetic evaluation. Harding

et al.[18] studied knee flexion and extension force and concluded that maximum reliability of torque measurements occurs with repetitive testing on more than one occasion to include all sources of error caused by patient variability. The best estimate would be a mean value of the test results. Likewise, Wessel et al.[35] recommended that patients be given a practice session. The actual testing session should be performed on a second testing session after the patient has familiarized himself/herself with the testing procedure and the isokinetic dynamometer. Eccentric testing especially involves a significant learning curve.

Testing of multiaxial joints, such as the shoulder and ankle, provides the sports therapist with difficulty in reproducing test results secondary to the complexity of set-ups, as well as the limitations in aligning the axis of rotation of the limb with the mechanical axis of rotation of the machine. Results have shown very poor reliability between repetitive trials of peak torque for ankle plantarflexion/dorsiflexion.[34] A suggestion to limit the error is to always test both extremities during a testing session. The sports therapist should limit comparisons between testing sessions. The sports therapist needs to recognize the limitations associated with testing multiaxial joints.

Retesting the athlete allows the sports therapist to evaluate the progress made with the rehabilitation program. Broad statements regarding the strength and functional ability of the tested musculature should be limited, since isokinetic evaluation is not correlated with the ability to perform functional activity.[1] However, retesting of the involved musculature does afford the sports therapist the ability to evaluate the effectiveness of the rehabilitation program. Improvements in test results that occur within 1 week of testing probably do not reflect changes in strength of the involved musculature but are indicative of either the athlete's familiarity with testing or possibly neuromuscular changes within the muscle.[3] True strength changes involving hypertrophic changes in the muscle usually require 4 to 6 weeks of training.[7] Both neuromuscular and hypertrophic strength changes are important to evaluate, but the sports therapist needs to understand that true strength changes of the involved musculature do not occur within a short period of time.

Interpretation of Graphs

Specific ratios of force, torque, work, or power are identified during isokinetic testing to determine differences between the two tested extremities. The most commonly used ratios are peak/average torque ratios between injured/noninjured extremities, agonist/antagonist ratios, and concentric/eccentric ratios. Normal peak and average force/torque ratios comparing the injured to the uninjured extremity typically use the 85% to 90% ratio to allow the athlete to return to competition.[26] Some authors are more specific with isokinetic discharge criteria. Engle and Canner[11] identified discharge criteria for anterolateral instability of the knee including a 50% ratio at 100 degrees/second for hamstring peak torque to body weight, equal bilateral hamstring peak torque and total work at different speeds, and no greater than a 10% deficit of quadriceps peak torque and total work. Eccentric testing is more variable than concentric testing with less available literature for normative data.

Agonist/antagonist ratios are another commonly used ratio in isokinetic evaluation. The hamstring/quadriceps ratio is the most analyzed ratio. Historically, based on Cybex evaluations, a 66% ratio between the hamstrings and the quadriceps at 60 degrees/second is described as the normative value.[9] This testing is only done in the concentric mode. The sports therapist needs to be careful in comparing the hamstring/quadriceps ratio. The 66% ratio is reflective of testing done in the concentric mode at 60 degrees/second. Likewise, agonist/antagonist ratios have been identified for other muscle groups such as shoulder internal/external rotation. The sports therapist does not need to know all the specifics of the data but does need to know which of the agonist/antagonist musculature is capable of producing the most force. The sports therapist can then evaluate the function of the opposing muscle groups without knowing the specific ratio numbers of the agonist/antagonist.

Finally, the eccentric/concentric ratio is another parameter to evaluate with isokinetic testing. Blacker[5] reports that eccentric testing should produce a 5% to 70% increase in force/torque as compared with concentric testing. Bennett and Stauber[3] identified eccentric to concentric quadriceps torque deficits in approximately 30% of their patients with anterior knee pain. The deficit was defined as less than an 85% peak torque ratio between eccentric and concentric activity. The researchers felt that the deficit may have been one cause of the subjects' increased pain. The symptoms and isokinetic deficits were reversed through a training program. Trudelle-Jackson et al.[31],

however, tested asymptomatic subjects concentrically and eccentrically. The researchers reported a significant percentage of healthy subjects who demonstrated the same percentage eccentric to concentric deficit as defined by Bennett and Stauber.[3] One reason for the difference is that eccentric testing involves a greater variability than concentric testing. The sports therapist needs to evaluate concentric and eccentric force production. The athlete should be able to produce more force eccentrically, but the sports therapist should be aware that a greater variance exists with eccentric testing.

Shape of the Curve

The information that evaluation of the curve provides varies depending on the researcher. Rothstein, Lamb, and Mayhew[28] state that the shape of the torque curve may be due to machine artifact and may not be related to patient performance. These researchers state that the sports therapist should not make specific conclusions regarding pathological conditions based on the shape of the torque curve. However, there is some evidence to support that the shape of the torque curve may be related to patient function.

Engle and Faust[12] tested patients with a history of shoulder subluxation. The testing involved performing traditional and diagonal patterns of shoulder motion. The researchers identified consistent torque defects in symptomatic and asymptomatic patients. Torque curve abnormalities were found from 70 to 110 degrees with flexion/abduction/external rotation diagonal in patients with rotator cuff weakness. The abnormalities were seen at 85 degrees in the extension/adduction/internal rotation diagonal in patients with posterior labral tearing. Dvir et al[10] tested patients with patellofemoral pain. The researchers identified a large percentage of patients who exhibited a break in the torque curve that lasted for 10 degrees at approximately 45 degrees of flexion. The break was associated with a load reduction of approximately 25% of the patient's weight. Pain inhibition was hypothesized to be the cause of the break in the curve. Stanton and Purdham[29] identified deficits in the shape of the torque curve in athletes with hamstring strains. The deficits in the curve occurred before, during, and after concentric/eccentric turnaround. The authors stated these deficits at concentric/eccentric turnaround may represent abnormality in firing patterns that may increase the athlete's risk of sustaining further hamstring injury. These authors

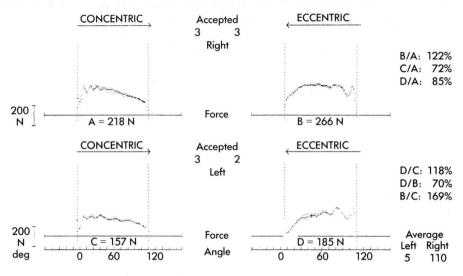

Fig. 5-7. Isokinetic torque curve abnormality.

developed specific concentric/eccentric exercises to attempt to correct these deficits.

Clinically, deficits in the shape of the curve should be identified. One repetition that produces a torque abnormality should not lead the sports therapist to conclude the athlete has altered function. Testing should include multiple repetitions to identify consistent torque curve deficits. The sports therapist should then design a specific rehabilitation program to attempt to correct for these deficits.

Figure 5-7 shows a torque curve abnormality. These graphs involve an isokinetic evaluation of a patient who had history of significant patellofemoral pain after an ACL reconstruction. The lower two graphs are of the involved side. Evaluation of the concentric force curve reveals consistent deficits between 25 and 60 degrees. The eccentric force curve is very inconsistent with a decrease in force production from 35 to 60 degrees. Pain inhibition was thought to be the contributing factor to these force curve abnormalities. A rehabilitation program was designed to attempt to correct for these deficits and to avoid painful ranges identified on the force curves.

Figure 5-8 shows an isokinetic evaluation of a decathlete with hamstring strain. This athlete had a history of recurrent hamstring strains of both extremities. The lower two graphs are of the involved side. Evaluation of the eccentric force curve reveals a divot bilaterally from 90 to 100 degrees of flexion. The athlete exhibits diminished eccentric control throughout the motion. The eccentric curve also reveals a decay of force from 30 to 50 degrees of flexion. A rehabilitation program was designed that included eccentric control of the hamstrings and eccentric/concentric quick reversals in the standing position for the leg curl motion in addition to traditional strengthening of the hamstrings.

ISOKINETIC TRAINING
Force-Velocity Curve

The use of isokinetic dynamometers should not be limited solely to evaluation purposes. Isokinetic training is a valuable rehabilitation tool and should not be overlooked in designing an exercise program. The force-velocity curve should be the basis for designing an isokinetic training program.

The force-velocity curve identifies two of the major components that sports therapists can control in a rehabilitation program—force and speed. Numerous research studies have been performed that identify the force production with concentric and eccentric activity with changes in velocity of motion. Figure 5-9 is a representation of the force-velocity curve.

Force production is located on the y axis and the velocity of motion (speed) is on the x axis. Concentric motion is located on the right side of the x axis, and eccentric motion is on the left side of the x axis. Velocity increases from left to right with concentric motion, and velocity increases from right to left with

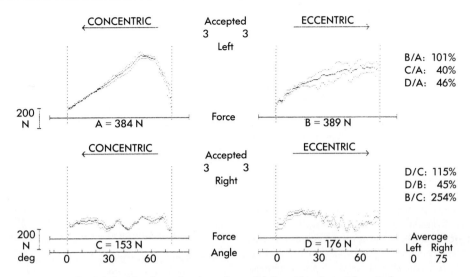

Fig. 5-8. Isokinetic evaluation of an athlete with a hamstring strain.

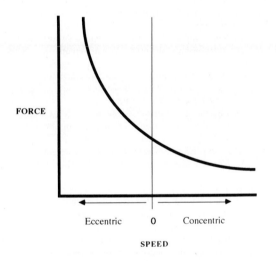

Fig. 5-9. Force-velocity curve.

eccentric motion. Force production decreases with increases in velocity with concentric motion.[6] Conversely, eccentric force production may increase with an increase in the velocity of motion.[17,32] However, some researchers disagree and feel eccentric torque remains the same with increases in velocity.[6,13] Research relating to the specificity of training for speed and mode of exercise is extremely variable and is beyond the scope of this text.

The sports therapist should use the force-velocity curve as the basis for designing a rehabilitation program. The velocity and the mode of exercise should be chosen with regard to the type of injury and the potential for force production with the different velocities and modes of exercise. In the acute phase of healing after injury, force production should be kept to a minimum to allow appropriate healing of the injured structures. Eccentric isokinetic training is not advised in this phase because of the potential for increased force production.

SAMPLE PROGRESSION

Some of the isokinetic dynamometers offer the ability to provide other types of resistance, such as isotonic, isometric, and passive motion, in the training mode, which allows the sports therapist more flexibility in the use of dynamometers in the rehabilitation program. Progression through the rehabilitation program should be based on the attainment of short-term goals and the phase of healing after injury. In the acute phase of injury, the goals should be related to regaining motion and maintenance of strength. The isokinetic dynamometer can be used in this phase to provide isometric and submaximal isotonic resistance and passive motion if needed. Positioning of the athlete for rehabilitation sessions may need to be altered to lessen the gravity effect torque. As the healing progresses and the injury enters the scar proliferation stage (7 to 21 days), graded resistive stresses can be applied to initiate the strengthening phase or rehabilitation. The isokinetic dynamometer can be used for submaximal to maximal isotonics and the initiation of submaximal concentric/eccentric isokinetics. As the injury progresses into the scar remodeling phase (21 days), more aggressive strengthening can be added to the rehabilitation program. The isokinetic dynamometer can be used to alter velocity and force production using traditional and diagonal planes of motion for maximal isotonic and isokinetic resistance.

The disadvantage of isokinetics as was previously mentioned is that motion is performed in an open isokinetic chain, which is not representative of functional activity. However, some dynamometers can be adjusted to provide closed kinetic resistance in the form of leg press motions and standing terminal knee extension. Biodex has also recently made a closed kinetic attachment for its dynamometer. The addition of closed kinetic activities makes the dynamometers more versatile in the rehabilitation setting. However, while isokinetic evaluation and training is a valuable tool for the sports therapist, isokinetic testing may not be representative of functional ability in sport-specific activity. The sports therapist needs to evaluate functional ability in the functional setting and use isokinetics as a guide for progression through the rehabilitation program.

SUMMARY

1. Isokinetic exercise is described as movement that occurs at a constant angular velocity with accommodating resistance.
2. Force can be best described as a push or pull produced by the action of one object on another.
3. Torque is defined as the moment of force applied during rotational motion.
4. Work is defined as force multiplied by displacement. Work is measured as the area under the torque curve.
5. Power is defined as the rate of performing work.
6. The sports therapist needs to be consistent with isokinetic testing from one session to another. Speed and position of the athlete should remain the same.
7. The athlete may need a practice session before isokinetic testing to be familiarized to the testing sequence and the isokinetic dynamometer.
8. Peak/average torque ratios, agonist/antagonist ratios, and eccentric/concentric ratios are commonly used to evaluate the results of isokinetic testing.
9. The sports therapist needs to evaluate the shape of the torque curve for consistent abnormalities. A rehabilitation program should be designed to correct specific deficits that are identified.
10. The force-velocity curve should be the basis for designing specific isokinetic training programs.

REFERENCES

1 Anderson M, Gieck J, Perrin D, et al.: The relationships among isometric, isotonic, and isokinetic concentric and eccentric quadriceps and hamstring force and three components of athletic performance, *JOSPT* 14(3):114–120, 1991.
2 Ariel Life Systems Informational Packet, La Jolla, Calif, Ariel Life Systems.
3 Bennett J, Stauber W: Evaluation and treatment of anterior knee pain using eccentric exercise, *Med Sci Sports Exerc* 18(5):526–530, 1986.
4 Biodex Informational Packet, Shirley, NY, Biodex Corp.
5 Blacker H: Measurements predicting outcome in pain treatment. In Kin-Com Clinical Resource Kit, Hixson, Tenn, Chattanooga Corp.
6 Chandler J, Duncan P: Eccentric versus concentric force-velocity relationships of the quadriceps femoris muscle, *Phys Ther* 68(5):800, 1988.
7 Coyle E, Feiring D, Rotkis T, et al.: Specificity of power improvements through slow and fast isokinetic training, *J Appl Physiol* 51(6):1437–1442, 1981.
8 Cybex Informational Packet, Ronkonkoma, NY, Cybex Corp.
9 Davies G: *A compendium of isokinetics in clinical usage*, LaCrosse, Wis, 1984, S and S Publishers.
10 Dvir Z, Halperin N, Snklar A, et al.: Quadriceps function and patellofemoral pain syndrome, *Isokinetics Exerc Sci* 1(1):31–35, 1991.
11 Engle R, Canner G: Rehabilitation of symptomatic anterolateral knee instability, *JOSPT* 11(6):237–244, 1989.
12 Engle R, Faust J: Isokinetic evaluation in posterior shoulder subluxation, *Isokinetics Exerc Sci* 1(2):72–74, 1991.
13 Hageman P, Gillaspie D, Hill L: Effects of speed and limb dominance on eccentric and concentric isokinetic testing of the knee, *JOSPT* 10(2):59–65, 1988.
14 Hageman P, Sorenson T: Eccentric isokinetics. In Albert M, editor: *Eccentric muscle training in sports and orthopaedics*, New York, 1991, Churchill Livingstone.
15 Hagood S, Solomonow M, Baratta R, et al.: The effect of joint velocity on the contribution of the antagonistic musculature to knee stiffness and laxity, *Am J Sports Med* 18(2):182–187, 1990.
16 Hall L, Williams J: The use of isokinetics in rehabilitation, *Physiotherapy* 75(12):737–740, 1989.
17 Hanten W, Wieding D: Isokinetic measurement of the force-velocity relationship of concentric and eccentric contractions, *Phys Ther* 68(5):801, 1988.
18 Harding B, Black T, Bruulsema A, et al.: Reliability of a reciprocal test protocol performed on the Kinetic Communicator:

an isokinetic test of knee extensor and flexor strength, *JOSPT* 10(6):218–223, 1988.

19 Highgenboten C, Jackson A, Meske N: Concentric and eccentric torque comparisons for knee extension and flexion in young adult males and females using the Kinetic Communicator, *Am J Sports Med* 16(3):234–237, 1988.

20 Hislop H, Perrine J: The isokinetic concept of exercise, *Phys Ther* 47(2):114–117, 1967.

21 Kin-Com Informational Packet, Hixson, Tenn, Chattanooga Corp.

22 Klopfer D, Greij S: Examining quadriceps/hamstring performance at high velocity isokinetics in untrained subjects, *JOSPT* 10(1):18–22, 1988.

23 Leveau B: *Williams and Lister's biomechanics of human motion,* ed 3, Philadelphia, 1992, WB Saunders.

24 LIDO Informational Packet, West Sacramento, Calif, Loredan Biomedical.

25 MERAC Informational Packet, Cedar Rapids, Iowa, Universal Gym Equipment.

26 Perrin D, Robertson R, Lay R: Bilateral isokinetic peak torque, torque acceleration energy, power, and work relationships in athletes and non-athletes, *JOSPT* 9(5):184–189, 1987.

27 Poulmedis P, Rondoyannis G, Mitsou A, et al.: The influence of isokinetic muscle torque exerted in various speeds on soccer ball velocity, *JOSPT* 10(3):93–96, 1988.

28 Rothstein J, Lamb L, Mayhew T: Clinical uses of isokinetic measurements, *Phys Ther* 67(12):1840–1844, 1987.

29 Stanton P, Purdham C: Hamstring injuries in sprinting—the role of eccentric exercise, *JOSPT* 10(9):343–349, 1989.

30 Taylor R, Casey J: Quadriceps torque production on the Cybex II dynamometer as related to changes in lever arm length, *JOSPT* 8(3):147–152, 1986.

31 Trudelle-Jackson E, Meske N, Highgenboten C, et al.: Eccentric/concentric torque deficits in the quadriceps muscle, *JOSPT* 11(4), 142, 1989.

32 Walmsley R, Pearson N, Stymiest P: Eccentric wrist extensor contractions and the force velocity relationship in muscle, *JOSPT* 8(6):288–293, 1986.

33 Weltman A, Tippett S, Janney C, et al.: Measurement of isokinetic strength in prepubertal males, *JOSPT* 9(10):345–351, 1988.

34 Wennerberg D: Reliability of an isokinetic dorsiflexion and plantarflexion apparatus, *Am J Sports Med* 19(5):519–522, 1991.

35 Wessel J, Mattison G, Luongo F, et al.: Reliability of eccentric and concentric measurements, *Phys Ther* 68(5):782, 1988.

36 Worrell T, Perrin D, Denegar C: The influence of hip position on quadriceps and hamstring peak torque and reciprocal muscle group ratio values, *JOSPT* 11(3):104–107, 1989.

37 Wyatt M, Edwards A: Comparisons of quadriceps and hamstring torque values during isokinetic exercise, *JOSPT* 3(2):48–56, 1981.

Plyometric Exercise in Rehabilitation

6

Michael Voight and Steve Tippett

OBJECTIVES

After completion of this chapter, the student should be able to do the following:

- Describe the mechanical, neurophysiological, and neuromuscular control mechanisms involved in plyometric training.

- Discuss how biomechanical evaluation, stability, dynamic movement, and flexibility should be assessed before beginning a plyometric program.

- Explain how a plyometric program can be modified by changing intensity, volume, frequency, and recovery.

- Discuss how plyometrics can be integrated into a rehabilitation program.

In sports training and rehabilitation of athletic injuries, the concept of specificity has emerged as an important parameter in determining the proper choice and sequence of exercise in a training program. The jumping movement is inherent in numerous sports activities such as basketball, volleyball, gymnastics, and aerobic dancing. Even running is a repeated series of jump-landing cycles. Therefore jump training should be used in the design and implementation in the overall training program.

Peak performance in sports requires technical skill and power. Skill in most activities combines natural athletic ability and learned specialized proficiency in an activity. Success in most activities is dependent upon the speed at which muscular force or power can be generated. Strength and conditioning programs throughout the years have attempted to augment the force production system to maximize the power generated. Since power combines strength and speed, it can be increased by increasing the amount of work or force that is produced by the muscles or by decreasing the amount of time required to produce the force. While weight training can produce increased gains in strength, the speed of movement is limited. The amount of time required to produce

muscular force is an important variable for increasing the power output. A form of training that attempts to combine speed of movement with strength is *plyometrics*.

While the term *plyometric training* may be relatively new, the concept of plyometric training is not new. The roots of plyometric training can be traced to eastern Europe, where it was known simply as jump training. The term *plyometrics* was coined by an American track and field coach, Fred Wilt.[33] The development of the term is confusing. *Plyo* comes from the Greek word *plythein*, which means to increase. *Plio* is the Greek word for more, and *metric* literally means to measure. The practical definition of plyometrics is a quick, powerful movement involving prestretching the muscle and activating the stretch-shortening cycle to produce a subsequently stronger concentric contraction. It takes advantage of the length-shortening cycle to increase muscular power.

In the late 1960s and early 1970s when the Eastern bloc countries began to dominate sports requiring power, their training methods became the focus of attention. After the 1972 Olympics, articles began to appear in coaching magazines outlining a strange new system of jumps and bounds that was used by the Soviets to increase speed. Valery Borzov, the 100-meter gold medalist, credited plyometric exercise for his success. As it turns out, the Eastern bloc countries were not the originators of plyometrics, just the organizers. This system of hops and jumps has been used by American coaches for years as a method of conditioning. Both rope jumping and bench hops have been used to improve quickness and reaction times. The organization of this training method has been credited to the legendary Soviet jump coach Yuri Verhoshanski, who during the late 1960s began to tie this method of miscellaneous hops and jumps into an organized training plan.[30]

The main purpose of plyometric training is to heighten the excitability of the nervous system for improved reactive ability of the neuromuscular system.[31] Therefore any type of exercise that uses the myotatic stretch reflex to produce a more powerful response of the contracting muscle is plyometric in nature. All movement patterns in both athletes and activities of daily living (ADL) involve repeated stretch-shortening cycles. Picture a jumping athlete preparing to transfer forward energy to upward energy. As the final step is taken before jumping, the loaded leg must stop the forward momentum and change it into an upward direction. As this happens, the muscle undergoes a lengthening eccentric contraction to decelerate the movement and prestretch the muscle. This prestretch energy is then immediately released in an equal and opposite reaction, thereby producing kinetic energy. The neuromuscular system must react quickly to produce the concentric shortening contraction to prevent falling and produce the upward change in direction. Most elite athletes will naturally exhibit with great ease this ability to use stored kinetic energy. The less gifted athlete can train this ability and enhance their production of power. Consequently, specific functional exercise to emphasize this rapid change of direction must be used to prepare patients and athletes for return to activity. Since plyometric exercises train specific movements in a biomechanically accurate manner, the muscles, tendons, and ligaments are all strengthened in a functional manner.

BIOMECHANICAL AND PHYSIOLOGICAL PRINCIPLES OF PLYOMETRIC TRAINING

The goal of plyometric training is to decrease the amount of time required between the yielding ec-

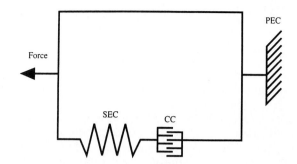

Fig. 6-1. Three component model.

centric muscle contraction and the initiation of the overcoming concentric contraction. Normal physiological movement rarely begins from a static starting position but rather is preceded by an eccentric prestretch that loads the muscle and prepares it for the ensuing concentric contraction. The coupling of this eccentric-concentric muscle contraction is known as the *stretch-shortening cycle*. The physiology of this stretch-shortening cycle can be broken down into two components: proprioceptive reflexes and the elastic properties of muscle fibers. While both of these components work together to produce a response, they will be discussed separately for the purpose of understanding.

Mechanical Characteristics

The mechanical characteristics of a muscle can best be represented by a three-component model (Figure 6-1). A contractile component (CC), series elastic component (SEC), and parallel elastic component (PEC) all interact to produce a force output. While the CC is usually the focal point of motor control, the SEC and PEC also play an important role in providing stability and integrity to the individual fibers when a muscle is lengthened. During this lengthening process, energy is stored within the musculature in the form of kinetic energy.

When a muscle contracts in a concentric fashion, most of the force that is produced comes from the muscle fiber filaments sliding past one another. Force is registered externally by being transferred through the SEC. When eccentric contraction occurs, the muscle lengthens like a spring. With this lengthening, the SEC is also stretched and allowed to contribute to the overall force production. Therefore the total force production is the sum of the force produced by the CC and the stretching of the SEC. An analogy would be the stretching of a rubber band. When a stretch is applied, potential energy is stored and applied as it returns to its original length when the stretch is released. Significant increases in concentric muscle force production have been documented when immediately preceded by an eccentric contraction.[2,4,9] This increase may be due in part to the storage of elastic energy since the muscles are able to use the force produced by the SEC. When the muscle contracts in a concentric manner, the elastic energy that is stored in the SEC can be recovered and used to augment the shortening contraction. The ability to use this stored elastic energy is affected by three variables: time, magnitude of stretch, and velocity of stretch.[17] The concentric contraction can only be magnified if the preceding eccentric contraction is of short range and performed quickly without delay.[2,4,9] Bosco and Komi proved this concept experimentally when they compared damped vs. undamped jumps.[4] Undamped jumps produced minimal knee flexion upon landing and were followed by an immediate rebound jump. With damped jumps, the knee flexion angle increased significantly. The power output was much higher with the undamped jumps. The increased knee flexion seen in the damped jumps decreased elastic behavior of the muscle, and the potential elastic energy stored in the SEC was lost as heat. Similar investigations produced greater vertical jump height when the movement was preceded by a countermovement as opposed to a static jump.[2,5,6,22]

Storage of elastic energy can also be affected by the type of muscle fiber involved in the contraction. Bosco et al. noted a difference in the recoil of elastic energy in slow-twitch vs. fast-twitch muscle fibers.[7] This study indicates that fast-twitch muscle fibers respond to a high-speed, small-amplitude prestretch. The amount of elastic energy used was proportional to the amount stored. When a long, slow stretch is applied to muscle, both slow- and fast-twitch fibers exhibit a similar amount of stored elastic energy; however, this stored energy is used to a greater extent with the slow-twitch fibers as compared to the fast-twitch fibers. This trend would suggest that slow-twitch muscle fibers may be able to use elastic energy more efficiently in ballistic movement characterized by long and slow prestretching in the stretch-shortening cycle.

Neurophysiological Mechanisms

The proprioceptive stretch reflex is the other mechanism by which force can be produced during the stretch-shortening cycle. Mechanoreceptors located within the muscle provide information about the degree of muscular stretch. This information is transmitted to the central nervous system and becomes capable of influencing muscle tone, motor execution programs, and kinesthetic awareness. The mechanoreceptors that are primarily responsible for the stretch reflex are the Golgi tendon organs and muscle spindles.[24] The muscle spindle is a complex stretch receptor that is located in parallel within the muscle fibers. Sensory information regarding the length of the muscle spindle and the rate of the applied stretch is transmitted to the central nervous system. If the length of the surrounding muscle fibers is less than that of the spindle, the frequency of the nerve impulses from the spindle is reduced. When the muscle spindle becomes stretched, an afferent sensory response is produced and transmitted to the central nervous system. Neurological impulses are in turn sent back to the muscle, causing a motor response. As the muscle contracts, the stretch on the muscle spindle is relieved, thereby removing the original stimulus. The strength of the muscle spindle response is determined by the rate of stretch.[24] The more rapidly the load is applied to the muscle, the greater the firing frequency of the spindle and resultant reflexive muscle contraction.

The Golgi tendon organ lies within the muscle tendon near the point of attachment of the muscle fiber to the tendon. Unlike the facilitory action of the muscle spindle, the Golgi tendon organ has an inhibitory effect on the muscle by contributing to a tension limiting reflex. Because the Golgi tendon organ is in series alignment with the contracting muscle fibers, they become activated with tension or stretch within the muscle. Upon activation, sensory impulses are transmitted to the central nervous system. These sensory impulses cause an inhibition of the alpha motor neurons of the contracting muscle and its synergists, thereby limiting the amount of force produced. With a concentric muscle contraction the activity of the muscle spindle is reduced because the surrounding muscle fibers are shortening. During an eccentric muscle contraction, the muscle stretch reflex generates more tension in the lengthening muscle. When the tension within the muscle reaches a potentially harmful level, the Golgi tendon organ fires, thereby reducing the excitation of the muscle. The muscle spindle and Golgi tendon organ systems oppose each other, and increasing force is produced. The descending neural pathways from the brain help to balance these forces and ultimately control which reflex will dominate.[26]

The degree of muscle fiber elongation is dependent upon three physiological factors. Fiber length is proportional to the amount of stretching force applied to the muscle. The ultimate elongation or deformation is also dependent upon the absolute strength of the individual muscle fibers. The stronger the tensile strength, the less elongation that will occur. The last factor for elongation is the ability of the muscle spindle to produce a neurophysiological response. A muscle spindle with a low sensitivity level will result in a difficulty in overcoming the rapid elongation and therefore produce a less powerful response. Plyometric training will assist in enhancing muscular control within the neurological system.

The increased force production seen during the stretch-shortening cycle is due to the combined effects of the storage of elastic energy and the myotatic reflex activation of the muscle.[2,5,8,9,23,27] The percentage of contribution from each component is unknown.[5] The increased amount of force production is dependent upon the time frame between the eccentric and concentric contractions.[9] This time frame can be defined as the *amortization phase*.[13] The amortization phase is the electromechanical delay between eccentric and concentric contraction during which time the muscle must switch from overcoming work to acceleration in the opposite direction. Komi found that the greatest amount of tension developed within the muscle during the stretch-shortening cycle occurred during the phase of muscle lengthening just before the concentric contraction.[21] The conclusion from this study was that an increased time in the amortization phase would lead to a decrease in force production.

Physiological performance can be improved by several mechanisms with plyometric training. While there has been documented evidence of increased speed of the stretch reflex, the increased intensity of the subsequent muscle contraction may be best attributed to better recruitment of additional motor units.[11] The force-velocity relationship states that the faster a muscle is loaded or lengthened eccentrically, the greater the resultant force output. Eccentric lengthening will also place a load on the elastic components of the muscle fibers. The stretch reflex may also increase the stiffness of the muscular spring by recruiting additional muscle fibers.[11] This additional stiffness may allow the muscular system to use more external stress in the form of elastic recoil.[11]

Another possible mechanism by which plyometric training can increase the force or power output involves the inhibitory effect of the Golgi tendon organs on force production. Since the Golgi tendon organ serves as a tension-limiting reflex, restricting the amount of force that can be produced, the stimulation threshold for the Golgi tendon organ becomes a limiting factor. Bosco and Komi have suggested that plyometric training may desensitize the Golgi tendon organ, thereby raising the level of inhibition.[4] If the level of inhibition is raised, a greater amount of force production and load can be applied to the musculoskeletal system.

Neuromuscular Coordination

The last mechanism in which plyometric training may improve muscular performance centers around neuromuscular coordination. The speed of muscular contraction may be limited by neuromuscular coordination. In other words, the body may only move within a set speed range, no matter how strong the muscles are. Training with an explosive prestretch of the muscle may improve the neural efficiency, thereby increasing neuromuscular performance. Plyometric training may promote changes within the neuromuscular system that allow the individual to have better control of the contracting muscle and its synergists, yielding a greater net force even in the absence of morphological adaptation of the muscle. This neural adaptation can increase performance by enhancing the nervous system to become more automatic.

In summary, effective plyometric training relies more on the rate of stretch rather than the length of stretch. Emphasis should center on the reduction of the amortization phase. If the amortization phase is slow, the elastic energy is lost as heat and the stretch reflex is not activated. Conversely, the quicker the individual is able to switch from yielding eccentric work to overcoming concentric work, the more powerful the response.

PROGRAM DEVELOPMENT

Specificity is the key concept in any training program. Sports-specific activities should be analyzed and broken down into basic movement patterns. These specific movement patterns should then be stressed in a gradual fashion based upon individual tolerance to these activities. Development of a plyometric program should begin by establishing an adequate strength base that will allow the body to withstand the large stress that will be placed upon it. A greater strength base will allow for greater force production due to increased muscular cross-sectional area. Additionally, a larger cross-sectional area can contribute to the SEC and subsequently store a greater amount of elastic energy.

Plyometric exercises can be characterized as rapid eccentric loading of the musculoskeletal complex.[11] This type of exercise trains the neuromuscular system by teaching it to more readily accept the increased strength loads.[3] Also, the nervous system is more readily able to react with maximal speed to the lengthening muscle by exploiting the stretch reflex. Since plyometric training attempts to fine tune the neuromuscular system, all training programs should be designed with specificity in mind.[25] This goal will help to ensure that the body is prepared to accept the stress that will be placed upon it during return to function.

Plyometric Prerequisites

BIOMECHANICAL EXAMINATION. Before beginning a plyometric training program, a cursory biomechanical examination and a battery of functional tests should be performed to identify potential contraindications or precautions. Lower quarter biomechanics should be sound to help ensure a stable base of support and normal force transmission. Biomechanical abnormalities of the lower quarter are not contraindications for plyometrics but may contribute to stress failure—overuse injury if not addressed. Before initiating plyometric training, an adequate strength base must be present. Functional tests are very effective to screen for an adequate strength base before initiating plyometrics. Poor strength in the lower extremities will result in a loss of stability when landing and also increase the amount of stress that is absorbed by the weight-bearing tissues with high impact forces, which will reduce performance and increase the risk of injury. The Eastern bloc countries arbitrarily placed a one repetition maximum in the squat at 1.5 to 2 times the individual's body weight before initiating lower quarter plyometrics.[3] If this were to hold true, a 200-pound individual would have to squat 400

Plyometric Static Stability Testing

- Single Leg Stance - 30 sec.
  - Eyes open
  - Eyes closed

- Single Leg 25% Squat - 30 sec.
  - Eyes open
  - Eyes closed

- Single Leg 50% Squat - 30 sec.
  - Eyes open
  - Eyes closed

Fig. 6-2. Stability testing.

pounds before beginning plyometrics. Unfortunately, not many individuals would meet this minimal criteria. Clinical and practical experience has demonstrated that plyometrics can be started without that kind of leg strength.[11] A simple functional parameter to use in determining if an individual is strong enough to initiate a plyometric training program has been advocated by Chu.[12] Power squat testing with a weight equal to 60% of the individual's body weight is used. The individual is asked to perform five squat repetitions in 5 seconds. If the individual cannot perform this task, emphasis in the training program should again center on the strength-training program to develop an adequate base.

Since eccentric muscle strength is an important component to plyometric training, it is especially important to ensure an adequate eccentric strength base is present. Before an individual is allowed to begin a plyometric regimen, a program of closed-chain stability training that focuses on eccentric lower quarter strength should be initiated. In addition to strengthening in a functional manner, closed chain—weight bearing exercises also allow the individual to use functional movement patterns. Once cleared to participate in the plyometric program, precautionary safety tips should be adhered to.

STABILITY TESTING. Stability testing before initiating plyometric training can be divided into two subcategories: static stability and dynamic movement testing. Static stability testing determines the individual's ability to stabilize and control the body. The muscles of postural support must be strong enough to withstand the stress of explosive training. Static stability testing (Figure 6-2) should begin with simple movements of low motor complexity and progress to more difficult high motor skills. The basis for lower quarter stability centers around single-leg strength. Difficulty can be increased by having the individual close his or her eyes. The basic static tests are one-leg standing and single-leg quarter squats that are held for 30 seconds. An individual should be able to perform one-leg standing for 30 seconds with eyes open and closed before the initiation of plyometric training. The individual should be observed for shaking or wobbling of the extremity joints. If there is more movement of a weight-bearing joint in one direction than the other, the musculature producing the movement in the opposite direction needs to be assessed for specific weakness. If weakness is determined, the individual's program should be limited and emphasis placed on isolated strengthening of the weak muscles. For dynamic jump exercises to be initiated, there should be no wobbling of the support leg during the quarter knee squats.

DYNAMIC MOVEMENT TESTING. Dynamic movement testing will assess the individual's ability to produce explosive, coordinated movement. Vertical or single-leg jumping for distance can be used for the lower quarter. Rus Paine and Dr. David Drez have investigated the use of single-leg hop for distance and a determinant for return to play after knee injury. A passing score on their test is 85% in regard to symmetry. The involved leg is tested twice, and the average between the two trials is recorded. The non-involved leg is tested in the same fashion, and then the scores of the noninvolved leg are divided by the scores of the involved leg and multiplied by 100. This provides the symmetry index score. Another functional test that can be used to determine if an individual is ready for plyometric training is the ability to long jump a distance equal to the individual's height. In the upper quarter, the medicine ball toss is used as a functional assessment.

FLEXIBILITY. Another important prerequisite for plyometric training is general and specific flexibility. This is due to the high amount of stress that is applied to the musculoskeletal system. Therefore all plyometric training sessions should begin with a general warm-up and flexibility exercise program. The warm-up should produce mild sweating.[19] The flexibility exercise program should address muscle groups involved in the plyometric program and should include static and short dynamic stretching techniques.[18]

When the individual can demonstrate static and dynamic control of their body weight with single-leg squats, low intensity in-place plyometrics can be initiated. Plyometric training should consist of low-intensity drills and progress slowly in deliberate fash-

Chu's Plyometric Categories

- In-place jumping
- Standing jumps
- Multiple response jumps and hops
- In-depth jumping and box drills
- Bounding
- High stress sport specific drills

Fig. 6-3. Six categories of plyometric training.

ion. As skill and strength foundation increase, moderate intensity plyometrics can be introduced. Mature athletes with strong weight-training backgrounds can be introduced to ballistic-reactive plyometric exercises of high intensity.[12] Once the individual has been classified into the category of either a beginner, intermediate, or advanced level, the plyometric program can be planned and initiated. Chu[10,11,13] has divided lower-quarter plyometric training into six categories (Figure 6-3).

PLYOMETRIC PROGRAM DESIGN

As with any conditioning program, the plyometric training program can be manipulated through four variables: intensity, volume, frequency, and recovery.

Intensity

Intensity can be defined as the amount of effort exerted. With traditional weight lifting, intensity can be modified by changing the amount of weight that is lifted. With plyometric training, intensity can be controlled by the type of exercise that is performed. Double leg jumping is less stressful than single leg jumping. As with all functional exercise, the plyometric exercise program should progress from simple to complex activities. Intensity can be further increased by altering the specific exercises. The addition of external weight or raising the height of the step or box will also increase the exercise intensity.

Volume

Volume is the total amount of work that is performed in a single workout session. With weight training, volume would be recorded as the total amount of weight that was lifted (weight times repetitions). Volume of plyometric training is measured by counting the total number of foot contacts. The recommended volume of foot contacts in any one session will vary inversely with the intensity of the exercise. A beginner should start with low-intensity exercise with a volume of approximately 75 to 100 foot contacts. As ability is increased, the volume is increased to 200 to 250 foot contacts of low-to-moderate intensity.

Frequency

Frequency is the number of times that an exercise session is performed during a training cycle. With weight training, the frequency of exercise has typically been performed on a three-time weekly basis. Unfortunately, research on the frequency of plyometric exercise has not been conducted. Therefore the optimum frequency for increased performance is not known. It has been suggested that 48 to 72 hours of rest are necessary for full recovery before the next training stimulus.[12] Intensity however plays a major role in determining the frequency of training. If an adequate recovery period does not occur, muscle fatigue will result with a corresponding increase in neuromuscular reaction times. The beginner should allow at least 48 hours between training sessions.

Recovery

Recovery is the rest time used between exercise sets. Manipulation of this variable will depend on whether the goal is to increase power or muscular endurance. Since plyometric training is anaerobic in nature, a longer recovery period should be used to allow restoration of metabolic stores. With power training, a work rest ratio of 1:3 or 1:4 should be used. This time frame will allow maximal recovery between sets. For endurance training, this work:rest ratio can be shortened to 1:1 or 1:2. Endurance training typically uses circuit training, where the individual moves from one exercise set to another with minimal rest in between.

The beginning plyometric program should emphasize the importance of eccentric vs. concentric muscle contractions. The relevance of the stretch-shortening cycle with decreased amortization time should be stressed. Initiation of lower quarter plyometric training begins with low intensity in-place and multiple response jumps. The individual should be instructed in proper exercise technique. The feet should be nearly flat in all landings, and the individual should be encouraged to "touch and go." An analogy would be landing on a hot bed of coals. The goal is to reverse the landing as quickly as possible, spending only a minimal amount of time on the ground.

Success of the plyometric program will depend on how well the four training variables are controlled, modified, and manipulated. In general, as the intensity of the exercise is increased, the volume is decreased. The corollary to this is as volume increases, the intensity is decreased. The overall key to successfully controlling these variables is to be flexible and listen to what the athlete's body is telling you. The body's response to the program will dictate the speed of progression. Whenever in doubt as to the exercise intensity or volume, it is better to underestimate to prevent injury.

GUIDELINES FOR PLYOMETRIC PROGRAMS

As the plyometric program is initiated, the individual must be made aware of several guidelines.[31] Any deviation from these guidelines will result in minimal improvement and increased risk for injury. These guidelines include the following:

1. Plyometric training should be specific to the individual goals of the athlete. Activity specific–movement patterns should be trained. These sport-specific skills should be broken down and trained in their smaller components and then rebuilt into a coordinated activity specific–movement pattern.
2. The quality of work is more important than the quantity of work. The intensity of the exercise should be kept at a maximal level.
3. The greater the exercise intensity level, the greater the recovery time.
4. Plyometric training may have its greatest benefit at the conclusion of the normal workout. This pattern will best replicate exercise under a partial to total fatigue environment that is specific to activity. Only low-to-medium stress plyometrics should be used at the conclusion of a workout because of the increased potential of injury with high-stress drills.
5. When proper technique can no longer be demonstrated, maximum volume has been achieved, and the exercise must be stopped.
6. The plyometric training program should be progressive in nature. The volume and intensity can be modified in several ways:
   a. Increase the number of exercises.
   b. Increase the number of repetitions and sets.
   c. Decrease the rest period between sets of exercise.
7. Plyometric training sessions should be conducted no more than three times weekly in the

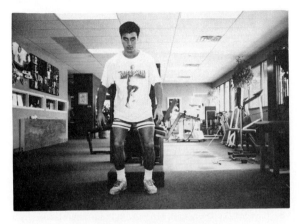

Fig. 6-4. Jump-down exercises.

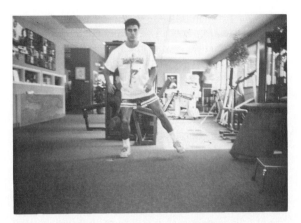

Fig. 6-5. Lateral bounding drills.

preseason phase of training. During this phase, volume should prevail. During the competitive season, the frequency of plyometric training should be reduced to twice weekly, with the intensity of the exercise becoming more important.

8. Dynamic testing of the individual on a regular basis will provide important progression and motivational feedback.

INTEGRATING PLYOMETRICS INTO THE REHABILITATION PROGRAM: CLINICAL CONCERNS

When used judiciously, plyometrics are a valuable asset in the sports rehabilitation program. As previously stated, the majority of lower quarter sport function occurs in the closed kinetic chain. Lower extremity plyometrics are an effective functional closed-chain exercise that can be incorporated into the sports rehabilitation program. According to Davis' law, soft tissue responds to stress imparted upon it to become more resilient along these same lines of stress. As previously mentioned, through the eccentric prestretch, plyometrics place added stress on the tendinous portion of the contractile unit. Eccentric loading is beneficial in the management of tendinitis.[32] Through a gradually progressed eccentric loading program, healing tendinous tissue is stressed, yielding an increase in ultimate tensile strength. This eccentric load can be applied through jump-downs (Figure 6-4). Simple jumping drills (bilateral activities) can be progressed to hopping (unilateral activities). Similar principles can be applied to medial soft tissues around

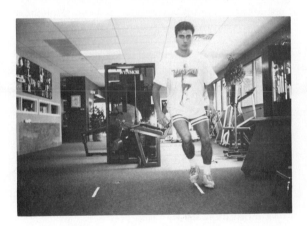

Fig. 6-6. Lateral sliding activities.

the knee after a valgus stress injury. By gradually imparting progressive valgus loads, tissue tensile strength is augmented.[34] In the rehabilitation setting, bilateral support drills can be progressed to unilateral valgus loading efforts. Specifically, lateral jumping drills are progressed to lateral hopping activities. However, the medial structures must also be trained to accept greater valgus loads sustained during cutting activities. As a prerequisite to full-speed cutting, lateral bounding drills should be performed (Figure 6-5). These efforts are progressed to activities that add acceleration, deceleration, and momentum. Lateral sliding activities that require the individual to cover a greater distance can be performed on a slide board. If a slide board is not available, the same movement pattern can be stressed with plyometrics (Figure 6-6). By manipulating volume, frequency, and intensity the program can be advanced appropriately. Proper progression is of prime importance when using plyometrics in the rehabilitation program. These progressive activities are reinjuries waiting to happen without allowing for adequate healing or with an inadequate strength base. A close working relationship fostering open communication and acute observation skills is vital in helping ensure that the program is not overly aggressive.

SUMMARY

1. While the effects of plyometric training are not yet fully understood, it still remains a widely used form of combining strength with speed training to functionally increase power. While the research is somewhat contradictory, the neurophysiological concept of plyometric training is on a sound foundation.
2. A successful plyometric training program should be carefully designed and implemented after establishing an adequate strength base.
3. The effects of this type of high intensity training can be achieved safely if the individual is supervised by a knowledgeable person who uses common sense and follows the prescribed training regimen.
4. The plyometric training program should use a large variety of different exercises, since year-round training often results in boredom and a lack of motivation.
5. Program variety can be manipulated with different types of equipment or kinds of movement performed.
6. Continued motivation and an organized progression are the keys to successful training.
7. Plyometrics are also a valuable asset in the rehabilitation program after a sports injury.
8. Used after lower quarter injury, plyometrics are effective in facilitating joint awareness, strengthening tissue during the healing process, and increasing sport-specific strength and power.
9. The most important considerations in the plyometric program are common sense and experience.

REFERENCES

1 Adams T: An investigation of selected plyometric training exercises on muscular leg strength and power, *Track and Field Quarterly Review* 84(1):36–40, 1984.

2 Asmussen E, Bonde-Peterson F: Storage of elastic energy in skeletal muscles in man, *Acta Physiol Scan* 91:385, 1974.
3 Bielik E, Chu D, Costello F, et al.: Roundtable: 1. practical considerations for utilizing plyometrics, *NSCA J* 8:14, 1986.
4 Bosco C, Komi PV: Potentiation of the mechanical behavior of the human skeletal muscle through prestretching, *Acta Physio Scan* 106:467, 1979.
5 Bosco C, Komi PV: Muscle elasticity in athletes. In: Komi, editor: *Exercise and sports biology,* Champaign, Ill, 1982, Human Kinetics.
6 Bosco C, Tarkka J, Komi PV: Effect of elastic energy and myoelectric potentiation of triceps surea during stretch-shortening cycle exercise, *Int J Sports Med* 2:137, 1982.
7 Bosco C, Tihanyia J, Komi PV, et al.: Store and recoil of elastic energy in slow and fast types of human skeletal muscles, *Acta Physio Scan* 116:343, 1987.
8 Cavagna GA, Dusman B, Margaria R: Positive work done by a previously stretched muscle, *J Appl Physiol* 24:21, 1968.
9 Cavagna G, Saibene F, Margaria R: Effect of negative work on the amount of positive work performed by an isolated muscle, *J Appl Physiol* 20:157, 1965.
10 Chu D: Plyometric exercise, *NSCA J* 6:56, 1984.
11 Chu D: *Conditioning/plyometrics.* Paper presented at 10th Annual Sports Medicine Team Concept Conference, San Francisco, Calif, December, 1989.
12 Chu D: *Jumping into plyometrics,* Champaign, Ill, 1992, Leisure Press.
13 Chu D, Plummer L: The language of plyometrics, *NSCA J* 6:30, 1984.
14 Curwin S, Stannish WD: *Tendinitis: its etiology and treatment,* Lexington, Mass, 1984, Collamore Press.
15 Dunsenev CI: Strength training for jumpers, *Soviet Sports Review* 14:2, 1979.
16 Dunsenev CI: Strength training of jumpers, *Track and Field Quarterly* 82:4, 1982.
17 Enoka RM: *Neuromechanical basis of kinesiology,* Champaign, Ill, 1988, Human Kinetics.
18 Javorek I: Plyometrics, *NSCA J* 11:52, 1989.
19 Jensen C: Pertinent facts about warming, *Athletic J* 56:72, 1975.
20 Katchajov S, Gomberaze K, Revson A: Rebound jumps, *Modern Athlete Coach* 14(4):23, 1976.
21 Komi PV: Physiological and biomechanical correlates of muscle function: effects of muscle structure and stretch-shortening cycle on force and speed. In: Terjung, editor: Exercise and sports sciences review, Lexington, 1984, Collamore Press.
22 Komi PV, Bosco C: Utilization of stored elastic energy in leg extensor muscles by men and women, *Med Sci Sports Exerc* 10(4):261, 1978.
23 Komi PV, Buskirk E: Effects of eccentric and concentric muscle conditioning on tension and electrical activity of human muscle, *Ergonomics* 15:417, 1972.
24 Lundon P: A review of plyometric training, *NSCA J* 7:69, 1985.
25 Rach PJ, Grabiner MD, Gregor RJ, et al.: Kinesiology and applied anatomy, ed 7, Philadelphia, 1989, Lea & Febiger.
26 Rowinski M: The role of eccentric exercise, Biodex Corp, 1988, Pro Clinica.
27 Thomas DW: Plyometrics—more than the stretch reflex, *NSCA J* 10:49, 1988.
28 Verhoshanski Y: Are depth jumps useful? *Yesis Review of Soviet Physical Education and Sport* 4:74-79, 1969.

29   Verkhoshanski Y: Perspectives in the improvement of speed-strength preparation of jumpers, *Yesis Review of Soviet Physical Education and Sports* 4(2):28–29, 1969.

30   Verhoshanski Y, Chornonson G: Jump exercises in sprint training. *Track and Field Quarterly* 9:1909, 1967.

31   Voight M, Draovitch P: Plyometrics. In Albert, editor: *Eccentric muscle training in sports and orthopedics,* New York, 1991, Churchill Livingstone.

32   Von Arx F: Power development in the high jump, *Track Technique* 88:2818–2819, 1984.

33   Wilt F: Plyometrics—what it is and how it works, *Athletic J* 55b:76, 1975.

34   Woo SL, Inoue M, McGurk-Burleson E, et al: Treatment of the medial collateral ligament injury: structure and function of canine knees in response to differing treatment regimens, *Am J Sports Med* 15(1):22–29, 1987.

Closed-Kinetic Chain Exercise

7

William E. Prentice

OBJECTIVES

After completion of this chapter, the student should be able to do the following:

- Differentiate between the concepts of the open kinetic chain and a closed kinetic chain.

- Describe the biomechanics of closed-kinetic chain exercise in the lower extremity.

- Identify the functional advantages of closed-kinetic chain exercises.

- Recognize that closed-kinetic chain exercises are particularly useful in rehabilitation of injuries involving the anterior cruciate ligament.

- Describe the various types of closed-kinetic chain exercises for the lower extremity.

- Explain how closed-kinetic chain exercises are used in rehabilitation of the upper extremity.

In recent years the concept of **closed-kinetic chain exercise** has received considerable attention as a useful and effective technique of rehabilitation, particularly for injuries involving the lower extremity. The ankle, knee, and hip joints comprise the kinetic chain for the lower extremity. When the distal segment of the lower extremity is stabilized or fixed, as is the case when the foot is weightbearing on the ground, the kinetic chain is said to be closed. Conversely, in an **open kinetic chain,** the distal segment is mobile and is not fixed. Traditionally, rehabilitation strengthening protocols have used open-kinetic chain exercises such as knee flexion and extension on a knee machine.

Closed-kinetic chain exercises have two distinct advantages over open-kinetic chain exercises. From a biomechanical perspective, they are safer and produce stresses and forces that are potentially less of a threat to healing structures. They are also more functional than open-kinetic chain exercises since they involve weight-bearing activities.

While closed-kinetic chain exercises are more often used in lower extremity rehabilitation, they may also be useful in rehabilitation protocols for certain upper extremity activities as well.

CONCEPT OF THE KINETIC CHAIN

The concept of the kinetic chain was first proposed in the 1970s and was initially referred to as the *link system* by mechanical engineers.[32] In this link system, pin joints connect a series of overlapping, rigid segments. If both ends of this system are connected to an immovable frame, translation of the proximal or distal ends is impossible. In this closed link system, movement at one joint produces predictable movement at all other joints.[12] This type of closed link system does not exist in either the upper or lower extremities. However, when the distal segment in the extremity (that is, the foot or hand) meets resistance, muscle recruitment patterns and joint movements are different than when the distal segment moves freely.[32]

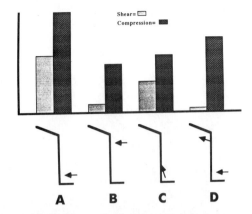

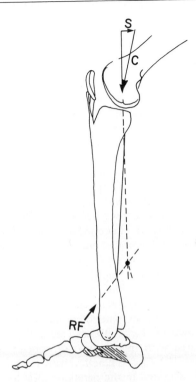

Fig. 7-1. Shear and compressive force vectors.
Mathematical model showing shear and compressive force vectors. S = shear, C = compressive.

Thus two systems, an open and a closed system, were proposed. Whenever the foot or the hand meets resistance, a closed kinetic chain exists. A true closed kinetic chain can only exist during isometric exercise, since neither the proximal nor distal segments can move in a closed system.

BIOMECHANICS OF CLOSED-KINETIC CHAIN EXERCISES IN THE LOWER EXTREMITY

Open- and closed-kinetic chain exercises have different biomechanical effects on the lower extremity and in particular on the knee joint. It is essential for the sports therapist to understand forces that occur around the knee joint. Palmitier et al. have proposed a biomechanical model of the lower extremity that quantifies two critical forces at the knee joint[25] (Figure 7-1). A **shear force** occurs in a posterior direction that would cause the tibia to translate anteriorly if not checked by soft tissue constraints (primarily the anterior cruciate ligament).[5] The second force is a **compressive force** directed along a longitudinal axis

Fig. 7-2. Resistive forces. Resistive forces applied in different positions alter the magnitude of the shear and compressive forces. **A,** Resistive force applied distally. **B,** Resistive force applied proximally. **C,** Resistive force applied axially. **D,** Resistive force applied distally with hamstring co-contraction.

of the tibia. Weight-bearing exercises increase joint compression, which enhances joint stability.

In an open-kinetic chain seated knee joint exercise, as a resistive force is applied to the distal tibia, the shear and compressive forces would be maximized (Figure 7-2, *A*). When a resistive force is applied more proximally, shear force is significantly reduced, as is the compressive force (Figure 7-2, *B*). If the resistive force is applied in a more axial direction, the shear force is also smaller (Figure 7-2, *C*). If a hamstring co-contraction occurs, the shear force is minimized (Figure 7-2, *D*).

Closed-kinetic chain exercises induce hamstring contraction by creating a flexion moment at both the hip and knee with the contracting hamstrings stabilizing the hip and the quadriceps stabilizing the knee. A **moment** is the product of force and distance from the axis of rotation. Also referred to as *torque,* it describes the turning effect produced when a force is exerted on the body that is pivoted about some fixed point (Figure 7-3). Co-contraction of the hamstring muscles helps to counteract the tendency of the quadriceps to cause anterior tibial translation. Co-contraction of the hamstrings is most efficient in reducing shear force when the resistive force is directed in an axial orientation relative to the tibia, as is the case in a weight-bearing exercise.[25] Several studies have shown that co-contraction is useful in stabilizing the knee joint and decreasing shear forces.[18,27,31]

The tension in the hamstrings can be further enhanced with slight anterior flexion of the trunk. Trunk

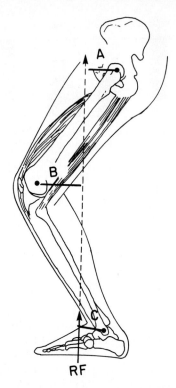

Fig. 7-3. Closed-kinetic chain exercises. Closed-kinetic chain exercises induce hamstring contraction by creating a flexion moment at both **A,** hip; **B,** knee; and **C,** ankle.

flexion moves the center of gravity anteriorly, decreasing the knee flexion moment and thus reducing knee shear force and decreasing patellofemoral compression forces.[24] Closed-kinetic chain exercises try to minimize the flexion moment at the knee while increasing the flexion moment at the hip.

A flexion moment is also created at the ankle when the resistive force is applied to the bottom of the foot. The soleus stabilizes ankle flexion and creates a knee extension moment, which again helps to neutralize anterior shear force (see Figure 7-3). Thus the entire lower extremity kinetic chain is recruited by applying an axial force at the distal segment.

In an open-kinetic chain exercise involving seated leg extensions, the resistive force is applied to the distal tibia, creating a flexion moment at the knee only. This negates the effects of a hamstring co-contraction and thus produces maximal shear force at the knee joint.

Shear forces created by isometric open-kinetic chain knee flexion and extension at 30 and 60 degrees of knee flexion are greater than with closed-kinetic chain exercises.[19] Decreased anterior tibial displacement during isometric closed-kinetic chain knee flexion at 30 degrees when measured by knee arthrometry has also been demonstrated.[34]

The effects of open- vs. closed-kinetic chain exercises on the patellofemoral joint must also be considered. In open-kinetic chain knee extension exercise, the flexion moment increases as the knee extends from 90 degrees of flexion to full extension, increasing tension in the quadriceps and patellar tendon. Thus the patellofemoral joint reaction forces are increased with peak force occurring at 36 degrees of joint flexion.[10] As the knee moves toward full extension, the patellofemoral contact area decreases, causing increased contact stress per unit area.[2,15]

In closed-kinetic chain exercise, the flexion moment increases as the knee flexes, once again causing increased quadriceps and patellar tendon tension and thus an increase in patellofemoral joint reaction forces. However, the patella has a much larger surface contact area with the femur, and contact stress is minimized.[2,10,15] Closed-kinetic chain exercises may be better tolerated in the patellofemoral joint since contact stress is minimized.

FUNCTIONAL ASPECTS OF CLOSED-KINETIC CHAIN EXERCISE

There is a second major advantage of using closed-kinetic chain strengthening exercises for the lower extremity in rehabilitation. The majority of activities performed in daily living, such as walking, climbing, and rising to a standing position, as well as in most sports activities, involve a closed-kinetic chain system. Since the foot is usually in contact with the ground, activities that make use of this closed system are more functional. With the exception of a kicking movement, there is no question that closed-kinetic chain exercises are more sport- or activity-specific, involving exercise that more closely approximates the desired activity. In a sports medicine setting, specificity of training must be emphasized to maximize carryover to functional activities on the playing field.[25]

With closed-kinetic chain exercises, the axis of motion is not isolated to a single joint, and movement occurs both proximal and distal to the joint. Closed-kinetic chain exercises also allow variable velocity of movement and depend on the functional speed of the exercise. They rely on posture for stabilization, which is more functional than some external strap or brace, as is the case with many exercise machines. Proprioceptive training occurs with the body having a more functional situation to which to react. Closed-kinetic chain exercises are not limited by equipment design, thus they can be altered or adapted to more sport-specific activities.[6,35]

Closed-kinetic chain exercises use varying combinations of isometric, concentric, and eccentric contractions that must occur simultaneously in different muscle groups within the chain. Isolation-type exercises typically use one specific type of muscular contraction to produce or control movement. Consequently there must be some neural adaptation to this type of strengthening exercise that will allow for synchronicity of more complex agonist and antagonist muscle actions.[16]

USE OF CLOSED-KINETIC CHAIN EXERCISE IN REHABILITATION OF LOWER EXTREMITY INJURIES

For many years, sports therapists have made use of open-kinetic chain exercises for lower extremity strengthening. This practice has been due in part to design constraints of existing resistive exercise machines. However, the current popularity of closed-kinetic chain exercises may be attributed primarily to a better understanding of the kinesiology and biomechanics involved in rehabilitation of lower extremity injuries.

The course of rehabilitation after injury to the anterior cruciate ligament (ACL) has changed drastically in recent years. (Specific rehabilitation protocols will be discussed in detail in Chapter 23.) Technological advances have created significant improvement in surgical techniques, which has allowed sports therapists to change their philosophy of rehabilitation. The current literature provides a great deal of support for accelerated rehabilitation programs that recommend the extensive use of closed-kinetic chain exercises.*

Because of the biomechanical and functional advantages of closed-kinetic chain exercises described earlier, these activities are perhaps best suited to rehabilitation of the ACL. The majority of these studies also indicate that closed-kinetic chain exercises may be safely incorporated into the rehabilitation proto-

*References 3, 6, 8, 9, 10, 20, 21, 30, 33, 36.

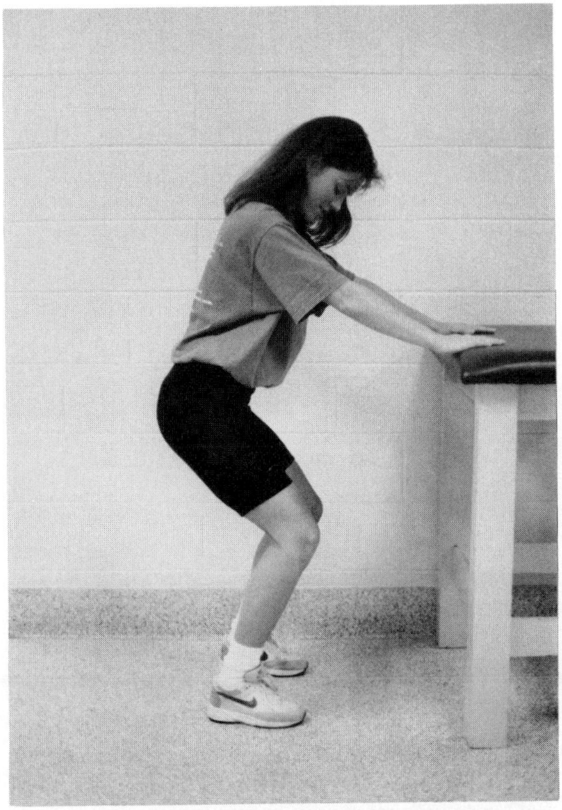

Fig. 7-4. Mini-squat performed in 0 to 40 degree range.

cols very early. Some sports therapists recommend beginning within the first few days after surgery.

SPECIFIC CLOSED-KINETIC CHAIN EXERCISES FOR THE LOWER EXTREMITY

In the sports medicine setting, several different closed-kinetic chain exercises have gained popularity and have been incorporated into rehabilitation protocols. Among those exercises commonly used are the mini-squat, leg press, stair climbing machines, lateral step-up, terminal knee extension using tubing, and stationary bicycling.

Mini-Squat

The mini-squat involves simultaneous hip and knee extension and is performed in a 0 to 40 degree range[36] (Figure 7-4). As the hip extends, the rectus femoris contracts eccentrically while the hamstrings contract

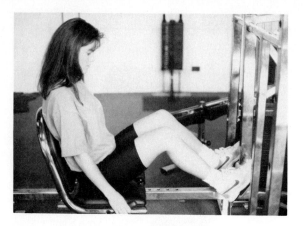

Fig. 7-5. Standard leg press exercise.

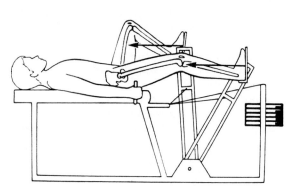

Fig. 7-6. Modified and recommended leg press positioning.

concentrically. Concurrently, as the knee extends, the hamstrings contract eccentrically while the rectus femoris contracts concentrically. Both concentric and eccentric contractions occur simultaneously at either end of both muscles, producing what has been called a **concurrent shift** contraction. This type of contraction is necessary during weight-bearing activities. It will be elicited with all closed-kinetic chain exercise and is impossible with isolation exercises.[32]

These concurrent shift contractions minimize the flexion moment at the knee. The eccentric contraction of the hamstrings helps to neutralize the effects of a concentric quadriceps contraction in producing anterior translation of the tibia. Henning et al. found that the half-squat produced significantly less anterior shear at the knee than did an open-chain exercise in full extension.[14] A full-squat markedly increases the flexion moment at the knee and thus increases anterior shear of the tibia. As mentioned previously, slightly flexing the trunk anteriorly will also increase the hip flexion moment and decrease the knee moment.

Leg Press

Theoretically the leg press takes full advantage of the kinetic chain and at the same time provides stability, which decreases strain on the low back. It also allows exercise with resistance lower than body weight and the capability of exercising each leg independently[25] (Figure 7-5). It has been recommended that leg press exercises be performed in a 0 to 60 degree range of knee flexion.[36]

It has also been recommended that traditional leg press machines be modified to allow full hip extension to take maximum advantage of the kinetic chain (Figure 7-6). Most leg press machines are designed to allow 45 degrees of hip flexion with the athlete in a sitting position. Full hip extension can only be achieved in a supine position. In this position full hip and knee flexion and extension can occur, thus reproducing the concurrent shift and ensuring appropriate hamstring recruitment.[25]

The foot plates should also be designed to move in an arc of motion rather than in a straight line. This movement would facilitate hamstring recruitment by increasing the hip flexion moment and decreasing the knee moment. Foot plates should be fixed perpendicular to the frontal plane of the hip to maximize the knee extension moment created by the soleus.

Stair Climbing

Stair climbing machines have gained a great deal of popularity not only as a closed-kinetic chain exercise device useful in rehabilitation but also as a means of improving cardiorespiratory endurance (Figure 7-7). Stair climbing machines have two basic designs: one involves a series of rotating steps similar to a department store escalator; the other uses two foot plates that move up and down to simulate a stepping type movement. With the latter type of stair climber, also sometimes referred to as a *stepping machine*, the foot never leaves the foot plate, making it a true closed-kinetic chain exercise device.

Stair climbing involves many of the same biomechanical principles identified with the leg press exercise. When exercising on the stair climber, the body

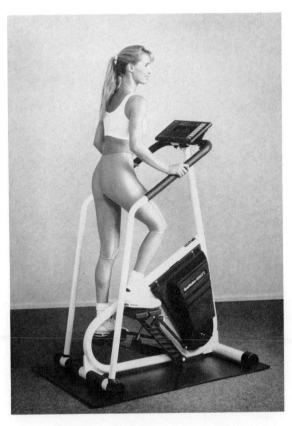

Fig. 7-7. Stairmaster stepping machine.

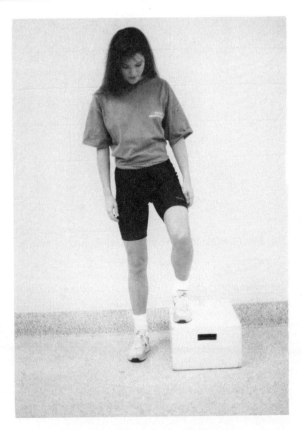

Fig. 7-8. Lateral step-up exercise.

should be held erect with only slight trunk flexion, thus maximizing hamstring recruitment through concurrent shift contractions while increasing the hip flexion moment and decreasing the knee flexion moment.

Exercise on a stepping machine produces increased electromyogram (EMG) activity in the gastrocnemius. Since the gastrocnemius attaches to the posterior aspect of the femoral condyles, increased activity of this muscle could produce a flexion moment of the femur on the tibia. This motion would cause posterior translation of the femur on the tibia, increasing strain on the ACL. Peak firing of the quadriceps may offset the effects of increased EMG activity in the gastrocnemius.[7]

Lateral Step-Ups

Lateral step-ups are another widely used closed-kinetic chain exercise (Figure 7-8). Lateral step-ups seem to be used more often clinically than do forward

step-ups. Step height can be adjusted to patient capabilities and generally progress up to about 8 inches. Heights greater than 8 inches create a large flexion moment at the knee, increasing anterior shear force and making hamstring co-contraction more difficult.[4,7]

Lateral step-ups elicit significantly greater mean quadriceps EMG activity than does a stepping machine. When performing a step-up, the entire body weight must be raised and lowered, while on the stepping machine the center of gravity is maintained at a relatively constant height. The lateral step-up may produce increased muscle and joint shear forces compared to stepping exercise.[7] Caution should be exercised by the sports therapist in using the lateral step-up in cases where minimizing anterior shear forces is essential. Contraction of the hamstrings appears to be of insufficient magnitude to neutralize the shear force produced by the quadriceps.[4] In situations where strengthening of the quadriceps is the goal, the lateral step-up has been recommended as a beneficial exercise. However, lateral stepping exercises

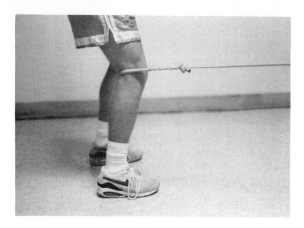

Fig. 7-9. Terminal knee extensions using rubber tubing.

have failed to increase isokinetic strength of the quadriceps muscle.[28]

Terminal Knee Extensions Using Surgical Tubing

It has been reported in numerous studies that the greatest amount of anterior tibial translation occurs between 0 and 30 degrees of flexion during open-kinetic chain exercise.* Avoiding terminal knee extension after surgery became a well accepted rule among sports therapists. Unfortunately, this practice led to quadriceps weakness, flexion contracture, and patellofemoral pain.[23,29]

Closed-kinetic chain terminal knee extensions using surgical tubing resistance have created a means of safely strengthening terminal knee extension (Figure 7-9). Application of resistance anteriorly at the femur produces anterior shear of the femur, which eliminates any anterior translation of the tibia. This type of exercise performed in the 0 to 30 degree range also minimizes the knee flexion moment, further reducing anterior shear of the tibia. The use of rubber tubing produces an eccentric contraction of the quadriceps when moving into knee flexion.

Stationary Bicycling

The stationary bicycle has been routinely used in sports medicine, primarily for conditioning purposes when the injured athlete cannot engage in running

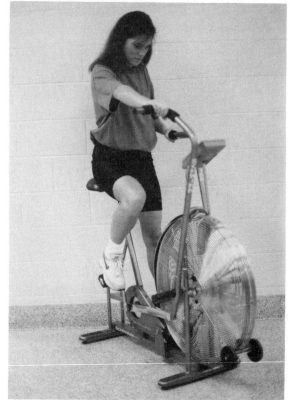

Fig. 7-10. Stationary bicycle.

activities (Figure 7-10). However, it also can be of significant value as a closed-kinetic chain exercise device.

The advantage of stationary bicycling over other closed-kinetic chain exercises for rehabilitation is that the amount of the weight-bearing force exerted by the injured lower extremity can be adapted within patient limitations. The seat height should be carefully adjusted to minimize the knee flexion moment on the downstroke. However, if the stationary bike is being used to regain range of motion in flexion, the seat height should be adjusted to a lowered position using passive motion of the injured extremity. Toe clips will facilitate hamstring contractions on the upstroke.

Isokinetic Closed-Kinetic Chain Exercise

Recently, Biodex has begun marketing an attachment for existing equipment that will allow for isokinetic conditioning and testing of the lower extremity in a

*References 1, 11, 13, 17, 22, 26, 27, 36.

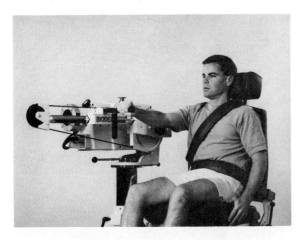

Fig. 7-11. Closed-kinetic chain isokinetic testing. Closed-kinetic chain isokinetic testing attachment from Biodex.

closed-kinetic chain seated position (Figure 7-11). Data on reliability, validity, and effectiveness of the particular piece of equipment are not yet available.

CLOSED-KINETIC CHAIN EXERCISES IN REHABILITATION OF UPPER EXTREMITY INJURIES

While it is true that closed-kinetic chain exercises are most often used in rehabilitation of lower extremity injuries, there are instances where closed-kinetic chain exercises should be incorporated into upper-extremity rehabilitation protocols. Unlike the lower extremity, the upper extremity is most functional as an open-kinetic chain system. Most sports activities involve movement of the upper extremity in which the hand moves freely. These activities are generally dynamic movements, often occurring at high velocities such as throwing a baseball, serving a tennis ball, or spiking a volleyball. In these movements, the proximal segments of the kinetic chain are used for stabilization while the distal segments have a high degree of mobility.

Push-ups, chinning exercises, and performing a handstand in gymnastics are all examples of closed-kinetic chain activities in the upper extremity. In these cases, the hand is stabilized, and muscular contractions around the more proximal segments, the elbow and shoulder, function to raise and lower the body.

For the most part in rehabilitation, closed-kinetic chain exercises are used primarily for strengthening and establishing neuromuscular control of those muscles that act to stabilize the shoulder girdle. In particular the scapular stabilizers and the rotator cuff muscles function at one time or another to control movements about the shoulder. It is essential to develop strength and control in these muscle groups, thus allowing them to provide a stable base for more mobile and dynamic movements that occur in the distal segments. Push-ups done in either the prone or seated positions and weight-shifting exercises are perhaps the two most typically used upper extremity closed-kinetic chain exercises used by sports therapists (Figure 7-12, A and B). To date, little information is available in the literature that discusses the efficacy and use of upper extremity closed-kinetic chain exercise.

A
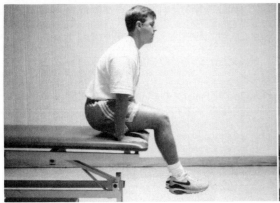
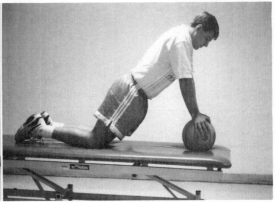
B

Fig. 7-12. Closed-kinetic chain exercises for upper extremity. A, Seated push-ups. **B,** Weight-shifting exercises.

SUMMARY

1. A closed-kinetic chain exercise is one in which the distal segment of the extremity is fixed or stabilized. In an open-kinetic chain, the distal segment is mobile and is not fixed.
2. Closed-kinetic chain exercises in the lower extremity decrease the shear forces, reducing anterior tibial translation, and increase the compressive forces, which increases stability around the knee joint.
3. Biomechanically, closed-kinetic chain exercises function to decrease the knee flexion moment and increase the hip flexion moment.
4. Closed-kinetic chain exercises induce co-contraction of the hamstrings, which helps to decrease the shear forces at the knee joint.
5. The majority of functional activities involve a closed-kinetic chain system.
6. Closed-kinetic chain exercises have become the recommended strengthening technique of injuries involving in particular the ACL.
7. Mini-squats, leg press, stepping exercise, lateral step-up, terminal knee extension using rubber tubing, and stationary bicycling are all examples of closed-kinetic chain activities for the lower extremity.
8. Closed-kinetic chain activities, such as push-ups and weight-shifting, are strengthening exercises used primarily for improving shoulder stabilization in the upper extremity.

REFERENCES

1   Arms S, Pope M, Johnson R, et al.: The biomechanics of anterior cruciate ligament rehabilitation and reconstruction, *Am J Sports Med* 4:285-290, 1986.
2   Baratta R, Solomonow M, Zhou B: Muscular coactivation: the role of the antagonist musculature in maintaining knee stability, *Am J Sports Med* 16(2):113-122, 1988.
3   Blair D, Willis R: Rapid rehabilitation following anterior cruciate ligament reconstruction, *Ath Training* 26(1):32-43, 1991.
4   Brask B, Lueke R, Soderberg G: Electromyographic analysis of selected muscles during the lateral step-up, *Phys Ther* 64(3):324-329, 1984.
5   Butler D, Noyes F, Grood E: Ligamentous restraints to anterior-posterior drawer in the human knee: a biomechanical study, *J Bone Joint Surg* 62[A]:259-270, 1980.
6   Case J, DePalma B, Zelko R: Knee rehabilitation following anterior cruciate ligament repair/reconstruction: an update, *Ath Training* 26(1):22-31, 1991.
7   Cook T, Zimmerman C, Lux K, et al.: EMG comparison of lateral

step-up and stepping machine exercise, *J Ortho Sports Phys Ther* 16(3):108-113, 1992.
8   DeCarlo M, Shelbourne D, McCarroll J, et al.: A traditional vs. accelerated rehabilitation following ACL reconstruction: a one-year follow-up, *J Ortho Sports Phys Ther* 15(6):309-316, 1992.
9   DePalma B, Zelko R: Knee rehabilitation following anterior cruciate ligament injury or surgery, *Ath Training* 21(3):200-206, 1986.
10 Fu F, Woo S, Irrgang J: Current concepts for rehabilitation following anterior cruciate ligament reconstruction, *J Ortho Sports Phys Ther* 15(6):270-278, 1992.
11 Fukubayashi T, Torzilli P, Sherman M: An in-vitro biomechanical evaluation of anterior/posterior motion of the knee. Tibial displacement, rotation, and torque, *J Bone Joint Surg* 64[B]:258-264, 1982.
12 Gowitzke B, Milner S: *Scientific basis of human movement,* Baltimore, 1988, Williams & Wilkins.
13 Grood E, Suntag W, Noyes F, et al.: Biomechanics of knee extension exercise, *J Bone Joint Surg* 66[A]:725-733, 1984.
14 Henning S, Lench M, Glick K: An in-vivo strain gauge study of elongation of the anterior cruciate ligament, *Am J Sports Med* 13:22-26, 1985.
15 Hungerford D, Barry M: Biomechanics of the patellofemoral joint, *Clin Orthop* 144:9-15, 1979.
16 Jones N, McCartney N, McComas A: *Human muscle power,* Champaign, Ill, 1986, Human Kinetics.
17 Jurist K, Otis V: Anteroposterior tibiofemoral displacements during isometric extension efforts. The roles of external load and knee flexion angle, *Am J Sports Med* 13:254-258, 1985.
18 Kaland S, Sinkjaer T, Arendt-Neilsen L, et al.: Altered timing of hamstring muscle action in anterior cruciate ligament deficient patients, *Am J Sports Med* 18(3):245-248, 1990.
19 Lutz G, Stuart M, Franklin H: Rehabilitative techniques for athletes after reconstruction of the anterior cruciate ligament, *Mayo Clin Proc* 65:1322-1329, 1990.
20 Malone T, Garrett W: Commentary and historical perspective of anterior cruciate ligament rehabilitation, *J Ortho Sports Phys Ther* 15(6):265-269, 1992.
21 Mangine R, Noyes F: Rehabilitation of the allograft reconstruction, *J Ortho Sports Phys Ther* 15(6):294-302, 1992.
22 Nisell R, Ericson M, Nemeth G, et al.: Tibiofemoral joint forces during isokinetic knee extension, *Am J Sports Med* 17:49-54, 1989.
23 Noyes F, Mangine R, Barber S: Early knee motion after open and arthroscopic anterior cruciate ligament reconstruction, *Am J Sports Med* 15:149-160, 1987.
24 Ohkoshi Y, Yasuda K, Kaneda K, et al.: Biomechanical analysis of rehabilitation in the standing position, *Am J Sports Med* 19(6):605-611, 1991.
25 Palmitier R, Kai-Nan A, Scott S, et al.: Kinetic chain exercise in knee rehabilitation, *Sports Med* 11(6):402-413, 1991.
26 Paulos L, Noyes F, Grood E: Knee rehabilitation after anterior cruciate ligament reconstruction and repair, *Am J Sports Med* 9:140-149, 1981.
27 Renstrom P, Arms S, Stanwyck T, et al.: Strain within the anterior cruciate ligament during hamstring and quadriceps activity, *Am J Sports Med* 14:83-87, 1986.
28 Reynolds N, Worrell T, Perrin D: Effect of lateral step-up ex-

ercise protocol on quadriceps isokinetic peak torque values and thigh girth, *J Ortho Sports Phys Ther* 15(3):151-1556, 1992.

29   Sachs R, Daniel D, Stone M, et al.: Patellofemoral problems after anterior cruciate ligament reconstruction, *Am J Sports Med* 17:760-765, 1989.

30   Shellbourne D, Nitz P: Accelerated rehabilitation after anterior cruciate ligament reconstruction, *Am J Sports Med* 18:292-299, 1990.

31   Solomonow M, Barata R, Zhou B, et al.: The synergistic action of the anterior cruciate ligament and thigh muscles in maintaining joint stability, *Am J Sports Med* 15:207-213, 1987.

32   Steindler A: *Kinesiology of the human body under normal and pathological conditions,* Springfield, Ill, 1977, Charles C. Thomas.

33   Tovin B, Tovin T, Tovin M: Surgical and biomechanical considerations in rehabilitation of patients with intra-articular ACL reconstructions, *J Ortho Sports Phys Ther* 15(6):317-322, 1992.

34   Voight M, Bell S, Rhodes D: Instrumented testing of tibial translation during a positive Lachman's test and selected closed chain activities in anterior cruciate deficient knees, *J Ortho Sports Phys Ther* 15:49, 1992.

35   Voight M, Tippett S: *Closed-kinetic chain.* Presented at 41st Annual Clinical Symposium of the National Athletic Trainers Association, Indianapolis, Ind, June 12, 1990.

36   Wilk K, Andrews J: Current concepts in the treatment of anterior cruciate ligament disruption, *J Ortho Sports Phys Ther* 15(6):279-293, 1992.

Maintenance of Cardiorespiratory Endurance

8

William E. Prentice

OBJECTIVES

After completion of this chapter, the student should be able to do the following:

- Explain the relationships between heart rate, stroke volume, cardiac output, and rate of oxygen use.

- Describe the function of the heart, blood vessels, and lungs in oxygen transport.

- Describe the oxygen transport system and the concept of maximal rate of oxygen use.

- Describe the principles of continuous, interval, fartlek, and par cours training and the potential of each technique for improving cardiorespiratory endurance.

- Describe the differences between aerobic and anaerobic activity.

- Identify methods for assessment of cardiorespiratory endurance.

- Demonstrate a method to assess one's level of cardiorespiratory endurance.

Although strength and flexibility are commonly regarded as essential components in any injury rehabilitation program, relatively little consideration is given toward maintaining levels of cardiorespiratory endurance. An athlete spends a considerable amount of time preparing the cardiorespiratory system to be able to handle the increased demands made upon it during a competitive season. When injury occurs and the athlete is forced to miss training time, levels of cardiorespiratory endurance may decrease rapidly. Thus the sports therapist must design or substitute alternative activities that allow the individual to maintain existing levels of fitness during the rehabilitation period.

By definition, cardiorespiratory endurance is the ability to perform whole body activities for extended periods of time.[10] The cardiorespiratory system provides a means by which oxygen is supplied to the various tissues of the body. Without oxygen the cells within the human body cannot possibly function, and

ultimately death will occur. Thus the cardiorespiratory system is the basic life-support system of the body.[10]

TRANSPORT AND USE OF OXYGEN

Basically, transport of oxygen throughout the body involves the coordinated function of four components: (1) the heart, (2) the blood vessels, (3) the blood, and (4) the lungs. The improvement of cardiorespiratory endurance through training occurs because of increased capability of each of these elements in providing necessary oxygen to the working tissues. It is well beyond the scope of this text to discuss the detailed anatomy and physiology involved in the cardiorespiratory system. However, a basic discussion of the training effects and responses to exercise that occur to the heart, blood vessels, blood, and lungs should make it easier to understand why the training techniques to be discussed should be

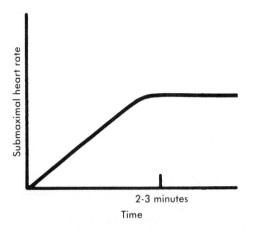

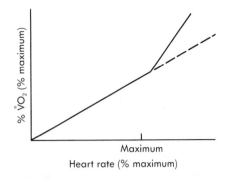

Fig. 8-2. Maximum heart rate. Maximum heart rate is achieved at about the same time as $\dot{V}O_2$max.

Fig. 8-1. Plateau heart rate. For the heart rate to plateau at a given level, 2 to 3 minutes are required.

incorporated into a rehabilitation program to maintain existing levels of cardiorespiratory endurance.

TRAINING EFFECTS ON THE CARDIOVASCULAR SYSTEM
Effects on the Heart

The heart is the main pumping mechanism that circulates oxygenated blood throughout the body to the working tissues. The heart receives deoxygenated blood from the venous system and then pumps the blood through the pulmonary vessels to the lungs, where carbon dioxide is exchanged for oxygen. The oxygenated blood then returns to the heart, from which it exits through the aorta to the arterial system and is circulated throughout the body, supplying oxygen to the tissues.

As the body begins to exercise, the muscles use the oxygen at a much higher rate, and the heart must pump more oxygenated blood to meet this increased demand. The heart can adapt to this increased demand through several mechanisms. *Heart rate* shows a gradual adaptation to an increased workload by increasing proportionally to the intensity of the exercise and will plateau at a given level after about 2 to 3 minutes (Figure 8-1).

Monitoring heart rate is an indirect method of estimating oxygen consumption.[15] In general, heart rate and oxygen consumption have a linear relationship, although at very low intensities and at high intensities this linear relationship breaks down (Figure 8-2). During higher intensity activities maximal heart rate

may be achieved before maximum oxygen consumption, which will continue to rise.[24] The greater the intensity of the exercise, the higher the heart rate. Because of these existing relationships it should become apparent that the rate of oxygen consumption can be estimated by taking the heart rate.[11]

A second mechanism by which the heart is able to adapt to increased demand during exercise is to increase the **stroke volume,** the volume of blood being pumped out with each beat. The heart pumps out approximately 70 milliliters of blood per beat. Stroke volume continues to increase only to the point at which there is simply not enough time between beats for the heart to fill up. This point occurs at about 40% of maximal heart rate, and above this level increases in the volume of blood being pumped out per unit of time must be caused entirely by increases in heart rate (Figure 8-3).

Stroke volume and heart rate together determine the volume of blood being pumped through the heart in a given unit of time. Approximately 5 liters of blood are pumped through the heart during each minute at rest, referred to as the *cardiac output,* which indicates how much blood the heart is capable of pumping in exactly 1 minute. Thus cardiac output is the primary determinant of the maximal rate of oxygen consumption possible (Figure 8-4). During exercise, cardiac output increases to approximately four times that experienced during rest in the normal individual and may increase as much as six times in the elite endurance athlete.

Cardiac Output = Stroke Volume × Heart Rate

A *training effect* that occurs with regard to cardiac output of the heart is that the stroke volume increases

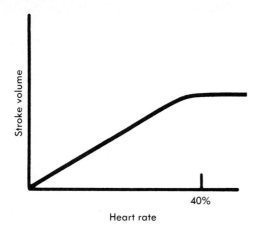

Fig. 8-3. Stroke volume plateaus. Stroke volume plateaus at about 40% of maximal heart rate.

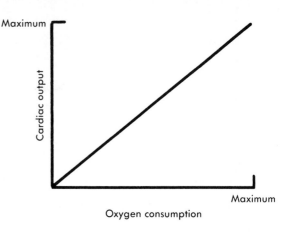

Fig. 8-4. Cardiac output limits $\dot{V}O_2$max.

while exercise heart rate is reduced by a given standard exercise load. The heart becomes more efficient because it is capable of pumping more blood with each stroke. Because the heart is a muscle, it will hypertrophy, or increase in size and strength to some extent, but this is in no way a negative effect of training.

Training Effect

Cardiac output = Increased stroke volume × Decreased heart rate

During exercise females tend to have a 5% to 10% higher cardiac output than males do at all intensities. This difference is likely due to a lower concentration of hemoglobin in the female, which is compensated for during exercise by an increased cardiac output.[5]

Blood Flow

The amount of blood flowing to the various organs increases during exercise. However, there is a change in overall distribution of cardiac output; the percentage of total cardiac output to the nonessential organs is decreased, whereas it is increased to active skeletal muscle. Volume of blood flow to the heart muscle or *myocardium* increases substantially because of exercise, even though the percentage of total cardiac output supplying the heart muscle remains unchanged. In skeletal muscle there is increased for-

mation of blood vessels or capillaries, although it is not clear whether new ones form or dormant ones simply open up and fill with blood. Blood pressure in the arterial system is determined by the cardiac output in relation to total peripheral resistance to blood flow. Blood pressure is created by contraction of the heart muscle. Contraction of the ventricles of the heart creates systolic pressure, and contraction of the atria creates diastolic pressure. During exercise, there is a decrease in total peripheral resistance and an increase in cardiac output. Systolic pressure increases in proportion to oxygen consumption and cardiac output, while diastolic pressure shows little or no increase.[24] Blood pressure falls below preexercise levels after exercise and may stay low for several hours. There is general agreement that engaging in consistent aerobic exercise will produce modest reductions in systolic and diastolic blood pressure at rest and during submaximal exercise.[24]

Blood

Blood transports oxygen throughout the system by binding it with *hemoglobin.* Found in red blood cells, hemoglobin is an iron-containing protein that can easily accept or give up molecules of oxygen as needed. Training for improvement of cardiorespiratory endurance produces an increase in total blood volume, with a corresponding increase in the amount of hemoglobin. The concentration of hemoglobin in circulating blood does not change with training. It may actually decrease slightly.

Lungs

As a result of training, pulmonary function is improved in the trained individual relative to the untrained individual. The volume of air that is inspired in a single maximal ventilation is increased. The diffusing capacity of the lungs is also increased, facilitating the exchange of oxygen and carbon dioxide. Pulmonary resistance to air flow is also decreased.[21]

The following list summarizes the effects of training on the cardiorespiratory system:

- Decreased resting heart rate
- Decreased heart rate at specific workloads
- Increased stroke volume
- Unchanged cardiac output
- Decrease in recovery time
- Increased capillarization
- Increased functional capacity in the lungs
- Decreased muscle glycogen use

MAXIMAL OXYGEN CONSUMPTION

The greatest rate at which oxygen can be taken in and used during exercise is referred to as **maximal oxygen consumption** ($\dot{V}O_2$max).[3] The performance of any activity requires a certain rate of oxygen consumption that is about the same for all persons, depending on the present level of fitness. Generally, the greater the rate or more intense the performance of an activity, the greater will be the oxygen consumption. Each person has his or her own maximal rate of oxygen consumption. That person's ability to perform an activity (or to fatigue) is closely related to the amount of oxygen required by that activity and limited by the maximal rate of oxygen consumption of which the person is capable. The greater percentage of maximal oxygen consumption required during an activity, the less time the activity may be performed (Figure 8-5).

Three factors determine the maximal rate at which oxygen can be used: (1) external respiration, involving the ventilatory process, or pulmonary function, (2) gas transport, which is accomplished by the cardiovascular system (that is, the heart, blood vessels, and blood), and (3) internal respiration, which involves the use of oxygen by the cells to produce energy. Of these three factors the most limiting is generally the ability to transport oxygen through the system, thus the cardiovascular system limits the overall rate of oxygen consumption. A high $\dot{V}O_2$max

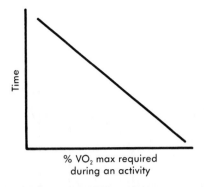

Fig. 8-5. $\dot{V}O_2$max required during activity. The greater the percentage of $\dot{V}O_2$max required during an activity, the less the time that activity can be performed.

within a persons's inherited range indicates that all three systems are working well.

The maximal rate at which oxygen can be used is a genetically determined characteristic; we inherit a certain range of $\dot{V}O_2$max, and the more active we are, the higher the existing $\dot{V}O_2$max will be in that range.[31] A training program can increase $\dot{V}O_2$max to its highest limit within our range.[31] $\dot{V}O_2$max is most often presented in terms of the volume of oxygen relative to body weight per unit of time (ml/kg/min). A normal $\dot{V}O_2$max for most collegiate level athletes would fall somewhere in the range of 50 to 60 ml/kg/min. A world-class male marathon runner may have a $\dot{V}O_2$max in the 70 to 75 ml/kg/min range.

The inherited range of maximal oxygen consumption is largely determined by the metabolic and functional properties of skeletal muscle fibers. Basically there are two distinct types of muscle fibers. Fast-twitch fibers (FT), or fast-contracting fibers, do not depend on oxygen for contraction and tend to fatigue very rapidly. Fast-twitch fibers are responsible for speed or power activities such as sprinting and weight lifting. Slow-twitch fibers (ST) are slow-contracting fibers that require oxygen for contraction and are more resistant to fatigue. Slow-twitch fibers are more useful in long-term, endurance activities such as marathon running or cross-country skiing. If an individual has a greater percentage of slow-twitch muscle fibers throughout the body, he or she will be more efficient in oxygen use and thus will have a higher $\dot{V}O_2$max.

Within a particular muscle are both types of fibers, and the ratio varies with each person. The average is about 50% slow-twitch and 50% fast-twitch fibers.

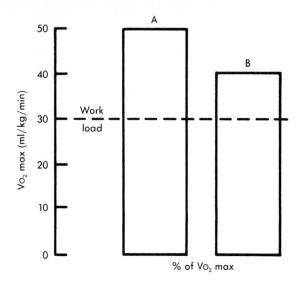

Fig. 8-6. Use of $\dot{V}O_2$max. Athlete *A* should be able to work longer than athlete *B* as a result of a lower percentage use of $\dot{V}O_2$max.

However, tremendous variations have been demonstrated in various athletes.

Because this ratio is genetically determined, it may play a large role in determining ability for a given sport activity. Sprinters, for example, have a large percentage of fast-twitch fibers in relation to slow-twitch fibers. One study has shown that they may have as many as 95% fast-twitch fibers in certain muscles. Conversely, marathon runners generally have a higher percentage of slow-twitch fibers.

Effects on Work Ability

Cardiorespiratory endurance plays a critical role in the ability to carry out normal daily activities.[1] Fatigue is closely related to the percentage of $\dot{V}O_2$max that a particular workload demands.[30] For example, Figure 8-6 presents two athletes, *A* and *B*. *A* has a $\dot{V}O_2$max of 50 ml/kg/min, whereas *B* has a $\dot{V}O_2$max of only 40 ml/kg/min. If *A* and *B* are exercising at the same intensity, then *A* will be working at a much lower percentage of $\dot{V}O_2$max than *B* is. Consequently, *A* should be able to sustain his or her activity over a much longer period of time. Everyday activities may be impaired if the ability to use oxygen efficiently is impaired. Thus improvement of cardiorespiratory endurance should be an essential component of any training program.[8]

Regardless of the training technique used for the improvement of cardiorespiratory endurance, one principal goal remains the same: **to increase the ability with which the cardiorespiratory system is able to supply a sufficient amount of oxygen to the working muscles.** Without oxygen, the body is incapable of producing energy for an extended time.

THE ENERGY SYSTEMS

Various sports activities involve specific demands for energy. For example, sprinting and jumping are high-energy output activities, requiring a relatively large production of energy for a short time. Long-distance running and swimming, on the other hand, are mostly low-energy output activities per unit of time, requiring energy production for a prolonged time. Other physical activities demand a blend of both high- and low-energy output. These various energy demands can be met by the different processes by which energy can be supplied to the skeletal muscles.

ATP: The Immediate Energy Source

Energy is produced from the breakdown of carbohydrates, fat, and protein. This energy is used to produce **adenosine triphosphate (ATP),** which is the ultimate usable form of energy for muscular activity. ATP is produced in the muscle tissue from blood glucose or glycogen. Glucose is derived from the breakdown of dietary carbohydrates. Glucose not needed immediately is stored as **glycogen** in the resting muscle and liver. Stored glycogen in the liver can later be converted back to glucose and transferred to the blood to meet the body's energy needs. Fats and proteins can also be metabolized to generate ATP.

Once much of the muscle and liver glycogen is depleted, the body relies more heavily on fats stored in adipose tissue to meet its energy needs. The longer the duration of an activity, the greater the amount of fat is used, especially during the later stages of endurance events. During rest and submaximal exertion, fat and carbohydrates are used as energy substrate in approximately a 60% to 40% ratio.[24]

Regardless of the nutrient source that produces ATP, it is always available in the cell as an immediate energy source. When all available sources of ATP are used, more must be regenerated for muscular contraction to continue.

AEROBIC VS. ANAEROBIC METABOLISM

Two major energy systems function in muscle tissue: anaerobic and aerobic metabolism. Each of these systems generates ATP. During sudden outbursts of activity in intensive, short-term exercise, ATP can be rapidly metabolized to meet energy needs. After a few seconds of intensive exercise, however, the small stores of ATP are used up. The body then turns to glycogen as an energy source. Glycogen can be metabolized within the muscle cells to generate ATP for muscle contractions. ATP and muscle glycogen can be metabolized without the need for oxygen. Thus this energy system involves **anaerobic metabolism** (occurring in the absence of oxygen).

As exercise continues, the body has to rely on the metabolism of carbohydrates (more specifically, glucose) and fats to generate ATP. The second energy system requires oxygen and is therefore referred to as *aerobic metabolism* (occurring in the presence of oxygen). In most activities aerobic and anaerobic systems function simultaneously. The degree to which the two major energy systems are involved is determined by the intensity and duration of the activity.[29] If the intensity of the activity is such that sufficient oxygen can be supplied to meet the demands of working tissues, the activity is considered to be **aerobic.** Conversely, if the activity is of high enough intensity and the duration is such that there is insufficient oxygen available to meet energy demands, the activity becomes **anaerobic.**[28] As the intensity of the exercise increases and insufficient amounts of oxygen are available to the tissues, lactic acid is formed. Consequently, an *oxygen debt* is incurred that must be paid back during the recovery period. Lactic acid is metabolized to eliminate this oxygen deficit. For example, short bursts of muscle contraction, such as in running or swimming sprints, use predominantly the anaerobic system. However, endurance events depend a great deal on the aerobic system. Most sports use a combination of anaerobic and aerobic metabolism.

TRAINING TECHNIQUES FOR MAINTAINING CARDIORESPIRATORY ENDURANCE

There are several different training techniques that may be incorporated into a rehabilitation program through which cardiorespiratory endurance can be maintained. Certainly, a primary consideration for the sports therapist would be whether the injury involves the upper or lower extremity. With injuries that involve the upper extremity, weight-bearing activities, such as walking, running, stair climbing, and modified aerobics, can be used. However, if the injury is to the lower extremity, alternative nonweight–bearing activities, such as swimming or stationary cycling, may be necessary. In a sport, such as soccer, that requires a considerable amount of running, training using appropriate nonweight–bearing activities will not keep the athlete "match fit." The only way to achieve match fitness is to engage in functional activities specific to that sport. The goal of the sports therapist in substituting alternative activities during rehabilitation is to try and maintain a cardiorespiratory endurance base so that the athlete may quickly regain match fitness once the injury has healed.

The principles of the training techniques discussed below can be applied with running, cycling, swimming, stair climbing, or any other activity designed to maintain levels of cardiorespiratory fitness.

Continuous Training

Continuous training involves four considerations:
- The *type* of activity
- The *frequency* of the activity
- The *intensity* of the activity
- The *duration* of the activity

TYPE. The type of activity used in continuous training must be aerobic. Aerobic activities elevate the heart rate and maintain it at that level for an extended time.[9] Aerobic activities generally involve repetitive, whole-body, large-muscle movements performed over an extended time.[22] Examples of weight-bearing aerobic activities are walking, running, jogging, rope skipping, stepping, aerobic dance exercise, roller blading, and cross-country skiing. Nonweight–bearing aerobic activities include cycling and swimming. The advantage of these aerobic activities as opposed to more intermittent activities, such as racquetball, squash, basketball, or tennis, is that aerobic activities are easy to regulate by either speeding up or slowing down the pace. Since the intensity of the work elicits a specific heart rate, these aerobic activities can maintain heart rate at a specified or target level. Intermittent activities involve variable speeds and intensities that cause the heart rate to fluctuate considerably. Although these intermittent activities will improve cardiorespiratory endurance, they are much more difficult to monitor in terms of intensity.

FREQUENCY. To see at least minimal improvement

in cardiorespiratory endurance, it is necessary for the average person to engage in no less than three sessions per week. A competitive athlete should be prepared to train as often as six times per week. Everyone should take off at least 1 day a week to give damaged tissues a chance to repair themselves.

INTENSITY. The intensity of exercise is also a critical factor, though recommendations regarding training intensities vary. This statement is particularly true in the early stages of training, when the body is forced to make a lot of adjustments to increased work-load demands. Because heart rate is linearly related to the intensity of the exercise and to the rate of oxygen consumption, it becomes a relatively simple process to identify a specific work load (pace) that will make the heart rate plateau at the desired level. By monitoring heart rate, we know whether the pace is too fast or too slow to get the heart rate into a target range.

Monitoring heart rate. There are several points at which heart rate is easily measured. The most reliable is the radial artery. The carotid artery is simple to find, especially during exercise. However, there are pressure receptors located in the carotid artery that if subjected to hard pressure from the two fingers will slow down the heart rate, giving a false indication of exactly what the heart rate is. Thus the pulse at the radial artery proves the most accurate measure of heart rate. Regardless of where the heart rate is taken, it should be monitored within 15 seconds after stopping exercise. Another factor must be considered when measuring heart rate during exercise. The athlete is trying to elevate heart rate to a specific target rate and maintain it at that level during the entire workout. Heart rate can be increased or decreased by speeding up or slowing down the pace. It has already been indicated that heart rate increases proportionately with the intensity of the work load and will plateau after 2 to 3 minutes of activity. Thus the athlete should be actively engaged in the workout for 2 to 3 minutes before measuring pulse.

There are several formulas that will easily allow the sports therapist to identify a *target training heart rate.* Exact determination of maximal heart rate involves exercising an athlete at a maximal level and monitoring the heart rate using an electrocardiogram. This process is difficult outside of a laboratory. However, an approximate estimate of maximal heart rate (MHR) for both males and females in the population is thought to be about 220 beats per minute. MHR is related to age. As you get older, your MHR decreases.[20] Thus a relatively simple estimate of MHR

would be MHR = 220 − age. For a 20-year-old athlete, MHR would be about 200 beats per minute (220 − 20 = 200). If you are interested in working at 70% of your maximal heart rate, the target heart rate can be calculated by multiplying 0.7 × (220 − age). Again using a 20-year-old as an example, a target heart rate would be 140 beats per minute (0.7 × [220 − 20] = 140).

Another commonly used formula that takes into account your current level of fitness is the Karvonen equation.[17,19]

Target training HR = Resting HR* +
(0.6 [Maximum HR − Resting HR])

Resting heart rate generally falls between 60 to 80 beats per minute. A 20-year-old athlete with a resting pulse of 70 beats per minute, according to the Karvonen equation, would have a target training heart rate of 148 beats per minute (70 + 0.6 [200 − 70] = 148).

Regardless of the formula used, to see minimal improvement in cardiorespiratory endurance, the athlete must train with the heart rate elevated to at least 60% of its maximal rate.[4] The American College of Sports Medicine (ACSM)[2] recommends that for the collegiate athlete it is more desirable to train in the 60% to 90% range when training continuously. Exercising at a 70% level is considered moderate, since activity can be continued for a long period of time with little discomfort and still produce a training effect. In a trained individual it is not difficult to sustain a heart rate at the 85% level.

Rating of perceived exertion. Rating of perceived exertion (RPE) can be used in addition to monitoring heart rate to indicate exercise intensity. During exercise, individuals are asked to rate subjectively on a numerical scale from 6 to 20 exactly how they feel relative to their level of exertion[6] (Table 8-1). More intense exercise that requires a higher level of oxygen consumption and energy expenditure is directly related to higher subjective RPE. Over time athletes can be taught to exercise at a specific RPE that relates directly to more objective measures of exercise intensity.[26]

DURATION. For minimal improvement to occur, the athlete must participate in at least 20 minutes of continuous activity with the heart rate elevated to its

---

*True resting heart rate should be monitored with the subject lying down.

TABLE 8-1
Rating of Perceived Exertion

Scale	Verbal Rating
6	
7	Very, very light
8	
9	Very light
10	
11	Fairly light
12	
13	Somewhat hard
14	
15	Hard
16	
17	Very hard
18	
19	Very, very hard
20	

From Borg GA: Psycophysical basis of perceived exertion, *Med Sci Sports Exerc* 14:377, 1982.

working level. ACSM recommends 20 to 60 minutes of workout/activity with the heart rate elevated to training levels.[2,16] Generally, the greater the duration of the workout, the greater the improvement in cardiorespiratory endurance.[27] The competitive athlete should train for at least 45 minutes.

Interval Training

Unlike continuous training, **interval training** involves activities that are more intermittent. Interval training consists of alternating periods of relatively intense work and active recovery. It allows for performance of much more work at a more intense work load over a longer period of time than if working continuously.[21]

For the athlete, it is most desirable in continuous training to work at an intensity of about 75% to 80% of MHR. Obviously, sustaining activity at a higher intensity over a 20-minute period would be difficult. The advantage of interval training is that it allows work at this 80% or higher level for a short period of time followed by an active period of recovery during which the athlete may be working at only 60% to 70% of MHR.[12] Thus the intensity of the workout and its duration can be greater than with continuous training.

Most sports are anaerobic, involving short bursts of intense activity followed by a sort of active recovery period (for example, football, basketball, soccer,

or tennis). The interval technique allows training to be more sport-specific during the workout. With interval training the overload principle should be applied, making the training period much more intense.[13]

There are several important considerations in interval training. The **training period** is the amount of time that continuous activity is actually being performed, and the **recovery period** is the time between training periods. A **set** is a group of combined training and recovery periods, and a **repetition** is the number of training/recovery periods per set. **Training time** or **distance** refers to the rate or distance of the training period. The training/recovery ratio indicates a time ratio for training vs. recovery.

An example of interval training would be a soccer player running sprints. An interval workout would involve running one set of ten 120-yard sprints in under 18 seconds, with a 45-second walking recovery period between each repetition. During this training session the soccer player's heart rate would probably increase to 85% to 95% of maximal level during the dash and should likely fall to the 60% to 70% level during the recovery period. Older athletes should exercise caution when using interval training as a method for improving cardiorespiratory endurance. The intensity levels attained during the active periods may be too high for the untrained individual.

COMBINED CONTINUOUS AND INTERVAL TRAINING. As discussed previously, most sports activities involve some combination of aerobic and anaerobic metabolism.[32] Continuous training is generally done at an intensity level that primarily uses the aerobic system. In interval training the intensity is sufficient to necessitate a greater percentage of anaerobic metabolism. Therefore the sports therapist should incorporate both training techniques into a rehabilitation program to maximize cardiorespiratory fitness.

Additional Training Techniques

For those athletes who are capable of weight bearing, two additional techniques for maintaining cardiorespiratory endurance may be useful.

FARTLEK TRAINING. Fartlek is a training technique that is a type of cross-country running originated in Sweden. Fartlek literally means "speed play." It is similar to interval training in that the athlete must run for a specified period of time; however, specific pace and speed are not identified. It is recommended that the course for a fartlek workout be some type of varied terrain with some level running, some uphill and downhill running, and some running through obstacles such as trees or rocks. The object is to put surges into a running workout, varying the length of the surges according to individual purposes.

One advantage of fartlek training is that because the pace and terrain always change, the training session is less regimented and allows an effective alternative in the training routine.

Again, if fartlek training is going to improve cardiorespiratory endurance it must elevate the heart rate to at least minimal training levels. Fartlek may best be used as an off-season conditioning activity or as a change-of-pace activity to counteract the boredom of training using the same activity day after day.

PAR COURS. Par cours is a technique for improving cardiorespiratory endurance that basically combines continuous training and circuit training. This technique involves jogging a short distance from station to station and performing a designated exercise at each station according to guidelines and directions provided on an instruction board located at that station. Par cours circuits provide an excellent means for gaining some aerobic benefits while incorporating some of the benefits of calisthenics. Par cours circuits are found most typically in parks or recreational areas within metropolitan areas.

EVALUATION OF CARDIORESPIRATORY ENDURANCE

Numerous tests have been developed to evaluate fitness levels.[14,18,25] Most of these tests are based on the idea that cardiorespiratory endurance capability is best indicated by the maximal capacity of the working tissues to use oxygen ($\dot{V}O_2$max). We know from an earlier discussion that $\dot{V}O_2$max can be predicted or estimated by measuring heart rates at varying work loads. You can easily perform the following tests so that specific levels of cardiorespiratory endurance may be identified. Each of the tests described below is based to a large extent on one or both of the following factors: (1) the motivation of the person and (2) the minimal level of cardiovascular endurance.

SUMMARY

1. The sports therapist should routinely incorporate activities that will help maintain levels of cardiorespiratory endurance into the rehabilitation program.
2. Cardiorespiratory endurance involves the coordinated function of the heart, lungs, blood, and blood vessels to supply sufficient amounts of oxygen to the working tissues.
3. The best indicator of how efficiently the cardiorespiratory system functions is the maximal rate at which oxygen can be used by the tissues.
4. Heart rate is directly related to the rate of oxygen consumption. It is therefore possible to predict the intensity of the work in terms of a rate of oxygen use by monitoring heart rate.
5. Aerobic exercise involves an activity in which the level of intensity and duration is low enough to provide a sufficient amount of oxygen to supply the demands of the working tissues.
6. In anaerobic exercise the intensity of the activity is so high that oxygen is being used more quickly than it can be supplied, thus an oxygen debt is incurred that must be repaid before working tissue can return to its normal resting state.
7. Continuous or sustained training for maintenance of cardiorespiratory endurance involves selecting an activity that is aerobic in nature and training at least three times per week for a time period of no less than 20 minutes with the heart rate elevated to at least 60% of maximal rate.
8. Interval training involves alternating periods of relatively intense work followed by active recovery periods. Interval training allows performance of more work at a relatively higher work load than continuous training.
9. During rehabilitation, continuous and interval training techniques should be incorporated.
10. Fartlek makes use of jogging or running over varying types of terrain at changing speeds.
11. Par cours is a training technique that combines continuous training with exercises done at stations along the course.

REFERENCES

1. Allsen E: Circulorespiratory endurance, *J Phys Educ Rec Dance* 52:36, 1981.
2. American College of Sports Medicine: *Guidelines for exercise testing prescription,* Philadelphia, 1986, Lea & Febiger.
3. Åstrand PO: Åstrand-Rhyming nomogram for calculation of aerobic capacity from pulse rate during submaximal work, *J Appl Physiol* 7:218, 1954.
4. Åstrand PO, Rodahl K: *Textbook of work physiology,* New York, 1986, McGraw-Hill.
5. Bar-Or O: Cardiac output of 10- to 13-year-old boys and girls during submaximal exercise, *J Appl Physiol* 30:219, 1971.
6. Borg GA: Psychophysical basis of perceived exertion, *Med Sci Sports Exerc* 14:377, 1982.

7   Cantwell JD: Cardiovascular aspects of running, *Clin Sports Med* 4(4):627, 1985 (review).

8   Chillag SA: Endurance athletes: physiologic changes and nonorthopedic problems, *South Med J* 79(10):1264, 1986 (review).

9   Convertino VA: Aerobic fitness, endurance training, and orthostatic intolerance, *Exerc Sport Sci Rev* 15:223, 1987 (review).

10 Cooper KH: *The aerobics program for total well-being,* New York, 1982, Bantam Books.

11 deVries H: *Physiology of exercise for physical education and athletics,* Dubuque, Iowa, 1986, William C. Brown.

12 Fox E, Bowers R, Foss M: *The physiological basis of physical education and athletics,* Philadelphia, 1981, WB Saunders.

13 Gaesser GA, Wilson LA: Effects of continuous and interval training on the parameters of the power-endurance time relationship for high-intensity exercise, *Int J Sports Med* 9(6):417, 1988.

14 Ghosh AK, Ahuja A, Khanna GL: Distance run as predictor of aerobic endurance ($\dot{V}O_2$max) of sportsmen, *Indian J Med Res* 85:680, 1987.

15 Greer N, Katch F: Validity of palpation recovery pulse rate to estimate exercise heart rate following four intensities of bench step exercise, *Res Q Exerc Sport* 53:340, 1982.

16 Hage P: Exercise guidelines: which to believe? *Phys Sports Med* 10:23, 1982.

17 Hickson RC, Foster C, Pollac M, et al.: Reduced training intensities and loss of aerobic power, endurance, and cardiac growth, *J Appl Physiol* 58(2):492, 1985.

18 How fit are you? *University of California, Berkeley, Wellness Letter* 1(9):7, 1985.

19 Karvonen MJ, Kentala E, Mustala O: The effects of training on heart rate: a longitudinal study, *Ann Med Exp Biol* 35:305, 1957.

20 Londeree B, Moeschberger M: Effect of age and other factors on maximal heart rate, *Res Q Exerc Sport* 53:297, 1982.

21 MacDougall D, Sale D: Continuous vs. interval training: a review for the athlete and coach, *Can J Appl Sport Sci* 6:93, 1981.

22 Mahon AD, Vaccaro P: Ventilatory threshold and $\dot{V}O_2$max changes in children following endurance training, *Med Sci Sports Exerc* 21(4):425, 1989 (review).

23 Marcinik EJ, Hogden K, Mittleman K, et al.: Aerobic/calisthenic and aerobic/circuit weight training programs for Navy men: a comparative study, *Med Sci Sports Exerc* 17(4):482, 1985.

24 McArdle W, Katch F, Katch V: *Exercise physiology: energy, nutrition, and human performance,* Philadelphia, 1991, Lea & Febiger.

25 Mead W, Hartwig R: Fitness evaluation and exercise prescription, *Fam Pract* 13:1039, 1981.

26 Monahan T: Perceived exertion: an old exercise tool finds new applications, *Phys Sports Med* 16:174, 1988.

27 President's Council on Physical Fitness and Sports: *Adult fitness manual,* Washington, D.C., 1980, U.S. Government Printing Office.

28 Rowland TW, Green GM: Anaerobic threshold and the determination of training target heart rates in premenarcheal girls, *Pediatr Cardiol* 10(2):75, 1989.

29 Vago P, Mercier M, Ramonatxo M, et al.: Is ventilatory anaerobic threshold a good index of endurance capacity? *Int J Sports Med* 8(3):190, 1987.

30 Weltman A, Weltman J, Ruh R, et al.: Percentage of maximal heart rate reserve, and $\dot{V}O_2$ peak for determining endurance training intensity in sedentary women, *Int J Sports Med* 10(3):212, 1989 (review).

31 Weymans M, Reybrouck T: Habitual level of physical activity and cardiorespiratory endurance capacity in children, *Eur J Appl Physiol* 58(8):803, 1989.

32 Wilmore JH: *Training for sport and activity,* Boston, 1985, Allyn & Bacon.

Reestablishing Proprioception, Kinesthesia, Joint Position Sense, and Neuromuscular Control in Rehabilitation

9

Scott Lephart

OBJECTIVES

After completion of this chapter, the student should be able to do the following:

- Relate the history of sensation and the terminology of joint sensation.
- Describe the neural anatomy and physiology of joint receptors and how they mediate neuromuscular joint stabilization.
- Discuss the results of functional proprioception studies and their implications.
- Design lower and upper extremity kinesthetic rehabilitation protocols.

Ligaments play a major role in normal joint kinematics, providing mechanical restraint to abnormal joint movement when a stress is placed on the joint. The primary concern of the orthopedic surgeon has been the biochemical restoration of these ligaments after injury in an attempt to restore the joint's stability and therefore its kinematics. In restoring normal joint kinematics it is speculated that recurrent injury will be minimized and progressive joint degeneration can be avoided.

Kennedy et al.[38] however, observed that in addition to their mechanical restraining function, articular ligaments provide important neurological feedback that directly mediates muscular reflex stabilization about the joint. The neuromuscular controlling mechanism is mediated by articular mechanoreceptors and provides the individual with the proprioceptive sensations of kinesthesia and joint position sense. The neurological feedback for the control of

muscular actions protects against excessive strain on passive joint restraints and provides a prophylactic mechanism to recurrent injury. After the joint injury, disruption to these articular mechanoreceptors inhibits normal neuromuscular reflex joint stabilization and contributes to repetitive injuries and the progressive decline of the joint.

A rehabilitation program that addresses the need for restoring joint stability cannot be designed until one has a total appreciation of both the mechanical and sensory function of articular structures. Simply restoring mechanical restraints or strengthening the associated muscles neglects the coordinated neuromuscular controlling mechanism required for joint stability during the sudden changes in joint position common to sports activity. A lag time in the neuromuscular reaction time can result in recurrent joint subluxation and deterioration.

This chapter will address the issues central to the

role of articular structures in providing neuromuscular control of joint stability. The role of joint mechanoreceptors will be specifically elucidated as it pertains to the mediation of the sensations of proprioception, kinesthesia, and joint position awareness.

HISTORY OF SENSATION

Awareness of the body and its relationship to the surrounding environment is mediated by the phenomenon of sensation.[2] The history of sensation dates back to the Greek philosopher Aristotle, who was the first to describe the five senses. Sir Charles Bell[9] termed sensation as it relates to limb position and motion as the "sixth sense." This chapter will address articular sensation in its entirety since it mediates the perception of joint position and joint motion that regulates muscle contraction for movement and joint stabilization.

The relevance of articular sensation has been observed by a select few scientists over the past two centuries. The French neurologists Duchenne and Charcot[2] drew attention to articular sensations in 1865, while Sherrington and Adrian received the Nobel prize in 1932 for their work on the mechanisms of sensation and were the first to describe proprioception.[54,55] Abbott et al.,[1] in 1944, were the first to suggest that knee articular sensations were the first step in a kinetic chain that accounted for dynamic joint stabilization. More recently, Palmer[51] demonstrated the role of proprioceptive input from knee ligaments in mediating the reflex contraction of the hamstrings and vastus medialis with resultant weakening of the reflex after ligament trauma. Also, current investigators, including Barrack et al.,[4,5] Barrett,[6] and Lephart et al.,[43,44] have demonstrated that joint position perception is altered after articular pathology.

Terminology of Joint Sensation

The terminology related to joint sensation is often misunderstood and used inappropriately, which has led to confusion and a lack of appreciation for these mechanisms during rehabilitation. Articular sensations are described as *proprioception* and *kinesthesia*.[48] There is considerable discrepancy in the definitions of these two terms as related to their physiological functions. Mountcastle and Willis[49] define proprioception as the conscious awareness of limb position, while they define kinesthesia as the awareness of joint motion. On the other hand, Bastian[7] defines the kinesthetic mechanism as a complex of sensations including those in which movement is not featured, while Sherrington[54,55] describes the proprioceptive sense as including vestibular sensations and inputs from muscles and joints that are not necessarily perceived. We define proprioception as a specialized variation of the sensory modality of touch that encompasses the sensations of joint movement (kinesthesia) and joint position (joint position sense).

Conscious proprioception is essential for proper joint function in sports, activities of daily living, and occupational tasks. Unconscious proprioception modulates muscle function and initiates reflex stabilization. Much effort has been dedicated to elucidate the mechanical function of articular structures and the corresponding mechanical deficits that occur secondary to disruption of these structures. Articular structures also have a significant sensory function that plays a role in dynamic joint stability, acute and chronic injury, pathological wearing, and rehabilitation training.

JOINT AND MUSCLE NEURAL RECEPTORS
Anatomy of Neural Receptors

The extrinsic innervation of joints follows Hilton's law,[34] which states that joints are innervated by articular branches of the nerves supplying the muscles that cross the joint. The afferent innervation of joints is based on peripheral receptors located in articular, muscular, and cutaneous structures. Articular receptors include nociceptive free nerve endings and proprioceptive mechanoreceptors.

Several authors have identified mechanoreceptors in the cruciate ligaments (CL) of the cat knee joint.[11,20,22] Schultz et al.[52] were the first to identify mechanoreceptors in the human CL. Using gold chloride,[47] Bielshowky,[28] and Bodian staining techniques, these investigators histologically examined ACL obtained from cadavers at the time of total knee arthroplasty and demonstrated the presence of mechanoreceptors in the CL. Using a modified gold chloride technique,[67] Schutte et al.[53] and Zimny et al.[65] further characterized these ACL receptors into three morphological types of mechanoreceptors (Ruffini endings, Ruffini corpuscles or Golgi tendon organs, and pacinian corpuscles) and free-nerve endings. Others have demonstrated similar mechanoreceptors in cat knee menisci.[38] In their extensive study of the innervation of joints, Freeman and Wyke[20] histologically identified the three types of mechanoreceptors in the capsular and ligamentous structures of cat ankle joints. The presence of mechanoreceptors in human ankle joints has not yet been demonstrated. Finally, the three distinct mechanoreceptors have recently been histologically identified by Vangsness and Ennes[62] in the glenoid labrum and the glenohumeral ligaments of the shoulder, suggesting that these structures possess the anatomical basis for perceiving joint position and motion.

Physiology of Neural Receptors

Mechanoreceptors transduce some function of mechanical deformation into a frequency-modulated neural signal that is transmitted via cortical and reflex pathways. An increased stimulus of deformation is coded by an increased afferent discharge rate or a rise in the population of activated receptors. Grigg and Hoffman have correlated mechanoreceptor afferent discharge with strain energy density and have calibrated mechanoreceptors as in vivo load cells in the posterior capsule of the feline knee.[31,32] Receptors demonstrate different adaptive properties based on their response to a continuous stimulus. Quick-adapting (QA) mechanoreceptors, such as the pacinian corpuscle, decrease their discharge rate to extinction within milliseconds of the onset of a continuous stimulus. Slow-adapting (SA) mechanoreceptors, such as the Ruffini ending, Ruffini corpuscles, and the Golgi tendon organ, continue their discharge in response to a continuous stimulus. QA mechanoreceptors are very sensitive to changes in stimulation and are therefore thought to mediate the sensation of joint motion. Different populations of SA mechanoreceptors are maximally stimulated at specific joint angles, and thus a continuum of SA receptors is thought to mediate the sensation of joint position and change in joint position.[14,33,37] In animal models, these mechanoreceptors respond to active or passive motion with maximal stimulation occurring at the extremes of knee motion.[29,30,36] Stimulation of these receptors results in reflex muscle contraction about the joint.[8,18,60] In addition to the joint receptors, the muscle spindle receptors are complex, fusiform, SA receptors found within skeletal muscle. Via afferent and efferent fibers to intrafusal muscle fibers, the muscle spindle receptor can measure muscle tension over a large range of extrafusal muscle length.

There is considerable debate over the relative contribution to proprioception of muscle receptors vs.

joint receptors, with traditional views emphasizing joint mechanoreceptors and more contemporary views emphasizing muscle receptors.* Recent work suggests that joint and muscle receptors are probably complementary components of an intricate afferent system in which each receptor modifies the function of the other.[8,19,30] With the identification of these receptor types in most joints and the knowledge of their function,[29-32] it appears that the ligamentous, cartilaginous, and muscular structures of joints contain the neural components necessary for the sensation of motion (rapidly adapting receptors, that is, pacinian corpuscles), joint position and acceleration (slowly adapting receptors, that is, Ruffini endings and Ruffini corpuscles), and pain (free-nerve endings). This would therefore support the contemporary view that both joint and muscle receptors contribute to the sensory appreciation of joint position.

FUNCTIONAL PROPRIOCEPTION STUDIES

Functionally, kinesthesia is assessed by measuring threshold to detection of passive motion (TTDPM),† while joint position sense is assessed by measuring reproduction of passive positioning (RPP)[43,59] and reproduction of active positioning (RAP).[59] TTDPM, when tested at slow angular velocity (0.5 to 2.5 degrees/second), is thought to selectively stimulate Ruffini or Golgi-type mechanoreceptors, and because the test is performed passively, it is believed to maximally stimulate joint receptors while minimally stimulating muscle receptors. In shutting down muscle activity, TTDPM is often chosen to assess afferent activity after ligament pathology. RAP, although usually performed at slow speed, stimulates joint and muscle receptors and provides a more functional assessment of the afferent pathways. TTDPM, RPP, and RAP do not provide an assessment of the unconscious reflex arc believed to provide dynamic joint stability. The assessment of reflex capabilities is usually performed using EMG interpretation of firing patterns of those muscles crossing the respective joint.[26] In patients with unilateral joint involvement, the contralateral uninvolved extremity serves as an internal control, while uninjured joints in a normative population serve as external controls.

We have designed a proprioception testing device

---

*References 14, 16, 25, 26, 29, 66.
†References 3-5, 41-44, 59.

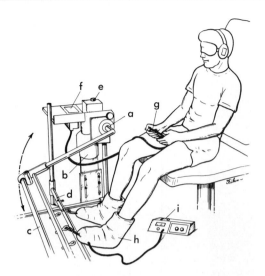

Fig. 9-1. Proprioceptive testing device. a = rotational transducer; b = motor; c = moving arm; d = stationary arm; e = control panel; f = digital microprocessor; g = hand-held disengage switch; h = pneumatic compression boot; i = pneumatic compression device; TTDPM is assessed by measuring the angular displacement until the subject senses motion in the knee.

(PTD) (Figure 9-1), similar to that described by Barrick and Skinner,[3-5] to assess TTDPM and RPP of the knee and shoulder. Proprioception is measured using a PTD, which is designed to assess kinesthetic awareness and joint position sense. The PTD measures the angular displacement of the joint being tested before detection of movement by the subject and measures the patient's accuracy in reproducing selected joint angles. The PTD moves the joint at a constant angular velocity ranging from 0.5 degrees/second to 2.5 degrees/second. A rotational transducer interfaced with a digital microprocessor counter provides angular displacement values.

Knee Proprioception Testing

With the demonstration of the neural framework necessary for joint sensation, investigators have just recently begun to perform functional studies of knee joint proprioception. Barrack and Skinner experimentally assessed proprioception by measuring TTDPM and RPP. They found decreased kinesthesia with increasing age[5] and ACL disruption.[4] Barrick and Skinner[3] also found enhanced kinesthesia in trained dancers. Barrett et al.[6] further demonstrated a decline

in joint position sense with osteoarthritis. It is hypothesized that ACL disruption, meniscal injury, and osteoarthritis damage articular structures containing mechanoreceptors and therefore result in deficits of kinesthesia and joint position sense.

Our laboratory has more recently revealed enhanced kinesthesia in intercollegiate gymnasts,[41] as well as some enlightening kinesthetic findings in individuals after ACL reconstruction.[44] Our studies on athletically active patients after arthroscopically assisted patellar-tendon autograft or allograft ACL reconstruction revealed the following: (1) kinesthetic deficits were present in the ACL-reconstructed knee compared with the uninvolved knee when tested at 15 degrees of knee flexion (near terminal extension), while moving into both flexion and extension (Figure 9-2); (2) there was no difference in TTDPM between the ACL-reconstructed knee and the contralateral uninvolved knee from a starting position of 45 degrees of knee flexion (midrange), while moving into either flexion or extension; (3) kinesthetic awareness was more sensitive from a starting position of 15 degrees of knee flexion than from a starting position of 45 degrees of knee flexion for both the ACL-reconstructed knee and the uninvolved knee while moving into both flexion and extension (Figure 9-3); and (4) kinesthetic awareness in the ACL-reconstructed knee was significantly enhanced with the use of a neoprene sleeve (Figure 9-4).

Although we were primarily focusing on joint receptors in knee injuries, muscle receptors are an integral component of a complex afferent system and may also play a role in kinesthetic awareness of slow, passive motion. In addition to reflex pathways, joint and muscle mechanoreceptors have cortical pathways that account for conscious appreciation of joint movement and position. Our finding of enhanced kinesthetic awareness in the near-terminal range of motion is commensurate with neurophysiological studies that have shown maximal response of joint mechanoreceptors at the extremes of motion.[29,30,36]

As previously stated, Barrack et al.[4] showed that a proprioceptive deficit exists after ACL disruption, and we have found that a deficit continues after reconstruction.[44] Knee articular structures, including the ACL, possess mechanoreceptors, and damage to these structures can result in partial deafferentation. Barrack et al. found a longer TTDPM in the ACL-disrupted knee compared to the contralateral uninvolved knee when tested at 30 to 40 degrees of knee flexion. In our study, we found a longer TTDPM in the ACL-

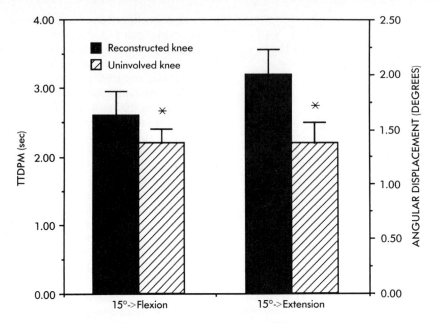

Fig. 9-2. Mean TTDPM. Mean TTDPM (in time and angular displacement) for reconstructed vs. uninvolved knee from a starting position of 15 degrees flexion moving into flexion and extension (± SE, $p < 0.05$).

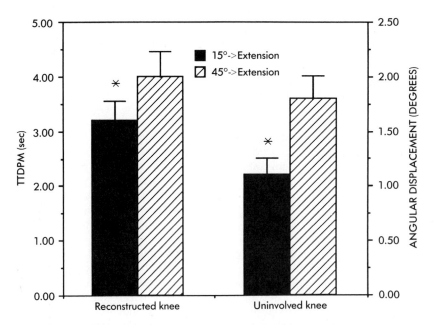

Fig. 9-3. Mean TTDPM. Mean TTDPM (in time and angular displacement) for reconstructed vs. uninvolved knee from a starting position of 15 and 45 degrees moving into extension (± SE, $p < 0.05$).

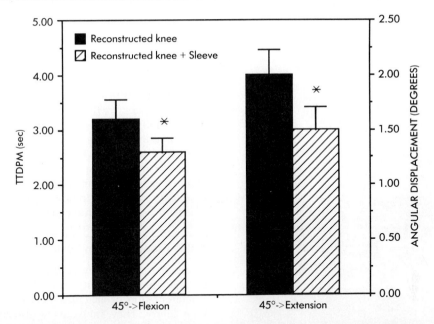

Fig. 9-4. Mean TTDPM. Mean TTDPM (in time and angular displacement) for reconstructed knee and reconstructed knee with neoprene sleeve from a starting position of 45 degrees flexion moving into flexion and extension ($\pm$ SE, $p < 0.05$).

reconstructed knee compared to the contralateral uninvolved knee when tested at 15 degrees knee flexion and no significant difference when tested at 45 degrees knee flexion.[44] Thus kinesthesia in the midrange of motion may have returned after ACL reconstruction. However, kinesthesia is more sensitive in the near-terminal range of motion, hence any difference between the involved and uninvolved knee would be more apparent.

For years, knee surgeons have postulated that the sensory loss associated with ACL injury may affect the results of ACL repair and reconstruction.[4] Du Toit,[17] Insall et al.,[35] and Noyes et al.[50] have advocated certain reconstructive techniques due, in part, to increased afferent preservation. Theoretically, operative techniques can restore proprioception directly through reinnervation of damaged structures or indirectly through restoration of appropriate tension in capsuloligamentous structures. Acute ACL repair may facilitate regeneration along with maintaining anatomical relationships. The extent of reinnervation in the reconstructed ligament and its relationship to revascularization needs to be addressed. Prosthetic grafts, vascularized grafts, free grafts, and allografts all may have different reinnervation potential.

Bracing and wrapping have been thought to serve a sensory function in addition to a mechanical function. Barrett et al.[6] found that an elastic bandage enhanced joint position sense in patients with osteoarthritic knees, as well as in patients after total knee arthroplasty. We found enhancement of kinesthesia with the use of a commercially available neoprene sleeve such as one from Pro Orthopedic Devices, Inc. (Figure 9-5).[44] Proprioception is mediated by afferent input from articular, muscular, and cutaneous structures. The neoprene sleeve could have augmented afferent input by providing increased cutaneous stimulation.

Proprioception may play a protective role in acute knee injury through reflex muscular splinting. The protective reflex arc initiated by mechanoreceptors and muscle spindle receptors occurs much more quickly than the reflex arc initiated by nociceptors (70 to 100 meters/second vs. 1 meter/second).[2] Thus proprioception may play a more significant role than pain sensation in preventing injury in the acute setting. Proprioceptive deficits, however, probably play more of a role in the etiology of chronic injuries and reinjury. Initial knee injury results in partial deafferentation and sensory deficits that can predispose

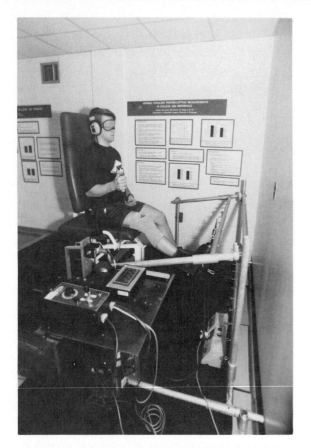

Fig. 9-5. Proprioception testing. Proprioception testing while wearing neoprene compression sleeve.

to further injury.[38] Proprioceptive deficits may also contribute to the etiology of degenerative joint disease through pathological wearing of a joint with poor sensation. It is unclear whether the proprioceptive deficits that accompany degenerative joint disease are a result of the underlying pathological process or contribute to the etiology of the pathological process.

It is clear that joint effusion, particularly in the knee, contributes to a decreased mechanoreceptor afference, resulting in the inhibition of muscular contractions. In the knee, this inhibition is mediated by slowly adapting mechanoreceptors and appears to provide long-term quadriceps shut down, particularly in the vastus medialis.[2] A 30% to 50% inhibition of the reflex-evoked quadriceps contraction can be observed with 60 cc of intraarticular effusion.[38] This muscular inhibition severely disrupts neuromuscular

training during rehabilitation and provides a fundamental basis for relief of joint effusions from a neurological basis. Any proprioceptive deficits resulting from chronic joint effusion may contribute to the inability to provide neuromuscular joint control and therefore result in joint degeneration.

A proprioceptive deficit may detract from the functional result of knee surgery, may inhibit complete rehabilitation, and may predispose the athlete to reinjury. Thus it is clear, based on the results of these studies, that any comprehensive rehabilitation program designed to return athletes to preinjury levels of activity after knee injuries should include an extensive proprioception element.

Ankle Proprioception Testing

Freeman and Wyke[20] were the first to postulate that chronic ankle instability was due, in part, to partial deafferention of articular mechanoreceptors with joint injury. They subjectively observed decreased stability in one-legged stance in the sprained ankle vs. the contralateral uninjured ankle. Konradsen and Ravn[39] studied the reaction of subjects with chronic ankle instability to sudden inversion using EMG and joint motion analysis. They found a prolonged peroneal reaction time in those patients vs. age-matched controls, suggestive of a partial deafferention of reflex stabilization. Garn and Newton[23] studied the ability of a subject to properly sense a passive movement or no movement state in the dorsiflexion-plantarflexion plane and found decreased kinesthetic awareness in the involved ankle of subjects with unilateral ankle sprains. Glenncross and Thornton[24] reported deficits in active replication of passive ankle/foot positioning in the dorsiflexion-plantarflexion plane while testing the sprained ankle vs. the contralateral uninjured ankle.

The results of studies using stabilometric techniques (force plate or opto-electronic joint analysis) to assess postural sway and balance in patients with chronic ankle instability has been equivocal. Tropp and Odenrick[61] found no increase in postural sway when comparing a group of soccer players with histories of ankle sprains with a control group of uninjured soccer players. Tropp and Odenrick[61] also compared the involved ankle with the uninvolved ankle in a group of soccer players with a history of unilateral, recurrent ankle sprains and found no differences in postural sway. Cornwall and Murrell,[15] however, found a significant increase in postural sway when comparing individuals with an acute ankle sprain to uninjured controls as much as 2 years after the injury.

"Proprioceptive training" techniques after acute and chronic ankle sprain injuries are the most widely used compared with other injuries, yet these techniques have only empirical evidence of effectiveness and remain untested. Ankle wrapping/bracing has also been suggested to carry a proprioceptive benefit, however this also remains unproven.

Shoulder Proprioception Testing

Although recent investigations involving the knee and ankle have drawn attention to the sensory role of articular structures and proprioception deficits after injury,[4,44] proprioceptive sensation of the shoulder, in contrast, has not been well studied. The perception of joint position and joint movement in the shoulder is essential for placement of the hand in upper limb function. In addition, proprioception may play an important role in dynamic shoulder stability and modulation of muscle function.

Symptoms of instability in the shoulder are commonly attributed to the loss of static and dynamic mechanical restraint provided by intact muscular and capsuloligamentous structures. Shoulder capsuloligamentous structures may contain receptors that, along with muscular and cutaneous receptors, provide the basis for a more active mechanism of protective joint restraint and joint position sense. With injury to these structures, partial deafferentation may occur with resultant proprioceptive deficits. These deficits, in turn, could lead to reinjury. The contribution of proprioceptive deficits to the vicious cycle of insidious microtrauma involved in impingement syndrome and recurrent instability is unclear (Figure 9-6). In addition, the protective role of proprioceptive initiated–reflex muscular splinting in acute traumatic instability is unknown.

It is unclear whether proprioceptive deficits occur after shoulder injury and how these deficits affect joint function and symptoms of instability. The role of proprioception in the pathogenesis of instability and impingement syndrome remains to be elucidated. In addition, the effect of surgical intervention on shoulder proprioception is unknown. Recent work by Smith and Brunolli has suggested that a sensory deficit occurs in patients with recurrent, atraumatic, anterior instability.[59]

The PTD discussed previously also permits us to assess both TTDPM and RPP of the shoulder (Figure

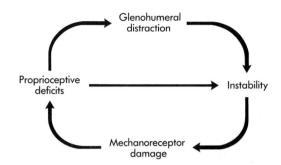

Fig. 9-6. Effect of mechanoreceptor deficits. Effect of mechanoreceptor deficits on shoulder instability.

9-7). Testing is performed with the subject positioned supine with the shoulder at 90 degrees abduction and the elbow in 90 degrees of flexion. TTDPM of internal and external rotary movements are measured from starting positions of neutral rotation and 30 to 75 degrees external rotation. In a population of college-aged individuals without any history of shoulder injury, we found minimal variation in kinesthesia and no differences between dominant and nondominant shoulders (Figure 9-8).[42]

In a group of male subjects with unilateral, traumatic, recurrent, anterior shoulder instability, we demonstrated both TTDPM and RPP deficits,[43] similar to the findings of Smith and Brunolli (Figure 9-9).[59] These two studies elucidate a pattern of proprioceptive deficits in unstable shoulders. The uninvolved shoulders in our study demonstrated proprioceptive measurements similar to those of the normative population without shoulder dysfunction. Although we have not yet had the opportunity to study it, one can hypothesize that altered proprioception in unstable shoulders may influence the dynamic mechanisms of joint restraint. This hypothesis would therefore indicate the necessity of integrating shoulder kinesthetic and joint position sense exercises as a part of shoulder rehabilitation. It is logical to assume that methods to improve proprioception in patients with shoulder disorders could improve shoulder function and decrease the risk of reinjury.

NEUROMUSCULAR/PROPRIOCEPTION REHABILITATION

Developing a rehabilitation program that incorporates proprioceptively mediated muscular control of

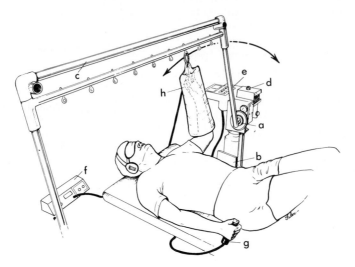

Fig. 9-7. Proprioception testing device for shoulder testing.

NORMAL SHOULDER PROPRIOCEPTION

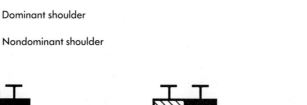

Fig. 9-8. Mean TTDPM. Mean TTDPM (degree of displacement) for normal dominant and nondominant shoulders, from starting positions of neutral rotation and 75 degrees external rotation moving into both internal and external rotation ($\pm$ SE).

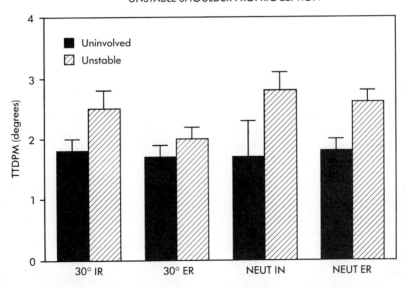

UNSTABLE SHOULDER PROPRIOCEPTION

Fig. 9-9. Mean TTDPM. Mean TTDPM (degree of displacement) for unilateral, traumatic, recurrent, anterior shoulder instability patients, from starting positions of neutral rotation and 30 degrees external rotation moving into both internal and external rotation (± SE).

joints necessitates an appreciation for the central nervous system's influence on motor activities. Joint afferents contribute to central nervous system function at three distinct levels of motor control.[62] At the spinal level, reflexes subserve movement patterns that are received from higher levels of the nervous system. This action provides for reflex splinting during conditions of abnormal stress about the joint and has significant implications for rehabilitation.[13,38,64] The muscle spindles play a major role in the control of muscular movement by adjusting activity in the lower motor neurons.[62] Partial deafferentation of joint afferent receptors has also altered the musculature's ability to provide cocontraction joint stabilization by antagonistic and synergistic muscles, thus resulting in the potential for reinjury.[38]

The second level of motor control is at the brain stem, where joint afference is relayed to maintain posture and balance of the body. The input to the brain stem about this information emanates from the joint proprioceptors, the vestibular centers in the ears, and from the eyes.[62]

The final aspect of motor control includes the highest level of central nervous system function (motor cortex, basal ganglia, and cerebellum) and is mediated by cognitive awareness of body position and movement. These higher centers initiate and program motor commands for voluntary movements. Movements that are repeated can be stored as central commands and can be performed without continuous reference to consciousness.[62] Although considerable controversy still exists relative to the role of joint and muscle receptors in the perception of joint movement, deep pressure, at the very least, can be consciously appreciated during joint motion.[12]

With these three levels of motor control in mind, mediated in part by joint and muscle afferents, one can begin to develop rehabilitation activities to address proprioceptive deficiencies. The objectives must be to stimulate the joint and muscle receptors to encourage maximum afferent discharge to the respective central nervous system level. At the spinal level, activities that encourage reflex joint stabilization should be addressed. Such activities include sudden alterations in joint positioning that necessitate reflex muscular stabilization. Balance and postural activities, both with and without visual input, will enhance motor function at the brain stem level. Consciously performed joint positioning activities, especially at joint end ranges, will maximally stimulate the conversion of conscious to unconscious motor programming.

Lower Extremity Training

Mechanoreceptors located in the joints of the lower extremities are most functionally stimulated when the extremity is positioned in a closed-kinetic chain orientation and perpendicular axial loading of the joint is permitted.[27] It is also important that these exercises are performed at various positions throughout the range of joint motion because of the differences in afferent response that have been observed.

Methods to improve proprioception after ankle and knee joint injury have been a staple in sports rehabilitation in an attempt to decrease the risk of reinjury. Afferent input is altered after joint injury and appears to remain altered after joint surgery.[4] The objectives of proprioceptive rehabilitation are to retrain altered afferent pathways, resulting in enhanced sensation of joint movement. Barrett et al. revealed a strong relationship between proprioception and knee joint function in patients after ACL injury.[6]

Kinesthetic training begins early in the rehabilitation program, with such simple tasks as balance training and joint repositioning, and becomes increasingly more difficult as the patient progresses. Activities should be structured to address all three of the previously discussed levels of afference mediated motor control. Once the athlete has reached the functional stage of rehabilitation,[40] the objectives of proprioception training are to refine joint sense awareness to initiate muscle reflex stabilization to prevent reinjury. Additionally, proprioceptive acuity plays an important role in the performance of those athletes requiring precise movement patterns.

The proprioceptive mechanism comprises both conscious and unconscious pathways. Therefore these exercises need to include not only consciously mediated patterned sequences but also sudden alterations of joint positions that initiate reflex muscle contraction. Kinesthetic training exercises that permit balancing on unstable platforms while enabling the athlete to perform a sport-specific skill integrate both of these neural pathways and maximally stimulate kinesthetic awareness. Therefore kinesthetic exercise progression should begin with balance training and joint position awareness and progress to highly complex, sport-specific activities.

The proprioception component of the rehabilitation program should correspond with the functional progression of the athlete. Proprioception activities can be initiated before weight bearing by having the athlete practice joint repositioning, and kinesthetic training can be started using an unstable platform while sitting. Once functional rehabilitation begins, kinesthetic activities concentrating on neuromuscular control of the joint should dominate activities.

The functional program begins with forward running and progresses to very complex maneuvers that require cutting, turning, and other highly agile maneuvers while running. The progression from forward running to cutting and turning is dictated by the refinement of kinesthetic acuity that permits dynamic joint stabilization when torsion and translatory forces are placed on the knee and ankle. Each phase of the rehabilitation program should attempt to refine kinesthetic acuity that will permit progression to more complex running maneuvers during the ensuing phases of the functional program. The following phases of kinesthetic training are designed to correspond with the functional progression of the athlete and increase in difficulty through the phases. Specific kinesthetic activities are provided in Table 9-1.

Kinesthetic Training: Phase I

Phase I of kinesthetic training concentrates on reestablishing balance, dynamic joint stabilization, and a kinesthetic running gait, which will permit the athlete to begin directional changes in phase II of the program. Joint repositioning, to enhance the conscious proprioceptive awareness, and balance training, to increase reflex stabilization and postural orientation, should be included in this phase. Walking and jogging straight ahead on flat surfaces are initiated during this phase. Finally, to allow for eccentric loading in an axial orientation, athletes should initiate forward and backward stair climbing and descent.

Balance training can begin by simply having the athlete perform a modified Rhomberg test (Figure 9-10) on both hard and soft surfaces such as foam. This exercise is frequently used in the clinical setting, since it is convenient and inexpensive. As the athlete's balance and reflex stabilization improve, unstable platform training can be integrated into the program. This activity is performed by having the athlete balance on the unstable platform with both feet, progressing to balancing on only the injured leg. These activities can be performed both with and without visual input (Figure 9-11, *A* and *B*).

There are a number of balance training devices that are commercially available for rehabilitation and research purposes. The kinesthetic ability training (KAT) (Breg, Inc., Vista, CA) device provides objec-

TABLE 9-1
Phases of Lower Extremity Kinesthetic Training

PHASE I

Walk/Run Series:

- Performed on flat/straight surfaces, progressing to continuous running

Kinesthetic Training:

- Two feet balancing on unstable platform, eyes open, multidirectional
- Two feet balancing on unstable platform, eyes closed, multidirectional
- One foot balancing on unstable platform, eyes open, unidirectional
- One foot balancing on unstable platform, eyes closed, unidirectional
- One foot balancing on unstable platform, eyes open, multidirectional
- One foot balancing on unstable platform, eyes closed, multidirectional

Passive and Active Joint Repositioning

Eccentric Loading

- Stair walking: forward and backward, up and down

PHASE II

Running:

- Figure eight: large to small circles, slow to fast speed

Kinesthetic Training:

- Cocontraction lateral slides
- Mini trampoline hopping and jogging
- Pogo ball balancing and hopping
- Sport activity of unstable platform
- Lateral slide board exercise

PHASE II cont'd

Active Joint Repositioning

Eccentric Loading:

- Plyometric exercises (6-12 inch height)
- Stair running (if tolerated)

PHASE III

Running:

- Shuttle run
- Cocontraction lateral slides

Kinesthetic/Agility Training:
(progress to normal speed)

- Shuttle run
- Carioca crossover maneuvers
- 4-corner running
- Reaction cutting drills

Eccentric Loading:

- Plyometrics (1-2 foot height)

PHASE IV

Sport-Specific Activities:
(performed at controlled speeds progressing toward normal speed)

- 4-corner running while dribbling
- Cutting off a minitrampoline while running pass route
- Cariocas while defending
- Sport-specific drills removed from team setting
  —basketball layups
  —fielding baseballs
  —running and receiving footballs
- Defensive maneuvers for respective sports

tive assessments of balance on an unstable platform similar to frequently used rehabilitation exercises (Figure 9-12). The Chattecx dynamic balance system (Chattanooga Group, Inc., Hixson, TN) provides objective assessments of a number of balance conditions including unilateral and bilateral stance with both a level and unlevel platform (Figure 9-13). However, balance training effectiveness, for the purpose of enhancing proprioception, has not been sufficiently studied especially relative to protocol prescription. It is postulated that these types of training activities provide proprioceptive feedback relative to joints and can therefore enhance the kinesthetic and joint position sense of injured hips, knees, and ankles.

Kinesthetic Training: Phase II

Phase II of the kinesthetic training program encourages turning and changing direction. To initiate turning activities, we recommend running figure-eights, beginning with large circles and progressively running smaller circles with increasing speed as the athlete's confidence and ability permit. The figure-eights should be performed in both directions. The kines-

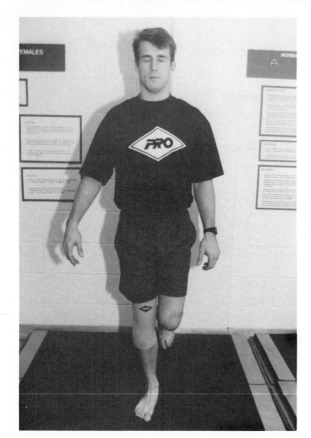

Fig. 9-10. Modified Rhomberg test. Modified Rhomberg test on foam surface for balance training wearing a neoprene compression sleeve.

A

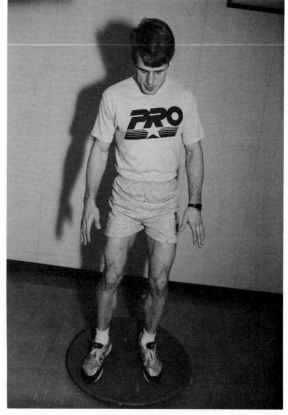

Fig. 9-11. Lower extremity kinesthetic training. Lower extremity kinesthetic training on an unstable platform. **A,** Both feet.

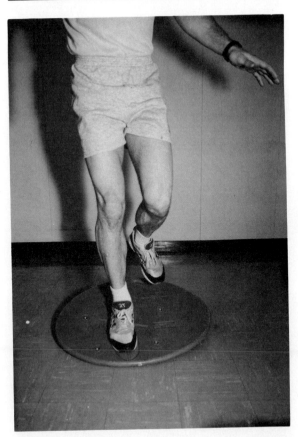

Fig. 9-11 cont'd. B, One foot.

B

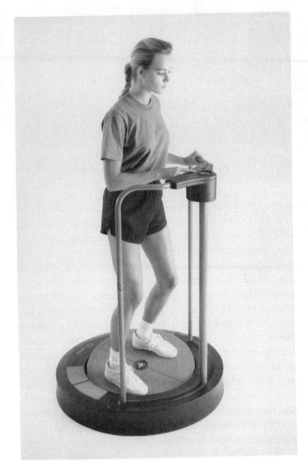

Fig. 9-12. Kinesthetic ability trainer (KAT).

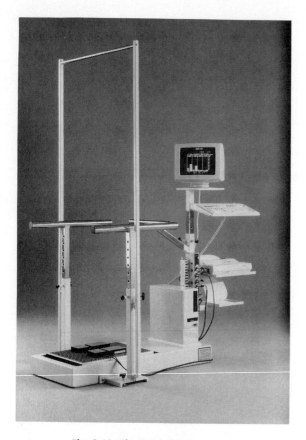

Fig. 9-13. Chattex balance system.

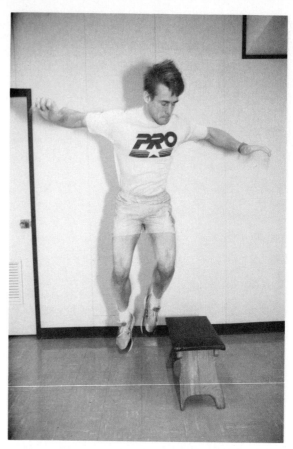

Fig. 9-14. Plyometric training.

thetic activities in phase II become more dynamic and encourage changing directions rapidly, landing, and performing balancing maneuvers while involved in sport-specific activities. Plyometrics should also be implemented during this phase to develop explosive contractile activities and permit eccentric deceleration of knee joint flexion.[1] Plyometrics should begin at a comfortable height (6 to 12 inches) and progressively increase as tolerated (Figure 9-14). Pogo bouncing exercises are an excellent form of plyometrics that integrate balance.[10] Lateral movements are also initiated during phase II with such activities as a slide board (Fitter, 321, 1021-10 Ave. F.W., Calgary, Alberta, Canada) (Figure 9-15) and the cocontraction maneuver[45,46] using resistance tubing (Sportcord, Pro Orthopedic Devices, Inc., Tucson, AZ) (Figure 9-16). These activities permit the development of balance while moving laterally and also develop

dynamic joint stabilization by cocontraction of the quadriceps and hamstring muscle groups.

Kinesthetic Training: Phase III

Phase III of the kinesthetic program prepares the athlete for return to sport-specific activities. Therefore phase III activities must reproduce the stress that will be placed on the knee upon return to sports. Cutting and agility/proprioception activities are initiated during this phase and should be progressed to near normal speed by the conclusion of the phase. Such activities as the shuttle run are used for acceleration and deceleration training, while agility is trained by activities including the 4-corner run, the carioca cross-over maneuver[45,46] (Figure 9-17), and reaction cutting maneuvers (Figure 9-18). Plyometrics are continued and advanced during this phase.

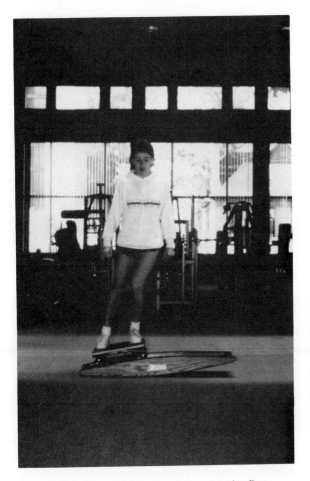

Fig. 9-15. Lateral slide exercised using the fitter.

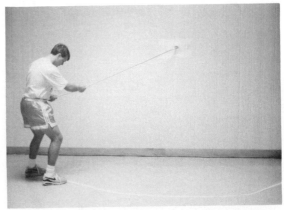

Fig. 9-16. Cocontraction lateral slide maneuver.

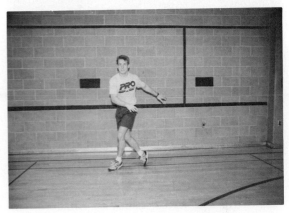

Fig. 9-17. Carioca cross-over maneuver.

Kinesthetic Training: Phase IV

The final phase of kinesthetic training focuses on integrating the kinesthetic elements refined in the first three phases of the program into sport-specific activities that are integral to the respective sport. Although the athlete is not returned to competition or team practice at this point, many of the drills and skills that are refined in phase IV are activities that are performed during practice sessions. The success of this phase of the program depends on appropriately defining the performance demands of the particular athlete within his or her sport and in some cases the position within the sport. Therefore the design of each phase IV of the kinesthetic program is unique to the individual athlete.

The effectiveness of the sport-specific kinesthetic program depends upon the clinician's understanding of the demands of the sport and the athlete's pathology. Many of the phase III agility and proprioception exercises can be performed with sport-specific objectives. Examples include shuttle runs and 4-corner running while dribbling a basketball (Figure 9-19), cutting off a mini-trampoline[10] while executing a pass route for a receiver in football, and performing carioca while defending an opponent. The last phase of the sport-specific program for the athlete is the integration of specific drills and programming performance activities. Examples include layup and defensive slide drills in basketball, fielding and base running in baseball, and pass receiving and defensive maneuvers in football. The athlete must perform the sport-

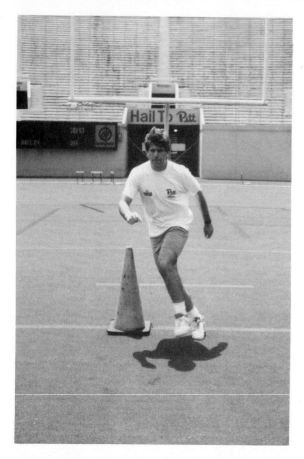

Fig. 9-18. Reaction cutting maneuver.

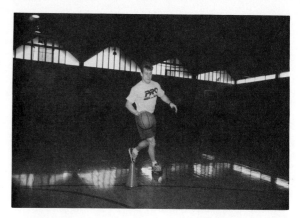

Fig. 9-19. Four-corner sport-specific dribbling drill.

specific functional activities in a controlled manner, and the speed and intensity of performance are determined by the athlete's motor skill development, functional joint stability, and confidence. Work at our laboratory has elucidated that the athlete's perception of his or her functional capacity is reasonably accurate and needs to be considered when progressing through functional activities.[45,46] One of the most devastating setbacks in a rehabilitation program is for the athlete to sustain reinjury during the rehabilitation process.

Upper Extremity Training

Proprioception training of the lower extremity is widely accepted and used in traditional athletic training and physical therapy settings during injury rehabilitation. To a lesser extent, proprioception training of the shoulder has been suggested after injury. Many strengthening and sport-specific activities incorporate proprioceptive activities, though none are directly designed for that purpose.

Because the throwing motion demands refined joint positioning and repositioning of the shoulder, it is logical to assume that mechanoreceptor activity plays a vital role in both performance and dynamic shoulder stabilization. The key to effective and efficient throwing is the ability to repeat the motion over a course of time. We have modified a lower extremity proprioceptive training device for upper extremity activity. The wobble board exercise stimulates both articular and muscular mechanoreceptors and is an effective means of training scapular stabilizers and joint receptors (Figure 9-20). This exercise is also of significant benefit to the athlete with an acute, traumatic, unilaterally unstable shoulder and provides a mechanism for developing dynamic shoulder stability. The activity is performed by having the athlete balance with one or both arms extended on the uneven platform. A series of patterns is performed by moving the platform, and thus sudden changes in joint position occur during the exercise. As joint position changes, dynamic stabilization must occur for the athlete to remain in balance. An oversized ball can also be used for this type of training (Figure 9-21).

The final proprioception training activity we suggest is active and passive shoulder repositioning. The athlete attempts to reposition given ranges of shoulder abduction—external rotation without visual input (Figure 9-22). When performed passively, with the assistance of a clinician or isokinetic device, the ar-

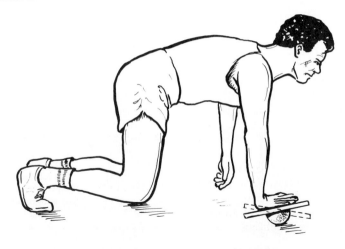

Fig. 9-20. Shoulder wobble board exercise.

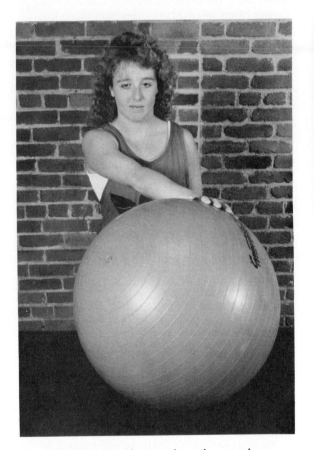

Fig. 9-21. Shoulder proprioception exercise.

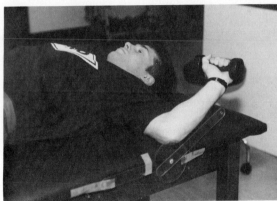

Fig. 9-22. Shoulder joint repositioning exercise.

ticular mechanoreceptors are maximally stimulated and relay afferent information relative to joint position. When performed actively, both articular and muscle mechanoreceptors provide joint position information. This training activity is designed to enhance neuromuscular controlling mechanisms relative to glenohumeral positioning during shoulder rotation.

SUMMARY

1. The sensory function of articular structures provides awareness of the body and its relationship

with the surrounding environment. This awareness is a specialized variation of the sensory modality of touch known as proprioception.

2. Proprioception encompasses the sensations of kinesthesia and joint position sense and is mediated by joint, muscle, and cutaneous mechanoreceptors responsible for afferent transmission of joint motion and position. These afferents modulate muscle function and initiate reflex joint stabilization.

3. After injury to articular structures, partial deafferentation has resulted in deficits in the proprioceptive mechanisms. These deficits may lead to an insidious pathological degeneration of joints because of the lack of muscle stabilization and resultant recurrence of injury.

4. The effects of training on the afferent deficits remain unclear, yet it seems reasonable that clinically stimulating these mechanisms should enhance the dynamics of joint kinematics and decrease the susceptibility to reinjury.

REFERENCES

1 Abbott JC, Saunders JB, Dec M, et al.: Injuries to the ligaments of the knee joint, *J Bone Joint Surg* 26:503-521, 1944.

2 Barrack RL, Skinner HB: The sensory function of knee ligaments. In Daniel D, editor: *Knee ligaments: structure, function, injury,* New York, 1990, Raven Press.

3 Barrack RL, Skinner HB, Brunet ME, et al.: Joint kinesthesia in the highly trained knee, *J Sports Med Phys Fitness* 24:18-20, 1983.

4 Barrack RL, Skinner HB, Brunet ME, et al.: Proprioception in the anterior cruciate ligament deficient knee, *Am J Sports Med* 17:1-6, 1989.

5 Barrack RL, Skinner HB, Cook SD, et al.: Effect of articular disease and total knee arthroplasty on knee joint–positioning sense, *J Neurophysiol* 50(3):684-687, 1983.

6 Barrett DS, Cobb AG, Bentley G: Joint proprioception in normal, osteoarthritic, and replaced knees, *J Bone Joint Surg* [Br]:73:53-56, 1991.

7 Bastian HC: The "muscular sense"; its nature and cortical localization, *Brain* 10:1-137, 1888.

8 Baxendale RA, Ferrell WR, Wood L: Responses of quadriceps motor units to mechanical stimulation of knee joint receptors in the decerebrate coat, *Brain Res* 453:150-156, 1988.

9 Bell C: The hand: its mechanism and vital endowments as evincing design, London, 1833, William Pickering.

10 Blair DF, Willis RP: Rapid rehabilitation following anterior cruciate ligament reconstruction, *JNATA* 26:32-44, 1991.

11 Boyd IA: The histological structure of the receptors in the knee-joint of the cat correlated with their physiologic response, *J Physiol* 124:476-488, 1954.

12 Burgess PR: Signaling of kinesthetic information by peripheral sensory receptors, *Annu Rev Neurosci* 5:171, 1982.

13 Cailliet R: *Low back pain syndrome,* ed 3, Philadelphia, 1981, FA Davis.

14 Clark FJ, Burgess PR: Slowly adapting receptors in cat knee joint: can they signal joint angle? *J Neurophysiol* 38:1448-1463, 1975.

15 Cornwall MW, Murrell W: Postural sway following inversion sprain of the ankle, *Podiatr Med Assoc* 81:243-247, 1991.

16 Cross MM, McCloskey DI: Position sense following surgical removal of joints in man, *Brain* 55:443-445, 1973.

17 Du Toit GT: Knee joint cruciate ligament substitution: the Lindemann (Heidelberg) operation, *S Afr J Surg* 5:25-30, 1967.

18 Ekholm J, Eklund G, Skoglund S: On the reflex effects from the knee joint of the cat, *Acta Physiol Scand* 50:167-174, 1960.

19 Ferrell WR: The response of slowly adapting mechanoreceptors in the cat knee joint to tetanic contraction of hind limb muscles, *Quart J Exp Physiol* 70:337-345, 1985.

20 Freeman MAR, Wyke B: The innervation of the knee joint: an anatomical and histological study in the cat, *J Anat* 101:505-532, 1967.

21 Freeman MAR, Wyke B: The innervation of the ankle joint: an anatomical and histological study in the cat, *Acta Anat* 68:321, 1967.

22 Gardner E: The distribution and termination of nerves in the knee-joint of the cat, *J Comp Neuro* 80:11-32, 1944.

23 Garn SN, Newton RA: Kinesthetic awareness in subjects with multiple ankle sprains, *Phys Ther* 68:1667-1671, 1988.

24 Glencross D, Thornton E: Position sense following joint injury, *J Sports Med Phys Fitness* 21:23-27, 1982.

25 Goodwin GM, McCloskey DI, Matthews PB: The contribution of muscle afferents to kinesthesia shown by vibration induced illusions of movement and by the effects of paralyzing joint afferents, *Brain* 95:705-748, 1972.

26 Goodwin GM, McCloskey DI, Matthews PB: The persistence of appreciable kinesthesia after paralyzing joint afferents but preserving muscle afferents, *Brain Res* 37:326-329, 1972.

27 Gray GW: *Chain reaction: a successful strategy for closed chain testing and rehabilitation,* Adrian, Mich, 1990, Wynn Market.

28 Gray P: *The microtomist's formulary and guide,* New York, 1954, Blakiston.

29 Grigg P: Mechanical factors influencing response of joint afferent neurons from cat knee, *J Neurophysiol* 38:1473-1484, 1975.

30 Grigg P: Response of joint afferent neurons in cat medial articular nerve to active and passive movements of the knee, *Brain Res* 118:482-485, 1976.

31 Grigg P, Hoffman AH: Ruffini mechanoreceptors in isolated joint capsule: responses correlated with strain energy density, *Somatosens Mot Res* 2:149-162, 1984.

32 Grigg P, Hoffman AH: Calibrating joint capsule mechanoreceptors as in vivo soft tissue load cells, *J Biomech* 22:781-785, 1989.

33 Heetderks WJ: Principle component analysis of neural population responses of knee joint proprioceptors in cat, *Brain Res* 156:51-65, 1978.

34 Hilton J: *On the influence of mechanical and physiological rest in the treatment of accidents and surgical diseases, and the diagnostic value of pain: a course of lectures,* London, 1863, Bell and Daldy.

35 Insall J, Joseph DH, Aglietta P, et al.: Bone-block iliotibial-band transfer for anterior cruciate insufficiency, *J Bone Joint Surg* 63[A]:560-569, 1981.

36 Johansson H, Sjolander P, Sojka P: A sensory role for the cruciate ligaments, *Clin Orthop* 268:161-178, 1991.

37 Johansson H, Sjolander P, Sojka P: Receptors in the knee joint ligaments and their role in the biomechanics of the joint, *Crit Rev Biomed Eng* 18:341-368, 1991.

38 Kennedy JC, Alexander IJ, Hayes KC: Nerve supply of the human knee and its functional importance, *Am J Sports Med* 10:329-335, 1982.

39 Konradsen L, Ravn JB: Ankle instability caused by prolonged peroneal reaction time, *Acta Orthop Scand* 61(5):388-390, 1990.

40 Lephart SM: *Functional rehabilitation,* Baltimore, 1993, Williams & Wilkins.

41 Lephart SM, Fu FH, Irrgang JJ, et al.: Proprioceptive characteristics of trained and untrained college females (abstract), *Med Sci Sports Exerc* 23:4 Supplement, 1991.

42 Lephart SM, Fu FH, Warner JP: *Normal shoulder proprioception measurements in college age individuals,* presented at the 1992 American Orthopaedic Society for Sports Medicine, San Diego, Calif.

43 Lephart SM, Fu FH, Warner JP: *Proprioception in the unstable shoulder,* presented at the 1993 Combined Congress of the International Arthroscopy Association and the International Society of the Knee, Copenhagen, Denmark.

44 Lephart SM, Kocher MS, Fu FH, et al.: Proprioception following ACL reconstruction, *J Sports Rehab* 1:186-196, 1992.

45 Lephart SM, Perrin DH, Fu F, et al.: Functional performance tests for the anterior cruciate ligament insufficient athlete, *JNATA* 26:44-51, 1991.

46 Lephart SM, Perrin DH, Fu FH, et al.: Relationship between selected physical characteristics and functional capacity in the ACL deficient athlete, *J Orthop Sports Phys Ther* 16:174-181, 1992.

47 Lillie RD: *Histopathological technic and practical histochemistry,* New York, 1954, McGraw-Hill.

48 McClowski DL: Kinesthetic sensibility, *Physiological Review* 58:763-820, 1978.

49 Mountcastle VS: *Medical physiology,* ed 14, St Louis, 1980, Mosby.

50 Noyes FR, Butler DL, Paulos LE, et al.: Intra-articular cruciate reconstruction, I. Perspectives on graft strength vascularization and immediate motion after replacement, *Clin Orthop* 172:71-77, 1983.

51 Palmer I: Pathophysiology of the medial ligament of the knee joint, *Acta Chir Scand* 115:312-318, 1958.

52 Schultz RA, Miller DC, Kerr CS, et al.: Mechanoreceptors in human cruciate ligaments: a histological study, *J Bone Joint Surg* 66[A]:1072-1076, 1984.

53 Schutte MJ, Dabezies EJ, Zimny ML, et al.: Neural anatomy of the human anterior cruciate ligament, *J Bone Joint Surg* 69[A]:243-247, 1987.

54 Sherrington CS: On the proprioceptive system, especially in its reflex aspects, *Brain* 29:467-482, 1906.

55 Sherrington CS: Observations on the sensual role of the proprioceptive nerve supply of the extrinsic ocular muscle, *Brain* 41:332-343, 1918.

56 Skinner HB, Barrack RL, Cook SD: Age-related decline in proprioception, *Clin Orthop* 184:208-211, 1984.

57 Skinner HB, Barrack RL, Cook SD, et al.: Joint position sense in total knee arthroplasty, *J Orthop Res* 1(3):276-283, 1984.

58 Skinner HB, Wyatt MP, Hodgdon JA, et al.: Effect of fatigue on joint position sense of the knee, *J Orthop Res* 4:112-118, 1986.

59 Smith RL, Brunolli J: Shoulder kinesthesia after shoulder dislocation, *Phys Ther* 69:106-112, 1989.

60 Sojka P, Sjolander P, Johansson H, et al.: Influence from stretch-sensitive receptors in the collateral ligaments of the knee joint on the gamma-muscle spindle systems of flexor and extensor muscles, *Neurosci Res* 11:55-62, 1991.

61 Tropp H, Odenrick P: Postural control in single-limb stance, *J Orthop Res* 6:833-839, 1988.

62 Vangsness CT, Ennis M: Neural anatomy of the human anterior glenohumeral joint dislocation, *AAOS,* presentation, 1992.

63 Vrettos XC, Wyke BD: Articular reflexogenic systems in the costovertebral joints, *J Bone Joint Surg* 56[Br]:382, 1974.

64 Williams WJ: A systems-oriented evaluation of the role of joint receptors and other afferents in position and motion sense, *Crit Rev Biomed Eng* 7:23-77, 1981.

65 Zimny ML, Albright DJ, Dabezies E: Mechanoreceptors in the human medial meniscus, *Acta Anatomica* 133:35-40, 1988.

66 Zimny ML, St. Onge M, Schutte M: A modified gold chloride method for demonstration of nerve endings in frozen sections, *Stain Technology* 60(5):305-306, 1985.

67 Zimny ML, Schutte M, Dabezies E: Mechanoreceptors in human anterior cruciate ligament, *Anat Rec* 214:204-209, 1986.

Mobilization and Traction Techniques in Rehabilitation

10

William E. Prentice

OBJECTIVES

After completion of this chapter, the student should be able to do the following:

- Discuss the role of manual therapy techniques in rehabilitation.

- Discuss joint arthrokinematics.

- Differentiate between physiological movements and accessory motions.

- Discuss how specific joint positions can enhance the effectiveness of the treatment technique.

- Discuss the basic techniques of joint mobilization.

- Identify Maitland's five oscillation grades.

- Discuss indications and contraindications for mobilization.

- Discuss the use of various traction grades in treating pain and joint hypomobility.

- Explain why traction and mobilization techniques should be used simultaneously.

- Demonstrate specific techniques of mobilization and traction for various joints.

Manual therapy techniques including mobilization and traction, as well as proprioceptive neuromuscular facilitation techniques, are being used more frequently in rehabilitation by the sports therapist. In recent years, the sports therapist has tended to get caught up in some of the technological advances that have been made available in rehabilitation equipment. These "high tech" devices have to a great extent taken the place of what many consider to be the greatest tool available in the rehabilitation repertoire, that being our hands. It seems however that the pendulum is beginning to swing back in the other direction, and more sports therapists are incorporating manual therapy techniques into their rehabilitation regimens. Thus in-depth discussions of mobilization and traction techniques in this chapter and PNF techniques in Chapter 11 are essential.

After injury to a joint, there will always be some associated loss of motion. That loss of movement may be attributed to a number of pathological factors including contracture of connective tissue (for example, ligaments and joint capsule); resistance of the musculotendinous unit (for example, muscle, tendon, and fascia) to stretch; or some combination of the two.[5]

In a postsurgical case, the limitation is almost always caused by capsular or ligamentous contracture. For example, the postoperative knee will typically demonstrate a position of comfort with the joint held in slight flexion. This position of comfort can very quickly become motion limiting if appropriate intervention measures are not initiated by the sports therapist. Certainly the advent of arthroscopy, the use of constant passive motion immediately after surgery,

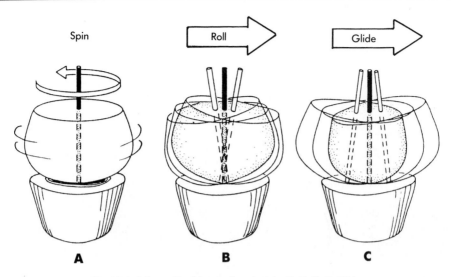

Fig. 10-1. Joint arthrokinematics. A, Spin. **B,** Roll. **C,** Glide.

and functional postoperative bracing have attempted to minimize loss of motion after surgery. Nevertheless, there still seems to be significant difficulty in many patients in regaining normal joint motion.[6]

JOINT ARTHROKINEMATICS

For the sports therapist who is supervising a rehabilitation program, some understanding of the biomechanics of joint movement is essential. There are basically two types of movement that govern motion about a joint. Perhaps the better known of the two types of movement are the **physiological movements** that result from an active muscle contraction that moves an extremity through traditional cardinal planes including flexion, extension, abduction, adduction, and rotation. The second type of motion is **accessory motion.** Accessory motions refer to the manner in which one articulating joint surface moves relative to another. Accessory motions are also referred to as **joint arthrokinematics,** which include **spin, roll,** and **glide**[1,9,11] (Figure 10-1).

Spin occurs around some stationary longitudinal mechanical axis and may be in either a clockwise or counterclockwise direction. An example of spinning is motion of the radial head at the humeroradial joint as occurs in forearm pronation/supination (Figure 10-1, *A*).

Rolling occurs when a series of points on one articulating surface comes in contact with a series of points on another articulating surface. An analogy would be to picture a rocker of a rocking chair rolling on the flat surface of the floor. An anatomical example would be the rounded femoral condyles rolling over a stationary flat tibial plateau (Figure 10-1, *B*).

Gliding occurs when a specific point on one articulating surface comes in contact with a series of points on another surface. Returning to the rocking chair analogy, the rocker slides across the flat surface of the floor without any rocking at all. Gliding is sometimes referred to as *translation*. Anatomically, gliding or translation would occur during an anterior drawer test at the knee when the flat tibial plateau slides anteriorly relative to the fixed rounded femoral condyles (Figure 10-1, *C*).

Pure gliding can occur only if the two articulating surfaces are congruent where either both are flat or both are curved. Since virtually all articulating joint surfaces are incongruent, meaning that one is usually flat while the other is more curved, it is more likely that gliding will occur simultaneously with a rolling motion. Rolling does not occur alone because this would result in compression or perhaps dislocation of the joint.

Although rolling and gliding usually occur together, they are not necessarily in similar proportion, nor are they always in the same direction. If the articulating surfaces are more congruent, more gliding will occur, whereas if they are less congruent, more rolling will occur.

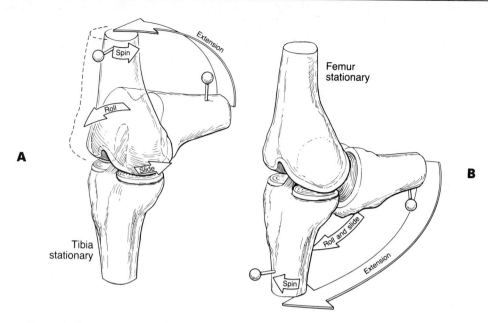

Fig. 10-2. Convex-concave rule. A, Convex moving on concave. **B,** Concave moving on convex.

Rolling will always occur in the same direction as the movement. For example, in the knee joint when the foot is fixed on the ground, the femur will always roll in an anterior direction when moving into knee extension and conversely will roll posteriorly when moving into flexion (Figure 10-2).

The direction of the gliding component of motion is determined by the shape of the articulating surface that is moving. If you consider the shape of two articulating surfaces, one joint surface can be determined to be convex in shape while the other may be considered to be concave in shape. In the knee, the femoral condyles would be considered the convex joint surface, while the tibial plateau would be the concave joint surface. In the glenohumeral joint, the humeral head would be the convex surface, while the glenoid fossa would be the concave surface.

This relationship between the shape of articulating joint surfaces and the direction of gliding is defined by the **Convex-Concave Rule.** If the concave joint surface is moving on a stationary convex surface, gliding will occur in the same direction as the rolling motion. Conversely, if the convex surface is moving on a stationary concave surface, gliding will occur in an opposite direction to rolling. Hypomobile joints are treated by using a gliding technique. Thus it is critical to know the appropriate direction to use for gliding.

JOINT POSITIONS

Each joint in the body has a position in which the joint capsule and the ligaments are most relaxed, allowing for a maximum amount of **joint play.**[9,10] This position is called the **resting position.** It is essential to know specifically where the resting position is since testing for joint play during an evaluation and treatment of the hypomobile joint using either mobilization or traction are both usually performed in this position. Table 10-1 summarizes the appropriate resting positions for many of the major joints.

Placing the joint capsule in the resting position allows the joint to assume a **loose-packed position** in which the articulating joint surfaces are maximally separated. A **close-packed position** is one in which there is maximal contact of the articulating surfaces of bones with the capsule and ligaments tight or tense. In a loose-packed position the joint will exhibit the greatest amount of joint play, while the close-packed position allows for no joint play. Thus the loose-packed position is most appropriate for mobilization and traction (Figure 10-3).

Both mobilization and traction techniques use a translational movement of one joint surface relative to the other. This translation may be in one of two directions; it may be either perpendicular or parallel to the **treatment plane.** The treatment plane falls

TABLE 10-1
Shape, Resting Position, and Treatment Planes of Various Joints

Joint	Convex Surface	Concave Surface	Resting Position	Treatment Plane
Sternoclavicular	Clavicle*	Sternum*	Anatomical position	In sternum
Acromioclavicular	Clavicle	Acromion	Anatomical position, in horizontal plane at 60 degrees to sagittal plane	In acromion
Glenohumeral	Humerus	Glenoid	Shoulder abducted 55 degrees, horizontally adducted 30 degrees, rotated so forearm is in horizontal plane	In glenoid fossa in scapular plane
Humeroradial	Humerus	Radius	Elbow extended, forearm supinated	In radial head perpendicular to long axis of radius
Humeroulnar	Humerus	Ulna	Elbow flexed 70 degrees, forearm supinated 10 degrees	In olecranon fossa, 45 degrees to long axis of ulna
Radioulnar (Proximal)	Radius	Ulna	Elbow flexed 70 degrees, forearm supinated 35 degrees	In radial notch of ulna, parallel to long axis of ulna
Radioulnar (Distal)	Ulna	Radius	Supinated 10 degrees	In radius, parallel to long axis of radius
Radiocarpal	Proximal carpal bones	Radius	Line through radius and third metacarpal	In radius, perpendicular to long axis of radius
Metacarpophalangeal	Metacarpal	Proximal phalanx	Slight flexion	In proximal phalanx
Interphalangeal	Proximal phalanx	Distal phalanx	Slight flexion	In proximal phalanx
Hip	Femur	Acetabulum	Hip flexed 30 degrees, abducted 30 degrees, slight external rotation	In acetabulum
Tibiofemoral	Femur	Tibia	Flexed 25 degrees	On surface of tibial plateau
Patellofemoral	Patella	Femur	Knee in full extension	Along femoral groove
Talocrural	Talus	Mortise	Plantarflexed 10 degrees	In the mortise in anterior/posterior direction
Subtalar	Calcaneus	Talus	Subtalar neutral between inversion/eversion	In talus, parallel to foot surface
Intertarsal	Proximal articulating surface	Distal articulating surface	Foot relaxed	In distal segment
Metatarsophalangeal	Tarsal bone	Proximal phalanx	Slight extension	In proximal phalanx
Interphalangeal	Proximal phalanx	Distal phalanx	Slight flexion	In distal phalanx

*In the sternoclavicular joint the clavicle surface is convex in a superior/inferior direction and concave in an anterior/posterior direction.

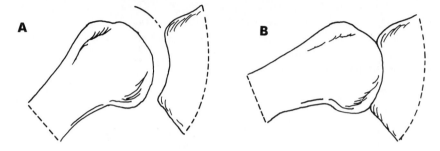

Fig. 10-3. Joint capsule resting position. A, Loose-packed position. **B,** Close-packed position.

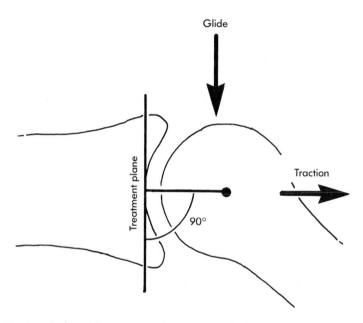

Fig. 10-4. Treatment plane. The treatment plane is perpendicular to a line drawn from the axis of rotation to the center of the articulating surface of the concave segment.

perpendicular to, or at a right angle to, a line running from the axis of rotation in the convex surface to the center of the concave articular surface[9,10] (Figure 10-4). Thus the treatment plane lies within the concave surface. If the convex segment moves, the treatment plane remains fixed. However, the treatment plane will move along with the concave segment. Mobilization techniques use glides that translate one articulating surface along a line parallel with the treatment plane. Traction techniques translate one of the articulating surfaces in a perpendicular direction to the treatment plane. Both techniques use a loose-packed joint position.[9]

RELATIONSHIP BETWEEN PHYSIOLOGICAL AND ACCESSORY MOTIONS

Physiological movement is voluntary, and accessory movements normally accompany physiological movement.[2] The two occur simultaneously. Although accessory movements cannot occur independently, they may be produced by some external force. Normal accessory component motions must occur for full-range physiological movement to take place. If any of the accessory component motions are restricted, normal physiological cardinal plane movement will not occur.[13,14]

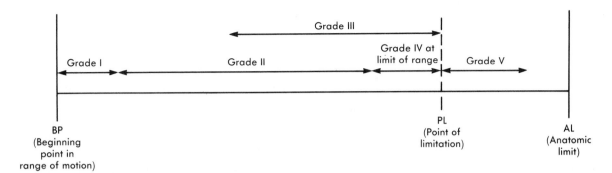

Fig. 10-5. Maitland's five grades of motion. *PL* (point of limitation); *AL* (anatomical limit).

Traditionally in rehabilitation programs we have tended to concentrate more on passive physiological movements without paying much attention to accessory motions. The question is always being asked, "How much flexion or extension is this patient lacking?" Rarely will anyone ask "How much is rolling or gliding restricted?"

It is critical for the sports therapist to closely evaluate the injured joint to determine whether motion is limited by physiological movement constraints involving musculotendinous units or by limitation in accessory motion involving the joint capsule and ligaments. If physiological movement is restricted, the athlete should engage in stretching activities designed to improve flexibility. Stretching exercises should be used whenever there is musculotendinous resistance to stretch. Stretching techniques are most effective at the end of physiological range of movement; they are limited to one direction, and they require some element of discomfort if additional range of motion is to be achieved. Stretching techniques make use of long lever arms to apply stretch to a given muscle.[8] Techniques of stretching have been discussed in Chapter 3, and PNF stretching techniques will be presented in Chapter 11.

If accessory motion is limited by some restriction of the joint capsule or the ligaments, the sports therapist should incorporate mobilization techniques into the treatment program. Mobilization techniques should be used whenever there are tight articular structures; they can be used effectively at any point in the range of motion, and they can be used in any direction in which movement is restricted. Mobilization techniques use a short lever arm to stretch ligaments and joint capsules, placing less stress on these structures, and consequently are somewhat safer to use than stretching techniques.[3]

JOINT MOBILIZATION TECHNIQUES

The techniques of **joint mobilization** are used to improve joint mobility or to decrease joint pain by restoring accessory movements to the joint and thus allowing full, nonrestricted, pain-free range of motion.[15,21]

Mobilization techniques may be used to attain a variety of treatment goals: reducing pain; decreasing muscle guarding; stretching or lengthening tissue surrounding a joint, in particular capsular and ligamentous tissue; reflexogenic effects that either inhibit or facilitate muscle tone or stretch reflex; and proprioceptive effects to improve postural and kinesthetic awareness.[1,7,14,16,18]

Movement throughout a range of motion can be quantified with various measurement techniques. Physiological movement is measured with a goniometer and composes the major portion of the range. Accessory motion is thought of in millimeters, although precise measurement is difficult.

Accessory movements may be hypomobile, normal, or hypermobile.[4] Each joint has a range of motion continuum with an anatomical limit (AL) to motion that is determined by both bony arrangement and surrounding soft tissue (Figure 10-5). In a hypomobile joint, motion stops at some point referred to as a *pathological point of limitation (PL),* short of the anatomical limit caused by pain, spasm, or tissue resistance. A hypermobile joint moves beyond its anatomical limit because of laxity of the surrounding structures. A hypomobile joint should respond well to techniques of mobilization and traction. A hypermobile joint should be treated with strengthening exercises, stability exercises, and, if indicated, taping, splinting, or bracing.[17]

Treatment techniques designed to improve accessory movement are generally small-amplitude movements, the amplitude being the distance that the joint is moved passively within its total range. Mobilization techniques use these small-amplitude oscillating motions that glide or slide one of the articulating joint surfaces in an appropriate direction within a specific part of the range.

Maitland has described various **grades of oscillation** for joint mobilization. The amplitude of each oscillation grade falls within the range of motion continuum between some beginning point (BP) and the AL.[13,14] Figure 10-5 shows the various grades of oscillation that are used in a joint with some limitation of motion. As the severity of the movement restriction increases, the PL will move to the left, away from the AL. However, the relationships that exist among the five grades in terms of their positions within the range of motion remain the same. The five mobilization grades are defined as follows:

GRADE I. A small-amplitude movement at the beginning of the range of movement. Used when pain and spasm limit movement early in the range of motion.[23]

GRADE II. A large-amplitude movement within the midrange of movement. Used when spasm limits movement sooner with a quick oscillation than with a slow one or when slowly increasing pain restricts movement halfway into the range.

GRADE III. A large amplitude movement up to the PL in the range of movement. Used when pain and resistance from spasm, inert tissue tension, or tissue compression limit movement near the end of the range.

GRADE IV. A small-amplitude movement at the very end of the range of movement. Used when resistance limits movement in the absence of pain and spasm.

GRADE V. A small-amplitude, quick thrust delivered at the end of the range of movement, usually accompanied by a popping sound, which is called a *manipulation*. Used when minimal resistance limits the end of the range. Manipulation is most effectively accomplished by the velocity of the thrust rather than by the force of the thrust.[19] Most authorities agree that manipulation should be used only by individuals trained specifically in these techniques because a great deal of skill and judgment is necessary for safe and effective treatment.[20]

Joint mobilization uses these oscillating gliding motions of one articulating joint surface in whatever direction is appropriate for the existing restriction. The appropriate direction for these oscillating glides is determined by the Convex-Concave Rule described previously. When the concave surface is stationary and the convex surface is mobilized, a glide of the convex segment should be in the direction opposite to the restriction of joint movement.[9,10,22] (Figure 10-6, *A*). If the convex articular surface is stationary and the concave surface is mobilized, gliding of the concave segment should be in the same direction as the restriction of joint movement (Figure 10-6, *B*). For example, the glenohumeral joint would be considered to be a convex joint with the convex humeral head moving on the concave glenoid. If shoulder abduction is restricted, the humerus should be glided in an inferior direction relative to the glenoid to alleviate the motion restriction. When mobilizing the knee joint, the concave tibia should be glided anteriorly in cases where knee extension is restricted. If mobilization in the appropriate direction exacerbates complaints of pain or stiffness, the sports therapist should apply the technique in the opposite direction until the patient can tolerate the appropriate direction.[22]

Typical mobilization of a joint may involve a series of three to six sets of oscillations lasting between 20 and 60 seconds each, with one to three oscillations per second.[13,14]

Indications for Mobilization

In Maitland's system, grades I and II are used primarily for treatment of pain, and grades III and IV are used for treating stiffness. Pain must be treated first and stiffness second.[14] Painful conditions should be treated on a daily basis. The purpose of the small-amplitude oscillations is to stimulate mechanoreceptors within the joint that can limit the transmission of pain perception at the spinal cord or brain stem levels.

Joints that are stiff or hypomobile and have restricted movement should be treated 3 to 4 times per week on alternating days with active motion exercise. The sports therapist must continuously reevaluate the joint to determine appropriate progression from one oscillation grade to another.

Indications for specific mobilization grades are relatively straightforward. If the athlete complains of pain before the sports therapist can apply any resistance to movement, it is too early, and all mobilization

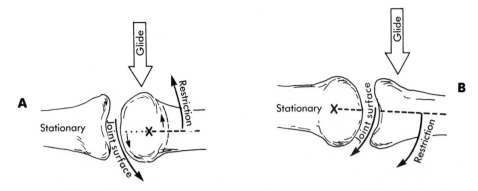

Fig. 10-6. Gliding motions. A, Glides of the convex segment should be in the direction opposite to the restriction. **B,** Glides of the concave segment should be in the direction of the restriction.

techniques should be avoided. If pain is elicited when resistance to motion is applied, mobilization using grades I and II is appropriate. If resistance can be applied before pain is elicited, mobilization can be progressed to grades III and IV. Mobilization should be done with both the athlete and the sports therapist positioned in a comfortable and relaxed manner. The sports therapist should mobilize one joint at a time. The joint should be stabilized as near one articulating surface as possible, while moving the other segment with a firm, confident grasp.

Contraindications for Mobilization

Techniques of mobilization and manipulation should not be used haphazardly. These techniques should generally not be used in cases of inflammatory arthritis, malignancy, bone disease, neurological involvement, bone fracture, congenital bone deformities, and vascular disorders of the vertebral artery. Again, manipulation should be performed only by those sports therapists specifically trained in the procedure because some special knowledge and judgment are required for effective treatment.[22]

JOINT TRACTION TECHNIQUES

Traction refers to a technique involving pulling on one articulating segment to produce some separation of the two joint surfaces. While mobilization glides are done parallel to the treatment plane, traction is performed perpendicular to the treatment plane (see Figure 10-4). Like mobilization techniques, traction may be used to either decrease pain or to reduce joint hypomobility.[24]

Kaltenborn has proposed a system using traction combined with mobilization as a means of reducing pain or mobilizing hypomobile joints.[9] As discussed earlier, all joints have a certain amount of joint play or looseness. Kaltenborn referred to this looseness as *slack.* Some degree of slack is necessary for normal joint motion. Kaltenborn's three traction grades are defined as follows (Figure 10-7):

- Grade I Traction (Loosen). Traction that neutralizes pressure in the joint without actual separation of the joint surfaces. The purpose is to produce pain relief by reducing the compressive forces of articular surfaces during mobilization and is used with all mobilization grades.
- Grade II Traction (Tighten or "Take Up the Slack"). Traction that effectively separates the articulating surfaces and takes up the slack or eliminates play in the joint capsule. Grade II is used in initial treatment to determine joint sensitivity.
- Grade III Traction (Stretch). Traction that involves actual stretching of the soft tissue surrounding the joint to increase mobility in a hypomobile joint.

Grade I traction should be used in the initial treatment to reduce the chance of a painful reaction. It is recommended that 10-second intermittent Grades I and II traction be used, distracting the joint surfaces up to a Grade III traction and then releasing distraction until the joint returns to its resting position.

Kaltenborn emphasizes that Grade III traction should be used in conjunction with mobilization glides to treat joint hypomobility.[9] Grade III traction stretches the joint capsule and increases the space between the articulating surfaces, placing the joint in a

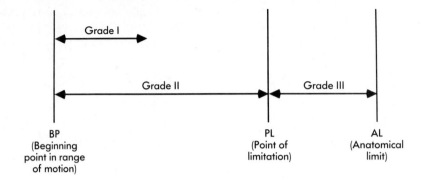

Fig. 10-7. Kaltenborn's grades of traction. *PL,* point of limitation; *AL,* anatomical limit.

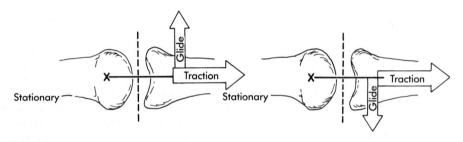

Fig. 10-8. Traction vs. glides. Traction should be perpendicular to the treatment plane, while glides are parallel to the treatment plane.

loose-packed position. Applying grade III and grade IV oscillations within the athlete's pain limitations should maximally improve joint mobility (Figure 10-8).

MOBILIZATION AND TRACTION TECHNIQUES

Figures 10-9 through 10-73 provide descriptions and illustrations of various mobilization and traction techniques.*

SUMMARY

1. Mobilization and traction techniques increase joint mobility or decrease pain by restoring accessory movements to the joint.
2. Physiological movements result from an active muscle contraction that moves an extremity through traditional cardinal planes.

*S = Stabilize, G = glide, T = traction, R = rotation.

3. Accessory motions refer to the manner in which one articulating joint surface moves relative to another.
4. Normal accessory component motions must occur for full-range physiological movement to take place.
5. Accessory motions are also referred to as *joint arthrokinematics,* which include spin, roll, and glide.
6. The Convex-Concave Rule states that if the concave joint surface is moving on the stationary convex surface, gliding will occur in the same direction as the rolling motion. Conversely, if the convex surface is moving on a stationary concave surface, gliding will occur in an opposite direction to rolling.
7. The resting position is one in which the joint capsule and the ligaments are most relaxed, allowing for a maximum amount of joint play.
8. The treatment plane falls perpendicular to a line running from the axis of rotation in the convex

Text continued on p. 163.

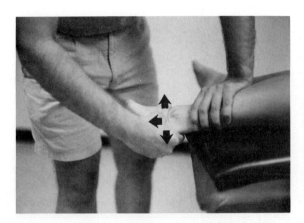

Fig. 10-9. Traction and mobilization. Traction and mobilization should be used together.

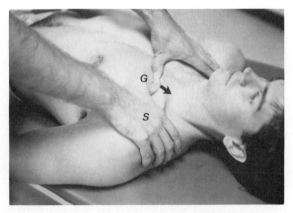

Fig. 10-10. Posterior and superior clavicular glides. When posterior or superior clavicular glides are done at the sternoclavicular joint, use the thumbs to glide the clavicle. Posterior glides are used to increase clavicular retraction, and superior glides increase clavicular retraction and clavicular depression.

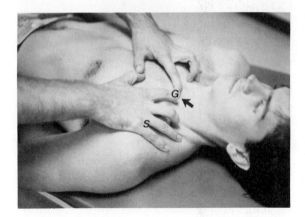

Fig. 10-11. Inferior clavicular glides. Inferior clavicular glides at the sternoclavicular joint use the index fingers to mobilize the clavicle, which increases clavicular elevation.

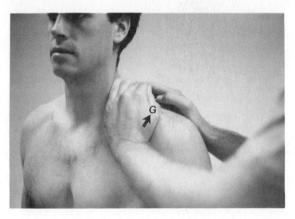

Fig. 10-12. Posterior clavicular glides. Posterior clavicular glides done at the acromioclavicular (AC) joint apply posterior pressure on the clavicle while stabilizing the scapula with the opposite hand. They increase mobility of the AC joint.

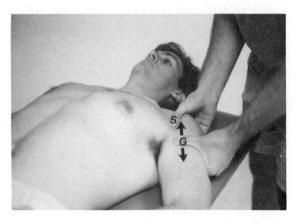

Fig. 10-13. Anterior/posterior glenohumeral glides.
Anterior/posterior glenohumeral glides are done with one
hand stabilizing the scapula, and the other gliding the
humeral head. They initiate motion in the painful shoulder.

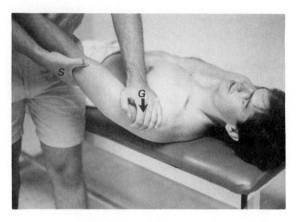

Fig. 10-14. Posterior humeral glides. Posterior humeral
glides use one hand to stabilize the humerus at the elbow
and the other to glide the humeral head. They increase
flexion and medial rotation.

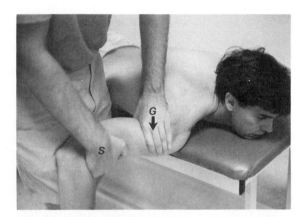

Fig. 10-15. Anterior humeral glides. In anterior humeral
glides the patient is prone. One hand stabilizes the humerus
at the elbow, and the other glides the humeral head. They
increase extension and lateral rotation.

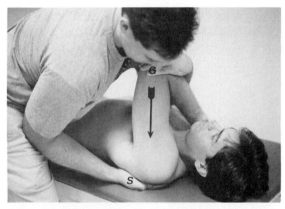

Fig. 10-16. Posterior humeral glides. Posterior humeral
glides may also be done with the shoulder at 90 degrees.
With the patient in supine position, one hand stabilizes the
scapula underneath while the patient's elbow is secured at
the sports therapist's shoulder. Glides are directed downward
through the humerus. They increase horizontal adduction.

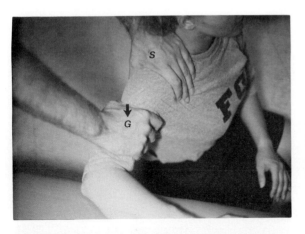

Fig. 10-17. Inferior humeral glides. For inferior humeral glides the patient is in the sitting position with the elbow resting on the treatment table. One hand stabilizes the scapula, and the other glides the humeral head inferiorly. These glides increase shoulder abduction.

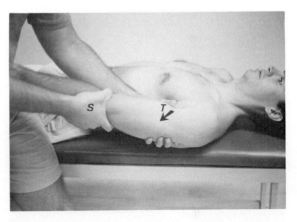

Fig. 10-18. Lateral glenohumeral joint traction. Lateral glenohumeral joint traction is used for initial testing of joint mobility and for decreasing pain. One hand stabilizes the elbow while the other applies lateral traction at the upper humerus.

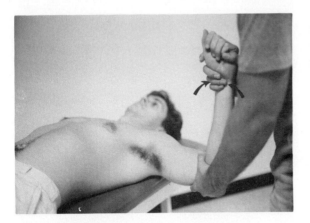

Fig. 10-19. Medial and lateral rotation oscillations. Medial and lateral rotation oscillations with the shoulder abducted at 90 degrees can increase medial and lateral rotation in a progressive manner according to patient tolerance.

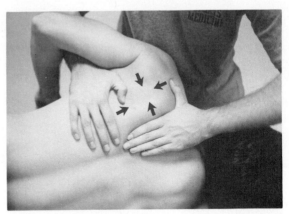

Fig. 10-20. General scapular glides. General scapular glides may be done in all directions, applying pressure at either the medial, inferior, lateral, or superior border of the scapula. Scapular glides increase general scapulothoracic mobility.

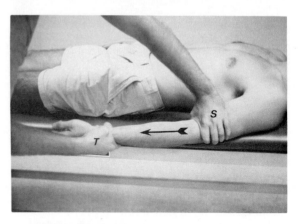

Fig. 10-21. Inferior humeroulnar glides. Inferior humeroulnar glides increase elbow flexion and extension. They are performed using the body weight to stabilize proximally with the hand grasping the ulna and gliding inferiorly.

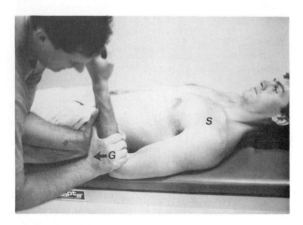

Fig. 10-22. Humeroradial inferior glides. Humeroradial inferior glides increase the joint space and improve flexion and extension. One hand stabilizes the humerus above the elbow; the other grasps the distal forearm and glides the radius inferiorly.

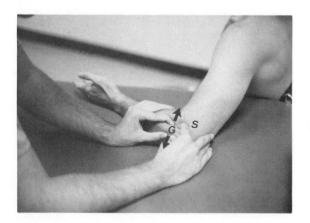

Fig. 10-23. Proximal anterior/posterior radial glides. Proximal anterior/posterior radial glides use the thumbs and index fingers to glide the radial head. Anterior glides increase flexion, while posterior glides increase extension.

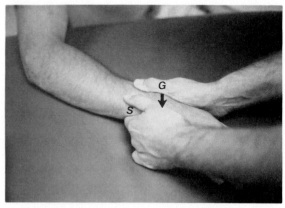

Fig. 10-24. Distal anterior/posterior radial glides. Distal anterior/posterior radial glides are done with one hand stabilizing the ulna and the other gliding the radius. These glides increase pronation.

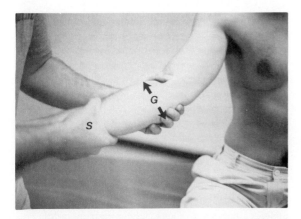

Fig. 10-25. Medial and lateral ulnar oscillations. Medial and lateral ulnar oscillations increase flexion and extension. Valgus and varus forces are used with a short lever arm.

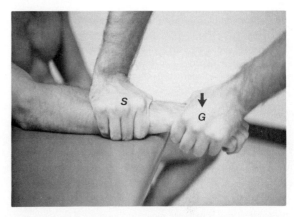

Fig. 10-26. Radiocarpal joint anterior glides. Radiocarpal joint anterior glides increase wrist extension.

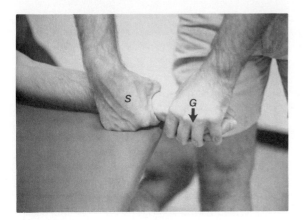

Fig. 10-27. Radiocarpal joint posterior glides. Radiocarpal joint posterior glides increase wrist flexion.

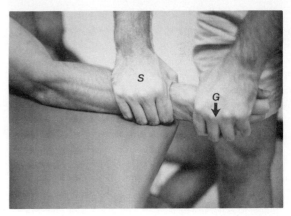

Fig. 10-28. Radiocarpal joint ulnar glides. Radiocarpal joint ulnar glides increase radial deviation.

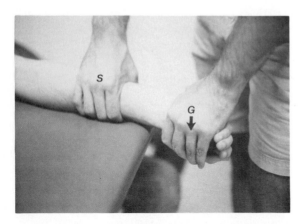

Fig. 10-29. Radiocarpal joint radial glides. Radiocarpal joint radial glides increase ulnar deviation.

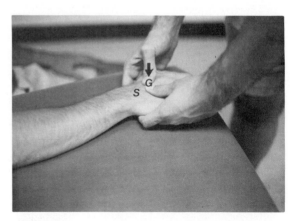

Fig. 10-30. Carpometacarpal joint anterior/posterior glides. Carpometacarpal joint anterior/posterior glides increase mobility of the hand.

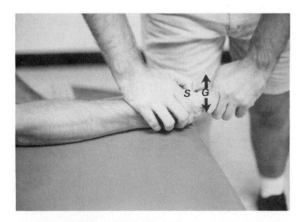

Fig. 10-31. Metacarpophalangeal joint anterior/posterior glides. In metacarpophalangeal joint anterior or posterior glides, the proximal segment, in this case the metacarpal, is stabilized and the distal segment is mobilized. Anterior glides increase flexion of the MP joint. Posterior glides increase extension.

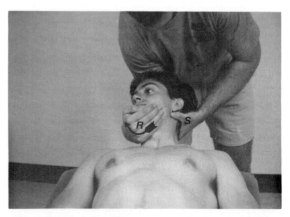

Fig. 10-32. Cervical vertebrae rotation oscillations. Cervical vertebrae rotation oscillations are done with one hand supporting the weight of the head and the other rotating the head in the direction of the restriction. These oscillations treat pain or stiffness when there is some resistance in the same direction as the rotation.

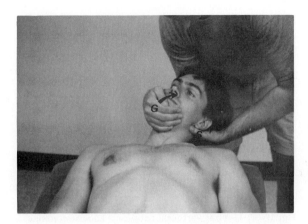

Fig. 10-33. Cervical vertebrae sidebending. Cervical vertebrae sidebending may be used to treat pain or stiffness with resistance when sidebending the neck.

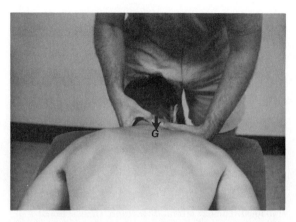

Fig. 10-34. Unilateral cervical facet anterior/posterior glides. Unilateral cervical facet anterior/posterior glides are done using pressure from the thumbs over individual facets. They increase rotation or flexion of the neck toward the side where the technique is used.

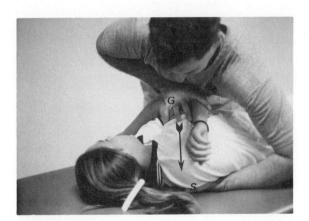

Fig. 10-35. Thoracic vertebral facet rotations. Thoracic vertebral facet rotations are accomplished with one hand underneath the patient providing stabilization and the weight of the body pressing downward through the rib cage to rotate an individual thoracic vertebrae. Rotation of the thoracic vertebrae is minimal, and most of the movement with this mobilization involves the rib facet joint.

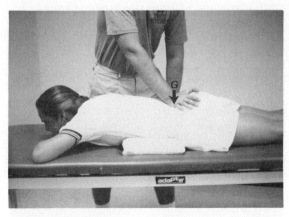

Fig. 10-36. Anterior/posterior lumbar vertebral glides. In the lumbar region, anterior/posterior lumbar vertebral glides may be accomplished at individual segments using pressure on the spinous process through the pisiform in the hand. These decrease pain or increase mobility of individual lumbar vertebrae.

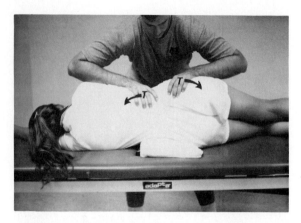

Fig. 10-37. Lumbar lateral distraction. Lumbar lateral distraction increases the space between transverse process and increases the opening of the intervertebral foramen. This position is achieved by lying over a support, flexing the patient's upper knee to a point where there is gapping in the appropriate spinal segment, then rotating the upper trunk to place the segment in a close-packed position. Then finger and forearm pressure are used to separate individual spaces. This pressure is used for reducing pain in the lumbar vertebrae associated with some compression of a spinal nerve.

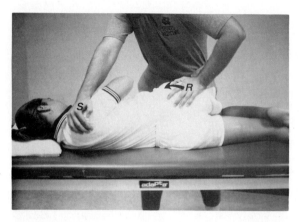

Fig. 10-38. Lumbar vertebral rotations. Lumbar vertebral rotations decrease pain and increase mobility in lumbar vertebrae. These rotations should be done in a sidelying position.

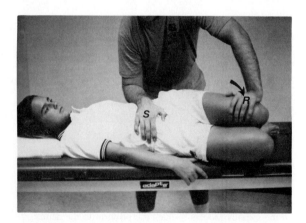

Fig. 10-39. Lateral lumbar rotations. Lateral lumbar rotations may be done with the patient in supine position. In this position, one hand must stabilize the upper trunk, while the other produces rotation.

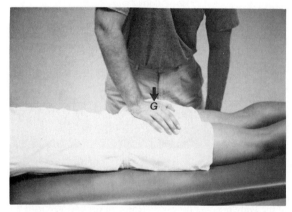

Fig. 10-40. Anterior sacral glides. Anterior sacral glides decrease pain and reduce muscle guarding around the sacroiliac joint.

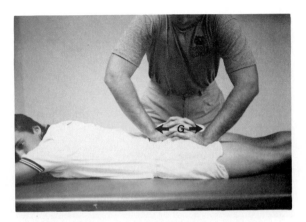

Fig. 10-41. Superior/inferior sacral glides. Superior/inferior sacral glides decrease pain and reduce muscle guarding around the sacroiliac joint.

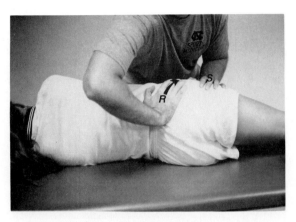

Fig. 10-42. Anterior innominate rotation. An anterior innominate rotation in a sidelying position is accomplished by extending the leg on the affected side then stabilizing with one hand on the front of the thigh while the other applies pressure anteriorly over the posterosuperior iliac spine to produce an anterior rotation. This technique will correct a unilateral posterior rotation.

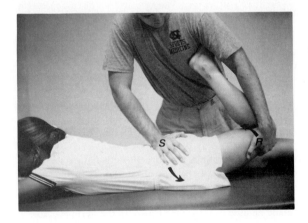

Fig. 10-43. Anterior innominate rotation. An anterior innominate rotation may also be accomplished by extending the hip, applying upward force on the upper thigh, and stabilizing over the posterosuperior iliac spine. This technique is once again used to correct a posterior unilateral innominate rotation.

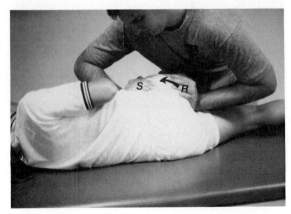

Fig. 10-44. Posterior innominate rotation. A posterior innominate rotation with the patient in sidelying position is done by flexing the hip, stabilizing the anterosuperior iliac spine, and applying pressure to the ischium in an anterior direction.

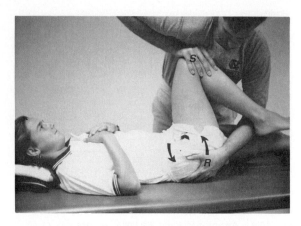

Fig. 10-45. Posterior innominate rotation. Another posterior innominate rotation with the hip flexed at 90 degrees stabilizes the knee and rotates the innominate anteriorly through upward pressure on the ischium.

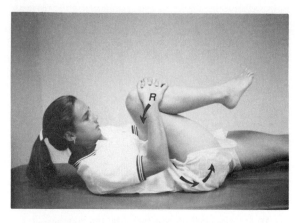

Fig. 10-46. Posterior innominate rotation self-mobilization (supine). Posterior innominate rotation may be easily accomplished using self-mobilization. In a supine position the patient grasps behind the flexed knee and gently rocks the innominate in a posterior direction.

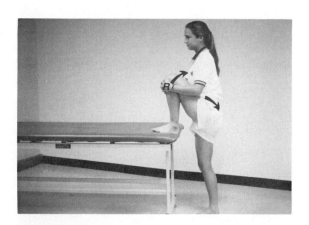

Fig. 10-47. Posterior rotation self-mobilization (standing). In a standing position the patient can perform a posterior rotation self-mobilization by pulling on the knee and rocking forward.

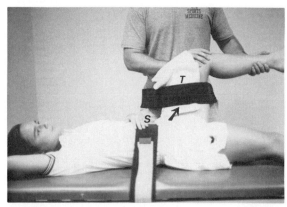

Fig. 10-48. Lateral hip traction. Since the hip is a very strong, stable joint, it may be necessary to use body weight to produce effective joint mobilization or traction. An example of this would be in lateral hip traction. One strap should be used to secure the patient to the treatment table. A second strap is secured around the patient's thigh and around the therapist's hips. Lateral traction is applied to the femur by leaning back away from the patient. This technique is used to reduce pain and increase hip mobility.

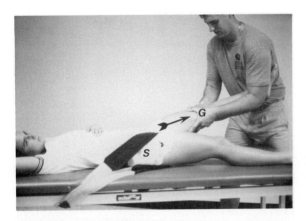

Fig. 10-49. Femoral traction. Femoral traction with the hip at 0 degrees reduces pain and increases hip mobility. Inferior femoral glides in this position should be used to increase flexion and abduction.

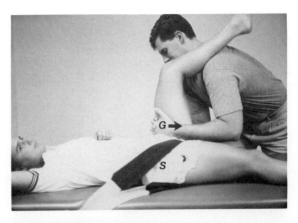

Fig. 10-50. Inferior femoral glides. Inferior femoral glides at 90 degrees of hip flexion may also be used to increase abduction and flexion.

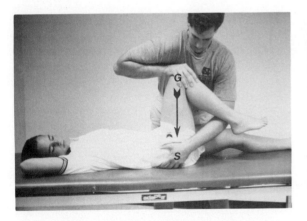

Fig. 10-51. Posterior femoral glides. With the patient supine, a posterior femoral glide can be done by stabilizing underneath the pelvis and using the body weight applied through the femur to glide posteriorly. Posterior glides are used to increase hip flexion.

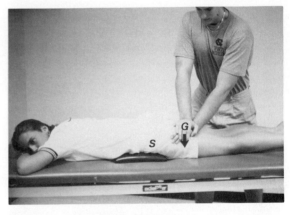

Fig. 10-52. Anterior femoral glides. Anterior femoral glides increase extension and are accomplished by using some support to stabilize under the pelvis and applying an anterior glide posteriorly on the femur.

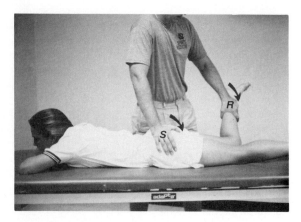

Fig. 10-53. Medial femoral rotations. Medial femoral rotations may be used for increasing medial rotation and are done by stabilizing the opposite innominate while internally rotating the hip through the flexed knee.

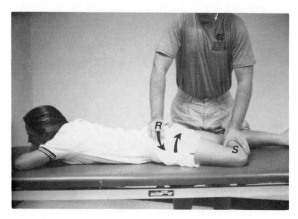

Fig. 10-54. Lateral femoral rotation. Lateral femoral rotation is done by stabilizing a bent knee in the figure 4 position and applying rotational force to the ischium. This technique increases lateral femoral rotation.

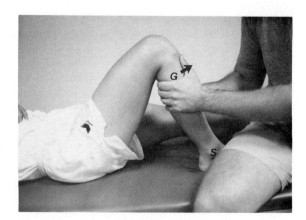

Fig. 10-55. Anterior tibial glides. Anterior tibial glides are appropriate for the patient lacking full extension. Anterior glides should be done in prone position with the femur stabilized. Pressure is applied to the posterior tibia to glide anteriorly.

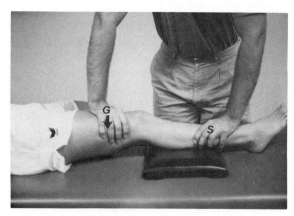

Fig. 10-56. Posterior femoral glides. Posterior femoral glides are appropriate for the patient lacking full extension. Posterior femoral glides should be done in supine position with the tibia stabilized. Pressure is applied to the anterior femur to glide posteriorly.

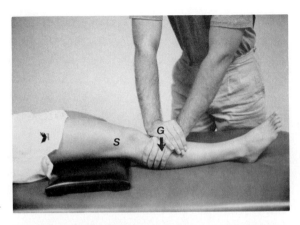

Fig. 10-57. Posterior tibial glides. Posterior tibial glides increase flexion. With the patient in supine position, stabilize the femur, and glide the tibia posteriorly.

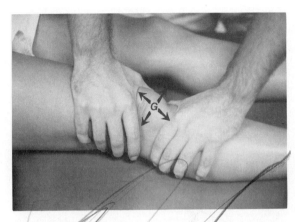

Fig. 10-58. Patellar glides. Superior patellar glides increase knee extension. Inferior glides increase knee flexion. Medial glides stretch the lateral retinaculum. Lateral glides stretch tight medial structures.

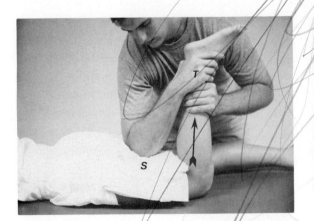

Fig. 10-59. Tibiofemoral joint traction. Tibiofemoral joint traction reduces pain and hypomobility. It may be done with the patient prone and the knee flexed at 90 degrees. The elbow should stabilize the thigh while traction is applied through the tibia.

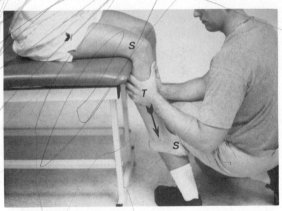

Fig. 10-60. Alternative techniques for tibiofemoral joint traction. In very large individuals an alternative technique for tibiofemoral joint traction uses body weight of the sports therapist to distract the joint once again for reducing pain and hypomobility.

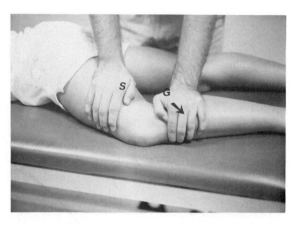

Fig. 10-61. Proximal anterior and posterior glides of the fibula. Anterior and posterior glides of the fibula may be done proximally. They increase mobility of the fibular head and reduce pain. The femur should be stabilized. With the knee slightly flexed, grasp the head of the femur, and glide it both anteriorly and posteriorly.

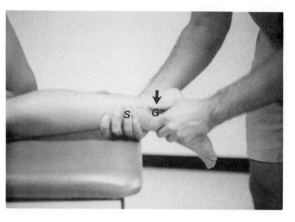

Fig. 10-62. Distal anterior and posterior fibular glides. Anterior and posterior glides of the fibula may be done distally. The tibia should be stabilized, and the fibular malleolus is mobilized in an anterior or posterior direction.

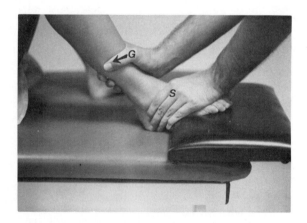

Fig. 10-63. Posterior tibial glides. Posterior tibial glides increase plantarflexion. The foot should be stabilized, and pressure on the anterior tibia produces a posterior glide.

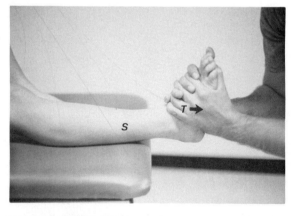

Fig. 10-64. Talocrural joint traction. Talocrural joint traction is performed using the patient's body weight to stabilize the lower leg and applying traction to the midtarsal portion of the foot. Traction reduces pain and increases dorsiflexion and plantarflexion.

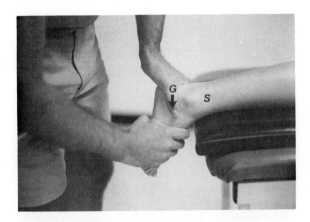

Fig. 10-65. Anterior talor glides. Plantarflexion may also be increased by using an anterior talar glide. With the patient prone the tibia is stabilized on the table, and pressure is applied to the posterior aspect of the talus to glide it anteriorly.

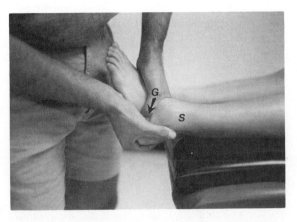

Fig. 10-66. Posterior talor glides. Posterior talar glides may be used for increasing dorsiflexion. With the patient supine the tibia is stabilized on the table, and pressure is applied to the anterior aspect of the talus to glide it posteriorly.

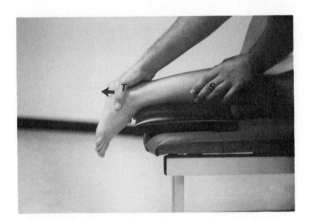

Fig. 10-67. Subtalor joint traction. Subtalar joint traction reduces pain and increases inversion and eversion. The lower leg is stabilized on the table, and traction is applied by grasping the posterior aspect of the calcaneus.

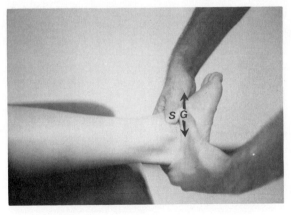

Fig. 10-68. Subtalor joint medial and lateral glides. Subtalar joint medial and lateral glides increase eversion and inversion. The talus must be stabilized while the calcaneus is mobilized medially to increase inversion and laterally to increase eversion.

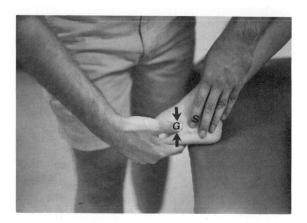

Fig. 10-69. Anterior/posterior calcaneocuboid glides.
Anterior/posterior calcaneocuboid glides may be used for increasing adduction and abduction. The calcaneus should be stabilized while the cuboid is mobilized.

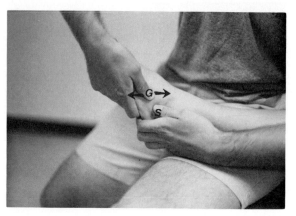

Fig. 10-70. Anterior/posterior cuboidmetatarsal glides.
Anterior/posterior cuboidmetatarsal glides are done with one hand stabilizing the cuboid and the other gliding the base of the fifth metatarsal. They are used for increasing mobility of the fifth metatarsal.

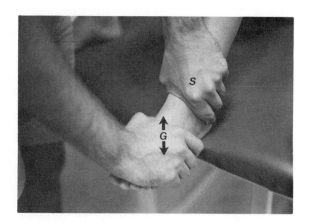

Fig. 10-71. Anterior/posterior carpometacarpal glides.
Anterior/posterior carpometacarpal glides decrease hypomobility of the metacarpals.

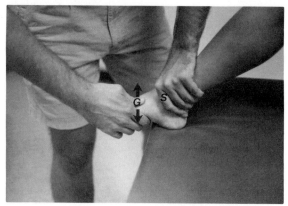

Fig. 10-72. Anterior/posterior talonavicular glides.
Anterior/posterior talonavicular glides also increase adduction and abduction. One hand stabilizes the talus while the other mobilizes the navicular bone.

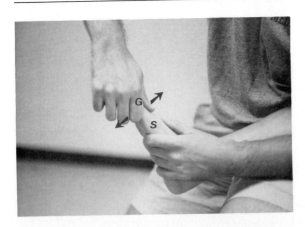

Fig. 10-73. Anterior/posterior metacarpophalangeal glides. With anterior/posterior metacarpophalangeal glides, the anterior glides increase extension, and posterior glides increase flexion. Mobilizations are accomplished by isolating individual segments.

surface to the center of the concave articular surface.

9. Maitland has proposed a series of five graded movements or oscillations in the range of motion to treat pain and stiffness.

10. Kaltenborn uses three grades of traction to reduce pain and stiffness.

11. Kaltenborn emphasizes that traction should be used in conjunction with mobilization glides to treat joint hypomobility.

REFERENCES

1 Barak T, Rosen E, Sofer R: Mobility: passive orthopedic manual therapy. In Gould J, Davies G, editors: *Orthopedic and sports physical therapy,* St Louis, 1990, Mosby.

2 Basmajian J: *Therapeutic exercise,* Baltimore, 1978, Williams & Wilkins.

3 Cookson J: Orthopedic manual therapy: an overview. II. The spine, *J Am Phys Ther Assoc* 59:259, 1979.

4 Cookson J, Kent B: Orthopedic manual therapy: an overview. I. The extremities, *J Am Phys Ther Assoc* 59:136, 1979.

5 Cyriax J: *Textbook of orthopedic medicine: treatment by manipulation, massage, and injection,* vol 2, Baltimore, 1974, Williams & Wilkins.

6 Donatelli R, Owens-Burkhart H: Effects of immobilization on the extensibility of periarticular connective tissue, *J Ortho Sports Phys Ther* 3:67, 1981.

7 Grimsby O: *Fundamentals of manual therapy: a course workbook,* Vagsbygd, Norway, 1981, Sorlandets Fysikalske Institutt.

8 Hollis M: *Practical exercise,* Oxford, 1981, Blackwell Scientific Publications.

9 Kaltenborn F: *Mobilization of the extremity joints: examination and basic treatment techniques,* Norway, 1980, Olaf Norlis Bokhandel.

10 Kisner C, Colby L: *Therapeutic exercise: foundations and techniques,* Philadelphia, 1985, FA Davis.

11 MacConaill M, Basmajian J: *Muscles and movements: a basis for kinesiology,* Baltimore, 1969, Williams & Wilkins.

12 Maigne R: *Orthopedic medicine,* Springfield, Ill, 1976, Charles C. Thomas.

13 Maitland G: *Extremity manipulation,* London, 1977, Butterworth Publications.

14 Maitland G: *Vertebral manipulation,* London, 1978, Butterworth Publications.

15 Mennell J: *Joint pain and diagnosis using manipulative techniques,* New York, 1964, Little, Brown.

16 Paris S: *The spine: course notebook,* Atlanta, 1979, Institute Press.

17 Paris S: Mobilization of the spine, *Phys Ther* 59:988, 1979.

18 Saunders D: *Evaluation, treatment and prevention of musculoskeletal disorders,* Bloomington, Minn, 1985, Educational Opportunities.

19 Schiotz E, Cyriax J: *Manipulation past and present,* London, 1978, Willian Heinemann Medical Books.

20 Stoddard A: *Manual of osteopathic practice,* London, 1969, Hutchinson Ross.

21 Taniqawa M: Comparison of the hold-relax procedure and passive mobilization on increasing muscle length, *Phys Ther* 52(7):725–735, 1972.

22 Wadsworth C: *Manual examination and treatment of the spine and extremities,* Baltimore, 1988, William & Wilkins.

23 Zohn D, Mennell J: *Musculoskeletal pain: diagnosis and physical treatment,* Boston, 1976, Little, Brown.

24 Zusman M: Reappraisal of a proposed neurophysiological mechanism for the relief of joint pain with passive joint movements, *Physiother Pract* 1:61–70, 1985.

Proprioceptive Neuromuscular Facilitation Techniques

11

William E. Prentice

OBJECTIVES

After completion of this chapter, the student should be able to do the following:

- Explain the neurophysiological basis of PNF techniques.

- Discuss the rationale for use of the techniques.

- Discuss the basic principles of using PNF in rehabilitation.

- Identify the various PNF strengthening and stretching techniques.

- Describe PNF patterns for the upper and lower extremity, for the upper and lower trunk, and for the neck.

Proprioceptive neuromuscular facilitation (PNF) is an approach to therapeutic exercise based on the principles of functional human anatomy and neurophysiology. It uses proprioceptive, cutaneous, and auditory input to produce functional improvement in motor output and can be a vital element in the rehabilitation process of many sports-related injuries. These techniques have been recommended for increasing strength, flexibility, and range of motion.* This discussion should guide the sports therapist using the principles and techniques of PNF as a component of a rehabilitation program.

THE NEUROPHYSIOLOGICAL BASIS OF PNF

The therapeutic techniques of PNF were first used in the treatment of patients with paralysis and neuromuscular disorders. Most of the principles underlying modern therapeutic exercise techniques can be attributed to the work of Sherrington,[19] who first

defined the concepts of facilitation and inhibition.

An impulse traveling down the corticospinal tract or an afferent impulse traveling up from peripheral receptors in the muscle causes an impulse volley, which results in the discharge of a limited number of specific motor neurons, as well as the discharge of additional surrounding (anatomically close) motor neurons in the subliminal fringe area. An impulse causing the recruitment and discharge of additional motor neurons within the subliminal fringe is said to be facilitory. Conversely, any stimulus that causes motor neurons to drop out of the discharge zone and away from the subliminal fringe is said to be inhibitory.[11] Facilitation results in increased excitability, and inhibition results in decreased excitability of motor neurons.[22] Thus the function of weak muscles would be aided by facilitation, and muscle spasticity would be decreased by inhibition.[8]

Sherrington attributed the impulses transmitted from the peripheral stretch receptors via the afferent system as being the strongest influence on the alpha motor neurons. Therefore the sports therapist should be able to modify the input from the peripheral re-

---

*References 7, 9, 12, 14, 15, 21.

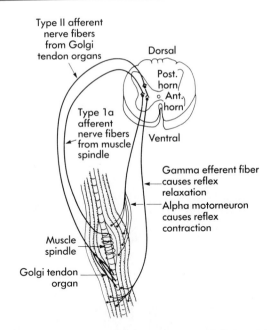

Fig. 11-1. Diagrammatical representation of the stretch reflex.

ceptors and thus influence the excitability of the alpha motor neurons. The discharge of motor neurons can be facilitated by peripheral stimulation, which causes afferent impulses to make contact with excitatory neurons and results in increased muscle tone or strength of voluntary contraction. Motor neurons can also be inhibited by peripheral stimulation, which causes afferent impulses to make contact with inhibitory neurons, thus resulting in muscle relaxation and allowing for stretching of the muscle.[19] To indicate any technique in which input from peripheral receptors is used to facilitate or inhibit, PNF should be used.[8]

The principles and techniques of PNF described here are based primarily on the neurophysiological mechanisms involving the stretch reflex. The **stretch reflex** involves two types of receptors: (1) muscle spindles that are sensitive to a change in length, as well as the rate of change in length of the muscle fiber, and (2) Golgi tendon organs that detect changes in tension (Figure 11-1).

Stretching a given muscle causes an increase in the frequency of impulses transmitted to the spinal cord from the muscle spindle, which in turn produces an increase in the frequency of motor nerve impulses returning to that same muscle, thus reflexively re-

sisting the stretch. However, the development of excessive tension within the muscle activates the Golgi tendon organs, whose sensory impulses are carried back to the spinal cord. These impulses have an inhibitory effect on the motor impulses returning to the muscles and thus cause that muscle to relax.

Two neurophysiological phenomena help to explain facilitation and inhibition of the neuromuscular systems. The first is known as *autogenic inhibition* and is defined as inhibition that is mediated by afferent fibers from a stretched muscle acting on the alpha motor neurons supplying that muscle, thus causing it to relax. When a muscle is stretched, motor neurons supplying that muscle receive both excitatory and inhibitory impulses from the receptors. If the stretch is continued for a slightly extended period of time, the inhibitory signals from the Golgi tendon organs eventually override the excitatory impulses and therefore cause relaxation. Because inhibitory motor neurons receive impulses from the Golgi tendon organs while the muscle spindle creates an initial reflex excitation leading to contraction, the Golgi tendon organs apparently send inhibitory impulses that last for the duration of increased tension (resulting from either passive stretch or active contraction) and eventually dominate the weaker impulses from the muscle spindle. This inhibition seems to protect the muscle against injury from reflex contractions resulting from excessive stretch.

A second mechanism known as *reciprocal inhibition* deals with the relationships of the agonist and antagonist muscles (Figure 11-2). The muscles that contract to produce joint motion are referred to as *agonists,* and the resulting movement is called an *agonistic pattern.* The muscles that stretch to allow the agonist pattern to occur are referred to as *antagonists.* Movement that occurs directly opposite to the agonist pattern is called the *antagonist pattern.*

When motor neurons of the agonist muscle receive excitatory impulses from afferent nerves, the motor neurons that supply the antagonist muscles are inhibited by afferent impulses.[2] Thus contraction or extended stretch of the agonist muscle must elicit relaxation or inhibit the antagonist. Likewise, a quick stretch of the antagonist muscle facilitates a contraction of the agonist. For facilitating or inhibiting motion, PNF relies heavily on the actions of these agonist and antagonist muscle groups.

A final point of clarification should be made regarding autogenic and reciprocal inhibition. The mo-

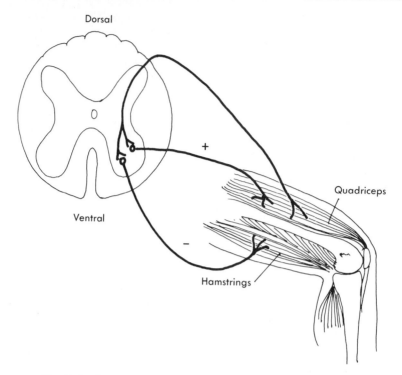

Dorsal

Ventral

Quadriceps

Hamstrings

Fig. 11-2. Diagrammatical representation of reciprocal inhibition.

tor neurons of the spinal cord always receive a combination of inhibitory and excitatory impulses from the afferent nerves. Whether these motor neurons will be excited or inhibited depends on the ratio of these incoming impulses.

Several different approaches to therapeutic exercise based on the principles of facilitation and inhibition have been proposed. Among these are the Bobath method,[3] Brunnstrom method,[4] Rood method,[18] and the Knott and Voss method,[10] which they called *proprioceptive neuromuscular facilitation*. Although each of these techniques is important and useful, the PNF approach of Knott and Voss probably makes the most explicit use of proprioceptive stimulation.[10]

Rationale for Use

As a positive approach to injury rehabilitation, PNF is aimed at what the patient can do physically within the limitations of the injury. It is perhaps best used to decrease deficiencies in strength, flexibility, and coordination in response to demands that are placed on the neuromuscular system.

The body tends to respond to the demands placed on it. The principles of PNF attempt to provide a maximal response for increasing strength, flexibility, and coordination. These principles should be applied with consideration of their appropriateness in achieving a particular goal. That continued activity during a rehabilitation program is essential for maintaining or improving strength or flexibility is well accepted. Therefore an intense program should offer the greatest potential for recovery.

The PNF approach is holistic, integrating sensory, motor, and psychological aspects of a rehabilitation program. It incorporates reflex activities from the spinal levels and upward, either inhibiting or facilitating them as appropriate.

The brain recognizes only gross joint movement and not individual muscle action. Moreover, the strength of a muscle contraction is directly proportional to the activated motor units. Therefore to increase the strength of a muscle, the maximum number of motor units must be stimulated to strengthen the remaining muscle fibers.[9,10] This "irradiation", or overflow effect, can occur when the stronger muscle groups help the weaker groups in completing a particular movement. This cooperation leads to the rehabilitation goal of return to optimal function.[2,10] The following principles of PNF should be applied to reach that ultimate goal.

Basic Principles of PNF

Margret Knott, in her text on PNF,[10] emphasized the importance of the principles rather than specific techniques in a rehabilitation program. These principles are the basis of PNF that must be superimposed on any specific technique. Application of the following principles may assist in promoting a desired response in the patient being treated.

1. The patient must be taught the PNF patterns regarding the sequential movements from starting position to terminal position. The sports therapist has to keep instructions brief and simple. The patterns should be used along with the techniques to increase the effects of the treatment.

2. When learning the patterns, the patient is often helped by looking at the moving limb. This visual stimulus offers the patient feedback for directional and positional control.

3. Verbal cues are used to coordinate voluntary effort with reflex responses. Commands should be firm and simple. Commands most commonly used with PNF techniques are "push" and "pull," which ask for an isotonic contraction; "hold," which implies an isometric contraction; and "relax."

4. Manual contact with appropriate pressure is essential for influencing direction of motion and facilitating a maximal response because reflex responses are greatly affected by pressure receptors. Manual contact should be firm and confident to give the patient a feeling of security. A movement response may be facilitated by the hand over the muscle being contracted to facilitate an increase in strength.

5. Proper mechanics and body positioning of the sports therapist are essential in applying pressure and resistance. The sports therapist should stand in a position that accommodates the diagonal movement pattern, with knees bent and close to the patient such that resistance can easily be applied throughout the range.

6. The amount of resistance given should facilitate a maximal response that allows smooth, coordinated motion. The appropriate resistance depends to a large extent on the capabilities of the patient. It may also change at different points throughout the range of motion. Maximal resistance may be used with those techniques that use isometric contractions to restrict motion to a specific point; it may also be used in isotonic contractions throughout a full range of movement.

7. Rotational movement is a critical component in all of the PNF patterns because maximal contraction is impossible without it.

8. Normal timing is the sequence of muscle contraction that occurs in any normal motor activity resulting in coordinated movement.[10] The distal movements of the patterns should occur first. The distal movement components should be completed by no later than halfway through the total PNF pattern. To accomplish this, appropriate verbal commands should be timed with manual commands. Normal timing may be used with maximal resistance or without resistance from the sports therapist.

9. Timing for emphasis is used primarily with isotonic contractions. This principle superimposes maximal resistance, at specific points in the range, upon the patterns of facilitation, allowing overflow or irradiation to the weaker components of a movement pattern. Thus the stronger components are emphasized to facilitate the weaker components of a movement pattern.

10. Specific joints may be facilitated by using **traction** or **approximation.** Traction spreads apart the joint articulations, and approximation presses them together. Both techniques stimulate the joint proprioceptors. Traction increases the muscular response, promotes movement, assists isotonic contractions, and is used with most flexion antigravity movements. Traction must be maintained throughout the pattern. Approximation increases the muscular response, promotes stability, assists isometric contractions, and is used most with extension (gravity-assisted) movements. Approximation may be quick or gradual and may be repeated during a pattern.

11. Giving a quick stretch to the muscle before muscle contraction facilitates a muscle to respond with greater force through the mechanisms of the stretch reflex. It is most effective

if all the components of a movement are stretched simultaneously. However, this quick stretch may be contraindicated in many orthopedic conditions because the extensibility limits of a damaged musculotendinous unit or joint structure may be exceeded, thus exacerbating the injury.

Techniques of PNF

Each of the principles described above should be applied to the specific techniques of PNF. These techniques may be used in a rehabilitation program either to strengthen or facilitate a particular agonistic muscle group or to stretch or inhibit the antagonistic group. The choice of a specific technique depends on the deficits of a particular patient. Specific techniques or combinations of techniques should be selected on the basis of the patient's problem.

STRENGTHENING TECHNIQUES. The following techniques are most appropriately used for the development of muscular strength, endurance, and coordination.

Repeated contraction is useful when a patient has weakness either at a specific point or throughout the entire range. It is used to correct imbalances that occur within the range by repeating the weakest portion of the total range. The patient moves isotonically against maximal resistance repeatedly until fatigue is evidenced in the weaker components of the motion. When fatigue of the weak components becomes apparent, a stretch at that point in the range should facilitate the weaker muscles and result in a smoother, more coordinated motion. Again, quick stretch may be contraindicated with some musculoskeletal injuries. The amount of resistance to motion given by the sports therapist should be modified to accommodate the strength of the muscle group. The patient is commanded to push by using the agonist concentrically and eccentrically throughout the range.

Slow reversal involves an isotonic contraction of the antagonist followed immediately by an isotonic contraction of the agonist. The initial contraction of the antagonist muscle group facilitates the succeeding contraction of the agonist muscles. The slow reversal technique can be used for developing active range of motion of the agonists and normal reciprocal timing between the antagonists and agonists, which is critical for normal coordinated motion. The patient should be commanded to push against maximal resistance by using the antagonist and then to pull by using the agonist. The initial antagonistic push facilitates the succeeding agonist contraction.

Slow reversal-hold is an isotonic contraction of the agonist followed immediately by an isometric contraction, with a hold command given at the end of each active movement. The direction of the pattern is reversed by using the same sequence of contraction with no relaxation before shifting to the antagonistic pattern. This technique can be especially useful in developing strength at a specific point in the range of motion.

Rhythmic stabilization uses an isometric contraction of the agonist, followed by an isometric contraction of the antagonist to produce cocontraction and stability of the two opposing muscle groups. The command given is always "hold," and movement is resisted in each direction. Rhythmic stabilization results in an increase in the holding power to a point where the position cannot be broken. Holding should emphasize cocontraction of agonists and antagonists.

The **rhythmic initiation** technique involves a progression of initial passive, then active-assistive, followed by active movement through the agonist pattern. Movement is slow, goes through the available range of motion, and avoids activation of a quick stretch. It is used for patients who are unable to initiate movement and who have a limited range of motion because of increased tone. It may also be used to teach the patient a movement pattern.

STRETCHING TECHNIQUES. The following techniques should be used to increase range of motion, relaxation, and inhibition.

Contract-relax is a stretching technique that moves the body part passively into the agonist pattern. The patient is instructed to push by contracting the antagonist (muscle that will be stretched) isotonically against the resistance of the sports therapist. The patient then relaxes the antagonist while the therapist moves the part passively through as much range as possible to the point where limitation is again felt. This contract-relax technique is beneficial when range of motion is limited by muscle tightness.

Hold-relax is very similar to the contract-relax technique. It begins with an isometric contraction of the antagonist (muscle that will be stretched) against resistance, followed by a concentric contraction of the agonist muscle combined with light pressure from the sports therapist to produce maximal stretch of the antagonist. This technique is appropriate muscle tension on one side of a joint and may be used with either the agonist or antagonist.

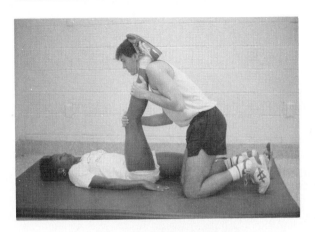

Fig. 11-3. PNF stretching technique.

Slow reversal-hold-relax technique begins with an isotonic contraction of the agonist, which often limits range of motion in the agonist pattern, followed by an isometric contraction of the antagonist (muscle that will be stretched) during the push phase. During the relax phase, the antagonists are relaxed while the agonists are contracting, causing movement in the direction of the agonist pattern and thus stretching the antagonist. The technique, like the contract-relax and hold-relax, is useful for increasing range of motion when the primary limiting factor is the antagonistic muscle group.

Because the goal of rehabilitation in most sports-related injuries is restoration of strength through a full, nonrestricted range of motion, several of these techniques are sometimes combined in sequence to accomplish this goal. Figure 11-3 shows a PNF stretching technique in which the sports therapist is stretching the injured athlete.

PNF PATTERNS. The PNF patterns are concerned with gross movement as opposed to specific muscle actions. The techniques identified previously may be superimposed on any of the PNF patterns. The techniques of PNF are composed of both rotational and diagonal exercise patterns that are similar to the motions required in most sports and in normal daily activities.

The exercise patterns are three component movements: flexion-extension, abduction-adduction, and internal-external rotation. Human movement is patterned and rarely involves straight motion because all muscles are spiral in nature and lie in diagonal directions.

The PNF patterns described by Knott and Voss[10] involve distinct diagonal and rotational movements of the upper extremity, lower extremity, upper trunk, lower trunk, and neck. The exercise pattern is initiated with the muscle groups in the lengthened or stretched position. The muscle group is then contracted, moving the body part through the range of motion to a shortened position.

The upper and lower extremities each have two separate patterns of diagonal movement for each part of the body, which are referred to as the *diagonal 1 (D1)* and *diagonal 2 (D2) patterns.* These diagonal patterns are subdivided into D1 moving into flexion, D1 moving into extension, D2 moving into flexion, and D2 moving into extension. Figures 11-4 and 11-5 diagram the PNF patterns for the upper and lower extremities respectively. The patterns are named according to the proximal pivots at either the shoulder or the hip (for example, the glenohumeral joint or femoralacetabular joint).

Tables 11-1 and 11-2 describe specific movements in the D1 and D2 patterns for the upper extremities. Figures 11-6 through 11-13 show starting and terminal positions for each of the diagonal patterns in the upper extremity.

Tables 11-3 and 11-4 describe specific movements in the D1 and D2 patterns for the lower extremities. Figures 11-14 through 11-21 show the starting and terminal positions for each of the diagonal patterns in the lower extremity.

Table 11-5 describes the rotational movement of the upper trunk moving into extension (also called **chopping**) and moving into flexion (also called **lifting**). Figures 11-22 and 11-23 show the starting and terminal positions of the upper extremity chopping pattern moving into flexion to the right. Figures 11-24 and 11-25 show the starting and terminal positions for the upper extremity lifting pattern moving into extension to the right.

Table 11-6 describes rotational movement of the lower extremities moving into positions of flexion and extension. Figures 11-26 and 11-27 show the lower extremity pattern moving into flexion to the left. Figures 11-28 and 11-29 show the lower extremity pattern moving into extension to the left.

The neck patterns involve simply flexion and rotation to one side (Figures 11-30 and 11-31) with extension and rotation to the opposite side (Figures 11-32 and 11-33). The patient should follow the direction of the movement with the eyes.

The principles and techniques of PNF, when used

Text continued on p. 179.

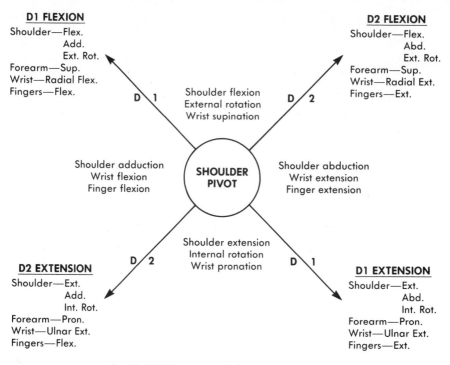

Fig. 11-4. PNF patterns of the upper extremity.

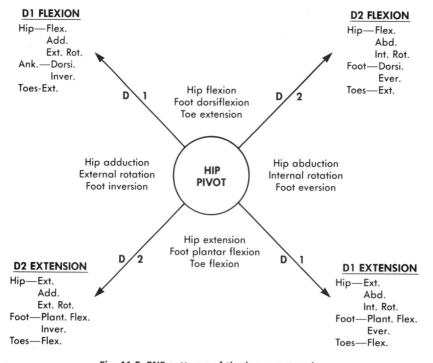

Fig. 11-5. PNF patterns of the lower extremity.

TABLE 11-1
D1 Upper Extremity Movement Patterns

Body Part	Moving into Flexion		Moving into Extension	
	Starting Position (Figure 11-6)	Terminal Position (Figure 11-7)	Starting Position (Figure 11-8)	Terminal Position (Figure 11-9)
Shoulder	Extended Abducted Internally rotated	Flexed Adducted Externally rotated	Flexed Adducted Externally rotated	Extended Abducted Internally rotated
Scapula	Depressed Retracted Downwardly rotated	Flexed Protracted Upwardly rotated	Elevated Protracted Upwardly rotated	Depressed Retracted Downwardly rotated
Forearm	Pronated	Supinated	Supinated	Pronated
Wrist	Ulnar extended	Radially flexed	Radially flexed	Ulnar extended
Finger and thumb	Extended Abducted	Flexed Adducted	Flexed Adducted	Extended Abducted
Hand position for sports therapist*	Left and inside volar surface of hand Right hand underneath arm in cubital fossa of elbow		Left hand on back of elbow on humerus Right hand on dorsum of hand	
Verbal command	Pull		Push	

*For athlete's right arm.

TABLE 11-2
D2 Upper Extremity Movement Patterns

Body Part	Moving into Flexion		Moving into Extension	
	Starting Position (Figure 11-10)	Terminal Position (Figure 11-11)	Starting Position (Figure 11-12)	Terminal Position (Figure 11-13)
Shoulder	Extended Adducted Internally rotated	Flexed Abducted Externally rotated	Flexed Abducted Externally rotated	Extended Adducted Internally rotated
Scapula	Depressed Protracted Downwardly rotated	Elevated Retracted Upwardly rotated	Elevated Retracted Upwardly rotated	Depressed Protracted Downwardly rotated
Forearm	Pronated	Supinated	Supinated	Pronated
Wrist	Ulnar flexed	Radially extended	Radially extended	Ulnar flexed
Finger and thumb	Flexed Adducted	Extended Abducted	Extended Abducted	Flexed Adducted
Hand position for sports therapist*	Left hand on back of humerus Right hand on dorsum of hand		Left hand on volar surface of humerus Right hand on cubital fossa of elbow	
Verbal command	Push		Pull	

*For athlete's right arm.

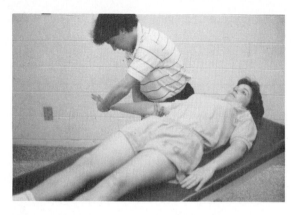

Fig. 11-6. D1 upper extremity movement pattern moving into flexion. Starting position.

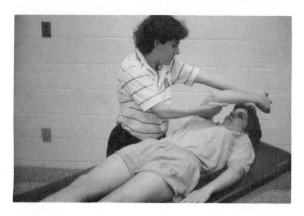

Fig. 11-7. D1 upper extremity movement pattern moving into flexion. Terminal position.

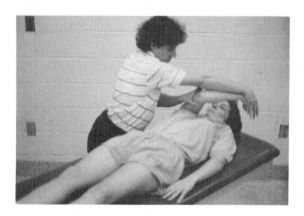

Fig. 11-8. D1 upper extremity movement pattern moving into extension. Starting position.

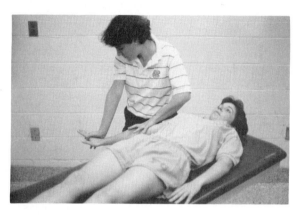

Fig. 11-9. D1 upper extremity movement pattern moving into extension. Terminal position.

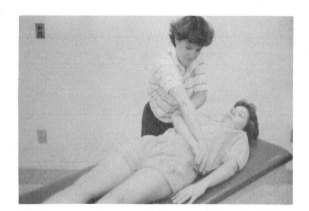

Fig. 11-10. D2 upper extremity movement pattern moving into flexion. Starting position.

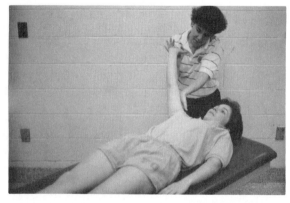

Fig. 11-11. D2 upper extremity movement pattern moving into flexion. Terminal position.

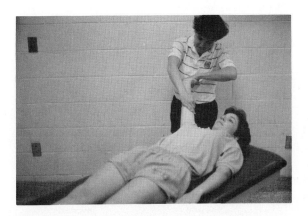

Fig. 11-12. D2 upper extremity movement pattern moving into extension. Starting position.

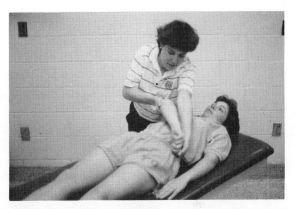

Fig. 11-13. D2 upper extremity movement pattern moving into extension. Terminal position.

TABLE 11-3
D1 Lower Extremity Movement Patterns

Body Part	Moving into Flexion		Moving into Extension	
	Starting Position (Figure 11-14)	Terminal Position (Figure 11-15)	Starting Position (Figure 11-16)	Terminal Position (Figure 11-17)
Hip	Extended Abducted Internally rotated	Flexed Adducted Externally rotated	Flexed Adducted Externally rotated	Extended Abducted Internally rotated
Knee	Extended	Flexed	Flexed	Extended
Position of tibia	Externally rotated	Internally rotated	Internally rotated	Externally rotated
Ankle and foot	Plantar flexed Everted	Dorsiflexed Inverted	Dorsiflexed Inverted	Plantar flexed Everted
Toes	Flexed	Extended	Extended	Flexed
Hand position for sports therapist*	Right hand on dorsimedial surface of foot Left hand on anteromedial thigh near patella		Right hand on lateralplantar surface of foot Left hand on posteriolateral thigh near popliteal crease	
Verbal command	Pull		Push	

*For athlete's right leg.

TABLE 11-4
D2 Lower Extremity Movement Patterns

Body Part	Moving into Flexion		Moving into Extension	
	Starting Position (Figure 11-18)	Terminal Position (Figure 11-19)	Starting Position (Figure 11-20)	Terminal Position (Figure 11-21)
Hip	Extended Adducted Externally rotated	Flexed Abducted Internally rotated	Flexed Abducted Internally rotated	Extended Adducted Externally rotated
Knee	Extended	Flexed	Flexed	Extended
Position of tibia	Externally rotated	Internally rotated	Internally rotated	Externally rotated
Ankle and foot	Plantar flexed Inverted	Dorsiflexed Everted	Dorsiflexed Everted	Plantar flexed Inverted
Toes	Flexed	Extended	Extended	Flexed
Hand position for sports therapist*	Right hand on dorsilateral surface of foot Left hand on anterolateral thigh near patella		Right hand on medialplantar surface of foot Left hand on posteriomedial thigh near popliteal crease	
Verbal command	Pull		Push	

*For athlete's right leg.

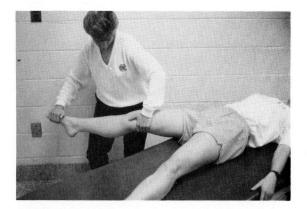

Fig. 11-14. D1 lower extremity movement pattern moving into flexion. Starting position.

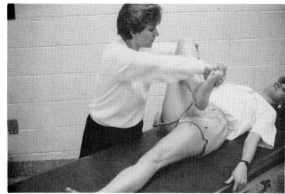

Fig. 11-15. D1 lower extremity movement pattern moving into flexion. Terminal position.

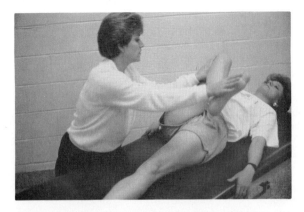

Fig. 11-16. D1 lower extremity movement pattern moving into extension. Starting position.

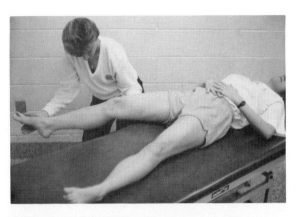

Fig. 11-17. D1 lower extremity movement pattern moving into extension. Terminal position.

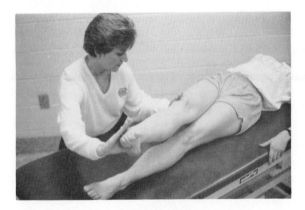

Fig. 11-18. D2 lower extremity movement pattern moving into flexion. Starting position.

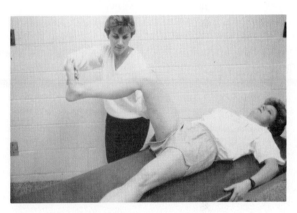

Fig. 11-19. D2 lower extremity movement pattern moving into flexion. Terminal position.

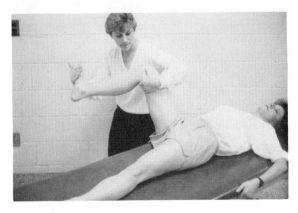

Fig. 11-20. D2 lower extremity movement pattern moving into extension. Starting position.

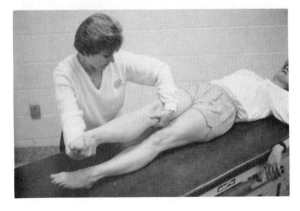

Fig. 11-21. D2 lower extremity movement pattern moving into extension. Terminal position.

TABLE 11-5
Upper Trunk Movement Patterns

| Body Part | Moving into Extension (Chopping)* | | Moving into Flexion (Lifting)* | |
	Starting Position (Figure 11-22)	Terminal Position (Figure 11-23)	Starting Position (Figure 11-24)	Terminal Position (Figure 11-25)
Right upper extremity	Flexed Adducted Internally rotated	Extended Abducted Externally rotated	Extended Adducted Internally rotated	Flexed Abducted Externally rotated
Left upper extremity (left hand grasps right forearm)	Flexed Abducted Externally rotated	Extended Adducted Internally rotated	Extended Abducted Externally rotated	Flexed Adducted Internally rotated
Trunk	Rotated and extended to left	Rotated and flexed to right	Rotated and flexed to left	Rotated and extended to right
Head	Rotated and extended to left	Rotated and flexed to right	Rotated and flexed to left	Rotated and extended to right
Hand position of sports therapist	Left hand on right anterolateral surface of forehead Right hand on dorsum of right hand		Right hand on dorsum of right hand Left hand on posteriolateral surface of head	
Verbal command	Pull down		Push up	

*Athletes rotation is to the right.

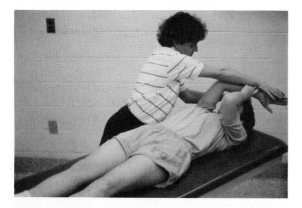

Fig. 11-22. Upper trunk pattern moving into extension or chopping. Starting position.

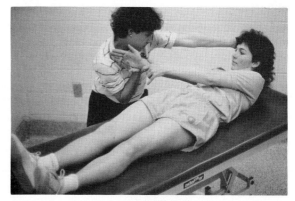

Fig. 11-23. Upper trunk pattern moving into extension or chopping. Terminal position.

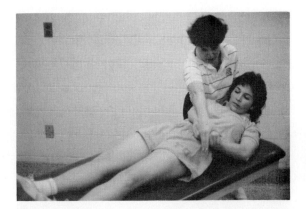

Fig. 11-24. Upper trunk pattern moving into flexion or lifting. Starting position.

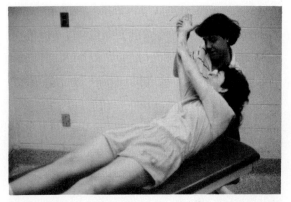

Fig. 11-25. Upper trunk pattern moving into flexion or lifting. Terminal position.

TABLE 11-6
Lower Trunk Movement Patterns

Body Part	Moving into Flexion*		Moving into Extension†	
	Starting Position (Figure 11-26)	Terminal Position (Figure 11-27)	Starting Position (Figure 11-28)	Terminal Position (Figure 11-29)
Right hip	Extended Abducted Externally rotated	Flexed Adducted Internally rotated	Flexed Adducted Internally rotated	Extended Abducted Externally rotated
Left hip	Extended Adducted Internally rotated	Flexed Abducted Externally rotated	Flexed Abducted Externally rotated	Extended Adducted Internally rotated
Ankles	Plantar flexed	Dorsiflexed	Dorsiflexed	Plantar flexed
Toes	Flexed	Extended	Extended	Flexed
Hand position of sports therapist	Right hand on dorsum of feet Left hand on anterolateral surface of left knee		Right hand on plantar surface of foot Left hand on posteriolateral surface of right knee	
Verbal command	Pull up and in		Push down and out	

*Athlete's rotation is to the left in flexion.
†Athlete's rotation is to the right in extension.

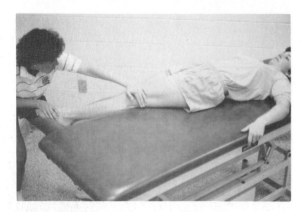

Fig. 11-26. Lower trunk pattern moving into flexion to the left. Starting position.

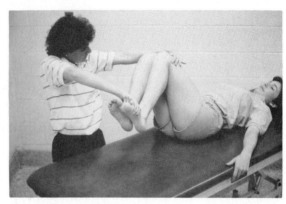

Fig. 11-27. Lower trunk pattern moving into flexion to the left. Terminal position.

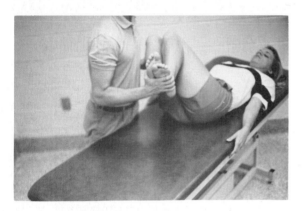

Fig. 11-28. Lower trunk pattern moving into extension to the left. Starting position.

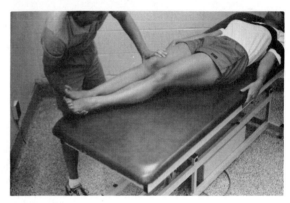

Fig. 11-29. Lower trunk pattern moving into extension to the left. Terminal position.

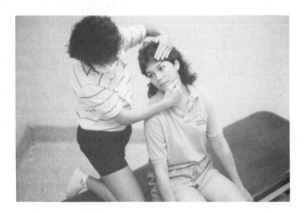

Fig. 11-30. Neck flexion and rotation to the left. Starting position.

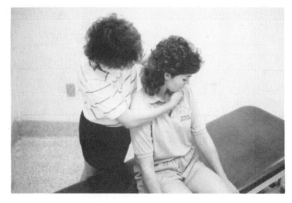

Fig. 11-31. Neck flexion and rotation to the left. Terminal position.

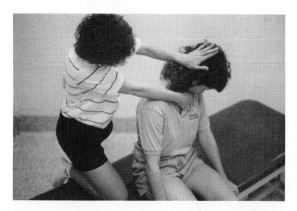

Fig. 11-32. Neck extension and rotation to the right.
Starting position.

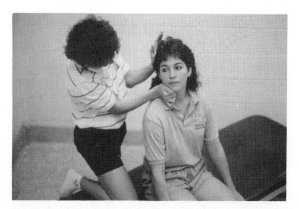

Fig. 11-33. Neck extension and rotation to the right.
Terminal position.

appropriately with specific patterns, can be an extremely effective tool for rehabilitation of sports-related injuries.[20] They may be used to strengthen weak muscles or muscle groups and to improve the range of motion about an injured joint. Specific techniques selected for use should depend on individual patient needs and may be modified accordingly.[5,6]

SUMMARY

1. The PNF techniques may be used to increase both strength and range of motion and are based on the neurophysiology of the stretch reflex.
2. The motor neurons of the spinal cord always receive a combination of inhibitory and excitatory impulses from the afferent nerves. Whether these motor neurons will be excited or inhibited depends on the ratio of the two types of incoming impulses.
3. The PNF techniques emphasize specific principles that may be superimposed on any of the specific techniques.
4. The PNF strengthening techniques include repeated contraction, slow-reversal, slow-reversal hold, rhythmic stabilization, and rhythmic initiation.
5. The PNF stretching techniques include contract-relax, hold-relax, and slow-reversal-hold-relax.
6. The techniques of PNF are rotational and diagonal movements in the upper extremity, lower extremity, upper trunk, and the head and neck.

REFERENCES

1 Barak T, Rosen E, Sofer R: Mobility: passive orthopedic manual therapy. In Gould J, Davies G, editors: *Orthopedic and sports physical therapy,* St Louis, 1985, Mosby.
2 Basmajian J: *Therapeutic exercise,* Baltimore, 1978, Williams & Wilkins.
3 Bobath B: The treatment of motor disorders of pyramidal and extrapyramidal tracts by reflex inhibition and by facilitation of movement, *Physiotherapy* 41:146, 1955.
4 Brunnstrom S: *Movement therapy in hemiplegia,* New York, 1970, Harper & Row.
5 Cookson J: Orthopedic manual therapy: an overview. II. The spine, *J Am Phys Ther Assoc* 59:259, 1979.
6 Cookson J, Kent B: Orthopedic manual therapy: an overview. I. The extremities. *J Am Phys Ther Assoc* 59:136, 1979.
7 Cornelius W, Jackson A: The effects of cryotherapy and PNF on hip extension flexibility, *Athletic Training* 19(3):184, 1984.
8 Harris F: Facilitation techniques and therapeutic exercise. In Basmajian J, editor: *Therapeutic exercise,* Baltimore, 1978, Williams & Wilkins.
9 Hollis M: *Practical exercise,* Oxford, 1981, Blackwell Scientific Publications.
10 Knott M, Voss D: *Proprioceptive neuromuscular facilitation: patterns and techniques,* New York, 1968, Harper & Row.
11 Lloyd D: Facilitation and inhibition of spinal motorneurons, *J Neurophysiol* 9:421, 1946.
12 Markos P: Ipsilateral and contralateral effects of proprioceptive neuromuscular facilitation techniques on hip motion and electromyographic activity, *Phys Ther* 59(11)P:1366-1373, 1979.
13 Osternig L, Robertson R, Troxel R, et al.: Differential responses to proprioceptive neuromuscular facilitation stretch techniques, *Med Sci Sports Exerc* 22:106-111, 1990.
14 Prentice W: An electromyographic analysis of heat and cold and stretching for inducing muscular relaxation, *J Orthop Sports Phys Ther* 3:133-140, 1982.

15 Prentice W: A comparison of static stretching and PNF stretching for improving hip joint flexibility, *Athletic Training* 18(1):56-59, 1983.

16 Prentice W: A manual resistance technique for strengthening tibial rotation, *Athletic Training* 23(3):230-233, 1988.

17 Prentice W, Kooima E: The use of proprioceptive neuromuscular facilitation techniques in the rehabilitation of sport-related injuries, *Athletic Training* 21:26-31, 1986.

18 Rood M: Neurophysiologic reactions as a basis of physical therapy, *Phys Ther Rev* 34:444, 1954.

19 Sherrington C: *The integrative action of the nervous system,* New Haven, 1947, Yale University Press.

20 Surberg P: Neuromuscular facilitation techniques in sportsmedicine, *Phys Ther Rev* 34:444, 1954.

21 Taniqawa M: Comparison of the hold-relax procedure and passive mobilization on increasing muscle length, *Phys Ther* 52(7):725-735, 1972.

22 Zohn D, Mennell J: *Musculoskeletal pain: diagnosis and physical treatment,* Boston, 1976, Little, Brown.

Functional Progression in Rehabilitation

12

Michael McGee

OBJECTIVES

After completion of this chapter, the student should be able to do the following:

- Define a functional progression.

- Indicate the proper position for a functional progression in the rehabilitation process.

- Identify and describe the physical benefits associated with a functional progression.

- Identify and describe the psychological benefits associated with functional progression.

- Identify and describe the disadvantages associated with a functional progression.

- Describe the components of a functional progression.

- Develop a functional progression for an athlete.

In the athletic community, injuries and subsequent disability frequently occur. Disabilities can be described as restrictive influences that "disease and injury exert upon neuromotor performances."[10] Thus, in an effort to reduce the lasting effects of injury, the sports therapist should direct rehabilitation toward improving neuromuscular coordination and agility, not simply to increasing strength and endurance. If rehabilitation is directed toward regaining range of motion, flexibility, strength, endurance, and perhaps primarily to increasing coordination and agility, a full return to activity is possible. However, if the program simply provides a means for the reduction of signs and symptoms associated with the injury, the athlete will not return to a safe and effective level of activity.[17] As a result, rehabilitation of athletic injuries needs to focus on the full preinjury fitness of the athlete.

ROLE OF FUNCTIONAL PROGRESSIONS IN REHABILITATION

Sports therapists must adapt rehabilitation to the sport-specific demands required by each sport and playing position. Rehabilitation conducted in a clinical setting cannot predict the effectiveness of the injured part to endure the imposed demands of full competition. For example, a solid, high-velocity tackle cannot be simulated in the clinical setting. The role of the functional progression is to improve and complete the clinical rehabilitation. A functional progression is a succession of activities that simulate actual motor and sport skills, enabling the athlete to acquire or reacquire the skills needed to perform athletic endeavors safely and effectively. The sports therapist takes the activities involved in a given sport and breaks them down into individual components. In this way the athlete concentrates on individual parts of the game or activity in a controlled environment before combining them together in an uncontrolled environment such as full competition. The functional progression places stresses and forces on each body system in a well-planned, positive, and progressive fashion, ultimately improving the athlete's overall ability to meet the demands placed upon him or her in daily activities, as well as in sports competition. The functional progression is indicated since tissues not placed under performance-level stresses do not adapt to the sudden return of such stresses with the resumption of full activity. Thus the functional progression is integrated into the normal rehabilitation scheme as one component of exercise therapy rather than replacing traditional rehabilitation altogether.[10]

Generally, rehabilitation of sports-related injuries has two goals: minimizing additional trauma to injured structures and safely and quickly returning injured athletes to prior levels of competition. The second rehabilitation goal is divided into three main stages: immediate, short-term, and long-term goals. The immediate goal stage begins at the time of injury and involves the treatment or management of the injury. This includes protection from further injury, restricted activity, and controls to minimize pain and swelling. The short-term goal stage deals with the healing process, enabling the symptoms and level of dysfunction to subside. Also during this stage, uninvolved body parts can be exercised to maintain normal function and fitness levels. The long-term goal stage overlaps the short-term goal stage and progresses to a point of full return to activity. Once the athlete meets criteria to return to controlled activity, exercise therapy is begun. The functional progression serves as a component of exercise therapy to help the athlete meet the preset criteria for return to play.

BENEFITS OF USING FUNCTIONAL PROGRESSIONS

Functional progressions provide physcial and psychological benefits to the injured athlete. Strength, endurance, mobility, flexibility, relaxation, coordination, and skill can be restored. At the same time the functional stability of the joint can be assessed, providing the physical benefits. Psychologically, the progression can reduce the feelings of anxiety, apprehension, and deprivation commonly observed in the injured athlete.

Muscular Strength

Increased strength is a physical benefit of the functional progression. Strength is the ability of the muscle to produce tension or apply force maximally against resistance and occurs statically or dynamically, in relation to the imposed demands. Strength increases are possible if the load imposed on a muscle

maximizes that muscle's capabilities to adapt during exercise. This is commonly referred to as the *overload principle* and is possible because of motor unit recruitment and muscle fiber hypertrophy.[11] To see these improvements, the muscle must be worked to the point of fatigue with either high or low resistance. The functional progression will develop strength using the SAID principle (specific adaptation to imposed demands). The muscles involved will be strengthened dynamically, under similar stresses encountered with competition.

Muscular Endurance

Muscular endurance, as well as cardiorespiratory endurance, can be enhanced with functional progression. Endurance is necessary for long duration activity whether it involves daily living or repeated motor functions found with sports participation. The functional progression will enhance muscular endurance through repetition of individual activities and by combining them into one general activity. The progression provides an environment for improving muscular strength and endurance without using more than one program. Cardiorespiratory endurance can be improved because of the repetition of motion found with the progression in the same way regular fitness levels improve with continuous exercise.

Flexibility

With injury, tissues will shorten or tighten in response to immobilization, which can inhibit proper function. With a functional progression, the injured area is stressed within a controlled range. This stress is significant enough to allow the tissue to elongate, thus returning to proper length. This improved mobility and flexibility is crucial to the athlete. Strength and endurance do not mean much if the injured body part cannot move through a full range of motion. Tissues also become stronger with consistent stresses, so tissues other than muscle can be improved with the functional progression.[11]

Muscle Relaxation

Relaxation involves the concerted effort to reduce muscle tension. The functional progression can teach an individual to recognize this tension and eventually how to control or remove it by consciously relaxing the muscles after exercise. This functional progression aids in total body relaxation and relaxing the injured area and may help relieve muscle guarding that inhibits the joint's full range of motion.[11]

Motor Skills

Coordination, agility, and motor skills are complex aspects of normal function requiring appropriate contraction at the most opportune time and with the appropriate intensity.[11] An athlete needs coordination, agility, and motor skills to transform strength, flexibility, and endurance into full-speed performance. This is especially important for an injured athlete. If he or she does not regain or improve coordination and agility, their performance is hampered and may in itself lead to further injury. Repetition and practice are important to learning motor skills. Regular motions that are consciously controlled develop into automatic reactions via motor learning. This control is possible because of the constant repetition and reinforcements of a particular skill.[11] To acquire these automatic reactions, one needs an intact and functional neuromuscular system. This system is disturbed with injury, therefore decreases in performance will occur, leading to injury susceptibility. The functional progression can be used to minimize the loss of normal neuromuscular control by providing exercises that stress proprioception, motor-skill integration, and proper timing. The functional progression is indicated for this improvement in agility and skill because of the constant repetition of sport-specific motor skills, use of sensory cues, and progressive increases in activity level. These are all components or general principles for enhancing coordination.[11] The practice variability seen with the functional progression allows athletes to relearn the various aspects of their sport that they may encounter in competition.

Traditional exercise programs cannot retrain the athlete to meet the demands of the sport because they lack the coordination and agility portion of the rehabilitation process. Increases in strength, endurance, and flexibility are definitely needed for safe and effective return to play, but without the neuromuscular coordination to integrate these aspects into proper function, little performance enhancement can occur. For this reason, functional progressions should become an integral part of the long-term rehabilitation stage so that each athlete receives every opportunity to get back in the game with preinjury status restored as much as possible.

Functional Stability

All of these factors combine to provide the athlete with physical benefits that will lead to the safe restoration of athletic ability. The functional progression not only helps with this restoration but also with the assessment of joint stability. The main concern of any rehabilitation program is whether the athlete can compete safely and effectively.[10] This concern constitutes the concept of functional stability as proposed by Noyes et al.[15] Functional stability is provided by (1) passive restraints of the ligaments, (2) joint geometry, (3) active restraints generated by muscles, and (4) joint compressive forces that occur with activity and force the joint together.[10] This stability is not always detectable by clinical examination. Therefore the functional progression can be used to evaluate the functional stability of athletes objectively and subjectively. Do they complete all tasks with no adverse effects? Do they appear to perform in the same or close to the same manner as before injury?

PSYCHOLOGICAL AND SOCIAL CONSIDERATIONS

Functional progressions can also provide psychological benefits to the athlete. Anxiety, apprehension, and deprivation are all common emotions found with injuries. The functional progression can aid the rehabilitation and the return to play by lessening these emotional restraints.

Anxiety

Uncertainty about the future is a prevalent reason many athletes give for their feelings of anxiety. Insecurity of this type is based on the vague understanding many athletes have of the severity of their injury and the length of time it will take for them to fully recover.[10] The progression can lessen anxiety since the athlete is gradually placed into progressively demanding situations. This progression allows the athlete to experience success and not be concerned as much with failure in the future.

Deprivation

The athlete may experience feelings of deprivation after being away from direct contact with his or her team and coaches for an extended period of time. The functional progression can limit deprivation

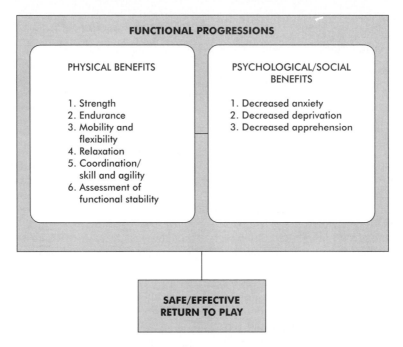

Fig. 12-1. Physical and psychological benefits of using functional progressions.

since the athlete can exercise during regular team practice times at the practice site. By providing some activity that can be completed during practice, the athlete remains close proximally and socially and feels little loss in team cohesion.[10]

Apprehension

Apprehension is often listed as an obstacle to performance and many times serves as a precursor to reinjury.[10] Functional progressions enable athletes to adapt to the imposed demands of their sports in a controlled environment, helping to restore confidence and thus decreasing apprehension. Each success builds on past success, allowing the athlete to feel in control and able to return to full activity.

Figure 12-1 provides a listing of all the benefits found with functional progressions. These benefits combine to allow the safe and effective return to play that all athletes and sports therapists desire.

COMPONENTS OF A FUNCTIONAL PROGRESSION: EXTERNAL CONSIDERATIONS

To provide a safe and effective return to play with the use of functional progressions, a variety of com-ponents should be addressed. First, what are the physician's expectations for the athlete's return to activity? Second, what are the athlete's expectations for his or her return to activity? Third, what is the total disability of the athlete? And fourth, what are the parameters of physical fitness for this athlete? Keeping the total well-being of the injured athlete in perspective is a significant concern.[19]

Activity Considerations

Exercise can be viewed from two perspectives. One is the single activity that comprises simple motor skills. The second involves the training and conditioning found with repetitive action.[8] Both definitions will apply to therapeutic exercise. Preinjury status can be regained only if similar activities with appropriate intensities are used to train and condition the athlete. To supply the athlete with these activities, four principles must be observed. First, individuality of the athlete, sport, and condition must be addressed. Second, the activities should be positive, not negative. No increased signs and symptoms should occur. Third, an orderly stair-step program should be used. And fourth, the program should be varied to avoid monotony.[11] Steps to minimize monotony include the following:

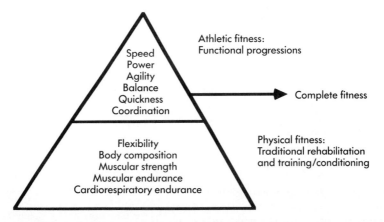

Fig. 12-2. Combining components of physical fitness with components of athletic fitness in functional progressions.

1. Vary exercise techniques used
2. Alter the program at regular intervals
3. Maintain fitness base to avoid reinjury with return to play
4. Set achievable goals; reevaluate and modify regularly
5. Use clinical, home, and on-the-field programs to vary activity.[11]

Traditional rehabilitation cannot meet these demands alone. Therefore functional therapeutic exercises, or more appropriately functional progressions, are used.

Athletes are continually exposed to situations that make reinjury likely; therefore every effort should be made to understand and incorporate the inherent demands of the sport into the rehabilitation program. With this in mind, the sports therapist can emphasize the importance of sport-specific activities to enhance the athlete's return to activity rather than simply concentrating on traditional rehabilitation methods involving only weight machines and analgesics. The components of rehabilitation are listed in Figure 12-2. As one can see, there are two distinct entities with which to work. The physical fitness items used in traditional rehabilitation should be merged with the athletic fitness items of functional progressions to give the athlete the best possible means of achieving preinjury status.

The components of a functional progression should aim to incorporate all the factors listed in Figure 12-2 under athletic fitness items. To meet this aim, certain steps should be followed.

Demand of the Sport

First, for proper program implementation, there should be a complete analysis of the demands placed on the athlete and the injured body part once return to play is achieved. After this step, all tasks involved in the activity should be placed on a continuum from easy to difficult. Primary concerns should include the intention of the activity, what activities should be included, and in what order the activities should occur.[8] For example, if throwing a baseball is the purpose, the action can be broken into an ordered sequence:

1. Grip the ball
2. Stance
3. Backswing of the upper limb
4. Forward swing of the upper limb
5. Release of the ball
6. Follow through[8]

Next, the sports therapist makes regular evaluation of the injured body part. This evaluation enables the sports therapist to assess the present functional status of the injury and to guide the progression safely.[10]

Factors Influencing Rehabilitation Goals

Along this same line, there are various considerations that may influence the rehabilitation goals.

1. What is the type of sport, and what position will be played? What demands will these place on the injury?
2. How much time is there remaining in the

season? An athlete at the end of the season has less time for full recovery to return to play. A decision has to be made as to whether the athlete realistically will return that season. All postseason play must be taken into account.

3. What other sports is the athlete involved in, and are they more important? For example, a sports therapist should not risk reinjury by hurrying a mediocre football player's rehabilitation and take the chance of having him miss basketball season when he has a chance to excel in basketball.

4. The sports therapist needs to know about injury rules pertaining to that sport. Can the athlete play with a splint, or does he or she need padding?

5. What is the psyche of the athlete? The sports therapist needs to measure the athlete's motivation, cooperation, compliance, competitiveness, and especially the individual's pain threshold.

6. Most importantly, the sports therapist needs to concentrate on the type of injury and type of rehabilitation. There is no "cookbook program" that is going to work well for each athlete. General treatment goals may be similar for a given injury, but the specific program has to be based on the goals of the individual athlete, the healing constraints, the extent of injury, progress to date, the athlete's tolerance to the program, and readiness to progress.[14] These factors not only affect rehabilitation, but should also be used to choose appropriate activities for the progression.

Program Evaluation

The progression should also be evaluated at regular intervals. This evaluation will allow the sports therapist to curtail any activity that results in immediate instability, pain, swelling, or patient anxiety in favor of less aggressive activities. The sports therapist can also use this evaluation to gauge the individual's progress. Completion of a certain skill in the progression occurs when the skill can be completed at functional speed with high repetitions with no associated increase in pain, swelling, or decreased range of motion. The sports therapist and athlete should realize that setbacks will occur and are common. Sometimes it takes two steps forward and one step back to achieve the needed level of improvement.

UPPER EXTREMITY PROGRESSION

1-Functional activity can begin early with assisted PNF techniques
2-Rubber tubing exercises simulating PNF patterns or sports motions
3-Swimming
4-Push-ups
5-Sports drills:
 -Interval Throwing Program
 45 foot phase

Step 1:	**Step 2:**
1-warm-up throwing	1-warm-up throwing
2-25 throws	2-25 throws
3-15 minute rest	3-rest 10 minutes
4-warm-up throwing	4-warm-up throwing
5-25 throws	5-25 throws
	6-rest 10 minutes
	7-warm-up throwing
	8-25 throws

Repeat steps 1 and 2 for 60, 90, 120, 150, and 180 feet, until full throwing from the mound or respective position is achieved.

Full Return to Play

Allowing the athlete to return to play at full participation is a difficult task. The decision requires a complete evaluation of the athlete's condition, including objective observations and subjective evaluation. The sports therapist should feel that the athlete is ready both physically and mentally before allowing a return to play.[6] Return to activity should not be attempted too soon to avoid exacerbation of the injury, which may interfere with healing and result in longer, more painful recovery or perhaps reinjury.[5] In a sports-medicine setting, the injured athlete is rarely completely healed when he or she returns to full competition. Hence the athlete is certainly susceptible to further injury. To release an athlete, a few criteria should be met:

1. Physician's release
2. Free of pain
3. No swelling
4. Normal range of motion
5. Normal strength (in reference to opposite extremity)
6. Appropriate functional testing completed with no adverse reactions.

TABLE 12-1
Interval Golf Rehabilitation Program

Day 1	Day 2	Day 3
WEEK 1:		
5 foot chipping/ putting	5 foot chipping/ putting	5 foot chipping/ putting
5 foot rest	5 foot rest	5 foot rest
5 foot chipping	5 foot chipping	5 foot chipping
	5 foot rest	5 foot rest
	5 foot chipping	5 foot chipping
WEEK 2:		
10 foot chipping	10 foot chipping	10 foot short iron
10 foot rest	10 foot rest	10 foot rest
10 foot short iron	10 foot short iron	10 foot short iron
	10 foot rest	10 foot rest
	10 foot short iron	10 foot short iron
WEEK 3:		
10 foot short iron	10 foot short iron	10 foot short iron
10 foot rest	10 foot rest	10 foot rest
10 foot long iron	10 foot long iron	10 foot long iron
10 foot rest	10 foot rest	10 foot rest
10 foot long iron	10 foot long iron	10 foot long iron
WEEK 4:		
Repeat week 3, day 2	Play 9 holes	Play 18 holes

TABLE 12-2
Interval Tennis Program

Day 1	Day 2	Day 3
WEEK 1:		
12 FH	15 FH	15 FH
8 BH	8 BH	10 BH
10 min rest	10 min rest	10 min rest
13 FH	15 FH	15 FH
7 BH	7 BH	10 BH
WEEK 2:		
25 FH	30 FH	30 FH
15 BH	20 BH	25 BH
10 min rest	10 min rest	10 min rest
25 FH	30 FH	30 FH
15 BH	20 BH	15 BH
		10 OH
WEEK 3:		
30 FH	30 FH	30 FH
25 BH	25 BH	30 BH
10 OH	15 OH	15 OH
10 min rest	10 min rest	10 min rest
30 FH	30 FH	30 FH
25 BH	25 BH	15 OH
10 OH	15 OH	10 min rest
		30 FH
		30 BH
		15 OH
WEEK 4:		
30 FH	30 FH	30 FH
30 BH	30 BH	30 BH
10 OH	10 OH	10 OH
10 min rest	10 min rest	10 min rest
Play 3 games	Play set	Play 1.5 sets
10 FH	10 FH	10 FH
10 BH	10 BH	10 BH
5 OH	5 OH	5 OH

Key—*FH* = Forehand, *BH* = backhand, *OH* = overhead.

EXAMPLES OF FUNCTIONAL PROGRESSIONS
The Upper Extremity

Now that the benefits and components of a functional progression have been addressed, some examples of functional progression activities are warranted. Functional activities that will enhance the healing and performance of the upper extremity might include PNF patterns, swimming (land or in water), or using pulley machines or rubber tubing to simulate sport activity (see Figure 12-16).[6] Specifically, to rehabilitate the throwing shoulder, a gradual progression to actual throwing should occur. First, a proper warm-up must be instructed and completed. Before the actual throwing exercise, the athlete must complete steps mimicking the motion with low stresses. The athlete can start with the techniques mentioned above. The progression will then flow into gradations of throwing, as indicated in the box on p. 186. Table 12-1 provides an example of a functional progression for hitting a golf ball, and Table 12-2 provides a program for return to hitting a tennis ball. Any upper extremity injury can benefit from one of these programs or can be exercised in similar fashion using any sports equipment needed.[2]

The Lower Extremity

The lower extremity follows the same basic pattern with different exercises. The activities used should provide a functional stress to the injured limb. The progression for the lower extremity is found in the box on p. 188.

Text continued on p. 192.

LOWER EXTREMITY FUNCTIONAL PROGRESSION

1-Functional Activity can begin early in the rehabilitation process with:
- -Assisted PNF techniques
- -Cycling
- -Nonweight bearing (NWB)-BAPS board or tilt board exercises
- -Partial-weight bearing (PWB)-BAPS board or tilt board exercises
- -Full-weight bearing (FWB)-BAPS board or tilt board exercise (Figure 12-3, *A* and *B*)
- -Walking
  - Normal
  - Heel
  - Side step/shuffle slides (Figure 12-4)

2-Lunges:
- -90 degree pivot (Figure 12-5)
- -180 degree pivot (Figure 12-6)

3-Step-ups:
- -Forward step-up 50%-75% max speed (Figure 12-7, *A*)
- -Lateral step-up 50%-75% max speed (Figure 12-7, *B*)

4-Jogging:
- -Straight-aways on track; walk in turns (Goal = 2 miles)
- -100 yards S course 50%-75% max speed (Figure 12-8)
- -100 yards figure 8 course 50%-75% max speed (Figure 12-9)
- -100 yards Z course 50%-75% max speed (Figure 12-10)
- -Side step/shuffle slides

5-Running:
- -Straight-aways on track; jog in turns (Goal = 2 miles)
- -Complete oval of track (Goal = 2-4 miles)

- -100 yards S course 75%-100% max speed with gradual increase in number of curves
- -100 yards figure 8 course 75%-100% max speed with gradual decrease in size of figure 8 to fit 5-10 yards
- -100 yards Z course 75%-100% max speed with gradual increase in number of Zs
- -Side step/shuffle slides

6-Lunges:
- -90 degree pivot with weight or increased speed
- -180 degree pivot with weight or increased speed

7-Sprints:
- -10 yards × 10
- -20 yards × 10
- -40 yards × 10
- -Acceleration/deceleration; 50 yards × 10 (Figure 12-11)
- -W sprints × 10 (Figure 12-12)

8-Box runs: (Figure 12-13)
- -5 yards clockwise/counterclockwise × 10

9-Carioca: (Figure 12-14, *A* and *B*)
- -30 yards × 5 right lead-off; 30 yards × 5 left lead-off

10-Jumping (Figure 12-15)
- -Rope
- -Lines
- -Boxes, balls, etc.

11-Hopping:
- -Two feet
- -One foot
- -Alternate

12-Cutting, jumping, hopping on command

13-Sports drills used for preseason or inseason practice

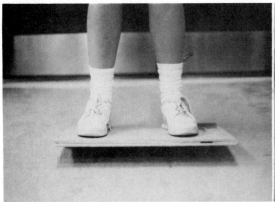 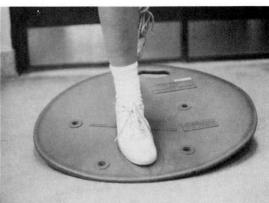

B

Fig. 12-3. Board exercises. A, Tilt board exercise. **B,** BAPS board exercise.

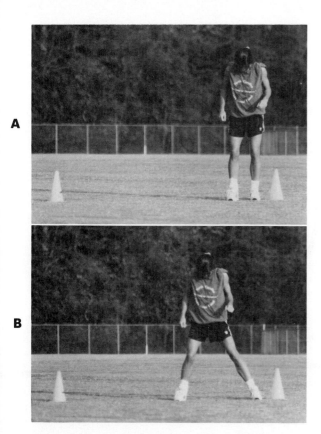

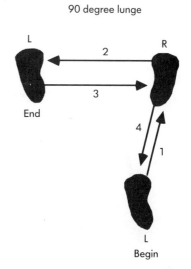

90 degree lunge

Fig. 12-4. Shuffle slides. A, Starting position. **B,** Finish position.

Fig. 12-5. 90 degree pivot. The athlete pushes off with the left foot, landing on the right foot directly in front, then steps immediately laterally landing on the left foot, then back laterally in the opposite direction landing on the right foot, then backwards onto the left foot.

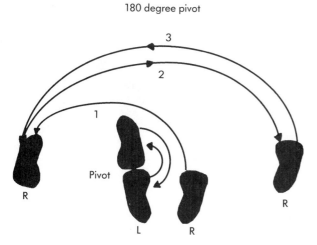

180 degree pivot

Fig. 12-6. 180 degree pivot. The athlete pushes off the right foot, pivoting on the left, thus rotating the body 180 degrees, landing on the right foot. Then pushing off the right foot, the body pivots on the left foot 180 degrees in the other direction, landing on the right foot.

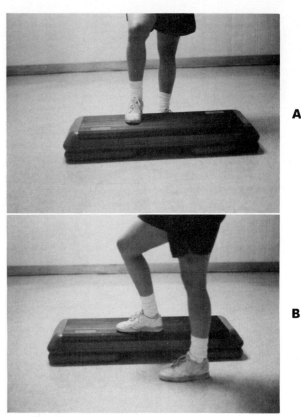

Fig. 12-7. Step-ups. The athlete steps **A,** forward or **B,** laterally onto a step.

"S" curve course

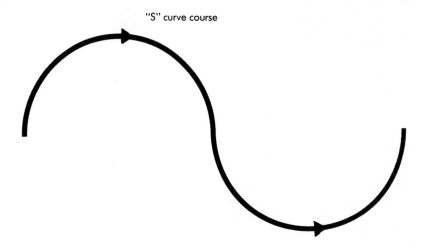

Fig. 12-8. S Curve. The athlete runs a set distance in a curving S pattern rather than straight ahead.

Figure "8" course

"Z" course (zig-zag)

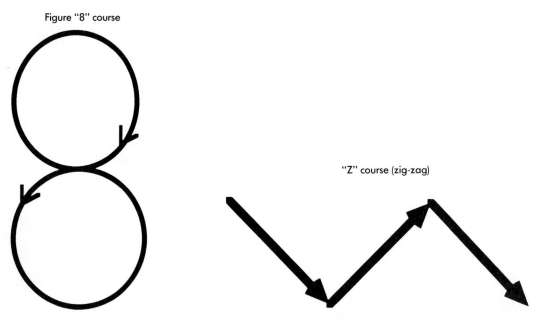

Fig. 12-9. Figure 8. The athlete walks, jogs, or runs a figure 8 pattern around cones or markers.

Fig. 12-10. Z course. The athlete runs a zig-zag course to emphasize sharp cutting motions and quick controlled directional changes.

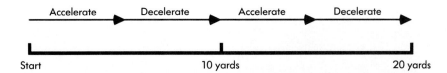

Fig. 12-11. Acceleration/deceleration. The athlete accelerates to a maximum then decelerates almost to a stop, then repeats this within a relatively short distance.

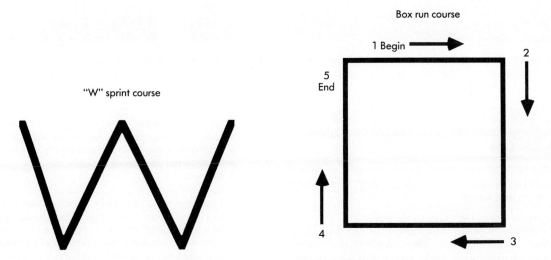

Fig. 12-12. W sprints. The athlete sprints forward to the first marker, then back pedals to the second, then forward to the third and so on.

Fig. 12-13. Box runs. Running both clockwise and counterclockwise, the athlete runs around four markers set in a box shape concentrating on abrupt directional changes at each corner.

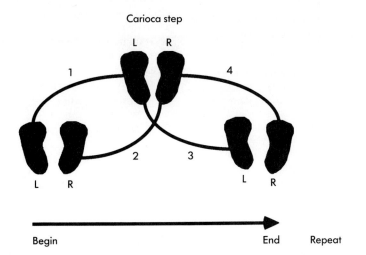

Fig. 12-14. Carioca. The athlete side steps onto the right foot, then steps across with the left foot in front of the right, then steps back onto the right foot, then the left foot steps across in back of the right, then back onto the right and so on.

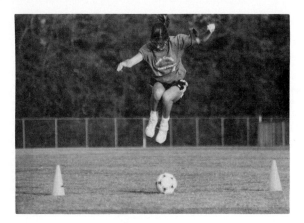

Fig. 12-15. Timed exercise. The athlete jumps side to side over a ball or other obstacle in a timed exercise.

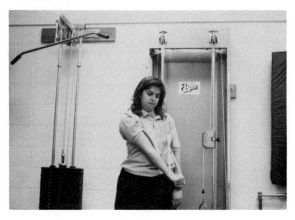

Fig. 12-16. Functional strengthening of upper extremity. Surgical tubing, THERABAND, or wall pulleys may be used in a D2 pattern for this activity.

Applying Functional Progressions to a Sport-Specific Case

The following case study is an example of how a functional progression may be applied to a specific sport-related injury:

Subject: 20-year-old female soccer player

History: Sustained ACL rupture of left knee while performing a cutting motion in practice. ACL reconstruction using an intraarticular patellar tendon graft was performed.

Rehabilitation for first 2 months was conducted both at home and in clinical setting. Emphasis of program concentrated on increasing range of motion and decreasing pain and swelling with some minor considerations to improving strength. At 2 months after surgery, athlete returned to school.

At this time, the rehabilitation protocol consisted of emphasizing general physical fitness, strengthening via traditional rehabilitation means and strength testing, and improving range of motion.

At approximately 3 months after surgery a functional progression was initiated. The progression included the following activities an average of three times per week:

- Walking
- PNF techniques using extremity D-1 and D-2 patterns
- Jogging on track with walking of curves
- Jogging full track
- Running on track with jogging of curves
- Running full track

This progression occupied the majority of the next 4 months coupled with traditional rehabilitation techniques to increase strength and maintain range of motion. At 7 months the progression intensified to a five-day-a-week program including the following:

- Running for fitness—²⁄₃ miles three times per week

- Lunges—90 degree, pivot, 180 degree
- Sprints—W, triangle, 6 second, 20, 40, and 120 yards
- Acceleration/deceleration runs (see Figure 12-12)
- Shuffle slides progressing to shuffle run
- Caricoca
- Ball work—turn/stop the pass, turn/mark opponent, mark/steal/shoot the ball, two-touch and shoot, one-touch and shoot, volley and shoot, passing, pass/knock/move, light drill work at practice, one vs. one, scrimmage (begin with short period and progress to full game), full active participation.

FUNCTIONAL TESTING

There are many ways to functionally test an athlete. The most common and often the simplest ways include timed performance. For the upper extremity, a throwing velocity test is often used. This test can be accomplished two ways, depending on the sports therapist's budget and availability of complex testing tools.

1. Test velocity in a controlled environment, preferably indoors, to decrease effects of the weather.
2. Set up a standard pitching distance (60 feet 6 inches).
3. Have athlete use a wind-up motion.
4. Maximum of five throws measured in mph with calibrated Magnum X ban radar gun (CMI Corporation, Owensburg, KY) placed 36 inches high and to the right of the catcher.
5. Compute mean of five throws, and compare to pretest value.

Many sports therapists may not have access to such

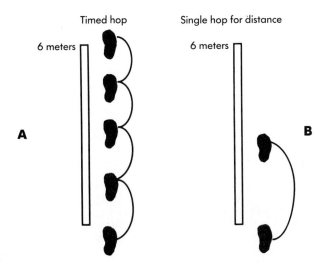

Timed hop   Single hop for distance

6 meters   6 meters

A   **B**

Fig. 12-17. Hop tests. A, In the timed hop test, time required to cover a 6-meter distance is measured in seconds. **B,** The single hop for distance test measures the distance covered in a single hop. Both tests use a percentage of the injured leg compared to the uninjured leg.

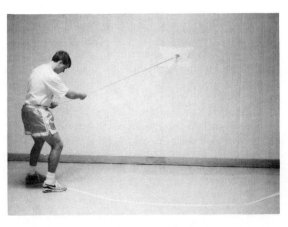

Fig. 12-18. Cocontraction test. The athlete moves in a side-step or shuffle fashion around the periphery of a semicircle with resistance applied using surgical tubing.

equipment. A second way to test the upper extremity using velocity is to use a similar set-up as above minus the radar gun. In this situation the therapist needs a stopwatch to time the flight of the ball. As the athlete releases the ball, the therapist begins timing and stops when the catcher receives the ball. Again, a mean of five throws should be computed to help decrease testing error. As one can see, the first method will be most accurate, but the second method can be used as an effective testing tool.[19]

The lower extremity can be tested in many different ways. Among these are sprint times, agility run times, jumping heights/distances, hop tests, cocontraction tests, carioca runs, and shuttle runs.

All of these cannot be covered in this test, but an attempt is made to cover a variety of tests. First, the sprint test is exactly what the name implies.

1. A set distance is measured.
2. The athlete then runs the distance with a time per run recorded.
3. Three to five sprints should be completed and the mean computed.
4. Comparison of pretest/posttest means is made.

Agility runs involve the same premise. The run is timed and a mean taken for 5 runs. The difference is the course. Rather than concentrating on straight ahead motion, the agility run incorporates changes of direction. For example, a simple figure 8 can be

set up with cones, and the athlete is instructed to travel the cones as fast as possible while being timed for performance.

The vertical jump test can also be used to evaluate the lower extremity. This test involves the athlete with chalked fingertips jumping and touching a white piece of paper. Three to five jumps should be attempted and the mean height recorded (measured from fingertips standing to the chalk mark).

The timed hop test or single hop test[15] can also be used to measure the functional limitations of the lower extremity. The athlete hops on the involved foot a distance of 6 meters against the clock. The fastest time can be recorded and compared to normative values or previous attempts to gauge the athlete's progress (Figure 12-17).

The cocontraction test involves securing the athlete to a resistance strap (THERABAND). The strap is then stretched to twice its recoil length, and the athlete completes 5 to 180 degree semicircles against the clock. The mean time to complete the test is then calculated (Figure 12-18).

Finally, carioca runs and shuttle runs can be attempted vs. time to measure the improvement in function.

Obviously, the budget and availability of equipment will determine the tests that the therapist can use, but simple timed sprints can give an effective indication of improved performance just as well as the more complicated tests that involve expensive equipment.[1,12]

Once athletes can perform all specific tasks leading up to the motor skill safely and effectively, they can return to activity. For example, an athlete might progress from cycling to walking to jogging to running before returning to sprinting activities and competition in the 4×400 relay.

The sports therapist must note that these are only examples, and no one program will benefit every athlete and every condition. Sports therapists should use these activities, along with others they develop, to help maximize the athlete's recovery. By providing athletes with every option available in rehabilitation, sports therapists can return the athlete to participation at preinjury status. The preinjury status achieved with the functional progression cannot only return the athlete to competition but can also ensure a safer, more effective return to play.

SUMMARY

1. Complete rehabilitation should strive to improve neuromuscular coordination and agility, as well as to improve strength, endurance, and flexibility.

2. The role of the functional progression is to improve and complete the traditional rehabilitation process by providing sport-specific exercise.

3. The functional progression is a sequence of activities that simulate sports activity. The progression will begin easily, increasing to full sports participation.

4. Each sports activity can be divided into smaller components, allowing the athlete to progress from easy to difficult.

5. Functional progressions are highly effective exercise therapy techniques found with the long-term rehabilitation stage.

6. Functional progressions allow for improvements in strength, endurance, mobility/flexibility, relaxation, coordination/agility/skill, and assessment of functional stability.

7. Functional progression can improve the athlete's psychology/social aspects by decreasing feelings of anxiety, deprivation, and apprehension.

8. Components of a functional progression that should be addressed include development, choice of activity, implementation, and termination.

REFERENCES

1 Anderson M: The relationships among isometric, isotonic, and isokinetic concentric and eccentric quadriceps and hamstring force and three components of athletic performance, *J Orthop Sports Phys Ther* 14(3):114-120, 1991.

2 Andrews JR: *Preventive and rehabilitative exercises for the shoulder and elbow,* Birmingham, 1990, American Sports Medicine Institute.

3 Andrews JR, McLeod WD, Ward T, et al.: The cutting mechanism, *Am J Sports Med* 5:111-121, 1977.

4 Bangerter BL: Contributive components in the vertical jump, *Res Q* 39:432-436, 1968.

5 Croce P, Greg J: Keeping fit when injured. In Nicholas A, Noble D, editors: *Clinics in Sports Medicine,* Philadelphia, 1991, WB Saunders/Harcourt Brace Jovanovich.

6 Davis M: *Rehabilitation: a practical approach.* In Bernhardt D, editor: *Sports physical therapy,* Philadelphia, 1986, Churchhill Livingstone.

7 Freeman M, Dean M, Hanham I: The etiology and prevention of functional instability of the foot, *J Bone Joint Surg* 47:678-685, 1965.

8 Galley J: *Human movement: an introductory test for physiotherapists,* London, 1991, UK Limited.

9 Jokl E: *The scope of exercise in rehabilitation,* Lexington, 1964, Charles C. Thomas.

10 Kegerreis S: The construction and implementation of functional progressions as a component of athletic rehabilitation, *J Orthop Sports Phys Ther* 63(4):14-19, 1983.

11 Kisner C, Colby L: *Therapeutic exercise foundations and techniques,* Philadelphia, 1985, FA Davis.

12 Lephart S: Relationship between selected physical characteristics and functional capacity in the anterior cruciate ligament-insufficient athlete, *J Orthop Sports Phys Ther* 16(4):174-181, 1992.

13 Lephart S, Perrin D, Minger K, et al.: Functional performance tests for the anterior cruciate ligament-insufficient athlete, *J Athletic Training* 26:44-50, 1991.

14 Melliam M: *Office management of sports injuries and athletic problems,* Philadelphia, 1988, Handy and Belfus.

15 Noyes F, Barber S, Mangine R: Abnormal limb symmetry determined by function hop tests after anterior cruciate ligament rupture, *Am J Sports Med* 19(5):513-518, 1991.

16 Shelbourne D: Functional ability in athletes with anterior cruciate ligament deficiency, *Am J Sports Med* 15:628, 1987.

17 Tegner Y, Lysholm J, Lysholm M, et al.: A performance test to monitor rehabilitation and evaluate anterior cruciate ligament injuries, *Am J Sports Med* 14:156-159, 1986.

18 Tibone JM, Antich MS, Fanton GS, et al.: Functional analysis of anterior cruciate ligament instability, *Am J Sports Med* 13:34-39, 1986.

19 Torg J, Vegso J, Torg E: *Rehabilitation of athletic injuries: an atlas of therapeutic exercise,* Chicago, 1987, Year Book.

20 Wooden M: Effects of strength training on throwing velocity and shoulder muscle performance in teenage baseball players. *J Orthop Sports Phys Ther* 15(5):223-228, 1992.

Aquatic Therapy in Rehabilitation

13

Gina Selepak

OBJECTIVES

After completion of this chapter, the student should be able to do the following:

- Explain the principles of buoyancy and specific gravity and the role they have in the aquatic environment.

- Identify and describe the three major resistive forces at work in the aquatic environment.

- Discuss the advantages and disadvantages of aquatic therapy in relation to traditional land exercises.

- Identify and describe the two prominent techniques of aquatic therapy.

In the past decade, widespread interest has developed in the area of aquatic therapy. It has rapidly become a popular rehabilitation technique among sports therapists. Aquatic therapy is beneficial in the treatment of everything from orthopedic injuries to spinal cord damage, chronic pain, cerebral palsy, multiple sclerosis, and many other conditions, making it useful in a variety of settings.[16]

Water healing techniques have been traced back through history as early as 2400 B.C., but it was not until the late nineteenth century that more traditional water exercise types of aquatic therapy came into existence. The development of the Hubbard tank in 1920 sparked the initiation of present-day therapeutic water exercise by allowing aquatic therapy to be conducted in a highly controlled, clinical setting.[4] Loeman and Roen took this a step further in 1924 and stimulated actual pool therapy interest. Only recently, however, has water come into its own as a therapeutic exercise medium.[17]

Aquatic therapy is believed to be successful because it lowers pain levels by decreasing joint compression forces. The perception of weightless-

ness experienced in the water seems to eliminate or drastically reduce the body's protective muscular guarding. This effect results in decreased muscular spasm and pain that may carry over into the patient's daily functional activities.[19] The primary goal of aquatic therapy is to teach the athlete how to use water as a modality for improving movement and fitness. Then, along with other therapeutic modalities and treatments, aquatic therapy can become one more link in the athlete's recovery chain.

PHYSICAL PROPERTIES AND RESISTIVE FORCES

The sports therapist must understand several physical properties of the water before designing an aquatic therapy program. Land exercise cannot always be converted to aquatic exercise because buoyancy rather than gravity is the major force. A thorough understanding of buoyancy, specific gravity, the resistive forces of the water, and their relationships must be the groundwork of any aquatics program. The program must also be specific and individualized to the athlete's particular injury if it is to be successful.

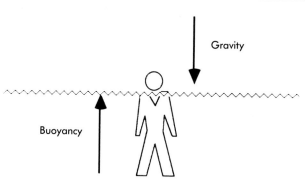

Gravity

Buoyancy

Fig. 13-1. The buoyant force.

TABLE 13-1
Weight Bearing Percentages

Body Level	Percentage of Weight Bearing	
	Male	Female
C7	8%	8%
Xiphisternal	28%	35%
ASIS	47%	54%

Buoyancy

Buoyancy is one of the primary forces involved in aquatic therapy. All objects, on land or in the water, are subjected to the downward pull of the earth's gravity. In the water, however, this force is counteracted to some degree by the upward buoyant force. According to the Archimedes' Principle, any object submerged or floating in water is buoyed upward by a counterforce that helps support the submerged or partially submerged object against the downward pull of gravity. In other words, the buoyant force assists motion toward the water's surface and resists motion away from the surface.[12] Because of this buoyant force, upon entering the water an apparent loss of weight is experienced.[8] The weight loss experienced is nearly equal to the weight of the liquid that is displaced when the object enters the water (Figure 13-1).

For example, a 100-pound individual, when almost completely submerged, displaces a volume of water that weighs nearly 95 pounds and therefore feels as though they weigh less than 5 pounds. This sensation occurs because when partially submerged, the individual only bears the weight of what is above the water. With immersion to the level of the seventh cervical vertebra, both males and females only bear approximately 8% of their total body weight (TBW). The percentages increase to 28% TBW for females and 35% TBW for males at the xiphisternal level and 47% TBW for females and 54% TBW for males at the anterosuperior iliac spine (ASIS) level (Table 13-1). The percentages differ for males and females because of the differences in centers of gravity. Males carry a higher percentage of their weight in the upper body, while females carry a higher percentage of their

weight in the lower body. The center of gravity on land corresponds with a center of buoyancy in the water.[17]

Specific Gravity

Because the weight of each body part is not a constant, the buoyancy of each part differs. Buoyant values can be determined by several factors. The bone to muscle weight, the amount and distribution of fat, and the depth and expansion of the chest all play a role in buoyancy.[17] Together, these factors determine the specific gravity of the individual body part. On average, humans have a specific gravity slightly less than that of water. Any object with a specific gravity less than that of water will float. A specific gravity greater than that of water will cause the object to sink. However, the specific gravity of all body parts is not uniform. Therefore, even with a total body, specific gravity is less than the specific gravity of water, and the individual may not float horizontally in the water. Furthermore, the lungs, when filled with air, can decrease the specific gravity of the chest area, allowing the head and chest to float higher in the water than the heavier, denser extremities. Therefore compensation with flotation devices at the extremities may be necessary for some treatments.

Resistive Forces

When an object moves in the water, just as on land, several resistive forces are at work that must be overcome. These forces include the cohesive force, the bow force, and the drag force.

COHESIVE FORCE. There is a slight but easily overcome cohesive force that runs in a parallel direction to the water surface. This resistance is formed by the water molecules loosely binding together, creating a surface tension. Surface tension can be seen in still

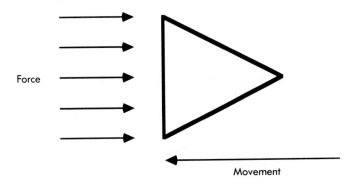

Fig. 13-2. The bow force.

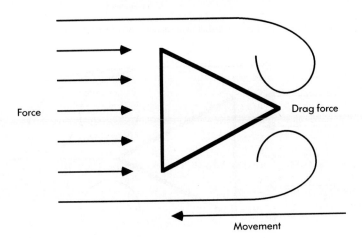

Fig. 13-3. Drag force.

water, since the water remains motionless with the cohesive force intact unless disturbed.

BOW FORCE. A second force is the bow force, or the force that is generated at the front of the object during movement. When the object moves, the bow force causes an increase in the water pressure at the front of the object and a decrease in the water pressure at the rear of the object. This pressure change causes a movement of water from the high pressure area in the front to the low pressure area behind the object. As the water enters the low pressure area, it swirls into the low pressure zone and forms eddies, or small whirlpool turbulences.[7] These eddies impede flow by creating a backward force, or drag force (Figure 13-2).

DRAG FORCE. This third force, the drag force, is very important in aquatic therapy. The drag force on an object can be controlled by changing the shape of the object or the speed of its movement (Figure 13-3).

Frictional resistance can be decreased by making the object more streamlined. This change causes less bow force and less of a change in pressure between the front and rear of the object, resulting in less drag force. In a streamlined flow, the resistance is proportional to the velocity of the object. Therefore, to decrease the resistance for a weak athlete, exercises should be performed slowly in the most streamlined position possible (Figure 13-4).

On the other hand, if the object is not streamlined, a turbulent situation exists. In a turbulent situation, drag is a function of the velocity squared. Therefore by increasing the speed of movement 2 times, the resistance the object must overcome is increased 4

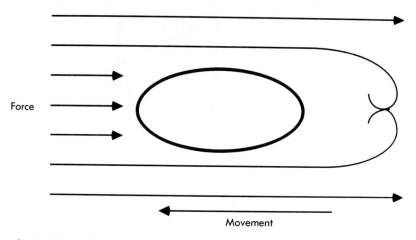

Fig. 13-4. Streamlined movement. This creates less drag force and less turbulence.

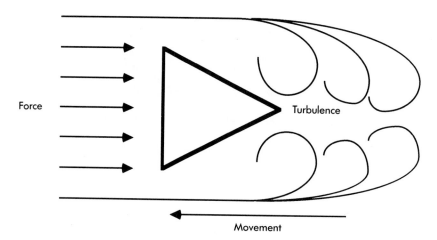

Fig. 13-5. Turbulent flow.

times.[8] This provides a method to increase resistance progressively during aquatic rehabilitation. However, increases in speed also affect stability adversely. Single limb movements are generally not as affected as trunk exercise by this loss of stability. Considerable turbulence can be generated when the speed of movement is increased, causing the muscles to work harder to keep the movement going. This is especially true when changes of direction take place. Therefore, by simply changing the shape of a limb through the addition of rehabilitation equipment or increasing the speed of movement, the sports therapist can modify the athlete's workout intensity to match strength increases (Figure 13-5).

ADVANTAGES OF AQUATIC REHABILITATION

An aquatic therapy program offers many advantages. Physiologically, aquatic therapy is similar to land exercises as blood supply, muscle temperature, metabolism, O_2 demand and CO_2 production increase just as they do in land exercises.[7] What makes aquatic therapy popular are the characteristics that separate it from traditional land exercises. Very fine gradation of exercise can be manipulated by using combinations of the different resistive forces. For instance, when using weights on land, the athlete is limited to the equipment available. If the 10-pound dumbell is too heavy but the 5-pound dumbell is too light, there

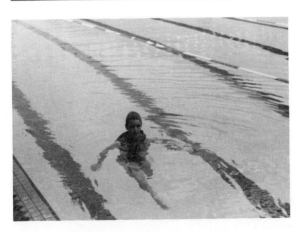

Fig. 13-6. Wet vest in deep water.

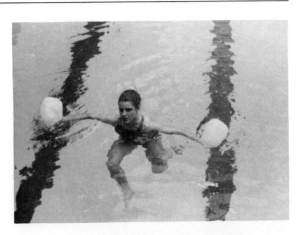

Fig. 13-7. Milk jugs in water for flotation.

is no middle ground. With aquatic therapy, however, extremely small gradations of intensity can be controlled by changing the body positioning or the equipment being used. Through water exercises, even individuals with minimal muscle contraction capabilities can do work and see improvement even though they are unable to do so on land.

A further advantage of aquatic therapy concerns weight-bearing principles. Locomotor activities after a lower extremity injury can safely begin earlier in the rehabilitation process by using the buoyant force to decrease the apparent weight and compressive forces. This advantage is of great importance to the athletic population in particular. Through careful use of Archimedes' Principle, a gradual increase in the percentage of weight bearing can be undertaken. Initially, the athlete would begin nonweight bearing in the deep end of the pool. A wet vest or similar buoyant device might be used to help the athlete remain afloat for the desired exercises (Figure 13-6). If such a device is unavailable, empty plastic milk jugs held in each hand are also a quite effective and very inexpensive method of flotation (Figure 13-7).

Once therapy has progressed, the athlete could be moved to neck-deep water to begin light weight bearing. Gradual increases in the percentage of weight-bearing are accomplished by systematically moving the athlete to more shallow water. Even when in waist-deep water, both male and female athletes are only bearing approximately 50% of their TBW. By placing a sinkable bench or chair in the shallow water, step-ups can then be initiated under partial weight-bearing conditions long before the athlete is capable

of performing the same exercise in full weight bearing on land. Thus the advantages of low weight bearing are coupled wtih the proprioceptive benefits of closed-kinetic chain exercise, making aquatic therapy an excellent functional rehabilitation activity.

Another advantage of aquatic therapy is increased range of motion , since the warmth of the water helps to induce muscular relaxation. The proprioceptive stimulation from the water may also serve as a gating mechanism in the decreasing pain. Muscular strengthening and reeducation can also be accomplished in the aquatic environment. Progressive resistive exercises can gradually be made more difficult as the athlete's strength increases. The water also serves as an accommodating resistance medium. Therefore the muscles are maximally stressed while the athlete works through the full range of motion available, helping to facilitate strength gains.[8] However, the extent of the gains depends on the effort exerted by the athlete and is not easily measured.

Strength gains through aquatic exercises are also brought about by the increased energy needs of the body working in an aquatic environment. Studies have shown that aquatic exercise requires a higher energy expenditure than the same exercise performed on land. The athlete not only has to perform the activity but must also maintain a level of buoyancy and overcome the resistive forces of the water. The energy cost for water running, for example, is four times greater than running the same distance on land.[7,8,14]

Psychologically, aquatic therapy increases confidence, since the athlete experiences increased success at locomotor, stretching, or strengthening activities in the water. Tension and anxiety are decreased and athlete morale increases, as well as postexercise vigor.[7,8,17]

DISADVANTAGES OF AQUATIC REHABILITATION

As with any therapeutic modality, aquatic therapy has its disadvantages. The cost of building and maintaining a rehabilitation pool, if there is no access to an existing facility, can be very high. Also, qualified pool attendants must be present, and the sports therapist involved in the treatment must be trained in aquatic safety and therapy procedures.[5,14]

Stabilization in the water is considerably more difficult than on land, and a patient who requires high stabilization will be more challenging to work with. Stabilization of the sports therapist is just as important as stabilization of the injured athlete. A wide stance in the water will help provide a solid base and better support of the athlete by the sports therapist. Flotation devices placed at the neck, hips, and extremities can also help support the athlete in the water (Figure 13-8).

The presence of any open wounds or sores on the patient is a contraindication to aquatic therapy, as are contagious skin diseases. This restriction is obvious for health reasons to reduce the chance of infection of the patient or of others who use the pool.[13,16] Because of this risk, all surgical wounds must be completely healed before the pool is accessed. An excessive fear of the water would also be a reason to keep an athlete out of an aquatic exercise program. Fever, urinary tract infections, allergies to the pool chemicals, cardiac problems, and uncontrolled seizures are also contraindications.

FACILITIES AND EQUIPMENT

When considering an existing facility or when planning to build one, certain characteristics of the pool should be taken into consideration. The pool should not be smaller than 10 feet × 12 feet. It can be in-ground or above-ground as long as athlete access is well planned for. Both a shallow (2-½ feet) and a deep (5 feet plus) area should be present to allow standing exercise and swimming or nonstanding exercise. The pool bottom should be flat and the depth gradations clearly marked. Water temperature will vary depending on the activity. For water exercise,

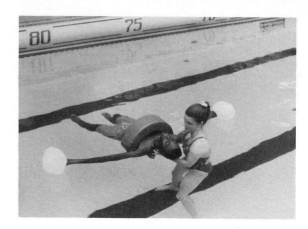

Fig. 13-8. Athlete and sports therapist using shallow water with floats.

92 to 95°F water temperature is appropriate; however, lower temperatures of 85 to 90°F are more suitable for active swimming.[17] Temperature is an important factor since water that is too warm can lead to fatigue or even heat exhaustion, and water that is too cool can cause shivering, increased muscular tension, or hypothermia.

Some prefabricated pools come with an inwater treadmill or current producing device (Figure 13-9). These devices can be beneficial but are not essential to treatment. Rescue tubes, inner tubes, or wet vests can be purchased to assist in flotation activities such as deep water running. Hand paddles and pull buoys are effective in strengthening the upper extremity, while kick boards and fins are useful for strengthening the lower extremity. Most of these products can be purchased from local sporting goods stores with no special ordering required. Equipment for aquatic therapy is limited only by the imagination of the sports therapist. Plastic milk jugs, balls, and other common items can be substituted for the more expensive commercial equipment with comparable results. What is important is to stimulate interest in therapy and to keep in mind what goals are to be accomplished (Figure 13-10).

TECHNIQUES

Designing an aquatic therapy program is very similar to designing a program for land exercises. A thorough history and evaluation of the injury is the first step. Once contraindications have been ruled out, the ath-

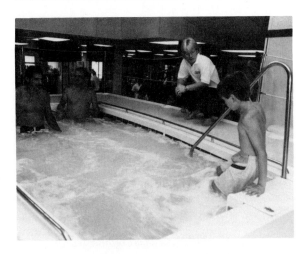

Fig. 13-9. The SwimEx pool. This pool's even, controllable water flow allows for the application of individualized prescriptive exercise and therapeutic programs. Up to three patients can be treated simultaneously.

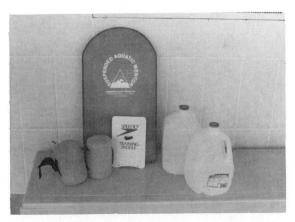

Fig. 13-10. Aquatic exercise equipment. Kickboard, fins, pull buoys, paddles, wet vest, and rescue tube are common forms of exercise equipment.

lete's water safety skills and swimming ability should be evaluated, as well as the general comfort level in the water. The athlete must be supervised at all times and should not be left unattended for any reason. From this point, an aquatic program that is specific and individualized can be developed using one of the aquatic therapy techniques.

Buoyancy Technique

Several popular aquatic therapy approaches are currently being used. The most common aquatic therapy technique seems to be the buoyancy technique. This technique is actually a three-part progression moving from buoyancy-assisted exercises to buoyancy-supported and finally to buoyancy-resisted exercises.[4] A rehabilitation progression would begin with the sports therapist assisting the athlete in the water through passive range of motion in any plane. Then the patient could move actively from below the water toward the surface in the buoyancy-assisted phase. The next phase would be to move parallel to the water surface while at the buoyant level. In this phase only the cohesive force is resisting motion. This would be a buoyancy-supported position. An intermediate stage would have movement start at the buoyant level and continue toward the surface. This stage is limited in use because some individuals' buoyant level is already at the surface. Therefore no move-

ment would be possible. In the buoyancy-resisted phase, the athlete would move downward from the buoyant level against the upward buoyant force. Finally, flotation devices could be used to increase the difficulty of moving against the buoyant force.[17] Thus every joint could be moved either actively or passively and with or without resistance or assistance through its full range of motion. Increasing the speed of movement or decreasing the streamline by changing the body positioning or adding rehabilitation equipment increases the drag force resistance as the patient gets stronger, making workouts more challenging.[16]

An example of a shoulder progression for flexion using this approach would begin with the sports therapist and the athlete together in neck-deep water. Passive range of motion of the injured extremity would be initiated in the flexion pattern by the sports therapist. In the next stage, the sports therapist would place the extremity below the buoyant level and allow the buoyant force to assist the athlete's active shoulder flexion. To accomplish this stage the athlete stands upright while the arm is passively moved to the athlete's side by the sports therapist. Then the athlete actively flexes the shoulder until the arm reaches the water surface. The flexion pattern for the next phase, the buoyancy-supported stage, begins with the athlete sidelying with the injured shoulder closest to the pool bottom. Support with floats would

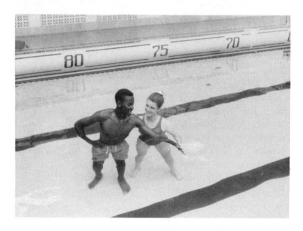

Fig. 13-11. Milk jugs used for resistance.

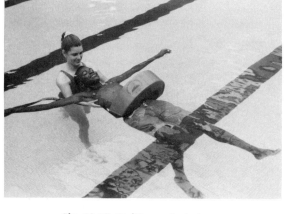

Fig. 13-12. Bad Ragaz technique.

be needed at the feet, hips, and neck, as well as additional support from the sports therapist at the torso. In this position, the athlete could work both flexion and extension while only encountering resistance from the cohesive force, allowing an excellent opportunity to increase active range of motion. Generally, two to three sets of 10 repetitions are appropriate depending on the athlete's tolerance.

In the strengthening phase, the buoyancy-resisted stage, the athlete is standing once again. Active flexion and extension of the shoulder begins at a starting position parallel to the water surface and progresses to the side of the thigh. From the thigh, the assistance of the buoyant force is resisted while the arm is returned to the starting position. When two to three sets of 10 repetitions can be completed without pain, equipment may be added to increase the difficulty. Hand paddles provide a greater surface area and therefore more resistance and a higher intensity. Plastic milk jugs partially filled with water are another excellent way to increase resistance. By placing less water in the jug, its buoyancy is increased, and the resistance on the arm increases correspondingly (Figure 13-11).

Bad Ragaz Technique

A second common technique in aquatic therapy is Bad Ragaz. In this method, buoyancy is used for flotation purposes only and not to assist or resist movement. The bow force ahead and drag force behind are the means for providing resistance. Three main positions apply in this method. The sports therapist

should be in waist-deep water to maintain optimal stability. In the first, the athlete actively moves while being fixated by the sports therapist (isokinetic). The athlete determines the resistance by controlling the speed of movement. For example, to work on knee flexion, the athlete could be stabilized sidelying with the involved leg closest to the surface. The buoyant force will act on that leg, and movement occurs, resulting in bow and drag forces. The bow force pushes the knee into flexion while the drag force pulls the knee in the same direction.

A second position has the athlete and sports therapist moving together in the direction of the desired motion (isotonic). To work on knee flexion in this position, the athlete is pushed forward, either sidelying or backlying. This position facilitates movement of the knee into flexion since the bow force helps the athlete's active contraction to push the knee into flexion. This position decreases the streamline of the leg and increases the drag force that also assists by pulling the knee into flexion. In this situation, the sports therapist controls the speed and therefore the resistance.

The third position in this technique has the athlete holding a fixed position while being pushed by the sports therapist (isometric). In this position, the athlete holds an isometric contraction against the bow and drag forces[4] (Figure 13-12).

Hold-relax, repeated contraction, and other PNF techniques can also be used in the water. They are very similar to those done on land but are performed in a buoyancy-assisted position to enhance results.[4,7] PNF techniques should be done carefully since research by Hurley and Turner[13] suggests the patient may have a reduced perception of stretch in the water. Once again, as the athlete's strength increases, resistive equipment should be added to make the workouts more challenging.

SUMMARY

1. The buoyant force counteracts the force of gravity as it assists motion toward the water's surface and resists motion away from the surface.
2. Because of differences in the specific gravity of the body, the head and chest tend to float higher in the water than the heavier, denser extremities, making compensation with flotation devices necessary.
3. The three forces that oppose movement in the water are the cohesive force, the bow force, and the drag force.
4. Aquatic therapy allows for fine gradation of exercise, increased control over the percentage of weight bearing, increased range of motion and strength, decreased pain, and increased confidence.
5. Cost, decreased stabilization, and athlete contraindications are some disadvantages of aquatic therapy.
6. Pool size, water temperature, and equipment will vary depending on the population using the facility.
7. The buoyancy technique consists of buoyancy-assisted, buoyancy-supported, and buoyancy-resisted phases.
8. The Bad Ragaz technique uses isokinetic, isotonic, and isometric holding positions.
9. Aquatic therapy is meant to complement, not replace, traditional land exercise.

REFERENCES

1 Arrigo C, editor: Aquatic rehabilitation, *Sports Medicine Update* 7(2), 1992.
2 Arrigo C, Fuller CS, Wilk KE: Aquatic rehabilitation following ACL-PTG reconstruction, *Sports Medicine Update* 7(2):22-27, 1992.
3 Bolton F, Goodwin D: *Pool exercises,* Edinburgh and London, 1974, Churchill Livingstone.
4 Campion MR: *Adult hydrotherapy: a practical approach,* Oxford, 1990, Heineman Medical.
5 Dioffenbach L: Aquatic therapy services, *Clinical Management* 11(1):14-19, 1991.
6 Dougherty NJ: Risk management in aquatics, *JOHPERD* May/June, 46-48, 1990.
7 Duffield NH: *Exercise in water,* London, 1976, Bailliere Tindall.
8 Edlich RF, Towler MA, Goitz RJ, et al.: Bioengineering principles of hydrotherapy, *J Burn Care Rehab* 8(6):580-584, 1987.
9 Fawcett CW: Principles of aquatic rehab: a new look at hydrotherapy, *Sports Medicine Update* 7(2):6-9, 1992.
10 Genuario SE, Vegso JJ: The use of a swimming pool in the rehabilitation and reconditioning of athletic injuries, *Contemp Orthop* 20(4):381-387, 1990.
11 Golland A: Basic hydrotherapy, *Physiotherapy* 67(9):258-262, 1961.
12 Haralson KM: Therapeutic pool programs, *Clinical Management* 5(2):10-13, 1985.
13 Hurley R, Turner C: Neurology and aquatic therapy, *Clinical Management* 11(1):26-27, 1991.
14 Kolb ME: Principles of underwater exercise, *Physical Therapy Review* 27(6):361-364, 1957.
15 McWaters JG: For faster recovery just add water, *Sports Medicine Update* 7(2):4-5, 1992.
16 Meyer RI: Practice settings for kinesiotherapy-aquatics, *Clinical Kinesiology* 44(1):12-13, 1990.
17 Moor FB, Peterson SC, Manueall EM, et al.: *Manual of hydrotherapy and massage,* Mountain View, Calif, 1964, Pacific Press.
18 Nolte-Heuritsch I: *Aqua rhythmics: exercises for the swimming pool,* New York, 1979, Sterling.
19 Triggs M: Orthopedic aquatic therapy, *Clinical Management* 11(1):30-31, 1991.

Therapeutic Modalities in Rehabilitation

14

William E. Prentice

OBJECTIVES

After completion of this chapter, the student should be able to do the following:

- Describe the approach of the sports therapist in using therapeutic modalities.

- Discuss the potential physiological responses of biological tissue to electrical stimulating currents.

- Discuss the use of diathermy in rehabilitation.

- Compare ultrasound with diathermy as a deep-heating modality.

- Discuss the physiological effects of thermotherapy and cryotherapy techniques.

- Describe the possible uses for the low-power laser in sports medicine.

- Discuss the progression of modality use as the healing process progresses through the different phases of healing.

- List indications and contraindications for use of the various modalities.

- Discuss the physiological effects associated with the use of the different modalities.

Therapeutic modalities, when used appropriately, can be extremely useful tools in the rehabilitation of the injured athlete. Like any other tool, their effectiveness is limited by the knowledge, skill, and experience of the person using them. For the sports therapist, decisions regarding how and when a modality may best be used should be based on a combination of theoretical knowledge and practical experience. Modalities should not be used at random nor should their use be based on what has always been done before. Instead, consideration must always be given to what should work best in a specific clinical situation.

In any program of rehabilitation, modalities should be used primarily as adjuncts to therapeutic exercise and certainly not at the exclusion of range-of-motion and strengthening exercises.

There are many different approaches and ideas regarding the use of modalities in injury rehabilitation. Therefore no "cookbook" exists for modality use. Instead, sports therapists should make their own decision from the options in a given clinical situation about which modality will be most effective.

ELECTRICAL STIMULATING CURRENTS

Electrical stimulating currents are among the therapeutic modalities most often used by the sports therapist.[25] The effects of electrical current passing through biological tissues may be physiological, chemical, or thermal. All biological tissue has some response to this current flow. The type and extent of the response depends on (1) the type of tissue and physiological response characteristics and (2) the parameters of the electrical current applied, that is, its intensity, duration, waveform, modulation, and po-

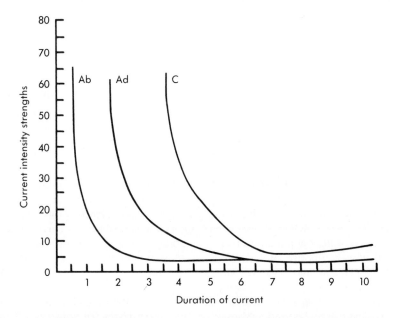

Fig. 14-1. Strength-duration curves. Curves represent the thresholds for depolarization of the various types of nerve fibers. *Ab,* Sensory nerves; *Ad,* motor fibers, *C,* pain fibers.

larity. Biological tissue responds to electrical energy in a manner similar to how it normally functions and grows.

Clinically, the sports therapist uses electrical currents for several purposes: (1) producing muscle contraction through stimulation of nerve muscle, (2) stimulating sensory nerves to help treat pain, (3) creating an electrical field on the skin surface to drive ions into tissues (iontophoresis), and (4) creating an electrical field within the tissues to stimulate or alter the healing process (medical galvanism). In a sports-medicine environment, the major therapeutic uses of electricity center on muscle contraction, sensory stimulation, or both.[15]

To produce any physiological response in the nerve and muscle fibers, an electrical current must be of sufficient intensity and last long enough to equal or exceed the nerve membrane's basic threshold for excitation. When this occurs, depolarization of the nerve fiber results in an action potential.[15]

Different types (sizes) of nerves have different thresholds for depolarization. The strength/duration curves in Figure 14-1 represent graphically the thresholds for depolarization of sensory, motor, and pain nerve fibers. If current intensity or duration is increased to a level great enough to reach the minimal threshold for depolarization of sensory fibers, the

electrical current can be felt. If current intensity or duration is increased further, a muscle contraction may be elicited by reaching the threshold for depolarization of the motor fibers. If the intensity/duration continues to increase, eventually a level is reached that causes depolarization of the smaller fibers and pain. By simply changing current intensity, current duration, or some combination of the two, very different physiological responses can be achieved.[2]

Traditionally, various types of electric currents have been classified by attaching specific names, such as high volt, low volt, alternating, direct, interferential, Russian, and microamperage (MENS). Electrical stimulators that output any of these varieties of current (with the possible exception of some new MENS units in which the intensity is not great enough) can produce any of these physiological responses if the current parameters are adjusted appropriately. Thus a discussion of the physiological effects of electrical current on the stimulation of sensory nerves and motor nerves is appropriate.[1]

Stimulation of Sensory Nerves

Transcutaneous electrical nerve stimulation (TENS) has been traditionally defined as a technique used to stimulate large-diameter sensory nerve fibers with electrodes placed on the skin specifically to relieve either chronic or acute pain. TENS is an effective, noninvasive, nonpharmacological method of pain modulation.[23]

Electrodes are placed on the skin surface generally in or over the area of pain. Electrodes placed at the painful region may be within the dermatome, on a specific point, or over a peripheral nerve supplying the painful region. Spinal cord segments that give rise to a specific nerve root conveying nociceptive input provide another choice for electrode placement. Electrodes are often placed along vertebrae or between spinous processes in conjunction with electrodes placed over specific dermatomal regions.[17] These stimulators are designed to deliver pulses with a waveform that generally differs depending on the manufacturer. Electrical currents are either direct (DC) or alternating (AC) and may take on sine, square, or triangular waveforms.[1] Various claims concerning the effectiveness of specific waveforms have been made by manufacturers and, although one type of waveform may be more effective for a particular patient, generalizations are difficult to make. These waveforms refer to the waveform produced by the stimulator and delivered to the patient and not the waveform of the current used to drive the generator.

The mechanism by which TENS produces pain relief is a matter for debate.[8] Certainly, the first units were designed and tried clinically on the basis of Melzack and Wall's gate control theory of pain, originally proposed in 1965 with several later modifications.[24] To summarize this theory, pain information is conveyed from the periphery to the spinal cord by small-diameter type-C fibers. These fibers directly or indirectly excite transmission cells in the spinal cord that transmit pain information to higher-conscious pain centers in the brain. By exciting large-diameter fibers (which innervate cutaneous receptors), synaptic transmission between the pain fibers and the transmission cells is inhibited, and thus pain is not consciously perceived.

Most recent theories concerning the mechanism of TENS in the relief of pain involve endogenously produced opiatelike substances called **enkephalins.** Enkephalins have been implicated in a pain-relief mechanism in the dorsal horn of the spinal cord. Stimulation of large-diameter afferent fibers locally releases enkephalins from small enkephalin interneurons that inhibit synaptic transmission of pain information to the brain, thus eliminating conscious appreciation of pain.[15]

Conventional TENS involves stimulation of large-diameter afferent fibers. How is this accomplished with commercially available TENS units? Peripheral nerves are actually bundles of a large number of large and small sensory and motor nerve fibers, innervating skin, muscle, and visceral structures. Because the electrodes connected to the TENS stimulator are placed on the skin (and thus in proximity to cutaneous sensory receptors), sensory fibers are preferentially stimulated. In addition, as stimulus intensity (or duration) is increased, large-diameter afferent fibers are excited (or recruited) before small ones. Of course, if the intensity or duration of the stimulus is increased sufficiently, motor and small-diameter sensory fibers (pain fibers) are excited. With TENS, the objective is to maximally stimulate the large-diameter afferent fibers without concomitant motor responses or pain.

Nerve and muscle tissues have characteristic strength-duration (S-D) curves. If S-D curves for single nerve fibers are constructed, that different sized nerve fibers have characteristic curves becomes apparent. Large fibers are more easily excited by an electrical stimulus than small fibers.[15,31] At very short pulse durations (on an order of 10 microseconds), the difference between the stimulus intensity necessary to excite large-diameter type A sensory fibers and that necessary to excite very-small-diameter type C pain fibers is maximized. Many commercial TENS units have variable adjustments for pulse duration, amplitude or intensity, and frequency. Optimal stimulation of large-diameter fibers (and therefore maximal pain relief) is obtained if a short-duration pulse is chosen and the intensity is gradually increased until a tingling sensation is perceived. Although optimal frequency of stimulation has not been determined, it is recommended that frequency be set at the maximum allowed by the stimulator.[15]

A second pain-control system is located in the brainstem and exerts a powerful inhibitory influence on transmission of impulses conveying pain information. These areas are located primarily in the periaqueductal gray matter, as well as in the Raphe nucleus and are preferentially activated by small-diameter fibers (C fibers). Intense electrical stimulation of peripheral pain fibers by either low-frequency, high-intensity TENS or electroacupuncture techniques results in **hyperstimulation analgesia.** Whereas in conventional TENS, the duration of relief is generally short because of the relatively short half-life of enkephalins, the duration of relief after hyperstimulation using high-intensity electrical stimulation is generally days or weeks, and in some cases the relief may be permanent.[15]

The Raphe nucleus appears to be a source of descending pain control. Descending neurons originating in the Raphe nucleus and descending in the dorsolateral tract to various levels of the spinal cord are activated by intense electrical stimulation. This descending inhibitory system acts at various levels of the spinal cord through stimulation of the enkephalin interneurons discussed earlier. The resulting inhibition of primary afferent pain fibers results in a reduction of pain sensation.

Hyperstimulation analgesia may result from intense electrical stimulation of acupuncture points and trigger points. The most effective type of stimulus is a high-intensity, DC pulse, which results in intense stimulation of pain fibers.

Another effect of such intense electrical stimulation is the release of another opiatelike polypeptide called **endorphin,** from the anterior pituitary gland. A large molecular complex known as ACTH/β-lipotropin is broken down to produce β-endorphin, certain types of enkephalins, and ACTH. This process is stimulated through low-frequency, high-intensity stimulation of peripheral pain fibers. The release of ACTH results in corticosteroid release from the adrenal glands. These antiinflammatory substances may affect pain reduction seen after high-intensity stimulation. The released endorphins may reduce pain locally by increasing the rate of degradation of prostaglandins and bradykinin. However, their most important function in the reduction of chronic and acute pain is through their direct stimulation of cells in the Raphe nucleus. This stimulation increases the activity of the descending pain-control mechanisms discussed earlier. One hypothesis is that β-endorphin is released in response to intense, low-frequency (1 to 5 Hertz) stimulation of specific acupuncture or trigger points. This technique has been referred to as *acustim* or *electroacutherapy.*[15]

Stimulation of Motor Nerves

Electrical stimulation of motor nerve fibers at sufficient intensity and duration to produce depolarization results in muscular contraction. Once a stimulus reaches the depolarizing threshold, an increase in the intensity of the stimulus does not alter the quality of the contraction. However, the frequency of stimulation is increased, the time for repolarization of the muscle fiber is decreased, and thus the contractions tend to summate. When the stimulation frequency reaches 50 Hertz or greater, the muscle exhibits a tetanic contraction.

Several therapeutic gains can be accomplished by electrically stimulating muscle contraction. Electrically induced contractions can facilitate circulation by pumping fluid and blood through the venous and lymphatic channels away from an area of swelling.[15]

Muscular inhibition after periods of immobilization or surgery or as a result of swelling is an indication for muscle reeducation. Electrically stimulating the muscle to contract produces an increase in the sensory input from the muscle and assists the patient in relearning a muscular response or pattern.[15]

Muscular strengthening may be accomplished using high-frequency AC current in conjunction with voluntary muscle contractions.[21,30] The exclusive use of electrical current does not appear to increase muscle strength.[10] Electrically stimulating the muscle to contract during periods of immobilization retards muscle atrophy and may potentially reduce the time required for rehabilitation after immobilization.

Electrical currents may also assist in increasing range of motion about a joint where contractures are limiting motion. Repeated contraction over an extended time appears to make the contracted joint structures and muscle modify and lengthen.[15]

Interferential Currents

Interferential current is a nonmodulated sine waveform alternating current produced by two simultaneously applied electrical generators that each produce this current at different frequencies. When the two currents intersect, the pulse intensities combine, and the difference in frequency produces a low-frequency "beat" pattern. Individual beats produce a physiological response that is essentially identical to a single pulse produced by a conventional electrical stimulator.

Proponents of interferential currents claim that this beating pulse lowers skin resistance and produces a more comfortable stimulation with a greater depth of penetration than other stimulators. However, they fail to realize that higher voltages also reduce tissue impedance; thus the relative comfort is no different than with high-volt stimulators. Interferential currents are simply a different electrical approach to achieve the same excitatory responses that traditional high-volt stimulators produce. The disadvantages of interferential units are that they are expensive and not as versatile as other high-volt generators. They can be used for pain modulation, edema reduction, and muscle relaxation. They are not suitable for muscle reeducation because there is no interrupt mode or modulation.

MENS Treatment

Microcurrent electrical neuromuscular stimulators (MENS) are one of the newer types of electrical stimulating units currently being used by the sports therapist. Certainly, the type of current being produced by these MENS generators is no different than current produced by other electrical stimulator generators. The majority of other electrical stimulating devices are capable of producing microcurrent. The only difference is that with MENS treatment the intensity of the current is at subsensory levels (below 1000 microamps) at a frequency of less than 1 pulse per second.

The majority of the literature dealing with microcurrents centers around research into stimulation of the healing process in fractures and skin wounds, and in pain modulation. The mechanism of their effectiveness is thought to be based on changes that occur at the cellular level rather than having to do with the effects of depolarization of sensory and motor nerve fibers.[15]

Microcurrent treatment may well be a useful addition to the electrical therapies. However, to date they are untested clinically, and claims of their effectiveness are based primarily on empirical rather than experimental evidence.[15]

Russian Current

Russian current is another relatively new type of current used by sports therapists. It uses an AC current at a high frequency (2500 to 10,000 PPS) produced in a series of "bursts." By putting the current in bursts, a greater intensity of current can be used, and the athlete will have a high tolerance to the current. As intensity of stimulation increases, more muscle fibers are stimulated and a stronger contraction occurs.

When used for muscle strengthening, this current is most effective when combined with active muscle contraction against resistance.

Iontophoresis

Electrical stimulating currents may also be used to produce chemical changes. Electricity is used in the clinic to cause chemical change in two important ways. The first is **iontophoresis** or **ion transfer,** defined as the introduction of chemical ions into superficial body tissues for medicinal purposes with the use of direct current. For iontophoresis to work, the chemical substance must be in an ionic form. Because like charges repel, chemical substances with a positive charge are introduced through the skin with the positive electrode, or anode, and substances with a negative charge must be introduced with the negative electrode, or cathode.[15]

The Phoresor is an electrical stimulating device designed specifically for iontophoresis. During recent years, this technique has gained significant popularity as a treatment modality.

If the drug is in solution form, it is generally applied to a gauze pad that is placed directly over the area to be treated. The active electrode of the same polarity as the charge of the ion is then placed on top of the drug-soaked gauze and secured firmly in place. The dispersive or indifferent electrode is generally placed at a remote area of the same extremity. Drugs in paste form are usually rubbed onto the skin surface, and a moist electrode with the proper polarity is then secured. In general, intensity is adjusted to tolerance. Treatment time is generally indicated by the physician, but 10 to 15 minutes is a typical treatment time.

Some care must be taken with very potent drugs that could potentially have deleterious systemic effects. However, iontophoretically applied medicinal ions generally do not migrate far below the surface of the skin or mucous membranes.

Some of the more common substances that may be iontophoretically applied are the following:

1. Heavy metal ions, such as zinc and copper, to fight certain types of skin infections
2. Chloride ions to loosen superficial scars
3. Local anesthetics
4. Vasodilating drugs
5. Magnesium ions for plantar warts

Medical Galvanism

The other major use of direct current that may be included under the general category of chemical effects has been termed **medical galvanism,** defined as the use of low-voltage galvanic or direct current for therapeutic purposes without the introduction of pharmacological substances. The therapeutic benefit is thought to result largely from local ionic changes that result in increased circulation to body parts between the electrodes. Presumably the improved circulation speeds up absorption of inflammatory products, such as accumulated metabolites, with subsequent pain relief. Low-volt electrical currents may speed wound healing, decrease edema, and help fight localized infection. Some conditions for which galvanic current has been used effectively include contusions, sprains, myositis, acute edema, certain forms of arthritis, tenosynovitis, and neuritis.[16]

Some other effects of long-duration, low-volt current, which seem to be polarity specific and result from local ionic and electrical changes are as follows:

Positive pole (anode)	hardening of tissues	decreases nerve excitability
Negative pole (cathode)	softening of tissues	increases nerve excitability

DIATHERMY

Direct currents and low-frequency alternating currents are not used to generate thermal effects clinically. The reason is not that such currents are incapable of generating thermal effects but that the intensities necessary would be prohibitively high and result in severe pain and cutaneous or subcutaneous tissue burns. Slight thermal effects, however, occur as a result of local circulation increases.

High-frequency currents may be used to produce a tissue temperature increase. Electrical current flowing through a conductor will generate an electrical field and a magnetic field. The ratio of electrical field to magnetic field depends on the characteristics of the generator and to a great extent on the type and set-up of the electrodes.

An electrical current that primarily generates an electrical field is used to produce electrostatic heating, which has its greatest heating effect on the more superficial skin and fat layers. Current that creates a magnetic field produces electromagnetic heating, which has greater thermal effect on the deeper tissues (that is, muscle and nerve).[9]

Primarily two forms of diathermy are used clinically today. The first is **shortwave diathermy** (Figure 14-2). The operating frequency of these devices is about 27 million cycles per second, with a wavelength of approximately 11 meters. Several types of electrodes transmit this shortwave energy to a patient, including pads, cuffs, air-spaced plates, drums, and induction field cables.[12]

In the case of shortwave diathermy units using air-spaced plates, the body part to be treated is placed

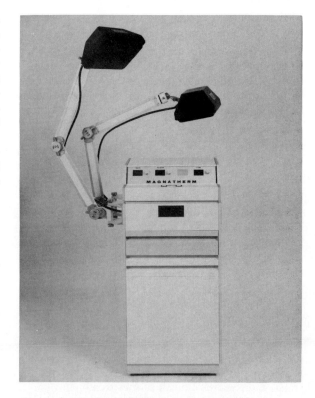

Fig. 14-2. Shortwave diathermy unit. Magnatherm is an example of a shortwave diathermy unit.

directly between the plates. Energy passing from plate to plate must therefore pass directly through the patient, who actually becomes part of the circuit. With a drum or induction field cable, the patient does not become a part of the circuit but rather is within the magnetic field resulting from current flow within the circuit.

The other type of diathermy unit used clinically is **microwave diathermy,** which has certain advantages over shortwave diathermy. The operating frequency of microwave diathermy is on the order of 2450 million cycles per second, yielding a wavelength of approximately 12 centimeters (as contrasted to a wavelength of 11 meters for shortwave diathermy). With microwave diathermy, the energy can be focused toward the body part to be treated. This focus allows for greater penetration because more of the energy strikes the skin perpendicularly. Scatter of the energy is minimized, and absorption is maximized. Because microwave energy can be focused, therapeutic tissue temperature increases can occur up to a depth of 5 centimeters, and microwave diathermy is probably as effective as shortwave diathermy in producing deep-tissue temperature rise.

Energy of clinical shortwave diathermy wavelengths is thought to cause deep-heating effect largely through the oscillation of polar molecules such as water. High-frequency microwaves result in intra-atomic vibrations or disturbances but probably have too high a frequency to result in molecular oscillation or spin. However, the increase in intramolecular vibration has the same effect as molecular oscillation, that is, the production of heat deep within the tissues.[22]

Neither type of diathermy is in as widespread use today as in past years. One major problem is that with significant subcutaneous fat the temperature of the fat may rise to dangerous levels, especially when the diathermy device produces its effects primarily with electrical fields. Furthermore, electrode choice and placement takes a significant amount of time, and areas needing treatment may not always be optimally accessible to available electrode types. Perhaps the main reason for the decline in the use of diathermy has been the development of ultrasound, which is cheaper, provides deep-tissue temperature rise, is safer, and requires a much shorter treatment time.

ULTRASOUND

By definition, **ultrasonic energy** is vibrational energy with a frequency above 20,000 Hertz. Unlike sound energy in the audible range, ultrasonic energy is for the most part absorbed by gases. For this reason, a liquid ointment must be used as a coupling agent to ensure significant transfer of energy from the source of ultrasound to the patient.[11]

Ultrasonic energy is generally produced in the clinic by a device that generates a high-frequency AC. This high-frequency current then sets a crystal (usually quartz or synthetic crystal), which is housed in a handheld transducer, into vibration (Figure 14-3). The most common clinical ultrasonic generators operate at a frequency of 1 million Hertz.

As used in the clinic, ultrasound is usually delivered at an intensity of about 1.5 watts per square centimeter of transducer surface. At this intensity, significant mechanical and deep-heating effects occur, caused primarily by absorption of high-frequency sound energy and the transduction of this energy into heat. Because of the considerable reflection of ultrasonic energy at tissue interfaces (for example, ten-

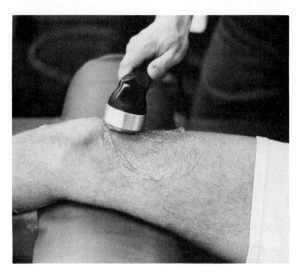

Fig. 14-3. Technique for applying ultrasound.

don-bone), sharply localized tissue temperature increases can occur at these junctions, particularly those junctions having limited vascularization. Such a temperature increase sometimes occurs at the junction of bone and periosteum. Because the periosteum is rich in sensory endings, a deep, dull ache of very sudden onset may occur.[32]

In addition to thermal effects, other physiological effects of ultrasound have been reported. Ultrasonic energy has been largely absorbed by proteins and caused changes in cell permeability to sodium and potassium. Ultrasound has also been effective in decreasing pain from neuromas, increasing range of motion limited by scar formation, and relieving pain resulting from tendinitis, bursitis, or fibrosis with or without evidence of mineral deposition. Whether ultrasound exerts these effects via thermal or nonthermal changes cannot yet be clearly determined. Ultrasonic energy is not transmitted efficiently through gas or, for that matter, through fluids containing high concentrations of gases because the energy is absorbed by the gas. Therefore an appropriate ultrasound conducting medium or coupling agent must be placed between the transducer or sonator and the patient. For fairly large and smooth body surfaces, a coating of commercial gel or mineral oil may be placed directly on the surface. The transducer is placed directly in contact with the oil or gel and is either continually moved in a circular or longitudinal motion or remains stationary with the unit set in either a pulsed mode or at a duty cycle of 50% or less. For very irregular body surfaces or areas with bony prominences, immersion techniques are often preferred. The body part is immersed in a container of fluid such as distilled water (previously boiled to remove gas bubbles). The transducer is then held 1 inch from the part to be treated and is usually moved continuously.

Ultrasound is sometimes also used to introduce pharmacological agents subcutaneously, possibly by causing changes in the permeability of the membrane. This technique is called **phonophoresis**. The medicinal agent is mixed with an ointment or liquid that serves as a coupling agent. The radiating surface of the transducer is placed into the coupling agent containing the pharmacological agent and energized using either the moving or stationary technique.[27]

Phonophoresis may be superior to iontophoresis as a method of introducing topically applied medication deep into underlying tissue. It has no danger of skin damage and no tendency to dissociate the introduced compound into ionized fragments. In addition, pharmacological agents may be introduced more deeply into subcutaneous tissues with phonophoresis than with iontophoresis without concern for the pH of the coupling agent. Treatment time may also be cut by as much as half.

Ultrasound has many advantages over the use of diathermy. In general, ultrasound can provide the deep-heating effects of diathermy and possibly useful nonthermal effects. Ultrasound units are generally much less expensive than diathermy units and usually much more portable. Another important clinical advantage is that ultrasound is poorly absorbed by homogeneous tissues such as fat, and therefore excessive heating of fat (which is superficial to tissues where deep heating is desired) is not a problem. Another advantage is that ultrasound can usually be used in the area of metal implants if they are deep enough. Metal, which is extremely homogeneous, does not absorb energy to as high a degree with ultrasound as with shortwave or microwave energy. Some reflection of ultrasound does occur, and some increase in temperature can occur at tissue-implant interfaces.

INFRARED MODALITIES

The superficial heating and cooling modalities used in a sports-medicine setting are all classified as infrared modalities.[4] Heat modalities are referred to as **thermotherapy**. Thermotherapy is used when a rise

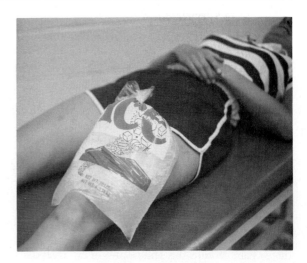

Fig. 14-4. Cryotherapy.

in tissue temperature is the goal of treatment. The use of cold, or **cryotherapy**, is most effective in the acute stages of the healing process immediately after injury when tissue temperature loss is the goal of therapy (Figure 14-4). Cold applications can be continued into the reconditioning state of athletic injury management. The term **hydrotherapy** can be applied to any cryotherapy or thermotherapy technique that uses water as the medium for heat transfer.[4]

Clinical Use of Heat and Cold

The physiological effects of heat and cold are rarely the result of direct absorption of infrared energy. There is general agreement that no form of infrared energy can have a depth of penetration greater than 1 centimeter. Thus the effects of the infrared modalities are primarily superficial and directly affect the cutaneous blood vessels and the cutaneous nerve receptors.[4]

Absorption of infrared energy cutaneously increases and decreases circulation subcutaneously in both the muscle and fat layers. If the energy is absorbed cutaneously over a long enough period to raise the temperature of the circulating blood, the hypothalamus will reflexively increase blood flow to the underlying tissue. Likewise, absorption of cold cutaneously can decrease blood flow via a similar mechanism in the area of treatment.

Thus if the primary treatment goal is a tissue temperature increase with corresponding increase in blood flow to the deeper tissues, a wiser choice is perhaps a modality, such as diathermy or ultrasound, that produces energy that can penetrate the cutaneous tissues and be directly absorbed by the deep tissues.

If the primary treatment goal is to reduce tissue temperature and decrease blood flow to an injured area, the superficial application of ice or cold is the only modality capable of producing such a response.

Perhaps the most effective use of the infrared modalities is for **analgesia,** that is, reducing the sensation of pain associated with injury. The infrared modalities primarily stimulate the cutaneous nerve receptors. Through one of the mechanisms of pain modulation, most likely the gate control theory, hyperstimulation of these nerve receptors by heating or cooling reduces pain. Within the philosophy of an aggressive program of rehabilitation, as is standard in most sports-medicine settings, the reduction of pain as a means of facilitating therapeutic exercise is a common practice. As emphasized earlier, therapeutic modalities are perhaps best used as an adjunct to therapeutic exercise. Certainly, this should be a prime consideration when selecting an infrared modality for use in any treatment program.[4]

Continued investigation and research into the use of heat and cold is warranted to provide useful data for the sports-medicine professional. Heat and cold applications, when used properly and efficiently, provide the sports therapist with tools to enhance recovery and provide the athlete with optimal health-care management. Thermotherapy and cryotherapy are only two of the tools available to assist in the well-being and reconditioning of the injured athlete.

Cryotherapy

Cryotherapy is the use of cold to treat acute trauma and subacute injury and to decrease discomfort after athletic reconditioning and rehabilitation. Tools of cryotherapy include ice packs, cold whirlpool, ice whirlpool, ice massage, commercial chemical cold spray, and contrast baths. Application of cryotherapy produces a three- to four-stage sensation. The first sensation of cold is followed by a stinging, then a burning or aching feeling, and finally numbness. Each stage is related to the nerve endings as they temporarily cease to function as a result of decreased blood flow. The time required for this sequence varies from 5 to 15 minutes. After 12 to 15 minutes, a reflex deep-tissue vasodilation called the **hunting response** is

sometimes demonstrable with intense cold ($10°$ C or $50°$ F). However, this response appears to occur only in the distal extremities, and its value as a protective mechanism is debatable.[18] A minimum of 15 minutes is necessary to achieve extreme analgesic effects.

Application of ice is safe, simple, and inexpensive. Cryotherapy is contraindicated in patients with cold allergies (hives, joint pain, nausea), Raynaud's phenomenon (arterial spasm), and some rheumatoid conditions.[14]

Depth of penetration depends on the amount of cold and the length of the treatment time. The body is well equipped to maintain skin and subcutaneous tissue viability through the capillary bed by reflex vasodilation of up to four times normal blood flow. The body can decrease blood flow to the body segment that is supposedly losing too much body heat by shunting the blood flow. Depth of penetration is also related to intensity and duration of cold application and the circulatory response to the body segment exposed. If the person has normal circulatory responses, frostbite should not be a concern. Even so, caution should be exercised when applying intense cold directly to the skin. If deeper penetration is desired, ice therapy is most effective with ice towels, ice packs, ice massage, and whirlpools.[19] Patients should be advised of the four stages of cryotherapy and the discomfort they will experience. The sports therapist should explain this sequence and advise the athlete of the expected outcome, which may include a rapid decrease in pain.[4]

Thermotherapy

Heat is still used as a universal treatment for pain and discomfort. Much of the benefit is derived because the treatment simply feels good. In the early stages after injury, however, heat causes increased capillary blood pressure and increased cellular permeability, which results in additional swelling or edema accumulation.[4] No athlete with edema should be treated with any heat modality until the reasons for edema are determined. The best interest of the sports therapist is to use cryotherapy techniques or contrast baths to reduce the edema before heat applications.

Superficial heat applications seem to feel more comfortable for complaints of the neck, back, low back, and pelvic areas and may be most appropriate for the athlete who exhibits some allergic response to cold application. However, the tissues in these areas are absolutely no different from those in the extremities. Thus the same physiological responses to the use of heat or cold are elicited in all body areas.

Primary goals of thermotherapy include increased blood flow and muscle temperature to stimulate analgesia, increased nutrition to the cellular level, reduction of edema, and removal of metabolites and other products of the inflammatory process.[4]

INTERMITTENT COMPRESSION

Intermittent compression units are used to control or reduce swelling after acute injury or pitting edema, which tends to develop in the injured area several hours after injury.

Intermittent compression uses a nylon pneumatic inflatable sleeve applied around the injured extremity (Figure 14-5). The sleeve can be inflated to a specific pressure that forces excessive fluid accumulated in the interstitial spaces into vascular and lymphatic channels, through which it is removed from the area of injury. Compression facilitates the movement of lymphatic fluid, which helps to eliminate the by-products of the injury process.[28]

Intermittent compression devices have essentially three parameters that may be adjusted: on-off time, inflation pressures, and treatment time. Recommended treatment protocols have been established through clinical trial and error with little experimental data currently available to support any protocol.[16]

On-off times include 1 minute on and 2 minutes off, 2 minutes on and 1 minute off, and 4 minutes on and 1 minute off. These recommendations are not based on research. Thus patient comfort should be the primary guide. Recommended inflation pressures have been loosely correlated with blood pressures. The Jobst Institute recommends that pressure be set at 30 to 50 mm Hg for the upper extremity and at 30 to 60 mm Hg for the lower extremity. Because arterial capillary pressures are approximately 30 mm Hg, any pressure that exceeds this rate should encourage the absorption of edema and the flow of lymphatic fluid.[16]

Clinical studies have demonstrated a significant reduction in limb volume after 30 minutes of compression.[16] Thus a 30-minute treatment time seems to be efficient in reducing edema.

Some intermittent compression units can combine cold along with compression. Electrical stimulating currents are not uncommonly used to produce muscle pumping and thus facilitate lymphatic flow.

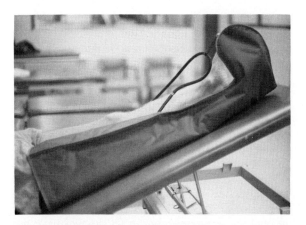

Fig. 14-5. Jobst full leg sleeve.

LOW-POWER LASER

Laser is an acronym that stands for light amplification of stimulated emissions of radiation.[3,25] Lasers are relatively new to the medical community and are certainly the newest of the modalities used by sports therapists. The principles of physics under which laser energy is produced are complex. Basically, an atom is excited when energy is applied and raises an orbiting electron to a higher orbit. When the electron returns to its original orbit, it releases energy (photons) through **spontaneous emission.** Stimulated emission occurs when the photon is released from the excited atom, and it promotes the release of an identical photon to be released from a similarly excited atom. For lasers to operate, a medium of excited atoms must be generated. This is termed **population inversion** and results when an external energy source or pumping device is applied to the medium.[29]

Laser light differs from conventional light in that laser light is monochromic (single color or wavelength), coherent (in phase), and collimated (minimal divergence). Laser can be thermal (hot) or nonthermal (low power, soft, cold). The categories include solid-state (glass or crystal), gas, semiconductor, dye, and chemical lasers.[29]

Helium-neon (HeNe gas) and gallium arsenide (GaAs semiconductor) lasers are two low-power lasers currently being investigated by the FDA for potential application in physical medicine. The HeNe lasers deliver a characteristic red beam with a wavelength of 632.8 nanometers. They are delivered in a continuous wave and have a direct penetration of 2 to 5 millimeters and an indirect penetration of 10 to 15 millimeters. The GaAs laser is invisible, with a wavelength of 904 nanometers. It is delivered in a pulse mode at a very low power output. It has a direct penetration of 1 to 2 centimeters and an indirect penetration of 5 centimeters.[29]

The proposed therapeutic applications of lasers in physical medicine include acceleration of collagen synthesis, decrease in microorganisms, increase in vascularization, and reduction of pain and inflammation.[6,9,10]

Laser application is ideally done with light contact to the surface and should be perpendicular to the target surface. Dosage appears to be the critical factor in eliciting a response, but exact dosages have not been determined. Dosage is altered by varying the pulse frequency and the treatment times. The treatment is applied by developing an imaginary grid over the target area. The grid comprises 1-centimeter squares, and the laser is applied to each square for a predetermined time. Trigger or acupuncture points are also treated for painful conditions.

The FDA considers low-power lasers as low-risk devices. Although no deleterious effects have been reported, certain precautions and contraindications exist, including lasing over cancerous tissue, directly into the eyes, and during the first trimester of pregnancy. Initial pain increases and episodes of syncope have been reported but do not warrant treatment cessation.

Future research for determining the efficacy and treatment parameters is needed to substantiate the application of low-power laser in a sports-medicine setting.

INJURY MANAGEMENT USING MODALITIES

Traditionally in a sports-medicine setting, injuries have been classified as being either acute injuries that result from trauma or chronic injuries that result primarily from overuse. This operational definition is not necessarily correct. If active inflammation is present, which includes the classic symptoms of tenderness, swelling, redness, and so on, the injury should be considered acute and must be treated accordingly using rest, compression, and elevation. Even if active inflammation persists for months after initial injury, it should still be considered acute. Classification of an injury should be made according to the existing signs and symptoms that indicate the various stages of the healing process and not according to time frames or mechanisms of injury. Once the signs of acute inflammation are no longer present, the injury may be considered to be chronic. As discussed in Chapter 1, inflammation may be considered chronic when the normal cellular response in the inflammatory process is altered by replacing leukocytes with macrophages and plasma cells, along with degeneration of the injured structure.

Based on these definitions of acute and chronic injury, the rehabilitation progression after injury may be loosely classified in four phases: initial acute injury, acute inflammatory response, fibroblastic-repair and maturation-remodeling. These phases overlap, and the estimated time frame for each phase shows extreme variability between patients. Table 14-1 summarizes the various modalities that may be used in each of the four phases.

Initial Acute Injury Phase

Modality use in the initial treatment phase should be directed toward limiting the amount of swelling and reducing pain that occurs acutely. The acute phase is marked by swelling, pain when touched, and pain on both active and passive motion. In general, the less initial swelling, the less the time required for rehabilitation. Traditionally, the modality of choice has been and still is **ice.**

Cryotherapy produces vasoconstriction, at least superficially and perhaps indirectly in the deeper tissues, and thus limits the bleeding that always occurs with injury. Ice bags, cold packs, and ice massage may all be used effectively. Cold baths should be avoided because the foot is placed in the gravity-dependent position. Cold whirlpools also place the foot in the gravity-dependent position and produce a massaging action that is likely to retard clotting. The importance of cryotherapy techniques for reducing acute swelling has probably been exaggerated. Cryotherapy is perhaps best used for producing analgesia, which most likely results from stimulation of sensory cutaneous nerves that, via the gating mechanism, blocks or reduces pain.

Compression is perhaps the most critical element in controlling swelling initially. An intermittent compression device may be used to provide even pressure around an injured extremity. The pressurized sleeve mechanically reduces the amount of space available for swelling to accumulate. Units that combine both compression and cold are extremely useful in this phase. Regardless of the specific techniques

TABLE 14-1

Clinical Decision Making on the Use of Various Therapeutic Modalities in Treatment of Acute Injury

Phase	Approximate Time Frame	Clinical Picture	Possible Modalities Used	Rationale for Use
Initial acute	Injury–day 3	Swelling, pain to touch, pain on motion	CRYO ESC IC LPL Rest	↓ Swelling, ↓ pain ↓ Pain ↓ Swelling ↓ Pain
Inflammatory response	Day 2–day 6	Swelling subsides, warm to touch, discoloration, pain to touch, pain on motion	CRYO ESC IC LPL Range of motion	↓ Swelling, ↓ pain ↓ Pain ↓ Swelling ↓ Pain
Fibroblastic-repair	Day 4–day 10	Pain to touch, pain on motion, swollen	THERMO ESC LPL IC Range of motion Strengthening	Mildly ↑ circulation ↓ Pain–muscle pumping ↓ Pain Facilitate lymphatic flow
Maturation-remodeling	Day 7–recovery	Swollen, no more pain to touch, decreasing pain on motion	ULTRA ESC LPL SWD MWD Range of motion Strengthening Functional activities	Deep heating to ↑ circulation ↑ Range of motion, ↑ strength ↓ Pain ↓ Pain Deep heating to ↑ circulation Deep heating to ↑ circulation

CRYO, Cryotherapy; *ESC,* electrical stimulating currents; *IC,* intermittent compression; *LPL,* low-power laser; *MWD,* microwave diathermy; *SWD,* shortwave diathermy; *THERMO,* thermotherapy; *ULTRA,* ultrasound; ↓ decrease; ↑ increase.

selected, cold and compression should always be combined with elevation to avoid any additional pooling of blood in the injured area from the effects of gravity.

Electrical stimulating currents may also be used in the initial phase for pain reduction. Parameters should be adjusted to maximally stimulate sensory cutaneous nerve fibers, again to take advantage of the gate control mechanism of pain modulation. Intensities that produce muscle contraction should be avoided because they may increase clotting time.

The low-power laser has also been demonstrated to be effective in pain modulation through the stimulation of trigger points and may be used acutely.

The injured part should be rested and protected for at least the first 48 to 72 hours to allow the inflammatory phase of the healing process to do what it is supposed to.

Inflammatory-Response Phase

The inflammatory-response phase begins as early as day 1 and may last as long as day 6 after injury. Clinically, swelling begins to subside and eventually stops altogether. The injured area may feel warm to the touch, and some discoloration is usually apparent. The injury is still painful to the touch, and pain is elicited on movement of the injured part. As in the initial injury stage, modalities should be used to control pain and reduce swelling. Cryotherapy should still be used during the inflammatory stage. Ice bags, cold packs, or ice massages provide analgesic effects. The use of cold also reduces the likelihood of swelling, which may continue during this stage. Swelling does subside completely by the end of this phase.

It must be emphasized that heating an injury too soon is a bigger mistake than using ice on an injury for too long. Many sports therapists elect to stay with cryotherapy for weeks after injury; some never switch to the superficial heating techniques. This procedure is simply a matter of personal preference that should be dictated by experience. Once swelling has stopped, the sports therapist may elect to begin contrast baths with a longer cold-to-hot ratio.

An intermittent compression device may be used to decrease swelling by facilitating resorption of the by-products of injury by the lymphatic system. Electrical stimulating currents and low-power laser can be used to help reduce pain.

After the initial stage, the athlete should begin to work on active and passive range of motion. Decisions regarding how rapidly to progress exercise should be determined by the response of the injury to that exercise. If exercise produces additional swelling and markedly exacerbates pain, then the level or intensity of the exercise is too great and should be reduced. Sports therapists should be aggressive in their approach to rehabilitation, but the approach will always be limited by the healing process.

Fibroblastic-Repair Phase

Once the inflammatory response has subsided, the fibroblastic-repair phase begins. During this phase of the healing process, fibroblastic cells lay down a matrix of collagen fibers and form scar tissue. This stage may begin as early as 4 days after the injury and may last for several weeks. At this point, swelling has stopped completely. The injury is still tender to the touch but is not as painful as during the last stage. Pain is also less on active and passive motion.

Treatments may change during this stage from cold to heat, once again using increased swelling as a precautionary indicator. Thermotherapy techniques, including hydrocollator packs, paraffin, or eventually warm whirlpool, may be safely used. The purpose of thermotherapy is to increase circulation to the injured area to promote healing. These modalities can also produce some degree of analgesia.

Intermittent compression can once again be used to facilitate removal of injury by-products from the area. Electrical stimulating currents can be used to assist this process by eliciting a muscle contraction and thus inducing a muscle pumping action. This aids in facilitating lymphatic flow. Electrical currents can once again be used for modulation of pain, as can stimulation of trigger points with the low-powered laser.

The sports therapist must continue to stress the importance of range-of-motion and strengthening exercises and progress them appropriately during this phase.

Maturation-Remodeling Phase

The maturation-remodeling phase is the longest of the four phases and may last for several years, depending on the severity of the injury. The ultimate goal during this maturation stage of the healing process is return to activity. The injury is no longer painful to the touch, although some progressively decreasing pain may still be felt on motion. The collagen fibers must be realigned according to tensile stresses and strains placed upon them. Virtually all modalities may be safely used during this stage; thus decisions should be based on what seems to work most effectively in a given situation.

At this point some type of heating modality is beneficial to the healing process. The deep-heating modalities, ultrasound, or shortwave and microwave diathermy should be used to increase circulation to the deeper tissues. Increased blood flow delivers the essential nutrients to the injured area to promote healing, and increased lymphatic flow assists in breakdown and removal of waste products. The superficial heating modalities are certainly less effective at this point.

Electrical stimulating currents can be used for a number of purposes. As before, they may be used in pain modulation. They may also be used to assist in increasing range of motion or muscular strength. Low-power laser can also assist in modulating pain. If pain is reduced, therapeutic exercises may be progressed more quickly. Range-of-motion and strengthening exercises can be increased relatively quickly and progress toward a full, pain-free return to levels required for successful participation in sports activities.

Other Considerations in Treating Injury

During the rehabilitation period after injury, athletes must alter their training and conditioning habits to allow the injury to heal sufficiently. The sports therapist must not neglect fitness training in designing a rehabilitation program. Consideration must be given to maintaining levels of strength, flexibility, and cardiorespiratory endurance.

Modality use should be combined with antiinflammatory medication, particularly during the initial acute and acute inflammatory phases of rehabilitation. A complete discussion of the effects of various medications on the rehabilitation process appears in Chapter 15.

INDICATIONS AND CONTRAINDICATIONS

Table 14-2 is a summary list of indications, contraindications, and precautions in using the various modalities. This list should aid the sports therapist in

TABLE 14-2
Indications and Contraindications for Therapeutic Modalities

Therapeutic Modality	Physiological Responses (Indications for Use)	Contraindications and Precautions
Electrical stimulating currents—high voltage	Pain modulation Muscle reeducation Muscle pumping contractions Retard atrophy Muscle strengthening Increase range of motion Fracture healing Acute injury	Pacemakers Thrombophlebitis Superficial skin lesions
Electrical stimulating currents—low voltage	Wound healing Fracture healing Iontophoresis	Malignancy Skin hypersensitivities Allergies to certain drugs
Electrical stimulating currents—interferential	Pain modulation Muscle reeducation Muscle pumping contractions Fracture healing Increase range of motion	Same as high-voltage
Electrical stimulating currents—Russian	Muscle strengthening	Pacemakers
Electrical stimulating currents—MENS	Fracture healing Wound healing	Malignancy Infections
Shortwave diathermy and microwave diathermy	Increase deep circulation Increase metabolical activity Reduce muscle guarding/spasm Reduce inflammation Facilitate wound healing Analgesia Increase tissue temperatures over a large area	Metal implants Pacemakers Malignancy Wet dressings Anesthetized areas Pregnancy Acute injury and inflammation Eyes Areas of reduced blood flow Anesthetized areas
Cryotherapy—cold packs, ice massage	Acute injury Vasoconstriction—decreased blood flow Analgesia Reduce inflammation Reduce muscle guarding/spasm	Allergy to cold Circulatory impairments Wound healing Hypertension
Thermotherapy—hot whirlpool, paraffin, hydrocollator, infrared lamps	Vasodilation—increased blood flow Analgesia Reduce muscle guarding/spasm Reduce inflammation Increase metabolical activity Facilitate tissue healing	Acute and postacute trauma Poor circulation Circulatory impairments Malignancy

Continued.

TABLE 14-2

Indications and Contraindications for Therapeutic Modalities—Cont'd

Therapeutic Modality	Physiological Responses (Indications for Use)	Contraindications and Precautions
Low-power laser	Pain modulation (trigger points)	Pregnancy
	Facilitate wound healing	Eyes
Ultraviolet	Acne	Psoriasis
	Aseptic wounds	Eczema
	Folliculitis	Herpes
	Pityriasis rosea	Diabetes
	Tinea	Pellagra
	Septic wounds	Lupus erythematosus
	Sinusitis	Hyperthyroidism
	Increase calcium metabolism	Renal and hepatic insufficiency
		Generalized dermatitis
		Advanced atherosclerosis
Ultrasound	Increase connective tissue extensibility	Infection
	Deep heat	Acute and postacute injury
	Increased circulation	Epiphyseal areas
	Treatment of most soft tissue injuries	Pregnancy
	Reduce inflammation	Thrombophlebitis
	Reduce muscle spasm	Impaired sensation
		Eyes
Intermittent compression	Decrease acute bleeding	Circulatory impairment
	Decrease edema	

making decisions regarding the appropriate use of a therapeutic modality in a given clinical situation.

SUMMARY

1. Modalities are best used by the sports therapist as adjuncts to other forms of therapeutic exercise. Decisions on how a particular modality may best be used should be based on both theoretical knowledge and practical experience.

2. Electrical stimulating currents may be used to stimulate sensory nerves to modulate pain, stimulate motor nerves to elicit a muscle contraction, introduce chemical ions into superficial tissues for medicinal purposes, and create an electrical field in the tissues to stimulate or alter the healing process.

3. The physiological response of the biological tissues to electrical stimulating currents is to a great extent determined by the treatment parameters of the current selected by the sports therapist.

4. Shortwave and microwave diathermy units use extremely high frequency electrical currents to produce a tissue temperature increase in the deeper tissues.

5. Ultrasound is vibrational acoustic energy that causes a tissue temperature increase in addition to other physiological effects that aid healing.

6. Ultrasound has a number of advantages over diathermy, including deeper penetration and more portable and less expensive equipment.

7. The effects of thermotherapy and cryotherapy are primarily superficial. These modalities are perhaps most effectively used to produce analgesia. They also have an indirect effect on circulation in the deeper tissues.

8. Low-powered lasers are the newest modality used in sports-medicine settings, primarily to promote wound healing and also pain modulation through stimulation of acupuncture and trigger points.

9. Modality use in the initial acute injury phase should be directed toward one goal, that being to reduce the amount of swelling that occurs. The less the amount of initial swelling, the less time will be required for rehabilitation.

10. During the inflammatory-response stage of healing, modalities should be used to reduce pain and limit the amount of swelling. The injured part should be rested to allow the healing process to work.

11. During the fibroblastic-repair phase, thermotherapy may be used to increase blood flow to the injured area. Also during this time, strengthening and range-of-motion exercises should begin.

12. The maturation-remodeling phase is a long-term process during which the athlete returns to activity. Deep-heating modalities that increase blood flow and assist in the breakdown and removal of the by-products of the healing process should be used. The quantity and intensity of therapeutic exercise should be progressively increased during this phase of healing.

REFERENCES

1 Alon G: *High voltage stimulation: a monograph,* Chattanooga Corporation, 1984.

2 Barr J: Transcutaneous electrical nerve stimulation characteristics altering pain perception, *Phys Ther* 66(10):1037-1048, 1987.

3 Beckerman H, deBierck R, Bouter L, et al.: The efficacy of laser therapy for musculoskeletal and skin disorders: a criteria based meta-analysis of randomized clinical trials, *Phys Ther* 72:483-491, 1992.

4 Bell G: Infrared modalities. In Prentice W, editor: *Therapeutic modalities in sports medicine,* St Louis, 1990, Mosby.

5 Benton L: *Functional electrical stimulation: a practical clinical guide,* Downet, Calif, 1980, Rancho Los Amigos Hospital.

6 Castel M: *A clinical guide to low-power laser therapy,* Downsview, Ont, 1985, Physiotechnology, Ltd.

7 Delitto A, Robinson A: Electrical stimulation of muscle: techniques application. In Snyder-Mackler L, editor: *Clinical electrophysiology: electrotherapy and electrophysiologic testing,* Baltimore, 1989, Williams and Wilkins.

8 Delitto A, Strube M, Schulman A, et al.: A study of discomfort with electrical stimulation, *Phys Ther* 72:410-424, 1992.

9 Donley P: Shortwave and microwave diathermy. In Prentice W, editor: *Therapeutic modalities in sports medicine,* St Louis, 1990, Mosby.

10 Enwemeka C: Laser biostimulation of healing wounds: specific effects and mechanisms of action, *J Orthop Sports Phys Ther* 9:333-338, 1988.

11 Eriksson E, Haggmark T: Comparison of isometric muscle training and electrical stimulation supplement: isometric training in recovery after major knee ligament surgery, *Am J Sports Med* 7:169-171, 1979.

12 Geick J, Bamford M, Stewart H, et al.: *Therapeutic ultrasound: technology, performance standards, biological effect, and clinical application,* HSH Publication, FOA 84-xxxx, August, 1984.

13 Griffin J, Karselis T: The diathermies. In Griffin J, Karselis T, editors: *Physical agents for physical therapists,* Springfield, Ill, 1982, Charles C Thomas.

14 Haar G: Basic physics of therapeutic ultrasound, *Physiotherapy* 64(4):100-102, 1978.

15 Hocutt J, Jaffe R, Rylander C, et al.: Cryotherapy in ankle sprains, *Am J Sports Med* 10(5):316-319, 1982.

16 Hooker D: Electrical stimulating currents. In Prentice W, editor: *Therapeutic modalities in sports medicine,* St Louis, 1990, Mosby.

17 Hooker D: Intermittent compression devices. In Prentice W, editor: *Therapeutic modalities in sports medicine,* St Louis, 1990, Mosby.

18 Howson D: Peripheral neural excitability, *Phys Ther* 58:1467-1473, 1978.

19 Knight K, Aquino J, Johannes S, et al.: A reexamination of Lewis cold induced vasodilation in the finger and ankle, *Ath Train* 15:248-250, 1980.

20 Knight K, Londeree B: Comparison of blood flow in the ankle of uninjured subjects during therapeutic applications of heat, cold, and exercise, *Med Sci Sports Exerc* 12(1):76-80, 1980.

21 Laughman RK: Strength changes in the normal quadriceps femoris muscle as a result of electrical stimulation, *Phys Ther* 63:494-499, 1983.

22 Lehmann J, Delauter B: Diathermy and superficial heat and cold. In Krusen F, editor: *Handbook of physical medicine and rehabilitation,* Philadelphia, 1982, WB Saunders.

23 Mannheimer J, Lampe G: *Clinical transcutaneous electrical nerve stimulation,* Philadelphia, 1984, FA Davis.

24 Melzack R: Prolonged relief of pain by brief intense transcutaneous electrical stimulation, *Pain* 1(4):357-373, 1975.

25 Mester E, Mester A, Mester A: Biomedical effects of laser application, *Laser Surg Med* 5:31-39, 1985.

26 Prentice W: Basic principles of electricity. In Prentice W, editor: *Therapeutic modalities in sports medicine,* St Louis, 1990, Mosby.

27 Quillen S: Phonophoresis: a review of the literature and technique, *Ath Train* 15(2):109-110, 1980.

28 Quillen W, Rouiller L: Initial management of acute ankle sprains with rapid pulsed pneumatic compression and cold, *J Orthop Sports Phys Ther* 4(1):39-43, 1982.

29 Saliba E: Low-power laser. In Prentice W, editor: *Therapeutic modalities in sports medicine,* St Louis, 1990, Mosby.

30 Selkowitz D: Improvement in isometric strength of the quadriceps femoris muscle as a result of electrical stimulation, *Phys Ther* 65:186, 1985.

31 Snyder-Mackler L: *Clinical electrophysiology: electrotherapy and electrophysiologic testing,* Baltimore, 1989, Williams and Wilkins.

32 Spiker J: Ultrasound. In Prentice W, editor: *Therapeutic modalities in sports medicine,* St Louis, 1990, Mosby.

Pharmacological Considerations in a Rehabilitation Program

15

William E. Prentice and Patsy Huff

OBJECTIVES

After completion of this chapter, the student should be able to do the following:

- Discuss the reasons for use of various analgesics, antiinflammatories, and antipyretics as an adjunct form of treatment in a rehabilitation program.

- Identify the potential side effects and reactions of medications that act on the respiratory tract, medications that affect the gastrointestinal tract, and antibiotics.

- Discuss the importance of record keeping when administering medications in a sports-medicine environment.

- Be aware of the legalities of dispensing vs. administering medications by sports-medicine personnel.

- Discuss the impact of drug testing programs on the use of various medications in a rehabilitation setting.

The use of medications prescribed for various medical conditions by qualified physicians may be of great value to the athlete as with any other individual in the population.[30] Under average circumstances an athlete would be expected to respond to medication just as anyone else would. However, because of the nature of physical activity, the athlete's situation is not average; with intense physical activity, special consideration should be given to the effects of certain types of medication.

For the sports therapist supervising a program of rehabilitation, some knowledge of the potential effects of certain types of drugs on performance during the rehabilitation program is essential. The sports therapist working under the direction of a team physician is responsible for keeping the athlete healthy and ready to train and compete under physically,

mentally, and emotionally demanding circumstances. The sports therapist should be concerned not only with rehabilitation but also with prevention, acute management, and evaluation of sports-related injuries. On occasion, the sports therapist must make decisions regarding the appropriate use of medications based on knowledge of the indications for use and the possible side effects in athletes who are involved in rehabilitation programs.

The sports therapist must be cognizant of the potential effects and side effects of over-the-counter and prescription medications on the athlete during rehabilitation, as well as during competition.

This chapter concentrates on the special considerations that must be given regarding those medications most commonly used in a sports-medicine environment.

COMMON MEDICATIONS

This section provides the sports therapist with some special considerations regarding those medications most commonly prescribed for and used by individuals involved in some sports-related activity. The classifications of medication discussed include (1) analgesics, antipyretics, and antiinflammatories; (2) drugs that affect the respiratory tract; (3) drugs that affect the gastrointestinal tract; and (4) antibiotic medications (Table 15-1).

Analgesics, Antipyretics, and Antiinflammatories

Perhaps medications are most commonly used in a sports-medicine environment for pain relief. The athlete is continuously in situations where injuries are very likely. Fortunately, most of the injuries that occur are not serious and lend themselves to rapid rehabilitation. However, pain is associated with even minor injury.

The three nonnarcotic analgesics most often used are aspirin (salicylate), acetaminophen, and ibuprofen. These belong to the group of drugs called *nonsteroidal antiinflammatory agents (NSAIDs)*. Aspirin is one of the most commonly used drugs in the world.[28] Because of its easy availability, it is also likely the most misused drug. Aspirin is a derivative of salicylic acid and is used for its analgesic, antiinflammatory, and antipyretic capabilities.

Analgesia may result from several mechanisms; aspirin may interfere with the transmission of painful impulses in the thalamus.[22] Soft tissue injury leads to tissue necrosis. This tissue injury causes the release of arachidonic acid from phospholipid cell walls. Oxygenation of arachidonic acid by cyclooxygenase produces a variety of prostaglandins, thromboxane, and prostacyclin that mediate the subsequent inflammatory reaction.[1] The predominant mechanism of action of aspirin and other NSAIDs is the inhibition of prostaglandin synthesis by blocking the cyclooxygenase pathway.[34] Pain and inflammation are reduced by the blockage of accumulation of proinflammatory prostaglandins in the synovium or cartilage.

Stabilization of the lysosomal membrane also occurs, preventing the efflux of destructive lysosomal enzymes into the joints.[18] Aspirin is the only NSAID that irreversibly inhibits cyclooxygenase; the other NSAIDs provide reversible inhibition. Aspirin also can reduce fever by altering sympathetic outflow from the hypothalamus, which produces increased vasodilation and heat loss through sweating.[22,31] Among the side effects of aspirin usage are gastric distress, heartburn, some nausea, tinnitus, headache, and diarrhea. More serious consequences can develop with prolonged use or high dosages.[2]

An athlete should be very cautious about selecting aspirin as a pain reliever for a number of reasons.[29] Aspirin decreases aggregation of platelets and thus impairs the clotting mechanism should injury occur.[24] Aspirin's irreversible inhibition of cyclooxygenase that leads to reduced production of clotting factors creates a bleeding risk not present with the other NSAIDs.[33] Prolonged bleeding at an injured site will increase the amount of swelling, which has a direct effect on the time required for rehabilitation.

Use of aspirin as an antiinflammatory should be recommended with caution. Other antiinflammatory medications do not produce many of the undesirable side effects of aspirin. Generally, prescription antiinflammatories are considered to be equally effective.

Aspirin sometimes produces gastric discomfort. In the case of an athlete, intense physical activity may exacerbate this side effect. Buffered aspirin is no less irritating to the stomach than is regular aspirin, but enteric-coated tablets resist aspirin breakdown in the stomach and may minimize gastric discomfort. Regardless of the form of aspirin ingested, it should be taken with meals or with large quantities of water (8 to 10 ounces/tablet) to reduce the likelihood of gastric irritation.

Ibuprofen is classified as a NSAID; however, it also has analgesic and antipyretic effects. Ibuprofen, like aspirin, has a number of side effects, including the potential for gastric irritation. It is not as likely to affect platelet aggregation as is aspirin. Ibuprofen administered at a dose of 200 mg does not require a prescription and at that dosage may be used for analgesia. At a dose of 400 mg, the effects are both analgesic and antiinflammatory. Dosage forms greater than 200 mg require a prescription. For names and recommended doses of prescription NSAIDs, refer to Table 15-2.

Acetaminophen, like aspirin, has both analgesic and antipyretic effects, but it does not have significant antiinflammatory capabilities.[2] Acetaminophen is indicated for relief of mild somatic pain and fever reduction through mechanisms similar to those of aspirin.[15]

The primary advantage of acetaminophen for the athlete is that it does not produce gastritis, irritation,

TABLE 15-1

Sports Therapists' Guide to Commonly Used Medications

Generic Name	Trade Name	Primary Use of Drug	Sports Medicine Considerations
ANALGESICS, ANTIPYRETICS, AND ANTIINFLAMMATORIES			
Aspirin	Many trade names	Analgesic, antipyretic, antiinflammatory	Gastric irritation, nausea, tinnitus, prolonged bleeding if injured in contact sports
Acetaminophen	Tylenol®, Datril®, others	Analgesic, antipyretic	None
(Nonsteroidal Antiinflammatories)			
Flurbiprofen	Ansaid®	All are analgesic, antipyretic, antiinflammatory	Gastric irritation less common than with aspirin except for indomethacin. These should be used on a long-term basis for reducing inflammation; should not be substituted for acetaminophen in cases of mild headache or low fever
Ketoprofen	Orudis®		
Indomethacin	Indocin®		
Ibuprofen	Advil®, Motrin®, Nuprin®		
Naproxen	Naprosyn®, Anaprox®		
Diflunisal	Dolobid®		
Piroxicam	Feldene®		
Tolmectin	Tolectin®		
Fenoprofen	Nalfon®		
Meclofenamate	Meclomen®		
Diclofenac	Voltaren®		
Ketrolac	Toradol®		
DRUGS THAT AFFECT THE RESPIRATORY TRACT			
Chlorpheniramine	Chlor-Trimeton®	Antihistamine for allergies	Used primarily for treatment of allergic reaction. Causes drowsiness, decreased coordination
Dimenhydrinate	Dramamine®	Antihistamine used for treatment of motion sickness, nausea, vomiting	Should be administered before travel begins, produces drowsiness
Oxymetazoline	Afrin®, Dristan Long Lasting®, Neosynephrine 12 Hour®, Nostrilla®, Sinex Long Lasting®, Allerest®	Adrenergic decongestant applied topically as spray	Do not exceed recommended dosage because of rebound congestion; may cause sneezing, dryness of nasal mucosa, and headache
Pseudoephedrine	Sudafed®, Cenafed®, Oranyl®, others	Adrenergic decongestant used orally	Produces stimulation of the central nervous system; topically applied decongestants work faster, but oral decongestants are preferred for long-term use
Diphenhydramine	Benlin cough syrup®, Benadryl®	Antihistamine used primarily for allergic reaction; also used for motion sickness and preventing nausea and vomiting	Produces drowsiness and dry mouth; found in over-the-counter sleeping medication
Dextromethorphan	Benylin DM®, Romilar CF®, Coughettes®, Sucrets Lozenge®, Robitussin DM®	Nonnarcotic antitussive used for suppression of cough	Very effective in case of unproductive cough; doesn't produce drowsiness and other side effects as commonly

TABLE 15-1—cont'd
Sports Therapists' Guide to Commonly Used Medications

Generic Name	Trade Name	Primary Use of Drug	Sports Medicine Considerations
Tertenadine	Seldane®	Antihistamine	Nonsedating
Benzonatate	Tessalon®	Peripherally acting antitussive that acts as an anesthetic	May produce dizziness and a chilled sensation
Codeine	Robitussin AC®	Narcotic antitussive that depresses the central cough mechanism	Used in combination with decongestant, an antihistamine, or expectorant; can produce sedation, dizziness, constipation, nausea
Guaifenesin	Robitussin®, Glyate®, Anti-tuss®	Expectorant used for symptomatic relief of unproductive cough	Used for treating a dry or sore throat; may cause drowsiness and nausea
DRUGS THAT AFFECT THE GASTROINTESTINAL TRACT			
Sodium bicarbonate	Soda Mint,®, Bell/ans®	Antacid used for quick relief of upset stomach	Produces gas belching and tension; may cause systemic alkalinity
Aluminum hydroxide	Amphogel®, Dialume®	Antacid used for upset stomach	May produce constipation; moderate acid neutralizer
Calcium carbonate	Mallamint®, Amitone®, Chooz®, Titralac®	Antacid used for upset stomach	May produce constipation and acid rebound; high acid neutralizing capability
Dihydroxyaluminum sodium carbonate	Rolaids®	Antacid used for upset stomach	May cause constipation; rapid neutralizing capabilities, but transient
Magnesium hydroxide, carbonate oxide	Milk of Magnesia®	Antacid used for upset stomach	May cause diarrhea and lasting neutralization of acid without rebound
Cimetidine	Tagamet®	Used for relief of upset stomach	May produce drowsiness and either constipation or diarrhea
Common combination antacids	Alka-Seltzer®, Di-Gel®, Gaviscon®, Gelusil®, Maalox®, Mylanta®, Tempo®, Titralac®, Wingel®, others	Over-the-counter combination drugs used for controlling gastric upset	May produce either diarrhea or constipation
Promethazine	Phenergan®	Antiemetic used for preventing motion sickness, nausea, and vomiting	Causes sedation and drowsiness
Diphenoxylate HCl	Lomotil®, Uni-Lom®	Narcotic antidiarrheal	Causes dry mouth, nausea, drowsiness
Loperamide	Imodium A-D®	Systemic antidiarrheal	Abdominal discomfort and drowsiness
Common over-the-counter antidiarrheals	Donnagel®, Kaopectate®, Pepto-Bismol®	Relief of diarrhea	All are relatively safe with few side effects, although their effectiveness is questionable

TABLE 15-2
Commonly Used NSAIDs Among Athletes

Drug	Initial Dosage	Maximum Daily Dose (mg)
Aspirin	325-650 mg every 4 hours	4000
Voltaren®	50-75 mg twice a day	200
Dolobid®	500-1000 mg followed by 250-300 mg 2-3 times a day	1500
Nalfon®	400-800 mg 3-4 times a day	3200
Advil®, Motrin®, Rufin®	400-800 mg 3-4 times a day	3200
Indocin®	75-150 mg a day in 3-4 divided doses	200
Orudis®	75 mg 3 times a day or 50 mg 4 times a day	300
Ponstel®	500 mg, followed by 250 mg every 6 hours	1000
Naprosyn®	500 mg, followed by 250 mg every 6-8 hours	1250
Anaprox®	550 mg, followed by 275-550 mg 3 times a day	1650
Feldene®	20 mg a day	20
Clinoril®	200 mg twice a day	400
Tolectin®	400 mg 3-4 times a day	1800
Ansaid®	50-100 mg 2-3 times a day	300
Toradol®	10 mg every 4-6 hours for pain	40

or gastrointestinal bleeding. Likewise, it does not affect platelet aggregation and thus does not increase clotting time after an injury.

For the athlete who is not in need of some antiinflammatory medication but who requires some pain-relieving medication or an antipyretic, acetaminophen should be the drug of choice. If inflammation is a consideration, the team physician may elect to use either aspirin or a type of NSAID. Most NSAIDs are prescription medications that, like aspirin, have not only antiinflammatory but also analgesic and antipyretic effects.[17] They are effective for patients who cannot tolerate aspirin because of gastrointestinal distress associated with aspirin use. Patients who have the aspirin allergy triad of (1) nasal polyps, (2) associated bronchospasm/asthma and (3) history of anaphylaxis should not receive any NSAID. Their antiinflammatory capabilities are thought to be equal to

those of aspirin, their advantages being that NSAIDs have fewer side effects and relatively longer duration of action. Perhaps the biggest disadvantage of the NSAIDs is that they tend to be expensive.[19] Even though NSAIDs have analgesic and antipyretic capabilities, they should not be used in cases of mild headache or increased body temperature in place of aspirin or acetaminophen. However, they can be used to relieve many other mild-to-moderately painful somatic conditions like menstrual cramps and soft tissue injury.[19]

The NSAIDs are used primarily for reducing the pain, stiffness, swelling, redness, and fever associated with localized inflammation, most likely by inhibiting the synthesis of prostaglandins.[9] The sports therapist must be aware that inflammation is simply a response to some underlying trauma or condition and that the source of irritation must be corrected or eliminated for these antiinflammatory medications to be effective.

Muscle spasm and guarding accompanies many musculoskeletal injuries. Elimination of this spasm and guarding should facilitate programs of rehabilitation. In many situations, centrally acting oral muscle relaxants are used to reduce spasm and guarding. However, to date the efficacy of using muscle relaxants has not been substantiated, and they do not appear to be superior to analgesics or sedatives in either acute or chronic conditions.[13]

Drugs That Affect the Respiratory Tract

ANTIHISTAMINES. Antihistamines reduce the effects of the chemical histamine on various tissues by selectively blocking receptor sites to which histamines attach. Histamine is abundant in the mast cells of the skin and lungs and in the basophils of blood. It is also found in the gastrointestinal tract and in the brain, where it acts as a neurotransmitter.[7] Histamine is released in response to some toxin, physical or chemical agent, drug, or antigen that has been introduced into the system. Thus it has a major function in many allergic or hypersensitivity reactions.[23]

Antihistamines are most typically used in the treatment of allergic reactions but may also be used as an antiemetic in the prevention of nausea and vomiting.[16] Histamine produces a number of systemic responses: (1) swelling and inflammation in the skin or mucous membranes (angioedema), (2) spasm of smooth bronchial muscle (asthma), (3) inflammation of nasal membranes (rhinitis), and (4) the possibility of anaphylaxis. These responses in varying degrees are typical of allergic reactions to insect stings, food reactions, drug hypersensitivities, and anything else that may facilitate the release of histamine.

Histamine produces these reactions by binding with the cells that compose the various tissues at specific receptor sites. An antihistamine medication can competitively block these receptor sites and thus prevent the typical histamine response. Antihistamines are classified as either H1 or H2 receptor blockers. The so-called true antihistamines affect the H1 receptors only; H2 blockers affect cells in the stomach that secrete hydrochloric acid. Antihistamines do not reverse the effects of histamine; they simply block the receptor sites. Newer nonsedating antihistamines, such as terfenadine (Seldane®) and astemizole (Hismanyl®), require a prescription. Because of the potential risk of drug interactions, these newer antihistamines should be used only under the supervision of a physician. An athlete would benefit from different types of antihistamine medications for (1) relief from various types of allergic reactions, (2) prevention of motion sickness, or (3) relief of rhinitis from colds or seasonal allergies.

Athletes, particularly those involved with fall and spring sports, practice outdoors where they are exposed to a number of allergens (such as pollen and insects) that potentially can produce a histamine response. Most cases are mild allergic reactions that may be treated by the sports therapist with an over-the-counter antihistamine. These medications are most effective in reducing the effects of histamine on the vascular system, which symptomatically include urticaria, rhinitis, and angioedema. These medications are effective in approximately 70% of the patients treated.[7] Chlorpheniramine is the antihistamine most commonly used to treat these mild allergic reactions.

A competitive schedule may require the athlete to do a great deal of traveling. People riding in a bus, car, or airplane often develop nausea and discomfort in response to motion. This motion sickness may be treated with a number of antihistamine medications. Dimenhydrinate and meclizine are the most commonly used drugs for the prevention of motion sickness. They are best used prophylactically before motion sickness occurs. Like other over-the-counter antihistamines, the major side effect is drowsiness and sedation.[5]

In the case of the athlete, antihistamines should be used with caution. The most common side effects of antihistamines are drowsiness and in some cases decreased coordination. Both of these side effects may adversely affect athletic performance and potentially predispose the athlete to unnecessary injury. Thus use of antihistamine medication immediately before athletic competition is not recommended. The athlete should also be reminded that use of any sedating antihistamine along with consumption of alcohol will markedly increase drowsiness.

DECONGESTANTS. Nasal congestion may be associated with a number of causes including pollinosis or hay fever; perennial rhinitis, a chronic inflammatory condition that occurs with constant exposure to an allergen; and infectious rhinitis, which is symptomatic of the common cold.[28] Antihistamines also have anticholinergic effects and can often help to dry up a runny nose. In addition, nasal congestion may be treated with sympathomimetic or decongestant medications that may be used topically or orally. Oxymetazoline is an adrenergic topical nasal decongestant that, when sprayed on the nasal mucosa, produces prolonged vasoconstriction and reduces edema and fluid exudation. Pseudoephedrine is also an adrenergic decongestant taken orally. Nose drops act more rapidly than do the oral decongestants, and oral medications cause more side effects such as stimulation of the central nervous system. However, oral medications are preferred in long-term use.[19]

Some medications combine both antihistamines and nasal decongestants into a single tablet taken orally, which produces relatively lower degrees of drowsiness and other side effects.

Drugs that may increase the rate of heat exhaustion. Heatstroke is a medical emergency associated with a mortality rate of 17% to 70%.[21] Patients of all ages may experience heatstroke. When the ambient temperature approaches body temperature and humidity approaches 100%, loss of heat from the body ceases. Physical exertion and stress, drug therapy, lack of nutrition, lack of acclimatization, alcohol intoxication, age, obesity, and other disease states may contribute to the precipitation of heatstroke.[21] Thermoregulation involves the central and peripheral nervous system and circulatory mechanisms. Drugs that affect neurotransmitters in these systems could affect temperature regulation. Table 15-3 lists drugs associated with heatstroke. Anticholinergics and antihistamines can decrease the peripheral mechanism of sweating and therefore eliminate the body's ability to lose heat from this mechanism. Sympathomimetic amines including decongestants are vasoconstrictors that may predispose an athlete to heatstroke. Phe-

TABLE 15-3
Drugs That May Predispose an Athlete to Heat Illness

Category	Specific Drugs
Neuroleptics	Thorazine®
	Haldol®
	Mellaril®
Antidepressants	Elavil®
	Nardil®
Anticholinergics	Atropine/Donnagel®
	Belladonna®
Antihistamines	Chlor-Trimeton®
Anti-Parkinsonism	Congentin®
Decongestants	Sudafed®
	Entex LA®
Diuretics	Oretic®

nothiazines affect both hot and cold temperature regulation. Tricyclic antidepressants have been shown to affect hypothalamic heat control, as well as having anticholinergic activity. Diuretics may prevent volume expansion and limit cutaneous vasodilation.[21]

Lithium carbonate may increase the risk of heatstroke by its effects on potassium levels. It is important that the sports therapist recognize medications that may increase the risk of heatstroke, especially when athletes are taking any of these medications and exercising in a warm climate.

ANTITUSSIVES AND EXPECTORANTS. Drugs that suppress coughing are **antitussives.** Coughing is a reflex response to some irritation of the throat or airway. A cough is productive if some material is brought up. This type of cough is beneficial in clearing excessive mucus or sputum. An unproductive cough may be caused by post-nasal drip, dry air, a sore throat, or anything else that may irritate the throat. An unproductive cough is of no benefit and should be treated with medication. If the cause of the cough is a dry or a sore throat, an expectorant medication may be used to increase production of fluid in the respiratory system to coat the dry and irritated mucosal linings.[19]

Antitussive drugs are divided into those that depress the central cough center in the medulla and may be either narcotic or nonnarcotic drugs and those that act peripherally to reduce irritation in the throat or trachea. Codeine is one of the more common narcotic antitussives that also has analgesic ef-

fects. They are relatively weak narcotics that are considered safe. Codeine is found primarily in liquid form and is often combined with a decongestant, an analgesic, an expectorant, or an antihistamine. Any liquid preparation that contains codeine is a prescription medication. The side effects of codeine include sedation, dizziness, constipation, and nausea.[7]

The most common nonnarcotic antitussives are diphenhydramine, dextromethorphan, and benzonatate. Perhaps their biggest advantage is that they have no analgesic effects and do not produce dependence. Diphenhydramine is an antihistamine-antitussive that produces both drowsiness and a drying effect. Dextromethorphan is the most widely used antitussive. It is as effective as codeine in medicating an unproductive cough but does not cause severe side effects. Benzonatate causes a local anesthetic action on the stretch receptors in the throat and thus dampens the cough reflex. Its side effects include drowsiness and a chilled sensation.[7] The peripherally acting antitussives are primarily expectorants. Although expectorants are thought to increase production of fluid in the throat, little experimental evidence suggests that the use of an expectorant is any more effective than drinking water or sucking a piece of hard candy. In many cases an expectorant is combined with some other medication such as an antihistamine or a decongestant.[6]

The athlete who is in need of antitussive or expectorant medication may benefit greatly from it. Physical activity tends to exacerbate the problem of a dry sore throat that may be responsible for an unproductive cough. The biggest consideration for the sports therapist would be the effects of other medications (that is, antihistamines or decongestants) that may also be contained in these fluids or lozenges. The drowsiness, gastric irritability, and lack of coordination that may occur will detract from athletic performance.

DRUGS FOR ASTHMA. Asthma, also known as exercise-induced bronchial obstruction, is one of the more common respiratory diseases. The problem may result from a number of respiratory stressors but is always characterized by spasm of smooth muscle, inflammation of mucous linings, and edema, each of which leads to shortness of breath. The medications used for the treatment of asthma are classified as sympathomimetic drugs administered most often as aerosols. Sympathomimetics are bronchodilators that generally reverse the symptoms. Perhaps the greatest side effect of the sympathomimetics is that they may cause some problems in hot environments.

Drugs That Affect the Gastrointestinal Tract

The gastrointestinal tract is subject to numerous disturbances and disorders that are probably among the most common human ailments. The ailments include indigestion, nausea, diarrhea, and constipation problems that virtually everyone has experienced at one time or another. Because of factors such as the stress associated with competition, inconsistent travel schedules, eating patterns on road trips, and even motion sickness during travel, the athlete is even more likely to experience gastric upset.

ANTACIDS. The primary function of an antacid is to neutralize acidity in the upper GI tract by raising the pH, inhibiting the activity of the digestive enzyme pepsin, and thus reducing its action on the gastric mucosal nerve endings.[11,32] Antacids are effective not only for relief of acid indigestion and heartburn but also in the treatment of peptic ulcer. Antacids available in the market possess a wide range of acid neutralizing capabilities and side effects. The sports therapist has to be aware of these side effects when selecting a specific antacid preparation.

One of the most commonly used antacid preparations is sodium bicarbonate or baking soda, which quickly neutralizes hydrochloric acid and yields carbon dioxide gas and water. Sodium bicarbonate is rapidly absorbed by the blood to produce systemic alkalinity. Belching is usually associated with sodium bicarbonate ingestion, and ingestion of excess sodium bicarbonate often produces a rebound effect in which gastric acid secretion increases in response to an alkaline environment.[20]

Other antacids include alkaline salts, which again neutralize hyperacidity but are not easily absorbed in the blood. They also produce disturbances in the lower GI tract. Many of these nonsystemic antacids slow absorption of other medications from the GI tract. Ingestion of antacids containing magnesium tends to have a laxative effect; those containing aluminum or calcium seem to cause constipation. Consequently, many antacid liquids or tablets are combinations of magnesium and either aluminum or calcium hydroxides.[7] If use of a specific antacid produces diarrhea, for example, it may be replaced by another antacid that is higher in aluminum or calcium content to counteract the effects of the magnesium. Conversely, an antacid high in magnesium content may reduce constipation. Simethicone is a silicone added to many of these preparations to reduce gas trapped in the upper GI tract through its antifoaming action.[28]

Sodium bicarbonate is best used on a short-term basis for rapid relief of heartburn or acid indigestion because of the subsequent rebound effect, but the hydroxide salt preparations may be used on a long-term basis.

Selection of specific antacids should be based on consideration of their potential side effects, such as tendency to produce diarrhea or constipation and on how well the patient tolerates their use in terms of taste, side effects, and finally cost.[19]

Calcium supplementation to increase calcium uptake by bone and hence increase bone density as a means of reducing the incidence of fractures is being recommended by some sports-medicine specialists. Caution should be exercised in ingesting large amounts of calcium carbonate from antacids because of the potential constipation that may accompany prolonged use.

Another medication used for relief of gastric discomfort is an antihistamine that is an H2 receptor blocker. Histamine2 receptor blockers inhibit the action of histamine on cells in the stomach that secrete hydrochloric acid and are most typically used to treat ulcers. However, its use in the treatment of indigestion is thought to be no more effective than other antacid preparations.[26]

ANTIEMETICS. This group of drugs is used to treat the nausea and vomiting that may result from a variety of causes. Vomiting serves as a means of eliminating irritants from the stomach before they can be absorbed. Most of the time, however, purging the stomach is not necessary, and vomiting serves only to make the athlete uncomfortable. Frequently, nausea may be treated by giving the individual carbonated soda, tea, or ice to suck. If nausea and vomiting persist, some medication may be beneficial.

Antiemetics are classified as acting either locally or centrally. The locally acting drugs such as most over-the-counter medications (for example, Pepto-Bismol® and Alka-Seltzer®) are topical anesthetics that reportedly affect the mucosal lining of the stomach. However, the effects of soothing an upset stomach may be more of a placebo effect.[28] The centrally acting drugs affect the chemoreceptor trigger zone in the medulla by making it less sensitive to irritating nerve impulses from the inner ear or stomach.

A variety of prescription antiemetics can be used for controlling nausea and vomiting, including phenothiazines, antihistamines, anticholinergic drugs for preventing motion sickness, and sedative drugs. The primary side effect of these medications is again extreme drowsiness.

The sports therapist should deal with nausea and vomiting first by using fluids, which have a calming effect on the stomach, followed by the administration of one of the locally acting medications. If vomiting persists, the athlete will become drowsy and thus may be unable to perform at competitive levels, and dehydration and the problems that accompany it are important considerations for an athlete who has been nauseated and vomiting. Antiemetics may also potentiate central nervous system depressants.

ANTIDIARRHEALS. Diarrhea may result from many causes, but it is generally considered to be a symptom rather than a disease. It can occur as a result of emotional stress, allergies to food or drugs, or many different types of intestinal problems. Diarrhea may be acute or chronic. Acute diarrhea, the most common, comes on suddenly and may be accompanied by nausea, vomiting, chills, and intense abdominal pain. It typically runs its course very rapidly, and symptoms subside once the irritating agent is removed from the system. Chronic diarrhea, which may last for weeks, may result from more serious disease states.

The athlete suffering from acute diarrhea may be totally incapacitated in terms of athletic performance. The major problem of diarrhea is potential dehydration. An athlete, particularly when exercising in a hot environment, depends on body fluids to maintain normal temperature. An individual who becomes dehydrated has difficulty with regulation of temperature and may experience some heat-related problem. The sports therapist's primary concern should be replacing lost body fluids and electrolytes. Medication may be used on a short-term basis for relief of the symptoms, but identifying and treating the cause of the problem are important as well.

Medications used for control of diarrhea are either locally acting or systemic. The locally acting medications most typically contain kaolin, which absorbs other chemicals, and pectin, which soothes the irritated bowel. Some contain substances that add bulk to the stool. The effectiveness of locally acting medications is questionable, but they are considered safe and inexpensive.[10]

The systemic agents, which are generally antiperistaltic or antispasmodic medications, are considered to be much more effective in relieving symptoms of diarrhea, but most except loperamide are prescription drugs. The systemic medications are either opiate derivatives or anticholinergic agents, both of which reduce peristalsis. Common side effects of the systemic antidiarrheals include drowsiness, nausea, dry mouth, and constipation. Long-term use of the opiate drugs may lead to dependence.[4]

If the cause of diarrhea is a noninvasive bacteria, a physician may choose to administer multispectrum antibiotics along with an antiperistaltic agent.

CATHARTICS. Laxatives may be used to empty the GI tract and eliminate constipation. In most cases, constipation may be relieved by proper diet, sufficient fluid intake, and exercise.[19] A cathartic medication is generally not necessary.

An athlete who complains of constipation should first be advised to consume those foods and juices that cause bulk in the feces and stimulate gastrointestinal peristalsis such as bran cereals, fresh fruits, coffee, and chocolate. Increased fluid intake also facilitates peristalsis in the bowel.

Generally speaking, athletes seem to suffer less from constipation than from diarrhea. This tendency may be attributed as much to activity levels as to any other single factor.

If a laxative medication is necessary, the bulk-forming laxatives are among the safest but should be used only for short periods, and dietary modifications should also be encouraged.

Antibiotic Medications

Many of the medications discussed have been over-the-counter medications that may be selected and administered by the sports therapist following strict guidelines and protocols for administration established by the team physician. In the case of infectious diseases, the team physician must be directly involved in the selection of specific antimicrobial agents. The sports therapist is often the individual who first recognizes an athlete's signs of developing infection, such as fever, redness, swelling, tenderness, purulent drainage, and swollen lymph nodes. The sports therapist should have the responsibility of referring the athlete with a suspected infection to the physician for a total assessment, including physical examination and laboratory tests. The team physician will then prescribe for the athlete an appropriate antibiotic medication that is selectively capable of destroying the invading microorganism without affecting the patient.[27] The sports therapist may be asked to provide adjunctive therapy such as applying hot compresses or soaks in antiseptic solutions in open infections.

In the case of an athlete who is using an antibiotic medication, the sports therapist's role should be to monitor the patient for signs and symptoms of allergic response or drug-induced toxicity. Many individuals exhibit hypersensitivity reactions to antimicrobial agents. Perhaps the most common reaction occurs with the use of penicillin. Antibiotics are also capable of damaging the tissues they contact. They may damage the mucosa of the stomach and cause diarrhea, nausea, and vomiting. They can also affect kidney function and may interfere with nervous system function. Should these reactions occur, the athlete should be sent back to the physician, who may elect to change to another type of antibiotic medication.[35]

An athlete who has an infection, be it localized or systemic, that requires use of an antibiotic will usually be advised not to train or compete until the infection is under control. The sports therapist should be certain that the athlete adheres to this recommendation both to benefit the infected athlete and to limit the possibility of the infection spreading or being transmitted to other athletes.

ADMINISTERING VS. DISPENSING MEDICATION

The methods by which drugs may be administered and dispensed vary according to individual state laws. Sports-medicine settings are subject to those laws. Administration of a drug is giving the athlete a single dose of a particular medication. Dispensing of medication is giving the athlete a drug in a quantity greater than would be used in a single dose. In most cases, the team physician is the individual ultimately responsible for prescribing medications. These prescription medications are then dispensed by either the physician, the physician extender licensed to dispense, or the pharmacist. The sports therapist may not dispense medication. However, in most states they may legally administer a single dose of a nonprescription medication. The sports therapist typically does not possess the background or the experience to make decisions about the appropriate use of medication and should be subject to strict protocols if and when administering medication.

On occasion over-the-counter medications are placed on a countertop in the sports-medicine clinic for use as the athlete sees fit. Although this method of administering medication saves time for the clinician, this somewhat indiscriminate use of even over-the-counter drugs by an athlete should be discouraged. The sports therapist who is administering over-the-counter medication of any variety should be knowledgeable about the possible effects of various drugs during exercise. Likewise, sports therapists should be subject to strict protocols established by the team physician for administering medication. Table 15-4 and the box on page 235 present a series of protocols for the administration of over-the-counter medications by the sports therapist for a number of minor illnesses or conditions seen commonly in the athletic population. Failure to follow these guidelines or protocols may make the sports therapist legally liable should something happen to the athlete that can be attributed to use or misuse of a particular drug.

Text continued on p. 235.

TABLE 15-4
Protocols for Use of Over-the-Counter Drugs by Sports Therapists

The sports therapist is often responsible for initial screening of athletes who present with various illnesses/injuries. Frequently, the sports therapist must make decisions regarding the appropriate use of over-the-counter medications for their athletes. Subjective findings such as onset, duration, medication taken, and known allergies must be included in the screening evaluation.

The following protocols should be viewed as guidelines to the disposition of the athlete. The protocols are aimed at clarifying the use of over-the-counter drugs in the treatment of common problems encountered by the sports therapist while covering or traveling with a particular team. These guidelines do not cover every situation the sports therapist encounters in assessing and managing the athlete's physical problems. Therefore physician consultation is recommended whenever there is uncertainty in making a decision regarding the appropriate care of the athlete.

Continued.

TABLE 15-4—cont'd
Protocols for Use of Over-the-Counter Drugs by Sports Therapists

Existing Illness/Injury	Appropriate Treatment Protocol

TEMPERATURE

(1) Greater than or equal to 102° F orally	Consult physician ASAP.
(2) Less than 102° F but more than 99.5° F	(1) Patient may be given acetaminophen. *See Acetaminophen Administration.*
	(2) Limit exercise of athlete. Do not allow participation in practice.
	(3) If fever decreases to less than 99.5° F the athlete may participate in practice.
	(4) If athlete is to be involved in an intercollegiate event, consult with a physician concerning participation.
(3) Less than or equal to 99.5° F orally	Follow management guidelines for fever less than 102° F but allow athlete to practice or compete.

THROAT

(1) History	(1) Advise saline gargles (½ tsp. salt in a glass of warm water).
(a) Sore throat No fever No chills	(2) Patient may also be given Cepastat®/Chloraseptic® throat lozenges. Before administering determine: a. Is the patient allergic to Cepastat®/Chloraseptic® (phenol containing) lozenges?*
(b) Sore throat Fever	b. Determine temperature. If fever, manage as outlined in temperature protocol, and consult physician ASAP.
(c) Sore throat and/or fever and/or swollen glands	Consult physician ASAP.

NOSE

(1) Watery discharge	Patient may be given Pseudoephedrine (Sudafed®) tablets. *See Pseudoephedrine Administration Protocols.*
(2) Nasal congestion	Patient may be given Oxymetazoline HCl (Afrin®) nasal spray. *See Oxymetazoline Administration Protocol.*

CHEST

(1) Cough (a) Dry hacking or (b) Clear mucoid sputum	Administer Robitussin DM® (generic guaifenesin with dextromethorphan). Before administering determine: Is the patient going to be involved in practice or game within 4 hours from administration of medication?† If indicated, you may administer one dose, 10 ml (2 tsp). Inform the patient that drowsiness may occur. Repeat doses may be administered every 6 hours. Push fluids, encourage patient to drink as much as possible.
(c) Green or rusty sputum	Consult physician ASAP.
(d) Severe, persistent cough	Consult physician ASAP.

EARS

(1) Discomfort from ears popping	Patient may be given Pseudoephedrine (Sudafed®) tablets and/or Oxymetazoline HCl (Afrin®) nasal spray. *See Pseudoephedrine Administration Protocol and/or Oxymetazoline Protocol.*
(2) Earache (or external otitis)	Patient may be given Acetaminophen. Consult physician ASAP. *See Acetaminophen Administration Protocol.*
(3) Recurrent earache	Consult physician ASAP.

*If yes, do not administer.
†If yes, do not give Robitussin DM®.

TABLE 15-4—cont'd
Protocols for Use of Over-the-Counter Drugs by Sports Therapists

Existing Illness/Injury	Appropriate Treatment Protocol

PREVENTION OF MOTION SICKNESS

(1) Complaint: History of nausea, dizziness, or vomiting associated with travel

Patient may be given dimenhydrinate (Dramamine®) or diphenhydramine (Benadryl®).
Before administering determine:

(a) Is the patient sensitive or allergic to Dramamine®, Benadryl® or any other antihistamine?*

(b) Has the patient taken any other antihistamines (Actifed®, Chlor-Trimeton®, various cold medications) or other medications that cause sedation within the last 6 hours?*

(c) Does the patient have asthma, glaucoma, or enlargement of the prostate gland?*

(d) Is the patient going to be involved in practice or game within 4 hours from administration of medication?†

Administer Dramamine® or Benadryl® dose based on body weight, 30 to 60 minutes before departure time:
Under 125 lb: one Dramamine® 50 mg tablet.
Over 125 lb: two Dramamine 50 mg tablets.

Benadryl® dose:
Under 125 lb: one 25 mg capsule.
Over 125 lb: two 25 mg capsules.

NAUSEA, VOMITING

(1) Prolonged, severe

Consult physician ASAP.

NAUSEA, GASTRIC UPSET, HEARTBURN, "BUTTERFLIES" IN THE STOMACH

(1) Associated with dietary indiscretion or tension.

You may administer an antacid as a single dose, as defined by label of particular antacid (Riopan®, Gelusil®, Maalox®, Pepto Bismol®, Titralac®).

(2) Associated with abdominal or chest pain

Consult physician ASAP.

(3) Vomiting, nausea; no severe distress

Monitor symptoms. Patient may be given dimenhydrinate (Dramamine®) or diphenhydramine (Benadryl®) orally. Same as instructions and precautions under motion sickness.

(4) Vomiting: projectile, coffee ground, febrile

Consult physician ASAP.

DIARRHEA

(1) Associated with abdominal pain or tenderness and/or dehydration, bloody stools, febrile, recurrent diarrhea

Consult physician ASAP.

(2) Frequent loose stools not associated with any of the above signs or symptoms

Encourage clear liquid diet. Encourage avoidance of dairy products and high-fat foods for 24 hours. If it persists consult physician ASAP.

Patient may be given kaolin-pectin (Kaopectate®) or loperamide (Immodium A-D®). Before administering, determine:

(a) How long has patient had diarrhea? If longer than 24 hours, see physician.

(b) Is patient taking any digitalis medication: digoxin, lanoxin, Lanoxicaps? If yes, see physician.

*If yes, do not administer.
†Inform the patient that drowsiness may occur for 4-6 hours after taking this medication. Avoid alcoholic beverages. Avoid driving for 6 hours after taking. If traveling time is extended, another dose may be administered 6 hours after the first dose.

Continued.

Existing Illness/Injury	Appropriate Treatment Protocol

DIARRHEA—cont'd

| | You may administer one dose of kaolin-pectin (Kaopectate®) (6-8 tsp). Shake well. Repeat dose after each loose bowel movement until diarrhea is controlled. Should not be used for more than 2 days. Discontinue use if fever develops or if diarrhea is not controlled within 24 hours of treatment, and consult physician. **OR** You may administer one dose (2 caplets) of loperamide (Immodium A-D® 2 mg per caplet). One caplet may be administered after each loose stool not to exceed 8 mg (4 caplets) per 24 hours. Inform the patient that dizziness or drowsiness may occur within 12 hours after taking this medication. Avoid alcoholic beverages. Use caution while driving or performing tasks requiring alertness. |

CONSTIPATION

| (1) Prolonged or severe abdominal pain or tenderness, nausea or vomiting | Consult physician ASAP. |
| (2) Discomfort associated with dietary change or decreased fluid intake | You may administer milk of magnesia 30 ml as a single dose. Before administering determine:
   Does the patient have chronic renal disease?*

Recommend increased fluid intake, increased intake of fruits, bulk vegetables, or cereals. |

HEADACHE

(1) Pain associated with elevated BP, temperature elevation, blurred vision, nausea, vomiting, or history of migraine.	Consult physician ASAP.
(2) Pain across forehead (mild headache)	Patient may be given Acetaminophen. *See Acetaminophen Administration Protocol.*
(3) Tension headache, occipital pain	Patient may be given Acetaminophen. *See Acetaminophen Administration Protocol.*
(4) Pain in antrum or forehead associated with sinus or nasal congestion.	Patient may be given Pseudoephedrine (Sudafed®) tablets and Acetaminophen. *See protocols for Pseudoephedrine and Acetaminophen Administration.*

MUSCULOSKELETAL INJURIES

(1) Deformity	Consult physician ASAP.
(2) Localized pain and tenderness, impaired range of motion	First aid to part as soon as possible. Ice Compression-Ace bandage Elevation Protection-crutches or sling and/or splint.
(3) Pain with swelling, discoloration, no impaired movement or localized tenderness	If this injury interferes with patient's normal activities, consult physician within 24 hours. Patient may be given Acetaminophen. *See Acetaminophen Administration Protocol.*

SKIN

| (1) Localized or generalized rash accompanied by elevated temperature, enlarged lymph nodes, sore throat, stiff neck, infected skin lesion, dyspnea, wheezing | Consult physician ASAP. |

*If yes, do not administer.

Existing Illness/Injury	Appropriate Treatment Protocol
SKIN—cont'd	
(2) Mild, localized, nonvesicular skin eruptions accompanied by pruritis	Hydrocortisone 0.5% cream may be applied. Before administering, determine: (a) Is the patient taking any medication?* (b) Are eyes or any large area of the body involved?* (c) Is there any evidence of lice infestation? The cream may be repeated every 6 hours if needed. Do not use more than three times daily.
(3) Abrasions	Control bleeding. Clean with antibacterial soap and water. Apply appropriate dressing and antibiotic ointment. Monitor for signs of infection. Dressing may be changed 2-3 times a day if needed.
(4) Localized erythema caused by ultraviolet rays	Advise application of compresses soaked in a solution of cold water.
(5) Jock itch or athlete's foot	Advise 10-15 minute application of compresses soaked in cool water to relieve intense itching. Patient may be given miconazole (Micatin®) cream topically. Before administering determine: (a) Is the patient sensitive or allergic to miconazole?† (b) Is the patient receiving other types of treatment for rash in same area?† Instruct patient to wash and dry area of rash, and then apply ¼-½ inch ribbon of cream (give patient the cream on a clean gauze pad), and rub gently on the infected area. Spread evenly and thinly over rash. The dose may be repeated in 8-12 hours (twice a day). Consult physician within 24 hours.
SKIN WOUNDS	
(1) Lacerations	Control bleeding. Cleanse area with antibacterial soap and water. Apply steristrips. Consult physician immediately if there is any question about the necessity for suturing.
(2) Extensive lacerations or other severe skin wounds	Control bleeding. Protect area with dressing. Refer to physician immediately.
WOUND INFECTION	
(1) Febrile, marked cellulitis, red streaks, tender or enlarged nodes	Consult physician ASAP.
(2) Localized inflammation, afebrile, absence of nodes and streaks	Warm soaks to affected area. Consult physician ASAP.
BURNS	
(1) First degree-erythema of skin, limited area	Apply cold compresses to affected area. Dressing is not necessary on first degree burns. If less than 45 minutes have elapsed since burn injury, clean gently with soap and water. Patient may be given acetaminophen. *See Acetaminophen Administration Protocol.*
(2) First degree with extensive involvement over body	Consult physician ASAP.
(3) Second degree-erythema with blistering	Consult physician ASAP.
(4) Third degree-pearly white appearance of affected area, no pain	Consult physician ASAP.

*If yes, do not administer. Refer to physician.
†If yes, do not administer. Consult physician ASAP.

Continued.

TABLE 15-4—cont'd
Protocols for Use of Over-the-Counter Drugs by Sports Therapists

Existing Illness/Injury	Appropriate Treatment Protocol
ALLERGIES	
Athlete with known seasonal allergies who forgot to bring own medication	Patient may be given chlorpheniramine (Chlor-Trimeton®) 4 mg tablets. Before administering determine:
	(a) Is the patient sensitive to chlorpheniramine?*
	(b) Does the patient have asthma, urinary retention, or glaucoma?*
	(c) Is patient going to be involved in training or game within 4 hours from administration of medication?*
	(d) Has the patient taken any other antihstamines (Actifed®, Dramamine®, various cold medications) or other medications that cause drowsiness within the last 6 hours?*
	Consult physician ASAP.
	You may administer 1 dose of chlorpheniramine 4 mg, ½ or 1 tablet. Repeat doses may be administered every 4 hours. Inform the patient that drowsiness may occur for 4-6 hours after taking this medication. Avoid alcoholic beverages. Avoid driving or operation of machinery for 6 hours after taking. Contact physician if symptoms do not abate.
CONTACT LENS CARE	
	Note: There are three types of contact lenses:
	(a) hard
	(b) gas permeable
	(c) soft
	Solutions are labeled for use with a *particular* type of lens and should not be used for any other type of lens.
	Do not use solutions preserved with thimersol or chlorhexidine because of possible allergy or irritation.
(1) Lens needs rinsing/wetting before insertion	(a) Hard lens: use all-purpose wetting/soaking solution (Wet-N-Soak®).
	(b) Gas permeable lens: use all-purpose wetting/soaking solution (Wet-N-Soak®).
	(c) Soft lens: use rinsing/soaking solution (Soft Mate ps®).
(2) Lens needs soaking/storage	(a) Hard lens: use all-purpose wetting/soaking solution (Wet-N-Soak®).
	(b) Gas permeable lens: use all-purpose wetting/soaking solution (Wet-N-Soak®).
	(c) Soft lens: use rinsing/soaking solution (Soft Mate ps®).
(3) Lens needs cleaning	(a) Hard lens: use cleaning solution (EasyClean®).
	(b) Gas permeable lens: use cleaning solution (EasyClean®).
	(c) Soft lens: use cleaning solution (Lens Plus Daily Cleaner®).
EYE CARE	
(1) Foreign body—Minor: sand, eyelash	Use eye wash irrigation solution (Dacriose®).
(2) Irritation—Minor	Use artificial tears. Do not use with contact lens in eye.
(3) Severe irritation, foreign body not easily removed, trauma	Consult physician ASAP.

*If yes, do not administer.

ADMINISTRATION PROTOCOLS FOR COMMON OVER-THE-COUNTER DRUGS USED IN SPORTS MEDICINE

ACETAMINOPHEN PROTOCOL (TYLENOL®)

Before administering, determine:

(a) Is the patient allergic to acetaminophen?*

You may administer Acetaminophen 325 mg, two tablets. Repeat doses may be administered every 6 hours if needed. If dispensing occurs, use labeled 2/pack only. Patient instructions must accompany dispensing.

IBUPROFEN PROTOCOL (ADVIL®)

Before administering, determine:

(a) Is the patient allergic to aspirin (asthma, swelling, shock, or hives associated with aspirin use)?
If yes, do not give ibuprofen because even though ibuprofen contains no aspirin or salicylates, cross reactions may occur in patients allergic to aspirin.

(b) Does the patient have renal disease or gastrointestinal ulcerations?*

You may administer ibuprofen 200 mg (Advil®), one or two tablets. Repeat doses may be administered every 4 to 6 hours if needed. Do not exceed 6 tablets in a 24-hour period without consulting a physician.

The patient should take ibuprofen with food if occasional and mild heartburn, upset stomach, or mild stomach pain occurs. Consult physician if these symptoms are more than mild or persist.

PSEUDOEPHEDRINE PROTOCOL (SUDAFED®)

Before administering, determine:

(a) Is the patient allergic or sensitive to pseudoephedrine?*
(b) Does the patient have high blood pressure, heart disease, diabetes, urinary retention, glaucoma, or thyroid disease?*
(c) Does the patient have problems with sweating?*
(d) Do not administer 4 hours before practice or game.
(e) Do not administer if patient is involved in postseason play.

You may administer pseudoephedrine (Sudafed®) 30 mg, two tablets. Repeat doses may be administered every 6 hours up to 4 times a day. If dispensing occurs use labeled 2/pack only. Patient instructions must accompany dispensing.

OXYMETAZOLINE PROTOCOL (AFRIN®)

Before administering, determine:

(a) Is the patient allergic or sensitive to Afrin® or Otrivin®?*
(b) Does the patient react unusually to nose sprays or drops?*

You may administer 2 to 3 sprays of Oxymetazoline (Afrin®) 0.05% nasal spray into each nostril. Repeat doses may be administered every 12 hours. (The container can be marked with the patient's name and maintained by the trainer for repeat administration or dispensed to the patient.) Patient instructions must accompany dispensing.
Do not use the same container for different patients.
Do not use for more than 3 days without physician supervision.
Use small package sizes to reduce risk of overuse/rebound congestion.

*If yes, do not administer.

Record Keeping

Those involved in any health-care profession are acutely aware of the necessity of maintaining complete up-to-date medical records. Again the sports-medicine setting is no exception. If medications are administered by a sports therapist, maintaining accurate records of the types of medications administered is just as important as recording progress notes, treatments given, and rehabilitation plans. The sports therapist may be dealing with a number of different patients simultaneously while trying to get a team ready for practice or competition. At times things become hectic, and stopping to record each time a medication is administered is difficult. Nevertheless, the sports therapist should include the following information on a type of medication administration log:

(1) name of the athlete, (2) complaint or symptoms, (3) type of medication given, (4) quantity of medication given, and (5) time of administration.

DRUG TESTING

Perhaps no other topic related to pharmacology has received more attention from the media during recent years than the use and abuse of drugs by athletes. Much has been written and discussed regarding the use of performance-enhancing drugs among Olympic athletes, the widespread use of "street drugs" by professional athletes, and the use of pain-relieving drugs by athletes at all levels.[8,12,14]

Although much of the information being disseminated to the public by the media may be based on hearsay and innuendo, the use and abuse of many different types of drugs can have a profound impact on athletic performance.

To say many experts in the field of sports medicine regard drug abuse among athletes with growing concern is a gross understatement. Drug testing of athletes at all levels for the purpose of identifying individuals who may have some problems with drug abuse is becoming commonplace. Both the NCAA and the International Olympic Committee have established lists of substances that are banned from use by athletes. The lists include performance-enhancing drugs and "street" or "recreational" drugs, as well as many over-the-counter and prescription drugs. The legality and ethics of testing only those individuals involved with sports are still open to debate. The pattern of drug usage among athletes may simply reflect that of our society in general.

The sports therapist who is working with an athlete who may be tested for drugs at the NCAA level or with world-class or Olympic athletes should be very familiar with the list of banned drugs. Having an athlete disqualified because of the indiscriminate use of some over-the-counter drug during a rehabilitation program would be most unfortunate.

SUMMARY

1. An athlete who requires an analgesic for pain relief should be given acetaminophen because aspirin may produce gastric upset and slow clotting time.

2. For treating inflammation, NSAIDs are recommended because they do not produce many of the side effects associated with aspirin use.

3. Antihistamines are used primarily in the treatment of allergic reactions and may produce drowsiness and sedation.

4. Decongestants are used to reduce nasal congestion and may be used orally or topically.

5. Antitussives and expectorants are used to suppress coughing and keep the throat moist. They generally produce drowsiness, gastric irritability, and some lack of coordination.

6. Antacids neutralize acidity in the upper GI tract and may produce diarrhea or constipation.

7. Antiemetics are used to treat nausea and vomiting and should be used with large quantities of fluid to prevent dehydration.

8. Antidiarrheals act to reduce peristaltic action in the lower GI tract and may produce drowsiness, nausea, dry mouth, and constipation.

9. Cathartics are used to empty the GI tract and reduce constipation.

10. Antibiotics are used to treat various infections and may produce hypersensitivity reactions in the athlete. Generally an athlete who is using an antibiotic should avoid training and competition until the infection subsides.

11. The use of medication in a sports-medicine setting should be subject to strict preestablished guidelines and protocols and monitored closely by the sports therapist supervising a rehabilitation program.

12. The sports therapist should maintain a log that documents all medications being administered during a rehabilitation program.

13. The sports therapist must be aware of medications commonly used in treatment of various disorders that may be detected in a drug test as banned substances.

REFERENCES

1 Almekinders L: The efficacy of nonsteroidal antiinflammatory drugs in the treatment of ligament injuries, *Sports Med* 9(3):137-142, 1990.

2 Beaver W: Aspirin and acetaminophen as constituents of analgesic combinations, *Arch Intern Med* 141:293-300, 1981.

3 Beaver W, Kantor T, Levy G: On guard for aspirin's harmful side effects, *Patient Care* 13:48, 1975.

4 Bertholf C: Protocol, acute diarrhea, *Nurse Pract* 3:8, 1980.

5 Black F, Correia M, Stucker F: Easing proneness to motion sickness, *Patient Care* 14(6):114, 1980.

6 Boyd E: A review of expectorants and inhalants, *Int J Clin Pharmacol Ther Toxicol* 3:55, 1970.

7 Clark J, Queener S, Karb V: *Pharmacologic basis of nursing practice*, St Louis, 1992, Mosby.

8 Clarke KS: Sports medicine and drug control programs of the US Olympic Committee, *J Allergy Clin Immunol* 73:740-744, 1984.

9 Clyman B: Role of the non-steroidal anti-inflammatory drugs in sports medicine, *Sports Med* 3:212-246, 1986.

10 Dahr G, Soergel K: Principles of diarrhea therapy, *Am Fam Physician* 19(1):165, 1979.

11 Dretchen K, Hollander D, Kirsner J: Roundup on antiacids and anticholinergics, *Patient Care* 9(6):94, 1975.

12 Drugs in the Olympics, *Med Lett Drugs Ther* 26:66, 1984.

13 Elenbaas JK: Centrally acting skeletal muscle relaxants, *Am J Hosp Pharm* 37:1313-1323, 1980.

14 Hill J: The athletic polydrug abuse phenomenon, *Am J Sports Med* 11:269-271, 1983.

15 Koch-Weser J: Acetaminophen, *N Engl J Med* 255:1297, 1976.

16 Krausen A: Antihistamines: guidelines and implications, *Ann Otol Rhinol Laryngol* 85:686, 1979.

17 Levy G: Comparative pharmacokinetics of aspirin and acetaminophen, *Arch Intern Med* 141:279-281, 1981.

18 Levy J, Smith D: Clinical differences among nonsteroidal an-

tiinflammatory drugs: implications for therapeutic substitution in ambulatory patients, DICP, *Ann Pharmacotherapy* 23:76-85, 1989.

19 Malseed R: *Pharmacology: drug therapy and nursing considerations,* Philadelphia, 1985, JB Lippincott.

20 Mehlisch DR: Review of the comparative analgesic efficacy of salicylates, acetaminophen and pyrazolones, *Am J Med* 75[A]:47-52, 1983.

21 Mirtallo J: Drug induced heat stroke, *Drug Intell Clin Pharm,* 12:652-657, 1978.

22 Moncada S, Vane J: Mode of action of aspirin-like drugs, *Adv Int Med* 24:1, 1979.

23 Pearlman D: Antihistamines: pharmacology and clinical use, *Drugs* 12:258, 1976.

24 Quick A: Salicylates and bleeding: the aspirin tolerance test, *Am J Med Sci* 252:265-269, 1966.

25 Reynolds RC, Floetz P, Thielke TS: Comparative analysis of drug distribution costs for controlled versus noncontrolled oral analgesics, *Am J Hosp Pharm* 41:1558-1563, 1984.

26 Rodman M: Antiinfectives you administer: choosing the right drug for every job, *RN* 40:73, 1977.

27 Rodman M: A fresh look at OTC drug interactions: antacid preparations, *RN* 46:84, 1981.

28 Rodman M, Smith D: *Clinical pharmacology in nursing,* Philadelphia, 1984, JB Lippincott.

29 Settipane GA: Adverse reactions to aspirin and related drugs, *Arch Intern Med* 141:328-332, 1981.

30 Strauss R: *Sports medicine,* Philadelphia, 1984, WB Saunders.

31 Szczeklik A: Antipyretic analgesics and the allergic patient, *Am J Med* 75[A]:82-84, 1983.

32 Texter E, Smart D, Butler R: Antiacids, *Am Fam Physician* 11(4):111, 1975.

33 Vane J: Inhibition of prostaglandin synthesis as a mechanism of action for aspirin like drugs, *Nature (New Biol)* 231:232-235, 1971.

34 Vane J: The evolution of nonsteroidal antiinflammatory drugs and their mechanism of action, *Drugs* 33(1):18-27, 1987.

35 Weinstein L: Some principles of antibiotic therapy, *Ration Drug Ther* 11(3):1, 1977.

Psychological Considerations for Rehabilitation

16

Joe Gieck

OBJECTIVES

After completion of this chapter, the student should be able to do the following:

- Discuss how different athletes deal with similar injuries.

- Describe the injury-prone athlete.

- Identify stressors in the athlete's life and effective methods with which to deal with them.

- Identify the four phases of injury and the athlete's perception of them.

- Explain the importance of athletes taking responsibility for their actions in regard to injury.

- Recognize irrational thinking and its resolution.

- Relate the importance, physically and mentally, of short-term goals in rehabilitation.

- Discuss strategies the athlete can use for gaining control of the injury situation.

- Recognize the importance of the relationship between the sports therapist and the athlete.

- Explain the importance of rehabilitation adherence and its deviations.

- Describe the coping skills necessary for successful rehabilitation.

- Identify the problems associated with long-term rehabilitation.

Sports medicine and athletic training are still inexact sciences, and nowhere within this area is this more evident than in the psychological phase of recovery from injury. Plato mentioned never attempting to cure the body without curing the soul. Current clinicians have found that people with negative self-concepts suffer more injuries.

Most athletes have the self-confidence to adapt to a mild or moderate injury, and most have the support, understanding, and proper encouragement to adapt to more severe injury, but even the most self-confi-dent have their doubts. One athlete put it this way:

> The best competitors like to compete and to me this is just a game—an inner game. It's an inner soul game. Can I beat my knee back? But he also expressed doubts about the real test when a tackler "takes a whack at the knee" and how I haven't thought about it, but I've had night-mares about it. My buddy told me he broke his ankle. He said once you get that real good hit and you pop up and it pops up with you, then everything is going to fall into place and you're going to be rolling. You're going to go out there like it's never been hurt and just play.

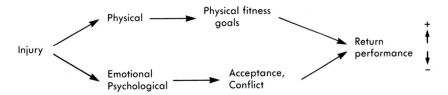

Fig. 16-1. Physical and emotional aspects of return to performance.

This quote expresses the positive aspects of return to competition but also some of the doubts involved.

With the emergence of sports psychology, more attention is paid to getting the mind ready to return to competition to match the adjustment of the body. Athletes have begun to describe the nightmares, fears, and anxiety of returning to competition. Also, in the current trend of high-salaried athletes, some describe their knee or other injuries and surgery as the most important things in their lives since they will either make or break them. These operations can allow the athletes to make either millions of dollars in a sports career or only thousands in a regular job if their careers end.

Athletes don't all deal with injury in the same manner. Rotella[11] describes how one may view the injury as disastrous, another may view it as an opportunity to show courage, and another athlete may relish the injury since it prevents his or her embarrassment over poor physical performance, provides an escape from a losing team, or discourages a pushy parent. If the injury is career-threatening, the athlete whose whole life has revolved around a sport may have an identity crisis.

Figure 16-1 demonstrates the physical and emotional aspects of return to performance. The return to performance is either enhanced or negated by the physiological and psychological results of both elements.

THE INJURY-PRONE ATHLETE

Some athletes seem to have a pattern of injury, whereas others in exactly the same position with the same physical makeup are injury-free. Certain researchers suggest that some psychological traits may predispose the athlete to a repeated injury cycle. No one particular personality type has been recognized as injury-prone. However, the individual who likes to take risks seems to represent the injury-prone athlete. This individual usually also lacks the ability to cope

LIFE STRESS EVENTS
Death of family member—100
Detention in jail—63
Injury—46
Death of close friend—37
Playing for new coach—35
Playing on new team—31
Outstanding personal achievements—28
Major change in living habits—25
Social readjustment—24
Change to new school—20
Major change in social activities—18
Sleep habit change—16

with the stresses associated with these risks and their consequences.

Much has been written about life's stress events and the likelihood of illness. These events are changes that require an adjustment, such as death of family members, divorce, school change, and job change. Sports researchers suggest that the inner thoughts and anxieties of the athlete create internal stresses, and these stresses increase the likelihood of injury and reinjury, especially for the athlete who is inflexible and resistant to change.

Stressors are both positive, such as making All-American, and negative, such as being arrested. Each requires a lifestyle adjustment.

Examples of life's stress events, including some related to football, are listed in the box above. The scale is based on a 0 to 100 rating, with 100 being the most stressful events.[4]

Obviously the staff of a smaller team is more familiar with the athletes and their problems and can more effectively deal with them, but larger teams' staffs should attempt to deal with the individual through the position coach, with the individual's problems being solved in the smaller unit. Unfortunately, many coaches do not have the interest or

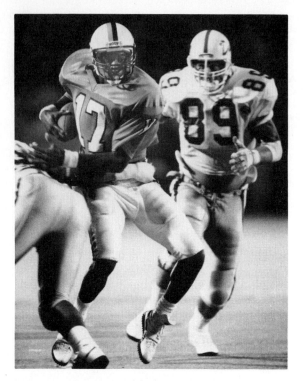

Fig. 16-2. Participation in sports and stress. Sports participation is often the one positive aspect of life that helps the athlete get through times of extreme stress.

ability to work with athletes needing help. Some sort of a screening device should be used to identify those individuals who are experiencing some of life's situations that they are unprepared to handle.

These individuals need someone to interact with to reduce the stress in their lives. In this way they can reduce the stress by talking about their feelings rather than holding them to themselves. Programs such as relaxation training, thought reorganization, simple support and empathy, or, in extreme stress situations, psychiatric intervention are necessary. In many instances the sport is the one positive thing in life that helps the athlete get through times of extreme stress (Figure 16-2). Areas outside sports are often stressful; intervention has to be within their comfortable emotional framework.

This life-stress information on the athlete is important for the sports therapist in rehabilitation work. Early detection of stresses and their relief are the avenues of choice for a more speedy rehabilitation after injury.

Each athlete copes with life stress differently. One athlete may adjust to a new coach with ease, especially if the coach is one in a long series, whereas another, who may have had only one or two coaches, may have a more difficult time with the adjustment, especially if the athlete goes from an easygoing coach to a strict disciplinarian. However, the individual with multiple coaches may have had difficulty adjusting to each new coach. Experience in the situation benefits the adjustment if the athlete has successfully handled the experience before.

Those with good support and, most important, perception of support from their friends, family, and athletic staff also have an easier time with life's stressful events. Often those with poor coping mechanisms and those who are inflexible are injury-prone.

Few athletes react to stress events by verbalizing them, yet most handle them very well by themselves. James Michener[8] makes the following point:

> For many athletes physical activity, rather than talking things out, appears to offer a means of expressing feelings and aggressions. Perhaps this substitution of actions for words contributes to the seeming reluctance of athletes to come to a service that requires that they articulate their feelings.

ATTITUDES SETTING UP INJURY

Certain attitudes toward sports have fostered injury and, more important, reinjury. The phrase "you have to play with pain" has been interpreted more literally to mean that the athlete has to play through an injury. The difference is that some injuries may be mild and only somewhat painful, resulting in no reinjury in competition, whereas a more severe injury is made worse by continuing to compete. The importance of a certified sports trainer to make this decision is obvious.

Unfortunately, untrained personnel, such as coaches, assume this responsibility when no sports therapist is present or when the sports therapist is easily intimidated by the coach and not backed up by the athletic director. Either situation results in poor medical care and leaves the management vulnerable to legal action as a result of negligence. Courts expect competent medical care to be provided to the athletes. That care can be provided only by a qualified sports therapist or a physician (Figure 16-3). Players who feel that a missed practice or game will relegate them to the bench for the year or those who have been encouraged to play no matter what

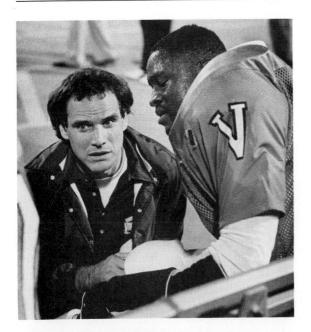

Fig. 16-3. Competent medical care. Courts expect competent medical care to be provided to athletes by a certified athletic trainer or physician.

are candidates for injury and reinjury. Usually what happens, however, is that they are performing poorly because they are not at full strength, thus they only reinforce the decision of the coach to play someone else. The role of the sports therapist is to determine when the player is functioning at top potential without risk of injury or reinjury and to keep the coach abreast of the player's status. A clear perception of the injury and its limitations by the athlete is important. An important role of the sports therapist is to inform the athlete of the difference between pain and injury.

The athlete who continues to play with an unhealed or repeated injury is constantly reducing the chances of a healthy life of activity. The athlete has to live past the few years of competition. Most athletes, however, have difficulty seeing past the present season or at best have the goal of participating in their sport until they can no longer compete, regardless of the consequences. The rewards of competition and the admiration of others take sports out of perspective and retard a healthy attitude toward sports. The attitude of the athlete is "Sacrifice everything for the sport; besides, I'm bulletproof." Lack of this attitude is viewed by some as weakness. These athletes

have difficulty adjusting to injury, especially a career-ending one.

Neglecting injured athletes or giving them the perception that they are "lepers" also can contribute to injury and reinjury. Coaches who foster this attitude are saying to the players that they have no self-worth if they are injured. Some coaches go so far as to prevent team contact until injured players are ready to return or to belittle them in front of their peers, believing that this will make the athlete want to get back to competition quicker. This tactic may work with some players with minor injuries but only causes major adjustment difficulties for athletes who suffer severe injury.

Some coaches refuse to talk to the athlete or tell others the athlete really doesn't want to play or isn't tough enough. The coach is experiencing frustration with the injury. Counseling the coach in this situation to point out the effects of such attitudes may be helpful. Fortunately, these coaches are in the minority.

During this period either the athletic staff shows its concern for the athlete and in return wins the athlete's loyalty and dedication down the road or they undermine the athlete's trust and set up a future situation to be let down when the athlete gets in the postion of controlling the outcome of a contest and may underperform in spite. Commitment is a two-way street. The athletic staff has to show its commitment to the athlete to receive the athlete's commitment.

PHASES OF INJURY

The athlete has to deal with four phases of injury: denial, anger, depression, and acceptance. These closely follow Elisabeth Kübler-Ross's model of the stages of death and dying.[7] After injury, the athlete faces three possible situations. The injury may be minimal and allow a speedy return, the athlete may have a prolonged period of rehabilitation, or the playing career may be at an end. The athlete must be encouraged along positive avenues to have the best opportunity to achieve complete rehabilitation, both emotionally and physically.

Early **denial** of the injury is commonplace, since the athlete attempts to rationalize that everything will be all right. The athlete feels that the injury will be fine the next day and that the early diagnosis is wrong. However, when the next day arrives and the injury is not better, the athlete begins to have difficulty dealing with recovery not being imminent. As a conse-

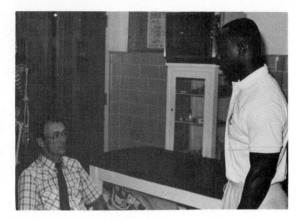

Fig. 16-4. The value of listening. Listen to determine how the athlete is feeling rather than to what he or she is saying.

quence, the athlete often feels anxious, isolated, and lonely.

Anger may soon replace this feeling of disbelief as the injured player vents feelings. Whoever happens to be around the athlete often bears the brunt of the anger. Anger cannot be reasoned with, and the athletic health-care personnel must understand and not react to the anger of the athlete. This response is merely emotional, a release of frustration. The sports therapist must act as an emotional blotter and, if possible, not further aggravate the situation by attempting to exert power to calm down the athlete. The sports therapist should listen to what the athlete is feeling rather than to what is said. This active listening requires time and effort. The athlete has lost control of the situation and is seeking to regain it (Figure 16-4).

Next, moods of anger, bargaining, and **depression** often are interrelated, with the athlete swinging from one to the other and back. Bargaining may also begin after the initial phase of denial, with the athlete saying the injury isn't real. The athlete may put a concentrated effort into treatment and rehabilitation for a brief period to get back into competition for the game. When this effort fails, the athlete often drops into depression and slacks off on rehabilitation effort.

In this phase the athlete has lost control of the physical situation and often the emotional control that goes with it. Team and individual identity are gone, and the athlete is an outsider watching from the sidelines or often from the stands. Being in the stands often further isolates the athlete. This action alone often solidifies the phase of depression and should be avoided wherever possible.

Success or failure of the team may produce anxiety within the injured athlete. If the team wins, the athlete wonders what role is left; if the team loses, the anxiety is great for the athlete to return to help the team.

Acceptance is a phase many well-managed athletes move into with ease. Fortunately, this group comprises most of the athletes with whom the competent sports therapist will work. The positive interest, energy, and empathy shown by the sports therapist make the transition from initial injury and denial to the acceptance phase a quicker recovery for the athlete. This explains why some rehabilitation personnel who rapidly get their athletes to acceptance rarely see the athlete who is not psychologically adjusting to injury, whereas some sports therapists who poorly manage their athletes continually see a great number of these individuals.

IT IS THE ATHLETE'S INJURY

The athlete who has reached the acceptance phase should take the responsibility for the injury. It is not the sports therapist's injury. The athlete has to accept the responsibility for the pain and the condition and deal with it. At this time the athlete is encouraged to transfer the time and energy given to the sport into the rehabilitation process. The athlete has to become an active and not a passive participant. The knee injury is now the competitor rather than the next week's opponent. Care should be taken so the athlete does not become a dependent patient. Some athletes want the sports therapist to be responsible for their welfare and to meet their every need at their whim and command. They demand more time be spent on them. Failure of one staff member to meet their demands results in their selecting a staff member who will meet their demands. Staff members with the greatest need to help others will be easily taken advantage of at the sacrifice of time needed for other athletes.

When these dependent patients no longer receive the special attention they feel they deserve, they often lash out in anger or frustration. The sports therapist needs to head off this response by firmly explaining the restrictions on time and what is required of the athlete in terms of rehabilitation. This response should be pointed out to the athlete as inappropriate and needs examination on the part of the sports therapist and the athlete if it becomes a continual problem, since it is only a detriment to recovery.

The athlete is guided in rehabilitation but must push within these guidelines. The athlete has to be encouraged and believe in future success. All efforts should point toward a positive result with the athlete working with what is available and not with wishful thinking.

IRRATIONAL THINKING

With injury a very real stressor in the life of the athlete, irrational thinking often sets in. Perceptions of situations that before have been rational now become irrational as self-destructive emotion colors the thought process. Emotional reaction is exacerbated, since the athlete fails to return to normal in a few days. The athlete's common sense and judgment become altered. This mood change may occur daily, so continual interaction with the athlete is necessary to restore rationality. The technique of restructuring perceptions helps the athlete become aware of these destructive, self-defeating behaviors. The athlete has often put in years of training and imposes pressures to return quickly. Fortunately, the certified sports trainer will prevent premature return and consequent reinjury by setting short-term goals and functional criteria before return.

The athlete, however, may fall into the mode of "I can't do it, I'll never get well." This irrational thinking produces anxiety, fear, and possibly depression that are detrimental to progress in rehabilitation. The athlete may be illogical, distort perceptions of events, or reach unrealistic decisions and conclusions. The athlete has replaced the old set of worries about simply playing well and helping the team win with the set of "woe is me," with its resultant anxiety. Obviously, these thought patterns are detrimental to the positive attitude necessary in the rehabilitation process. Some examples of irrational thinking are shown in the box above.

The sports therapist must recognize and intervene in this irrational thinking and challenge these thoughts with the athlete. Examination of these thoughts with athletes reassures them that it is "normal" to feel unhappy, frustrated, angry, insecure, or depressed, but the injury is not hopeless, they do not lack courage, and all is not lost and life is not over.

EXAMPLES OF IRRATIONAL THINKING TOWARD INJURY

Exaggeration: athletes exaggerate the severity of the injury.
Disregard: athletes pay no attention to the aspects of the injury that are important for healing and rehabilitation to occur.
Oversimplification: athletes think of the injury as good, bad, right, or wrong.
Overgeneralization: athletes tend to complicate the simple facts of the injury.
Unwarranted conclusions: athletes draw conclusions about the injury based on unsound or erroneous facts.

The athlete should be challenged to replace irrational thoughts with positive and rational ones. In short, the injury is aggravating and unfortunate, but it can be handled and overcome. The injury is placed in perspective and viewed the same as the athlete would consider preparation for the next contest.

The athlete has to identify faulty thinking, gain understanding of it, and actively work for its change. Research indicates that the self-thoughts, images, and attitudes during the recovery period determine the length and quality of the rehabilitation.

The many concerns on the mind of the athlete often prevent listening to the sports therapist until the acceptance phase of injury. Thus the sports therapist spends a lot of time repeating and reinforcing goals and exercise regimens (Figure 16-5).

This process is important but often frustrating to the sports therapist, especially for those with no insight into the personality of the athlete. During this phase, close observation of the exercise routines is necessary to make sure the athlete is following instructions and performing the exercises correctly. Injury is a major stressor, and the trainer-therapist needs patience. Texts such as Gordon's *Teacher Effectiveness Training*[3] can help the sports therapist understand the athlete's problem. Athletes in the adjustment phase do not have this problem and thus do not need the close supervision.

Obviously, the sports therapist must note any deviation in mood or personality from normal and counsel the athlete as to its cause. Often the athlete simply has become discouraged because the rehabilitation is taking too long, even though the athlete has been advised that the whole process requires even more weeks or months of rehabilitation.

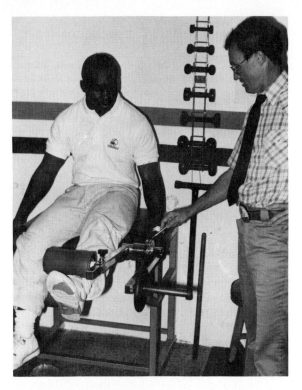

Fig. 16-5. The need for reinforcement. The athlete may not be listening to the sports therapist until the acceptance phase of the injury, thus the sports therapist may have to repeat and reinforce goals and exercise regimens.

During this time the athlete is often experiencing peaks and valleys in the recovery process. The athlete is used to two speeds: nothing and full speed. The athlete is frustrated to have to spend time in the crutch phase, then the walking phase, then the fast walk phase, then the walk-jog phase, then the jog phase, then the jog-run phase, then the run phase, and then finally the full-speed activity phase.

The athlete ends up with two problems: the physical injury and, what is often worse, the emotional frustration of the injury. The frustration often overshadows the injury since the athlete cannot adjust to restrictions. Adaptation to the frustration is hard work in the rehabilitative process. The work the athlete is doing is not producing the same rewards as participation in the sport; plus the athlete is becoming anxious about becoming further behind in the sport. Mind and body are out of sync, with the mind going ahead at a rapid pace while the body falls behind expectations.

At this point reinjury often occurs. The athlete skips the intermediate goals because of frustration and thus ends up with a setback because of reinjury. The athlete desperately wants to return to previous form. The sports therapist often has to explain over and over the purpose of the intermediate goals and the setbacks that occur without their attainment. The athlete must understand that this phase has to be gone through and that frustration, hopelessness, and self-pity are part of the adjustment process. Athletes often describe this inactivity during injury as harder than playing. When they are playing, all their energy is directed toward the goal of running plays and completing their assignments.

With an injury that requires weeks or months of rehabilitation before the athlete's return to competition, the athlete often feels that the coaches have ceased to care, which reinforces the depression. The athlete must understand that the coach cares but has to spend time to get a replacement ready for competition.

STRATEGIES FOR GAINING CONTROL

The athlete will be unable to return to play successfully without gaining the emotional self-control to think rationally about the injury and cope successfully with it. Several strategies used by sports psychologists to aid with those who need this help are as follows:

- Relaxation training
- Thought stoppage
- Imagery
- Visual rehearsal
- Emotional rehearsal
- Body rehearsal

A strategy suggested for getting the athlete over the passive phase of injury is a model of regaining an active role in the injury. The model outlines four tasks in the strategy:

1. Accept the reality of the loss.
2. Experience the pain of grief.
3. Adjust to the new environment that is void of the loss.
4. Withdraw emotional energy, and refocus it into another direction or activity.

Questions such as "How are you coping with your knee injury and the time you now have on your hands?" and "How do you perceive your rehabilitation is coming?" give the sports therapist a guide to the athlete's phase. Athletes should be encouraged to express their feelings. Athletes who are successfully coping with their injuries are rational in their assessments and thoughts. Fortunately, these athletes make up the great majority of clients encountered if they are managed properly.

Relaxation Training

Pain, lack of confidence, and anxiety may prevent athletes from achieving their potential in the rehabilitation setting. Relaxation training allows athletes to control these feelings with a series of deep breathing, voluntary muscular contractions, and relaxation exercises, in combination with thought control. In this manner, athletes may concentrate more on the tasks at hand.

Negative Thought Stoppers

One of the most difficult aspects of adjusting to injury is the stoppage of negative thoughts. They become detrimental to the return to competition. These thoughts have to be recognized by the athlete and controlled. Teaching athletes to control their inner thoughts helps to determine their future behavior. This technique is an ongoing process of awareness, education for removing negative thoughts, and encouragement for ultimate change.

Early education stresses that negative thoughts have a detrimental effect on both mental and physical performance. Keeping a daily record of when these thoughts take place and the circumstances in which they occur is helpful. Then athletes are helped to stop these negative thoughts and instill a positive regimen. This step is followed by an evaluation of the whole negative thought-stopping program on a regular basis. In this manner, athletes have the practice and feedback to begin their own positive outlook in terms of constructive thoughts, concentration, cues, images, and calming responses to change inappropriate attitudes. This positive outlook can assist athletes in returning more quickly to competition with better abilities to perform.

The reinforcement of phrases such as "You will get better" and "This too will pass" aids in the blockage of the negative thoughts that often occur. Negative thoughts block the athlete's road to recovery by increasing pain, anxiety, and anger. Athletes should be encouraged to put their efforts into recovery rather than into the downward spiral of self-pity. Thoughts create emotions, therefore these negative thoughts have to be recognized and dealt with for a more rapid recovery. The athlete should never be allowed to say "I can't" but rather substitute "I'll try."

Imagery

Imagery is used by athletes to reduce the anxieties associated with the return procedure. Visual images used in the process include visual rehearsal, emotive imagery rehearsal, and body rehearsal. Visual rehearsal uses both coping and mastery rehearsal. Coping rehearsal has athletes visually rehearsing problems they feel may stand in their way to return to competition. They then rehearse how they will overcome these problems.

Mastery rehearsal aids in gaining the confidence and motivational skills necessary. Athletes visualize their successful return to competition from the early drills of the sport to practice to the game situation.

Emotional rehearsal aids the athlete in gaining confidence and security by visualizing scenes relating to positive feelings of enthusiasm, confidence, and pride, in other words, the emotional rewards of praise and success from participating well in competition.

Body rehearsal empirically helps athletes in the healing process. Athletes visualize their bodies healing internally both during the rehabilitation process and during the day. To do this, they have to have a good understanding of the injury and of the type of healing occurring in relation to the rehabilitation procedures.

Care should be taken to explain the healing and rehabilitative process clearly but not to overwhelm athletes with so much information that they become intimidated and fearful. This mistake is often made by the inexperienced counselor who wants to impress the athletes. Educate athletes only to the amount of knowledge required. By the same token, don't hold back information athletes require for this imagery.

INTERPERSONAL RELATIONSHIPS OF THE ATHLETE AND THE SPORTS THERAPIST

The sports therapist is often the first person athletes interact with after injury and the one who will direct the recovery. As a result, the sports therapist has to deal with the athlete as a person and not as just as a patient. When athletes enter the treatment setting, they should get the perception that the sports therapist cares for the athlete as a person and not just as part of the job. Their perception of the sports therapist makes a difference in terms of recovery time and effort. First they have to respect the sports therapist as a person before they can trust the therapist-trainer in the rehabilitative setting. Successful communication between the sports therapist and the athlete is essential for effective rehabilitation. Taking an interest in athletes before injuries have occurred enables the sports therapist to know the athletes' personalities and be able to work with them in helping to build their confidence.

Active listening is one of the sports therapist's most important skills. One must learn to listen to the athlete beyond the complaining. The sports therapist should listen for fear, anger, depression, or anxiety in the athlete's voice. With fear, the athlete may be wondering what the pain means in terms of function and if he or she will be accepted by peers.

Anger is often a feeling of being victimized by the injury and the unfairness of it. In depression, the athlete may have an overwhelming feeling of hopelessness or loneliness. With anxiety the athlete wonders how he or she can survive the injury and what will happen if he or she cannot return to full competition.[10]

Body language is important as well. The sports therapist who continues to work on paperwork while talking to the athlete is sending a noncaring message. The therapist needs to be concerned, and look the athlete in the eye with a genuine interest in their problems. This will go a long way toward gaining confidence and respect.

It is important for the sports therapist to consider the athlete as an individual instead of the "sprained ankle." If the injury is the only consideration, the athlete becomes just an injury and not a person. As a result the attitude projected to the athlete is just that, thus the sports therapist is perceived as caring for the athlete superficially.

The relationship between the sports therapist and the athlete should be one of person to person and not of a coach to a player or one of a judgmental nature. When the athlete is treated as an equal the relationship is improved, and it helps the athlete accept responsibility for his or her own rehabilitation. With injury athletes lose control over their physical efforts. They have gone from 4 to 5 hours a day of practice or competition to no activity. They are in a temporary lifestyle change. Their feelings are going to affect the success or failure of the rehabilitation process. The sports therapist must establish rapport and a sense of genuine concern and caring for the

athlete, who is not fooled by the superficial concerns of the sports therapist.

During an injury evaluation, the sports therapist should allow the athlete to provide as much input about his or her injury as possible. Paraphrasing or restating the information to the athlete will be invaluable to the sports therapist who is unsure of the mechanism of injury or its results. Statements such as "I see" or "Go ahead" or simple silence to allow athletes to fully express themselves are of value. One of the most important bits of information can be the question posed at the end of gathering subjective information—"What else have I not asked you or do I need to know about this injury?"

The sports therapist is often the person who effectively explains the injury to the athlete. Care should be taken to explain the situation to the athlete in understandable terms. In most cases the simplest explanation acceptable to the athlete is the best. With mild and moderate injuries, the use of *sprain, strain,* or *bruise* suffices. The example of a sprained knee and torn ligaments of the knee can be descriptions of the same grade-II injury, but the athlete may interpret the two terms altogether differently.

With the more severe grade-III injuries, care should be taken to inform athletes accurately, while at the same time not frightening them. Knowledge of the injury, its healing mechanism, and the rehabilitation process and progression gives athletes an orderly timetable within which to proceed. If information is broken down this way, athletes do not become overwhelmed by the whole process. In this manner the anxiety and uncertainty manifested in the early denial and anger phases may be lessened. Athletes thus can put all their efforts into the rehabilitation process, with actions replacing anxiety.

Athletes must have injuries explained to them to their satisfaction. Disseminating injury information appropriate to athletes' emotional and intellectual level can be a real challenge. The rate and degree of acceptance is not the same with all athletes. Severity of injury is certainly important, but the athlete's perception of that severity is what matters in the rehabilitation process. Thus the physiological must be interrelated with the psychological. In working with athletes, the sports therapist should be not only empathetic but also nonjudgmental (Figure 16-6).

Athletes are expected to report for rehabilitation, but the coach is the disciplinarian, not the sports therapist, and the coach institutes punishment for lack of participation in the rehabilitation process. The

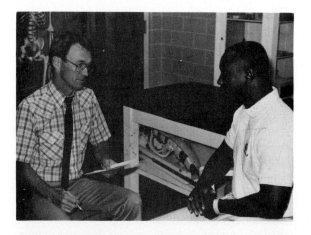

Fig. 16-6. Valuable characteristics of the sports therapist. In working with the athlete, the sports therapist has to be not only empathetic but also nonjudgmental.

coach must support the rehabilitation concept, or athletes soon know that this is not a priority with the coach and begin to lose interest if they are not highly motivated to return to competition.

The real challenge of rehabilitation is how to motivate athletes to do their best in the rehabilitation process. Athletes who are not reporting for rehabilitation have a reason.

Everything is done for some need. The rehabilitation program must be established within these needs. If athletes are not reporting for rehabilitation, either something is more important to them than a hastened recovery, or they have not had the importance of the process adequately explained to them. Reexamine the program and the athlete's goals. If the program has not been well explained and the athlete is not committed to the program, the program either is doomed to failure or will be less than successful. Motivation must come from within, but the sports therapist can provide the encouragement and positive reinforcement necessary for the athlete to make a commitment.

Lack of commitment may indicate frustration, boredom, or feelings of a lack of progress. In this case, further explanations or changes in routine are necessary. The athlete may need the opportunity to comment on the program and make a commitment to the rehabilitation before being structured into a strict regimen of rehabilitative procedures.

An angry, hostile, or surly attitude toward the personnel or program should not offend the sports ther-

apist. With anger the athlete is usually reacting to the situation and not necessarily to the individual. Whenever possible, anger should not be challenged, since no one can reason with anger. Instead, the sports therapist should wait until the individual is in control to discuss inappropriate behavior that cannot be tolerated in the rehabilitation setting. Then the sports therapist and the athlete can work out the cause of the anger and its solution.

As stressed before, knowing the personality of the athlete enables the sports therapist to have a better understanding of what the athlete is going through. This insight can make all the difference in getting the athlete into a proper frame of mind for successful completion of the rehabilitation process.

ADHERENCE TO THE REHABILITATION PROCESS

Shank[14] found that athletes who are committed to the rehabilitation program work harder and thus return to competition more quickly with better results than those who are nonadherents. Their pain tolerance is greater and of less concern, and they are more self-motivated, as opposed to the apathy of the nonadherents.

Also support from peers, coaches, and rehabilitation staff is important in influencing adherence. Those athletes with support show a greater effort to fit the rehabilitation effort into their schedules. They are more likely to keep commitments to those who support them than they are to themselves. Those athletes who are nonadherents respond better to support and motivation from their support group than do the adherents. Thus extra encouragement from this support group for the nonadherent athletes can really pay dividends in getting them motivated for successful completion of their rehabilitation.

The sports therapist should keep in mind that athletes may have many activities in their daily schedules, and fitting the rehabilitation to their schedules rather than the reverse can also encourage compliance. The more the athlete is allowed input and flexibility, the more successful the compliance will be.

As mentioned, pain is better tolerated by the compliant athlete. Rehabilitation programs should be examined to determine the aspects that may be painful. Almost all rehabilitation should be pain-free, and what is not is usually detrimental to the return to competition. Painful exercise, therefore, is not only harmful but also reduces compliance, especially in the nonadherent athlete.

Another aspect of compliance has to do with athletes' perception of their ability. Athletes who perceive themselves as ready to continue to a more advanced level of competition tend to shirk rehabilitation. They usually are the better athletes who do not have to work as hard as but perform better than their peers, so they assume the same attitude about rehabilitation. With this attitude, these good athletes never become truly great athletes because of their lack of commitment to their sport. Once they have risen to the top level where most athletes have the same skills, the work habit is not there to put them in the top of the elite athletic group.

Other factors of compliance for student athletes are the length of time at a particular school, semester grade-point average, perception of class load, career goals, amount of participation time in contests, perception of time available for treatments, and previous experience with rehabilitation programs. The more formal education a person has, the higher the level of compliance to treatments; the higher the semester grade-point average, the higher the treatment compliance. Interestingly enough, an inverse relationship exists between athletes' perception of difficulty of their class load and compliance. Often athletes do better academically during the season than at other times, possibly because they budget their time with better discipline during the season, and this approach carries over into the rehabilitation setting.

Those athletes who have better-defined career goals and those who have the greatest amount of participation time have higher levels of compliance, as do those who perceive they have a greater amount of time available for treatments and those who have previous experience with rehabilitation programs.

COPING WITH INJURY

The sports therapist has to remember that a big part of rehabilitation is to help the athlete cope with the injury. A mild physical injury can be a severe emotional one. At this time the athlete's abilities to cope with the situation are impaired or overwhelmed. The sports therapist must assist the athlete in getting through this time of crisis until the athlete becomes more in control of the situation. This situation may last from several hours to several days.

Athletes feel helpless because their whole lives may revolve around sports, and now they have lost the ability to perform. After this period, injured athletes take either the positive and recovering attitude or one of self-defeat and negativism. This period of limbo should be managed positively to benefit the athlete both on and off the field. Athletes often cope more successfully than the average person because they have self-discipline, emotional control, and better coping skills as a result of their years of competing and adjusting to these demands.

Moos and Tsu[9] talk about major adaptive tasks for the athlete and divide them into eight areas. The first adaptive task has the athlete responding to pain and loss of function and control. Second, the athlete copes with the stresses of the foreign situation of emergency rooms, surgical conditions, casts, braces, or crutches. Also with this coping is the unfamiliar situation of the tremendous amount of effort required of the rehabilitative process, in terms of both time and energy, all without the satisfaction of performing in a competitive setting. Stress is further added since athletes are no longer in the inner circle of their sport with their friends.

The third area has athletes reaching out to establish relationships with the rehabilitative staff. This step is often difficult for athletes who have been catered to when healthy and are now in a reversed role. At this time athletes question many of the aspects of the rehabilitation procedure. They question the doctor's diagnosis, the trainer for working them possibly too much, and the coach for not paying attention to them. They question whether they are malingerers and the rehabilitation personnel as to whether they know how important competition is to them.

The fourth stage requires athletes to acquire emotional balance. Before, they may have had many emotional outbursts to coaches, doctors, sports therapists, and friends as part of the anger mentioned earlier. This frustration is often the result of having been dedicated to a single sport or activity. Many top athletes are emotionally immature, which is one of the disadvantages of sports. Olympic and other top-caliber athletes are often emotionally and socially years behind their chronological peers because they have spent so much time in their sport that their social interactions have suffered. Therefore many top or single-minded athletes have difficulty with emotional control when they sustain a serious injury.

Next, athletes enter the fifth stage, that of maintaining a healthy self-image. This phase has athletes sustaining a sense of competence and mastery. Athletes have had to undergo a change in identity that is often difficult. They have had to remain upbeat and positive while at the same time revising their expectations. This phase is difficult for athletes who have had high expectations and lack the ability to attain these goals.

Athletes who are injured and do not regain their previous form are faced with the same problem. Athletics now takes on a different perspective, and a healthy self-image is required for successful adaptation. At this time athletes have to adjust to dependence on others for their rehabilitation needs, since their independence and self-control have been compromised.

The sixth phase is that of injured athletes maintaining or regaining normal relationships with peers, family, coaches, and rehabilitation personnel. The athletes may have had little support from this group, since everyone is concerned with the results of the team. Injured athletes feel neglected because their communication lines revolve around the sport, and they are no longer part of the sport. When athletes are involved around the team, however, they feel less isolated and guilty.

The seventh area requires athletes to get ready for future competition. This phase is often difficult for athletes, since the time necessary is constantly being reduced by surgical and rehabilitation philosophies and techniques. This reduced time may not allow the athletes adequate mental preparation for the return to competition. Prospective return dates should be discussed with athletes, so they may begin to anticipate their return.

Accepting the limitations of injury and fitting into the athletic lifestyle's restrictions and limitations is the eighth and final task area of adaptation. It can range from the athlete who continues a normal lifestyle with the exception of sports competition to the athlete who is a quadriplegic.

In the area of coping, the sports therapist needs to help athletes with short-term problems rather than with what may happen in the future. Trying to see the total picture right away may be too overwhelming for athletes. This emphasis is important from the time the injury is first assessed on the sidelines. In most cases this situation is foreign and hostile for athletes, and care should be taken to make them as much at ease as possible. How this situation is handled can determine their future attitude toward recovery. Sports therapists should accept their present conceptions, but direct them toward a more positive outlook of the situation.

As soon as possible, the athlete should begin sport-specific drills during practice time with his or her athletic team. The athlete thus feels more a part of the team and is not isolated from the team environment. Thus more effort is put into sport-specific functional situations that are generally less boring to the athlete. In so doing, the athlete gains a more realistic appreciation of the skills needed to attain preinjury performance levels. The rehabilitation routine is more easily tolerated by the athlete if they can see some carryover to their particular sport.

After injury, athletes need the support of those people who have been important and around them. To prevent possible feelings of negative self-worth and problems of loss of identity for athletes, their support groups need to stress that they are interested in the athlete as a person rather than as a team member. Friendships based on athletic identification are now compromised, since the athletic identification is gone, and they can be related to in athletic terms only by what they did yesterday or as injured teammates and not as individuals. If the rehabilitation personnel have established prior personal contact with the athlete as a worthwhile person, this transition can be easier.

GOALS

Goal setting is an important aspect of the rehabilitation of the athlete. First, the goal must be mutually acceptable to both athlete and sports therapist. If the goal is not acceptable to the athlete, the rehabilitation will fail. A goal of return to competitive athletics requires a different program than the goal of leisure athletics or one of just casual exercise.

The time in the season determines certain goals. The individual injured early in the season may be held out for the year as a redshirt or may have an accelerated rehabilitation program for return as soon as possible. The Little League player will have different goals than the high school participant, who will have different goals than the professional player. Remember, the injury belongs to the athlete, who has to accept the goals and be responsible for them if the program is to be a success. Short-term goals emphasize progress and help to maintain motivation better than long-term goals that will often seem unobtainable. The completion of short-term goals gives the athlete experience with success and helps to maintain a positive attitude. An increase in range of motion, lifting another set of weights, and walking without crutches are such short-term goals. Progress is easier to see when the goal is to walk

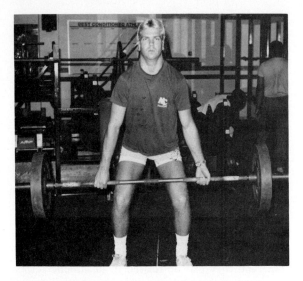

Fig. 16-7. Recognizing the attainment of short-term goals. Attainment of short-term goals emphasizes to the athlete that they are regaining physical control of their situations and that they are getting better.

without crutches than when the goal is to play competitive basketball.

Attainment of short-term goals emphasizes to athletes that they are regaining physical control of the situation once more and that they are getting better (Figure 16-7). Athletes should be kept busy working toward the attainment of these goals to help prevent negative thinking about the negative aspects of the injury.

At this time, the trainer-therapist should reassess the strengths and weaknesses of the athlete who will be disabled for several weeks or more. Strength, power, endurance, speed, agility, and flexibility indexes should be evaluated, as well as the percentage of body fat. Past physical fitness tests should be evaluated and their results integrated into the "new" program. Dietary habits should be investigated and corrected if necessary. With this positive approach toward the rehabilitation program, athletes may return to active status in better condition than before they were injured. The sports therapist must clarify what is expected from the athlete in terms that are within the athlete's ability. The athlete must make a commitment to the rehabilitation process and comply with its demands. However, the goal must be important enough to the athlete to make the commitment.

Here often lies the challenge for the sports therapist: making the goals of the athlete compatible with those of complete recovery.

Care must be taken not to promise more than is possible. A promise that "your knee will be as good as new after surgery" is not possible, but "we have a goal of 90% to 100% result for your knee after surgery" says much of the same without overstating the result.

Mastery of short-term goals allows athletes to feel they are regaining control of the situation. Written short-term goals are desirable because athletes can see their progress. For the same reason, athletes should be encouraged to keep workout journals that give them a more orderly sense of progression about the recuperation.

Return criteria must be explained to the athlete. All concerned—sports therapist, physician, coach, and, most of all, the athlete—must be in agreement about the readiness to return to competition. Positive reinforcement and successful completion of functional short-term goals should have reduced any fears, and the athlete should have relaxed and gained the confidence needed to put all the external factors out of mind. With successful rehabilitation the athlete's instincts return to replace the hesitation the athlete previously had in earlier phases of recovery after the injury.

PROBLEMS IN THE REHABILITATION PROCESS

Some athletes are problems who tax even the most empathetic and understanding of personnel. The better the athlete is dealt with before injury in terms of positive personal interaction, the more successful will be the result. The sports therapist spends 95% of the time with 5% of the athletes. Within this group are the athletes who do not seem to be getting better.

With treatment and rehabilitation, athletes are expected to improve. When they do not, the athlete, physician, sports therapist, and coach become anxious. The self-esteem of the rehabilitation team is based on its ability to cure the athlete, and the athlete is denying it that achievement. By the same token the athlete usually lacks or has lost his or her self-esteem, and it is a problem for him or her as well. Anxiety turns to frustration, antagonism, and hostility on the part of all involved. Often the athlete is described as crazy or unmotivated to explain the lack of improvement. "It certainly can't be the fault of the medical staff or coach."

This indirect communication to players tells them they are not worthwhile in the eyes of the staff. Lack of improvement may be a way that athletes, especially those with low self-esteem, get back at the coach or the system. Athletes may feel that they are not cared for and therefore not getting the attention they deserve. This is the environment for a lawsuit. Often the *perception* of poor care rather than actual poor care fosters most of these hostile feelings toward the athletic and rehabilitation staff.

During this time athletes may often be able to give some insight to the staff as to the reason why they are not improving. Maybe a change in routine, a missed diagnosis, or improper treatment is the cause. The more athletes are involved in their rehabilitation, the more they will move toward a speedy recovery. Athletes may be afraid to return or have other hidden reasons for not returning. The hypochondriac and the malingerer present two types of returning problems. The hypochondriac is often nervous and irritable and seems to be eccentric but often competes with a high tolerance to pain upon returning to the sport. These athletes perceive their lives to be extremely complicated, and they feel they have lost control of their lives both athletically and emotionally.

Many people are taught that all things can be overcome, which is not true. Athletes must be helped to perform within the limits of what they can control. Often hypochondriacs are used to a great deal of support that is suddenly gone. They face a new coach, new environment, new peers, a new athletic philosophy—all situations of change. Their only support is their self-confidence and coping skills, both of which are infantile.

Malingerers, however, claim nothing works in relieving their pain and symptoms. Everything is directed to a constant emphasis of symptoms. "Good morning" may be met with the response, "My ankle still hurts today; yesterday's treatment didn't help a bit." Bizarre symptoms, glove paresthesia, and the like are often tips. Malingerers often have reasons, whether it's saving face because they lack the athletic ability or hostility toward someone involved in the sport. They may fear loss of scholarship aid but not want to do the work required to maintain it, or they may be concerned with litigation at some future time because of some perceived injustice imposed by someone in the system.

Attacks on these individuals result in lowering their self-esteem and further exaggerating their problems. Only by active support and empathy can these individuals be helped, and professional counseling or psychiatric attention may be necessary.

The rehabilitation staff may be partially responsible for some of the problems experienced in the rehabilitation setting. The sports therapist who becomes more sympathetic than empathetic may be reinforcing behavior that is detrimental to the athlete. Chronic pain behaviors, complaining, dependence on the sports therapist, focusing only on the injury, and lack of desire to compete are examples of situations when the attention of the staff may reinforce this aberrant behavior. In this period, the athlete may be in a mood of self-pity just before entering the acceptance phase of the injury.

Hard work in the rehabilitation process should be praised, so the athlete is rewarded for positive responses as opposed to overconcern for the athlete's condition, which results in reinforcement of negative responses. The athlete who increases 5 degrees in range of motion or increases the amount of weight lifted by 5 pounds should be praised to reassure him or her of improvement.

REHABILITATION PERSONNEL

Sports therapists should examine their motives for being in the field, especially when problems are continually cropping up in day-to-day operations. Are they in it for the power or to help people? Some thrive on the following they get from the athletes and thus boost their egos.

Techniques and philosophies should be continually examined to judge their effectiveness. Outdated or invalid theories need to be eliminated to maintain a current rehabilitation program. Sports therapists must remember that many of the athletes will get well anyway if they do not mess the athletes up. Table 16-1 explains the effectiveness of the sports therapist. Without rapport or perceived concern, programs often fail since the athlete loses confidence in the sports therapist.

CONCLUSION

Injury is a foreign, emotional, and unpleasant experience for the athlete. Tradition says that injuries are to be shrugged off and the battle continued. When injuries cannot be ignored, the athlete can become psychologically upset. For this reason all teams should have access to the skills of a sports psychologist, when and if needs arise above the abilities of the coach,

TABLE 16-1
Effectiveness of the Sports Therapist

Type of Therapist	Knowledgeable	Convincing	Sincerely Concerned
Great sports therapist	x	x	x
Good sports therapist	x	x	o
Fair sports therapist	x	o	o
Quack	o	x	o
Bad sports therapist	o	o	o

team physician, or sports therapist. Rehabilitation is a physical and mental process. No two injuries are alike, and no two individuals necessarily react alike. Often attitudes and strategies for a rehabilitation process must be addressed for the troubled athlete. Only the sports therapist, with the necessary commitment, skills, and empathy, will be able to guide the athlete to a successful resolution of the symptoms and to a successful return to active status.

SUMMARY

1. Athletes do not deal with injuries in the same way. The sports therapist has to understand their views of injury. The manner in which the sports therapist manages these athletes often determines their time away from the sport.
2. Life's stressful events play an important role in the adjustment to a certain system or coach. The successful program takes this factor into consideration and adjusts to the individual player whenever possible.
3. Attitudes on the part of coaches and staff have a direct bearing on the performance of the athlete. These personnel direct the athlete in the right direction for successful maturation and athletic competition.
4. After injury the athlete must adjust to denial, anger, depression, and acceptance. Each phase requires empathy on the part of all rehabilitation personnel.
5. The athlete must take responsibility for the injury and deal with it as such. Guiding the athlete toward this goal is an integral part in injury management.
6. Irrational thinking on the part of the athlete is natural after injury. The role of rehabilitation personnel is to change this thinking through such strategies as relaxation training, thought stoppage,

visual rehearsal, emotional rehearsal, and body rehearsal.
7. The interpersonal relationships of the athlete and sports therapist are highly important and often the key to the return for the athlete.
8. Coping with the injury and adherence to the rehabilitation program are extremely important, as is the establishment of short- and long-term realistic goals.

REFERENCES

1   Fisher AC: Adherence to sports injury rehabilitation programs, *Phys Sports Med* 16(7):47-53, 1988.
2   Gieck J: Stress management and the athletic trainer, *Athletic Training* 19(2):115-119, 1984.
3   Gordon T: *Teacher effectiveness training,* New York, 1974, David McKay.
4   Holmes TH, Rahe RH: The social readjustment rating scale, *J Psychosom Res* 11:213, 1967.
5   *J Phys Ed Phys Fit* 48(4):66-69, 1987.
6   *J Sports Med Phys Fitness,* 279-284, 1987.
7   Kübler-Ross E: *On death and dying,* New York, 1969, MacMillian.
8   Michener J: *Sports in America,* New York, 1976, Random House.
9   Moos RH, Tsu VD: *Coping with physical illness,* New York, 1984, Plenum Medical Books.
10 Pitt R: *Phys Ther Forum,* September 16, 1992.
11 Rotella RJ: The psychological care of the injured athlete. In Bunker L, Rotella RJ, Reilly A, editors: *Sport psychology: psychological considerations in maximizing sport performance,* Michigan, 1985, Movement Publications.
12 Rotella RJ: Psychological care of the injured athlete. In Kulund D, editor: *The injured athlete,* Philadelphia, 1988, JB Lippincott.
13 Rotella RJ, Heyman S: Stress, injury and the psychological rehabilitation of athletes. In Williams J, editor: *Applied sport psychology: personal growth to peak performance,* Palo Alto, Calif, 1986, Mayfield.
14 Shank R: *Academic and athletic factors related to predicting compliance by athletes to treatments, dissertation,* Charlottesville, 1987, University of Virginia.

The Evaluation Process in Rehabilitation

17

David H. Perrin

OBJECTIVES

After completion of this chapter, the student should be able to do the following:

- Discuss the important components of a preparticipation physical examination.

- Explain the differences between an on-field and off-field injury evaluation.

- Outline the protocol to be followed for an on-field injury evaluation.

- Describe the usefulness of upper- and lower-quarter screening in the off-field evaluation.

- Describe the components and appropriate sequence for a comprehensive off-field evaluation.

- Discuss the importance and provide a format for documentation of injury evaluation findings.

To be effective in supervising programs of rehabilitation the sports therapist must be skillful in evaluating the status of the athlete. In a sports-medicine setting, several different types of evaluations exist.

Injuries may be prevented to some extent by including a preparticipation examination that must be done long before injury occurs. Information gathered during the preparticipation examination will allow the sports therapist to incorporate intervention strategies to correct existing deficits. The examination is not only helpful for injury prevention but also establishes baseline information that may be useful in determining the severity of an injury.

After acute injury, the sports therapist typically performs an initial evaluation either on the field or court of competition or later in the athletic training room. In the first case, the sports therapist is at a distinct advantage over other health-care providers. First, the sports therapist may have viewed the mechanism of injury, a component of injury evaluation that lends a great deal of insight into the anatomical structures involved. Second, the sports therapist is able to assess the nature of the injury before the onset of muscle spasm and swelling; both factors can confound the accurate assessment of severity. In either the on- or off-field setting, the examiner frequently has the advantage of knowing the athlete's personality, injury history, and pain threshold. Effective management of acute on-field injuries necessitates establishing an emergency plan that clarifies roles and responsibilities of the personnel involved.

The sports therapist cannot design an effective program of rehabilitation without conducting a thorough, detailed, sequential injury evaluation in the clinic or the training room. Throughout the rehabilitation process, the sports therapist must continuously reevaluate the status of the injured athlete and modify or adjust the program as necessary based on an understanding of the healing process.

Finally, accurate documentation of significant findings both during initial evaluation and throughout the rehabilitation program is critical.

PREPARTICIPATION EXAMINATION

Preparticipation examinations are an essential component of a comprehensive sports medicine healthcare plan. The National Collegiate Athletic Association (NCAA) lists it as the first component of a safe athletic program and recommends a thorough evaluation upon a student athlete's initial entrance into an institution's intercollegiate athletic program.[10] A survey of the 50 states and the District of Columbia conducted to assess the requirements for scholastic preparticipation physical examinations showed that 35 states require a yearly examination of some type.[6]

The ideal preparticipation examination incorporates the expertise of medical doctors and sports therapists. The role of the physician is to assess the status of the cardiorespiratory and musculoskeletal systems and review potential contraindications to participation. The team physician ultimately authorizes the athlete's participation in competitive sports. The nature and details of the medical evaluation are beyond the scope of this text.

The role of the sports therapist is to assess the strength, flexibility, and fitness of an athlete relative to the specific demands of the sport. The examination should be designed to screen for potential problem areas. A more definitive evaluation of problem areas should be conducted and referral made to appropriate medical specialists if necessary.

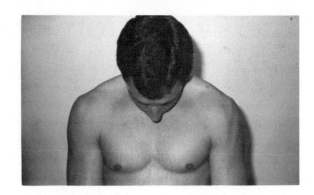

Fig. 17-1. Cervical flexion range of motion.

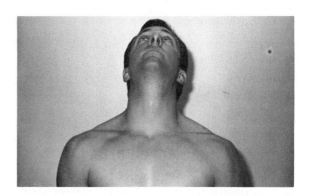

Fig. 17-2. Cervical extension range of motion.

History

The preparticipation examination should begin with a complete medical history that includes questions pertaining to prior illnesses, injuries, surgery, allergies, and immunizations, as well as any current medication therapy. An accurate family history should also be obtained, including any cardiovascular disease, diabetes, allergies, sudden death, or orthopedic problems experienced by members of the athlete's immediate family. Details about affirmative responses on the medical history form frequently need to be confirmed or explored through personal interview.

Flexibility

In determining normal flexibility, the requirements of the sport in question must be considered. For example, inflexibility by the standards of a gymnast is likely very flexible for an offensive lineman.

Assessment of flexibility should begin at the cer-

vical region, include the trunk and all extremities, and focus especially on muscles frequently injured during athletic participation. Normal cervical motion should permit the athlete to place the chin on the chest, look at the ceiling, nearly align the chin with the shoulder on right and left sides, and form a 45 degree angle while laterally flexing to the right and left (Figures 17-1 to 17-4). Shoulder motion may be screened with Apley's range-of-motion tests, which assess abduction and external rotation (Figure 17-5, A and B) and adduction and internal rotation (Figure 17-6, A and B). Inability to perform these tests would necessitate careful evaluation of each motion inherent to the shoulder girdle-joint complex. Elbow, forearm, and wrist range of motion can quickly be assessed by actively performing the motions inherent to these joints.

Evaluation of lower extremity flexibility should include motions about the hip, knee, and ankle joints.

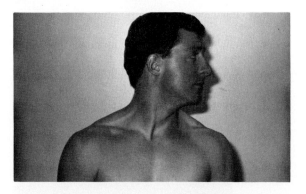

Fig. 17-3. Left cervical rotation range of motion.

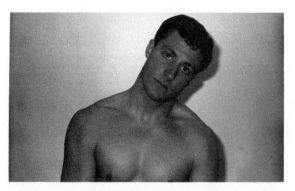

Fig. 17-4. Left lateral cervical flexion range of motion.

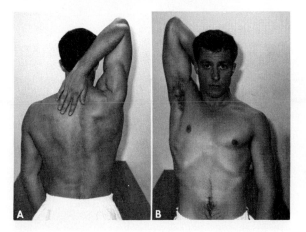

Fig. 17-5. Apley's range-of-motion test—abduction and external rotation.

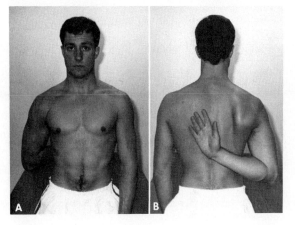

Fig. 17-6. Apley's range-of-motion test—adduction and internal rotation.

Figures 17-7 and 17-8 illustrate simple tests for evaluating flexibility of the hip flexors and adductor muscle groups. Hamstring flexibility can be assessed from a supine position with the hip stabilized at a 90 degree angle (Figure 17-9). Normal flexibility of the hamstring muscle group should permit the athlete to completely extend the knee. Low back and hamstring flexibility can be assessed by the sit-and-reach test (Figure 17-10). Tautness of the iliotibial band is frequently a cause of disability and can be assessed through use of the Ober test, as illustrated in Figure 17-11. Finally, flexibility of the triceps surae complex should be assessed with the knee first extended (gastrocnemius) and then flexed to a 90 degree angle (soleus).

Any limitations in flexibility detected by the examiner should be confirmed and documented through the use of standard goniometry.[11] Only in this way can limitations in motion be confirmed and the usefulness of prescribed stretching programs be ascertained.

Strength

Manual muscle testing should be performed to assess strength of the cervical spine muscles and the major muscle groups of the extremities. Several resources describe the technique of manual muscle testing for all major muscle groups of the body.[1,4]

Athletes presenting with obvious deficiencies in strength or with history of musculoskeletal injury should be evaluated by any one of several commer-

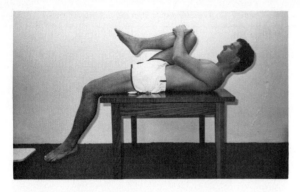

Fig. 17-7. Negative Thomas test for tightness of the left hip flexors.

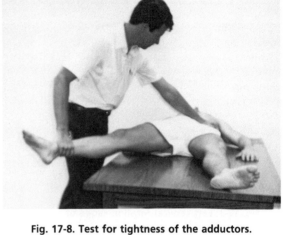

Fig. 17-8. Test for tightness of the adductors.

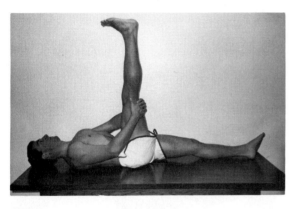

Fig. 17-9. Test for hamstring flexibility. Inability to completely extend the knee indicates a positive test.

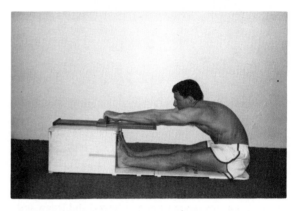

Fig. 17-10. Sit-and-reach test for low back and hamstring flexibility.

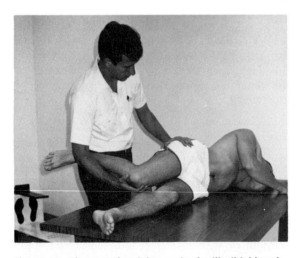

Fig. 17-11. Ober test for tightness in the iliotibial band.

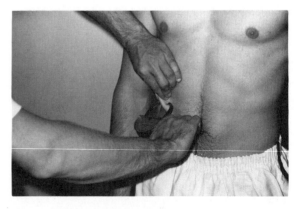

Fig. 17-12. Measurement of subcutaneous fat.

cially available strength dynamometers. Isokinetic testing enables the accurate evaluation of single muscle group performance and their relationship to bilateral and reciprocal muscle groups.[12] As with flexibility, the neuromuscular demands of a sport may dramatically influence the strength capacity of single muscle groups. This influence must be considered when establishing normal bilateral and reciprocal muscle group values for athletes in different sports. An extensive listing of normative isokinetic data for a variety of athletic and sedentary populations in both males and females can be found elsewhere.[12]

Body Composition

Assessment of body composition involves prediction of body density, from which the amount of body fat can be determined. The most accurate method for measuring body composition is hydrostatic weighing. Anthropometric techniques, which include a combination of height-weight indexes, skinfold fat, body circumference, and body diameters, are also available.[8]

When many athletes must be assessed, skinfold measurement of subcutaneous fat provides a rapid and reliable predictor of body density[8] (Figure 17-12). Jackson and Pollock[8] have recommended using the sum of three skinfold measurements to evaluate body composition in adults ranging from 18 to 61 years of age. Subcutaneous fat is distributed differently in men and women, so different sites are used for each group. For men, the sum of chest, abdomen, and thigh skinfolds are used, and for women, the triceps, suprailium, and thigh skinfolds are recommended.

The generalized approach for determination of body composition proposed by Jackson and Pollock is appropriate for a large, heterogeneous population (18 to 61 years of age) but may not be appropriate for the high school athlete. Sports therapists dealing with prepubescent and pubescent athletes are encouraged to read the work of Slaughter et al.[15]

The purpose of determining body composition during the preparticipation examination is to provide the athlete with guidelines relative to desirable levels of body fat. Optimal levels of body fat vary considerably between sports. In general, highly trained athletes range from 4% to 10% body fat for men and 13% to 18% body fat for women.[8]

Fitness

Aerobic fitness is a measure of the long-term energy system's efficiency and is most accurately determined through measurement of oxygen consumption during exhaustive work. However, this measurement also requires expensive laboratory equipment and is impractical for determining fitness of many athletes during the preparticipation examination. Several techniques have been used that predict fitness from recovery heart rates after vigorous stepping or cycling exercise. However, perhaps the most practical method for preparticipation screening of many athletes is the 12-minute run developed by Cooper[2] or a 2 mile run. These techniques predict maximal oxygen consumption from distance covered during a 12-minute run or time required to run 2 miles. From this information, athletes are categorized as having fitness levels falling somewhere between very poor and excellent. Based on test results and determined by the specific physiological demands of the sport, a conditioning program can be prescribed.

Anaerobic fitness assesses the immediate and short-term energy system's efficiency and can be assessed through a Wingate bicycle test, the Margaria stair climbing test, a vertical jump, or 40-yard dash. Most exercise physiology textbooks provide the details of these anerobic power tests. A review of the work of Wilmore[17] will be helpful in designing conditioning programs appropriate for athletes in many different sports.

ON-FIELD EVALUATION

Although most on-field injuries in athletics are not of a life-threatening nature, the first responsibility of a sports therapist is to establish an emergency plan in the event one does occur. The important components of such a plan include the acquisition of appropriate emergency care supplies and equipment such as airway devices, stretchers, spine board, and splints.[14] Accessibility to a telephone, whether competition is occurring indoors or outdoors, is essential. A mechanism for unlocking doors and gates along the path to the injured athlete is also a must. Finally, the lines of authority should be established early with regard to staff and student sports therapists, physicians, and coaches.

Prior knowledge of community rescue squad and hospital emergency room facilities and personnel can be very useful in ensuring the appropriate disposition of the injured athlete. Voluntary in-service training on athletic injuries for the community emergency medical technicians (EMT) and paramedics can be invaluable in establishing the expertise of the sports therapist. On-field management of a suspected cervical spine injury on Saturday afternoon is not the time to debate removal of a football helmet with an EMT.[7]

Another responsibility of the sports therapist is to be aware of the rules of each sport as they pertain to injury management. For example, intercollegiate wrestling permits only 2 minutes for evaluation of an athletic injury before a decision to either continue wrestling or forfeit must be made. Stepping on a basketball court to evaluate an injured player necessitates either removing the player from the game or taking a team timeout. The implication of these rules to the sports therapist, especially in the final moments of a close contest, make injury evaluation an even greater challenge.

Primary Injury Evaluation

The first responsibility during an on-field evaluation is to rule out serious and life threatening injury via a primary survey. Such injuries on the athletic field are generally those in which the athlete is not breathing or has sustained trauma to the vital organs (that is, central nervous system or internal organs). The components of a primary survey include the *ABCs* of emergency care: ensuring that there is an open *Airway*, *Breathing* is taking place, and *Circulation* is present. Once the *ABCs* have been established, injury to the cervical spine must be ruled out before the athlete is moved in any way. Should injury to the cervical spine be suspected, extreme care must be taken to avoid further injury from inappropriate movement. Several excellent sources have outlined the proper immobilization technique for an athlete with an injured spinal cord.[5,16]

Injuries to the chest and abdomen may also pose a threat to the athlete's life. Signs of serious injury to the chest may include pain at the site, difficulty breathing, coughing up of blood, cyanosis of the lips, and a rapid, weak pulse and low blood pressure.

Signs of injury to the abdomen may include tenderness when palpated, pain within the abdomen, difficulty in moving, low blood pressure, rapid pulse, and shallow respiration. Occasionally pain from injury to an internal structure may be referred else-

where, such as with pain in the left shoulder from injury to the spleen (Kehr's sign).

If injury to the chest or abdomen is suspected, the examiner should monitor the athlete's pulse, blood pressure, and respiration. Treatment should be directed toward the prevention of shock until emergency medical personnel arrive.

Secondary Injury Evaluation

The first task of the sports therapist in on-field evaluation of an athlete is to gain access to the athlete and establish control of the situation. Fellow teammates should be instructed never to touch or move an injured teammate; a non-displaced cervical spine fracture could become crippling or fatal by the act of a well intentioned teammate. Also, the sports therapist must never feel pressured by game officials or coaches to hasten the evaluation process.

The very early phase of acute injury evaluation may very well be simply to comfort the athlete and wait for the initial surge of pain to subside. Attempts to evaluate an injured athlete writhing in pain generally prove useless. Athletes usually gain control of their faculties within a few moments, at which time the evaluation may continue.

The next phase of the evaluation is to determine the mechanism of injury. Athletes can frequently describe the position of the body part or the point of contact by another player at the time of injury. Occasionally fellow teammates, game officials, or a coach can provide useful information about the mechanism of injury.

The athlete should next be asked to identify the site of pain as precisely as possible. Occasionally the site of pain is quite diffuse immediately after injury but tends to become more circumscribed within a few minutes. Early in the on-field situation, the sports therapist should palpate the site of injury to rule out gross and obvious deformity and to determine the anatomical structures involved. The athlete's willingness to move the injured part can also be indicative of the severity of the injury.

Should the injury be determined to be ligamentous, stress tests should be used immediately. Transporting an athlete even to the sideline can often lead to muscle spasm and guarding, which can confound the accurate assessment of joint laxity.

At this point in the evaluation, a determination should be made about transporting the athlete from the field of play. In most cases of upper extremity injury and with some lower extremity injuries the athlete is capable of ambulating to the sideline. If any question exists, however, the athlete should be transported without bearing weight until a more definitive sideline evaluation can be conducted.

Once on the sideline, the injury evaluation should follow the guidelines described for the off-field evaluation. The sports therapist should note several important features of the injury that may become useful in determining severity. In particular, the degree and onset of swelling is noteworthy. For example, a knee joint that swells rapidly and substantially usually indicates significant ligamentous injury. Conversely, swelling that occurs slowly and overnight might suggest injury to a meniscal structure.

The amount of motion of the part after injury should also be noted. A knee injury possessing full range of motion after injury but lacking complete extension the next day is probably from muscle spasm or joint effusion rather than from a displaced intra-articular structure.

Finally, the degree of laxity about a joint immediately after injury can be far more revealing than that observed the next day. Such information can be essential to the team physician's evaluation even several hours later and especially the next day.

Perhaps the most difficult questions the sports therapist must answer immediately after many injuries concern classifying the severity and predicting the length of disability. For the reasons stated earlier, the course an injury follows over a 24-hour period can be very revealing relative to its severity and to the period of time before full return to competition can be expected. Thus sports therapists should resist the attempts of others (coaches and press) to predict the period of disability associated with an injury immediately after its occurrence.

OFF-FIELD EVALUATION

Off-field evaluations are usually conducted in the athletic training room and allow the sports therapist the opportunity to perform a detailed and uninterrupted assessment of the injury. Two scenarios seem prevalent in athletics. The first is that of the injured athlete who knows exactly what hurts and can vividly describe the mechanism of injury. The second situation is the athlete who reports pain of an insidious onset and who has difficulty localizing the site of pain. In the first case, the evaluation may be more focused to the region where mechanism of injury and site of

pain are known. In the latter situation, the injury evaluation protocol should begin with a series of range-of-motion, muscle, and neurological tests known as *upper- or lower-quarter screening.*

Quarter Screening

The purpose of upper- or lower-quarter screening is to isolate the site of pain and to establish that the site of pain and location of injury are the same. Embryology of the human body occurs in a longitudinal manner through development of dermatomes and myotomes. Dermatomes are areas of sensation on the skin supplied by a single spinal segment, and myotomes are groups of muscles innervated by a single spinal segment. This formation is especially true in the extremities. The implication to the clinician is that pain from injury within a particular dermatome can be experienced at a point other than the actual site of injury. Also, injury to a nerve may manifest itself through sensory or motor deficit distally along the distribution of the nerve. This phenomenon of referred pain can confound the accurate assessment of injury to either an upper or lower extremity.

Deficits in strength, sensation, or tendon reflexes of specific spinal segments can also indicate pathology at the corresponding nerve root or spinal cord level. For example, impingement of a nerve root from a protruding disk can produce deficits in strength and loss of sensation at the myotome and dermatome that correspond to the spinal segment where the lesion exists. Table 17-1 summarizes the dermatomes, myotomes, and deep tendon reflexes for the upper and lower extremities.

Upper-quarter screening involves the quick assessment of the neck, shoulder girdle region, and arm. Lower-quarter screening involves similar assessment of the low back, hip region, and leg.

UPPER-QUARTER SCREENING. Upper-quarter screening should begin with the athlete in a seated position. Visual inspection to assess posture of the head and shoulder girdle complex should precede the evaluation. The evaluation includes a series of range-of-motion and manual muscle tests of the cervical region and proceeds distally along the upper extremity. Cervical spine motion is first assessed actively (see Figures 17-1 to 17-4) and then with slight overpressure, should active range-of-motion produce no pain or limitation of motion (Figure 17-13). (**Note:** In no instance should a suspected neck injury in the on-field situation include this assessment.) The muscles

TABLE 17-1
Upper and Lower Extremity Dermatomes, Myotomes, and Deep Tendon Reflexes

Spinal Level	Muscle Testing	Sensation	Deep Tendon Reflex
C5	Deltoid and biceps	Lateral arm	Biceps
C6	Wrist extensors	Lateral forearm	Brachioradialis
C7	Wrist flexors	Middle finger	Triceps
C8	Finger flexors	Medial forearm	None
T1	Finger abductors	Medial arm	None
L4	Anterior tibial	Medial foot	Patellar tendon
L5	Extensor muscle of toes	Dorsum of foot	None
S1	Long and short peroneal	Lateral foot	Achilles tendon

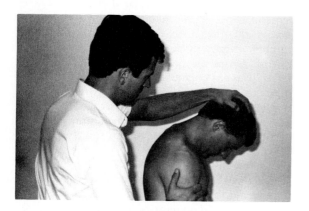

Fig. 17-13. Cervical flexion with overpressure.

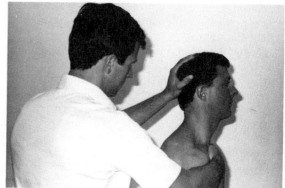

Fig. 17-14. Resisted cervical extension.

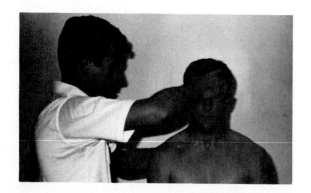

Fig. 17-15. Resisted cervical flexion.

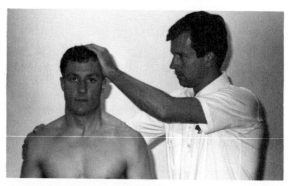

Fig. 17-16. Resisted left lateral flexion.

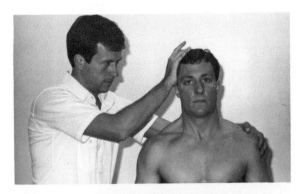

Fig. 17-17. Resisted right lateral flexion.

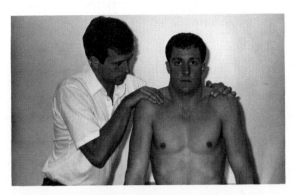

Fig. 17-18. Resisted shoulder elevation (C2, 3, 4).

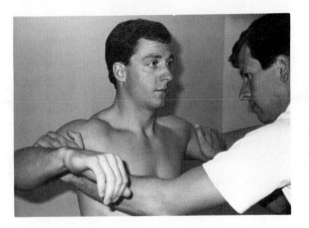

Fig. 17-19. Resisted shoulder abduction (C5).

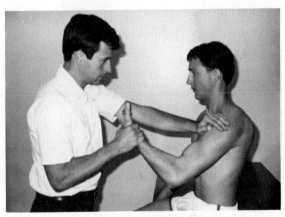

Fig. 17-20. Resisted elbow flexion (C6).

surrounding the cervical spine are then assessed with isometric resistance to examine for either neurological involvement or injury to a muscle (Figures 17-14 to 17-17). During assessment of the cervical region, the sports therapist should look for locally produced signs and symptoms and for pain that may emanate from the cervical region but refer distally elsewhere in the upper extremity.

Next the screening proceeds to the shoulder region and begins with range-of-motion tests (see Figures 17-5 and 17-6) for active motion of the shoulder girdle and glenohumeral joints. Resisted shoulder elevation (Figure 17-18) and abduction (Figure 17-19) are then tested to assess the C2 to C5 neurological levels. The screening continues along the upper extremity with testing in a similar manner at the

elbow, wrist, and hand, as illustrated in Figures 17-20 to 17-27.

As the upper-quarter screening proceeds distally from the cervical spine, the sports therapist should note pain or weakness. Should none be encountered, the site of injury is suspected elsewhere, and the procedure continues until the entire upper extremity has been examined. Should pain, weakness, or asymmetry be found, a more detailed evaluation should be performed focusing on the region of pain.

LOWER-QUARTER SCREENING. Lower-quarter screening involves a series of range-of-motion and manual muscle tests, beginning at the lumbar region and proceeding distally to include the entire lower extremity. As with the upper-quarter screening, the evaluation is preceded by a visual assessment of posture. The

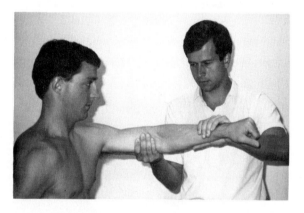

Fig. 17-21. Resisted elbow extension (C7).

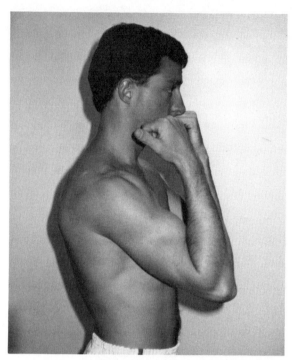

Fig. 17-22. Elbow flexion range of motion.

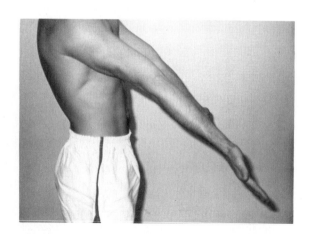

Fig. 17-23. Elbow extension range of motion.

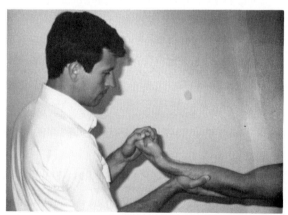

Fig. 17-24. Resisted wrist flexion (C7).

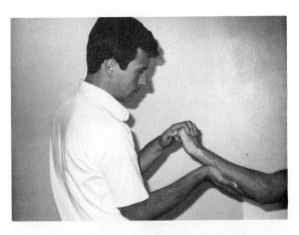

Fig. 17-25. Resisted wrist extension (C6).

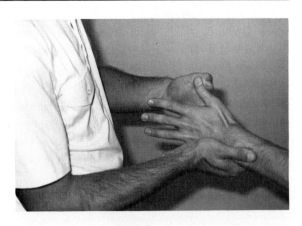

Fig. 17-26. Resisted thumb extension (C8).

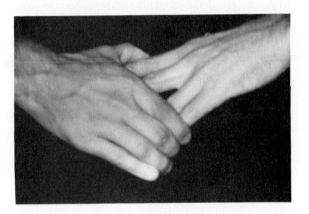

Fig. 17-27. Resisted finger abduction (T1).

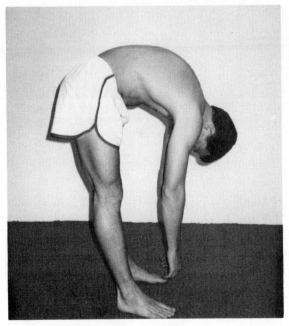

Fig. 17-28. Lumbar flexion range of motion.

evaluation is conducted first while the athlete is standing and then from the sitting, supine, and prone positions.

While standing, the athlete is asked to perform active motion of the lumbar spine (Figures 17-28 to 17-31). Locally or distally produced pain or limitation of lumbar motion should be noted. Heel and toe walking should also be performed to assess neurological levels L4 and L5 (anterior tibial and long extensor of great toe; Figure 17-32) and S1 (gastrocnemius and soleus; Figure 17-33). Additional range-of-motion and manual muscle tests are performed while the athlete is sitting, supine, and prone (Figures 17-34 to 17-42).

As with the upper-quarter screening, pain or weakness should be noted. A region free from pain, weakness, or asymmetry is considered screened and thus not the site of injury. Should pain or weakness be found, a more detailed evaluation that focuses on the region of injury should follow.

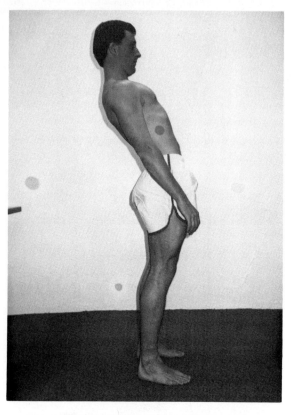

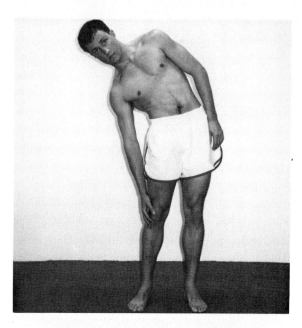

Fig. 17-29. Lumbar extension range of motion.

Fig. 17-30. Lumbar right lateral flexion.

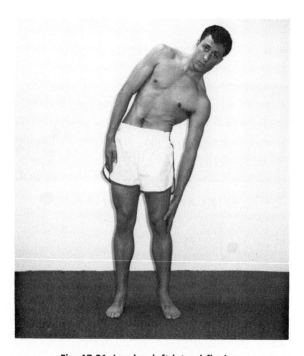

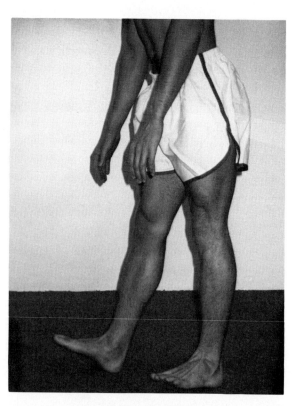

Fig. 17-31. Lumbar left lateral flexion.

Fig. 17-32. Heel walking (L4, L5).

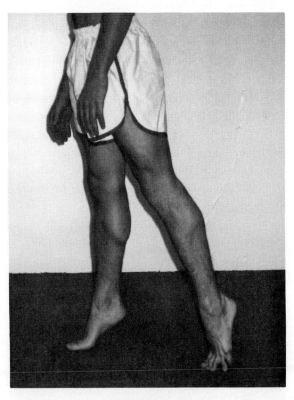

Fig. 17-33. Toe walking (S1).

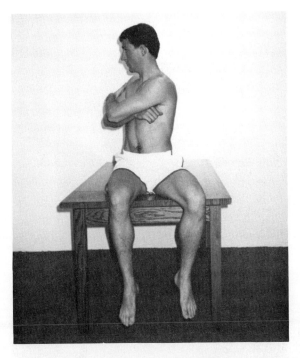

Fig. 17-34. Trunk right rotation.

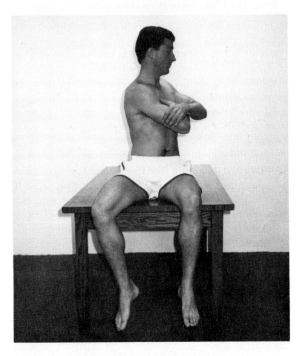

Fig. 17-35. Trunk left rotation.

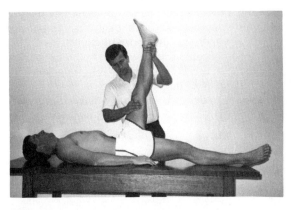

Fig. 17-36. Straight leg raise for sciatic nerve involvement.

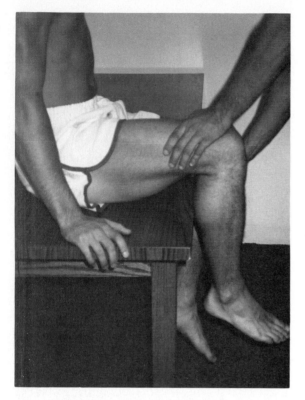

Fig. 17-37. Resisted hip flexion (L1, L2).

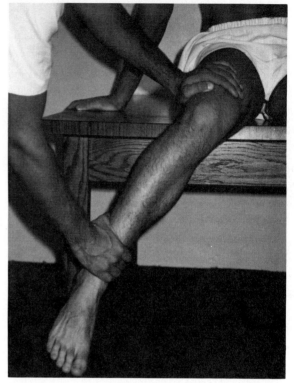

Fig. 17-38. Hip internal rotation range of motion.

CLINICAL EVALUATION SCHEME

The key to successful injury evaluation is to establish a sequential and systematic approach that is followed in every case. Only through a systematic approach can the sports therapist be confident that an important component of evaluation will not be forgotten. Every injury is different and may present with unique signs and symptoms. Thus, although a systematic approach is important, the sports therapist must take care not to become robotized during the evaluation process. With this in mind, the boxes on pp. 268-269 show examples of injury evaluation formats for the knee and shoulder to assist the beginning sports therapist in establishing a sequential injury evaluation plan.

History

Perhaps the single most revealing component of injury evaluation is the history. The primary goals of

the history are to determine the mechanism and site of injury. History taking includes recounting recent events leading to the injury and detailing previous injuries to the body part in question. The sports therapist should also refer to the injury profile obtained from the athlete during the preparticipation examination.

The role of the sports therapist in obtaining an accurate and pertinent history is to ask the right questions and listen carefully. Questions must be asked in a nonleading manner. For example, "What activities cause your knee to hurt?" is more likely to elicit an unbiased response than "Your knee probably hurts when you sit at the movies, right?"

From the athlete's responses, the evaluator must note the pertinent and disregard the irrelevant. Each response provides a key to the nature of the next question.

From the history, the sports therapist should determine whether the injury episode is acute or recurrent. If acute, knowledge of the athlete's posture

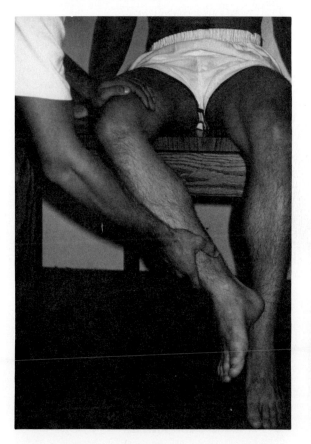

Fig. 17-39. Hip external rotation range of motion.

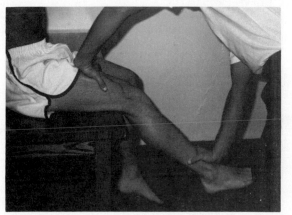

Fig. 17-40. Resisted knee extension (L3, L4).

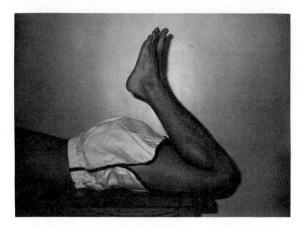

Fig. 17-41. Knee flexion range of motion.

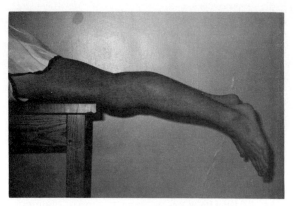

Fig. 17-42. Knee extension range of motion.

KNEE INJURY EVALUATION CHECKSHEET

I. HISTORY

   1. Ask what happened   _____
   2. Ask for description of mechanism   _____
   3. Ask for site of pain   _____
   4. Ask if any previous history   _____

II. INSPECTION

   1. Look for obvious deformity   _____
   2. Look for swelling and effusion   _____
   3. Compare bilaterally   _____

III. PALPATION

  A. Medial aspect

    1. MCL—femoral attachment   _____
    2. MCL—tibial attachment   _____
    3. Joint line   _____

  B. Lateral aspect

    1. LCL—femoral attachment   _____
    2. LCL—fibular attachment   _____
    3. Joint line   _____
    4. Fibular head   _____

  C. Anterior aspect

    1. Suprapatellar pouch   _____
    2. Quadriceps tendon   _____
    3. Patella (superior pole)   _____
    4. Patella (inferior pole)   _____
    5. Patellar tendon   _____
    6. Tibial tuberosity   _____

  D. Posterior aspect

    1. Popliteal fossa   _____
    2. Hamstring tendons   _____

IV. ACTIVE RANGE OF MOTION

   1. Knee flexion   _____
   2. Knee extension   _____
   3. Compare bilaterally   _____

V. PASSIVE RANGE OF MOTION

   1. Knee flexion   _____
   2. Knee extension   _____
   3. Compare bilaterally   _____

VI. RESISTIVE RANGE OF MOTION

   1. Knee extension   _____
   2. Knee flexion   _____
   3. Ankle plantar flexion   _____

VII. SPECIAL TESTS

  A. Menisci

    1. Check for terminal extension   _____
    2. McMurray test   _____

  B. MCL valgus stress test

    1. Correct hand placement   _____
    2. Ensure muscular relaxation   _____
    3. Stressed with terminal extension   _____
    4. Stressed with slight flexion   _____
    5. Compare bilaterally   _____

  C. LCL varus stress test

    1. Correct hand placement   _____
    2. Ensure muscular relaxation   _____
    3. Stressed with slight flexion   _____
    4. Compare bilaterally   _____

  D. ACL anterior drawer stress test

    1. Correct hand placement   _____
    2. Ensure hamstring relaxation   _____
    3. Stressed at 90 degree flexion   _____
    4. Compares bilaterally   _____

  E. ACL Lachman stress test

    1. Correct hand placement   _____
    2. Ensure muscular relaxation   _____
    3. Stressed at 20 degree flexion   _____
    4. Compare bilaterally   _____

---

at the moment of injury is important in determining the mechanism of injury. If swelling is present, the sports therapist should determine if the onset was immediate or slow. The athlete's ability to continue playing or need to stop immediately after the injury can be indicative of severity.

If chronic, the course of the injury should be ascertained relative to an increase or decrease of symptoms and the efficacy of previous treatment regimens. Asking whether the injury is getting better, getting worse, or staying the same provides the evaluator with information relative to the anatomical structures involved and the usefulness of previous or current treatments.

From the history, the evaluator should have a visual image of the injury mechanism and a general impression of the injury. With this information the evaluator is ready to proceed with a specific injury evaluation plan.

SHOULDER INJURY EVALUATION CHECKSHEET

I. HISTORY

1. Ask what happened _____
2. Ask for description of mechanism _____
3. Ask for site of pain _____
4. Ask if any previous history _____

II. INSPECTION

1. Gain visual access to region while maintaining athlete's modesty _____
2. Look for obvious deformity _____
3. Look for swelling _____
4. Compare bilaterally _____

III. PALPATION

A. Anterior aspect

1. Sternoclavicular joint _____
2. Clavicle _____
3. Subacromial bursa _____
4. Coracoid process _____

B. Posterior aspect

1. Scapula and scapular spine _____
2. Supraspinatus muscle _____
3. Infraspinatus muscle _____
4. Teres minor muscle _____
5. Rhomboid muscle _____

C. Lateral aspect

1. Deltoid muscle _____
2. Biceps tendon _____
3. Greater tuberosity _____
4. Lesser tuberosity _____

D. Superior aspect

1. Acromioclavicular joint _____
2. Trapezius muscle _____

E. Inferior aspect

1. Axilla _____
2. Pectoralis major muscle _____
3. Latissimus dorsi muscle _____

IV. ACTIVE RANGE OF MOTION

1. Cervical flexion _____
2. Cervical extension _____
3. Cervical right and left lateral flexion _____
4. Cervical right and left rotation _____
5. Shoulder flexion _____
6. Shoulder extension _____
7. Shoulder abduction _____
8. Shoulder adduction _____
9. Shoulder internal rotation _____
10. Shoulder external rotation _____
11. Shoulder horizontal flexion _____
12. Shoulder horizontal extension _____
13. Shoulder girdle elevation _____
14. Shoulder girdle depression _____
15. Check for normal glenohumeral/scapular motion _____
16. Compare bilaterally _____

V. PASSIVE RANGE OF MOTION

1. Shoulder flexion _____
2. Shoulder extension _____
3. Shoulder abduction _____
4. Shoulder adduction _____
5. Shoulder internal rotation _____
6. Shoulder external rotation _____
7. Shoulder horizontal flexion _____
8. Shoulder horizontal extension _____
9. Compare bilaterally _____

VI. RESISTIVE RANGE OF MOTION

1. Shoulder flexion _____
2. Shoulder extension _____
3. Shoulder abduction _____
4. Shoulder adduction _____
5. Shoulder internal rotation _____
6. Shoulder external rotation _____
7. Shoulder horizontal flexion _____
8. Shoulder horizontal extension _____
9. Shoulder girdle elevation _____
10. Shoulder girdle depression _____

VII. SPECIAL TESTS

A. Yergason's bicipital tendinitis and subluxing biceps tendon test

1. Correct hand placement _____
2. Maintain elbow at 90 degrees _____
3. Ask patient to supinate against resistance _____

B. Drop-arm test for rotator cuff involvement

1. Passively place patient's shoulder at 90 degrees _____
2. Ask patient to hold position or lower slowly _____

C. Empty-can test for supraspinatus strain

1. Places shoulder at 90 degree abduction and 30 degree horizontal flexion _____
2. Has patient internally rotate shoulder _____
3. Attempts to adduct patient's shoulder _____

D. Apprehension test for anterior dislocation/subluxation

1. Ensures muscular relaxation _____
2. Slowly abducts and externally rotates patient's shoulder _____

E. Adson maneuver for thoracic outlet syndrome

1. Has patient hold fully inspired breath _____
2. Has patient extend and turn head toward side being examined _____

Inspection

Visual inspection of the injury begins as the athlete enters the training room. Of special interest is the athlete's gait in the case of lower extremity injury. If an upper extremity is involved, the carrying position of the part should be noted.

A bilateral comparison of the anatomical region in question must be made. This comparison will necessitate removal of clothing in many cases. In all instances, the modesty of the athlete must be protected. Shorts alone may be worn by the male athlete; females should wear sleeveless shirts or halter tops for evaluation of upper extremity injury. As the athlete removes clothing, limitations in motion and weight bearing should be observed.

The primary purpose of the visual inspection is to first rule out the presence of gross or obvious deformity. Articular dislocations, such as those of the finger or shoulder, are easily visualized with careful inspection. Fractures of superficially located bones may also be noted in some cases, although non-displaced fractures of a bone, such as the clavicle, may be impossible to ascertain from physical examination. Swelling at the injury site should also be noted, as should the nature of its onset, that is, rapid and immediate or gradual and slow. Finally, in the case of chronic injury, the presence of atrophy of muscles surrounding the region should be noted. For example, an athlete experiencing patellofemoral pain over an extended period may present with a substantial deficit in thigh girth.

Palpation

Palpation of the injury site should occur early in the on-field evaluation for reasons previously described. During the more detailed off-field evaluation, palpating later in the injury evaluation process may be better. The disadvantage of palpating the injury site early is that such manual probing may elicit a pain response that will detract from the findings of the active, passive, and resistive motions that follow. Furthermore, the phenomenon of referred pain may make localization of the injury site difficult until other components of the evaluation have been performed.

The purpose of palpation is to identify as closely as possible the exact anatomical structures involved with the injury. Palpation may be quite revealing at some regions (ankle, knee, or elbow) but may be far less helpful at others (shoulder or hip). From palpation the presence of excessive heat from infection or inflammation should be noted. The volume and consistency of swelling may indicate effusion or hemarthrosis at a joint, and calcification may be identified in the residual hematoma from a soft tissue contusion. Rupture of a muscle or tendon may present as a gap at the point of separation. Some sports therapists believe malalignment of a skeletal structure, such as a vertebrae, can be ascertained through careful palpation.

Assessment of Motion

The goal of testing the motion of the injured part is to determine the nature of the anatomical structures involved. Cyriax has developed a method for locating and identifying a lesion by applying tension selectively to each of the structures that might potentially produce this pain.[3] Tissues are classified as being either contractile or inert. **Contractile** tissues include muscles and their tendons; **inert** tissues include bones, ligaments, joint capsules, fascia, bursae, nerve roots, and dura mater.

If a lesion is present in contractile tissue, pain occurs with active motion in one direction and with passive motion in the opposite direction. Thus a muscle strain would cause pain on both active contraction and passive stretch. Contractile tissues are tested through the midrange by an isometric contraction against maximum resistance. The specific location of the lesion within the musculotendinous unit cannot be specifically identified by the isometric contraction.

A lesion of inert tissue elicits pain on active and passive movement in the same direction. A sprain of a ligament results in pain whenever that ligament is stretched, through either active contraction or passive stretching. Again, a specific lesion of inert tissue cannot be identified by looking at movement patterns alone. Other special tests must be done to differentiate injured structures.

ACTIVE RANGE OF MOTION. Movement assessment should begin with active motion. The sports therapist should evaluate the quality of movement, range of movement, motion in other planes, movement at varying speeds, and strength throughout the range but in particular at the endpoint. A complaint of pain on active motion does not distinguish contractile pain from inert pain. Thus the sports therapist must proceed with an evaluation of both passive and resistive motion. An athlete who seems to be free of pain in each of these tests throughout a full range of motion should be tested by applying passive pressure at the endpoint.

CATEGORIZATION OF ENDPOINT "FEELS"

NORMAL ENDPOINTS

Soft tissue approximation	Soft and spongy, a gradual painless stop (for example, knee flexion)
Capsular feel	An abrupt, hard, firm endpoint with only a little give (for example, endpoint in hip rotation)
Bone-to-bone	A distinct and abrupt endpoint where two hard surfaces come in contact with one another (for example, elbow extension)
Muscular	Springy feel with some associated discomfort (for example, end of shoulder abduction)

ABNORMAL ENDPOINTS

Empty feel	Movement is definitely beyond the anatomical limit, and pain occurs before the end of the range (for example, a complete ligament rupture)
Spasm	Involuntary muscle contraction that prevents motion because of pain; should also be called *guarding* (for example, back spasms)
Loose	Occurs in extreme hypermobility (for example, previously sprained ankle)
Springy block	A rebound at the endpoint (for example, meniscus tear)

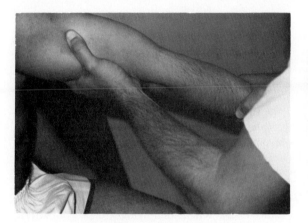

Fig. 17-43. Passive elbow extension illustrating bone-to-bone end feel.

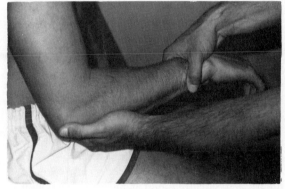

Fig. 17-44. Passive elbow pronation illustrating capsular end feel.

PASSIVE RANGE OF MOTION. When passive range of motion is being assessed, the athlete must relax completely and allow the sports therapist to move the extremity to reduce the influence of the contractile elements. Particular attention should be directed toward the sensation of the athlete at the end of the passive range of motion. The sports therapist should categorize the "feel" of the endpoints as indicated in the box above.[3] Figures 17-43 to 17-45 illustrate normal end-feels typically encountered during assessment of passive motion at the elbow. Common abnormal end-feels experienced during passive motion are the resistance encountered from a muscle in spasm or the springy block sensation resulting from a displaced intraarticular cartilage.

End-feel may also be quite revealing in assessment

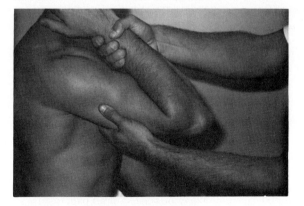

Fig. 17-45. Passive elbow flexion illustrating tissue approximation end feel.

of ligamentous integrity. For example, the sensation of end-feel is probably more revealing than the amount of instability when performing the Lachman test to assess integrity of the anterior cruciate ligament of the knee.

Also of significance during passive motion is the presence of crepitus or clicking. Crepitus may indicate roughening of one or more articular surfaces such as found in advanced patellofemoral disease. Clicking may result from a subluxing tendon or displaced intraarticular cartilage. A biceps tendon subluxing from the intertubercular groove of the humerus and a torn meniscus catching between tibia and femur during knee motion are two forms of clicking.

Throughout the passive range of motion, the sports therapist is looking for limitation in movement and the presence of pain. Occasionally the sports therapist may encounter a phenomenon during passive motion known as a **painful arc.** A painful arc is pain that occurs at some point in the midrange but disappears as the limb passes this point in either direction. It occurs from pinching or impingement of sensitive structures between two surfaces, which can be caused either by a biomechanical fault in the articulating bones or by swollen tissue pinched between two normally aligned bony surfaces. Painful arcs are most typically associated with active motion but can also occur in passive motions in which a tissue is being stretched. A classic example of a painful arc is an impingement of the supraspinatus muscle. A painful arc is frequently found at the shoulder region as the subacromial bursa or supraspinatus tendon is pinched during movements inherent to activities such as swimming and throwing.

Pain that occurs at the endpoint in the range of motion is usually caused by shortening or contracture of the capsule and ligaments. This tightness in the capsule places the joint in a close-packed position that abnormally compresses structures surrounding the joint. This problem may be eliminated by stretching the capsule in a neutral pain-free position. If the athlete reports pain before the end of the available range of motion, acute inflammation is likely indicated, in which stretching and manipulation are both contraindicated as treatments. Pain occurring synchronous with the end of the range of motion indicates that the condition is subacute and has progressed to some inert tissue fibrosis. During this stage, gentle stretching may be started. If no pain occurs at the end of the range of motion, the condition is

TABLE 17-2
Capsular Patterns for Major Joints

Joint	Capsular Pattern
Neck	Equal limitation side bending and rotation, full range flexion painful, extension limited
Glenohumeral	Limited external rotation greater than abduction greater than internal rotation
Elbow	Greater limitation of flexion than extension
Hip	Gross limitation of flexion, abduction, and internal rotation, slight limitation of extension, little or no limitation of external rotation
Knee	Gross limitation of flexion, slight limitation of extension, rotation unlimited
Talocrural	More limitation of plantarflexion than dorsiflexion
Subtalar	Inversion progressively limited

chronic, and contractures have replaced inflammation. At this point, mobilization, stretching, and exercise are all indicated.[3]

Capsular patterns of motion. A lesion that exists in the joint capsule or the synovial lining limits active movement in proportion to the extent of the various motions possible about that joint. This **capsular pattern** manifests as a characteristic pattern of decreased movements at a joint and occurs only in synovial joints. Each joint exhibits its own capsular pattern (Table 17-2). When identifying a capsular pattern, movement restrictions are listed in sequence with the first being the most limited. For example, the hip exhibits gross limitation of flexion, abduction, and internal rotation; slight limitation of extension; and little or no limitation of external rotation.[3] These capsular patterns exist whenever the entire capsule is affected. However, there are many situations where only one part of the capsule may be affected by trauma. In this case, limitation of motion will only be evident when that part of the capsule is stretched.

Noncapsular patterns of motion. In a **noncapsular pattern,** the limitation of motion does not follow the normal capsular pattern. It generally indicates the presence of a lesion outside the capsule. Cyriax has classified the following lesions as noncapsular.[3]

A **ligamentous adhesion** occurs after injury and may result in a movement restriction in one plane, with a full pain-free range in other planes.

Internal derangement involves a sudden onset of

TABLE 17-3
Results of Resistive Motion

Interpretation	Possible Pathology
Strong and painless	Healthy muscle-tendon unit
Strong and painful	Muscle-tendon unit injury
Weak and painful	Fracture or tendon avulsion
Weak and painless	Muscle rupture or nerve palsy
Pain on repetition	Single contraction is strong and pain-less, but repetition produces pain as in some vascular disorders
All muscles painful	May indicate serious emotional or psychological problem

TABLE 17-4
Numerical Isometric Grading System[1]

Numeral	Description
5	Maintains the test position against gravity and maximal resistance
4	Maintains the test position against gravity and moderate resistance
4−	Maintains the test position against gravity and less-than-moderate resistance
3+	Maintains the test position against gravity and minimal resistance
3	Maintains the test position against gravity

localized pain resulting from the displacement of a loose body within the joint. The mechanical block restricts motion in one plane while allowing normal, pain-free motion in the opposite direction. Movement restrictions may change as the loose body shifts its position in the joint space.

An **extraarticular lesion** results from adhesions occurring outside the joint. Movement in a plane that stretches that adhesion results in pain, whereas motion in the opposite direction is pain-free and non-restricted.

RESISTIVE MOTION. Resistive motion is movement performed by the athlete but against the opposite and equal resistance of the examiner. The goal of resistive motion is to assess the state of the contractile unit. Injury to any component of the muscle-tendon unit can result in pain or weakness during resistive motion. Also, injury to a component of the nervous system can manifest itself through muscular weakness, a situation that can confound the injury evaluation. Only through an integration of findings during active, passive, and resistive motion can the injured structure accurately be identified. Cyriax has designed a system for differentiating lesions through assessment of muscular contraction as indicated in Table 17-3.[3]

Resistive motion must be performed from a stationary joint position and while in the midrange of motion. Resistive motion assessed dynamically and allowed to progress to an extreme in the range of motion not only tests contractile capacity of the muscle in question but also stretches the antagonist muscle and inert tissue. Several excellent resources are available that illustrate manual muscle examination.[1,4] Table 17-4 indicates a numerical isometric grading

system for rating the quality of the resisted movement.

Figures 17-20 and 17-40 illustrate the resistance, counterpressure, and joint positions for an upper and lower extremity muscle group.

Special Tests

At this point in the evaluation, the examiner should have identified the structures involved in the injury. Depending on the examiner's findings, special tests are used to confirm suspicions or to assess severity of injury. For example, suspicion of recurrent anterior shoulder dislocation may be confirmed through use of an apprehension test designed to reproduce the typical mechanism of injury (Figure 17-46). Stress testing of knee ligaments is performed to confirm the structures involved and to determine the degree of laxity and thus severity of injury (Figure 17-47).

In some cases it may be appropriate to have the athlete perform a series of sport-specific functional drills to help determine readiness to return to competition.[9] A progression of functional tests might include straight-ahead running, large-to-small circles and figure-eights, carioca running, and other agility drills specific to the sport in question.

ARRIVING AT AN IMPRESSION

Only through a complete and systematic evaluation can a valid impression of an injury be made. One component of the evaluation alone usually provides insufficient information. Only through an integration of findings from the history and physical examination

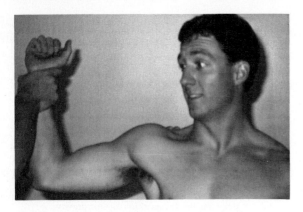

Fig. 17-46. Apley's apprehension test for anterior shoulder dislocation.

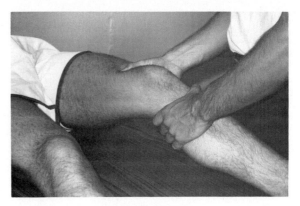

Fig. 17-47. Lachman's test for anterior cruciate ligament insufficiency.

can the examiner arrive at a reasonable impression of injury. With this information, an appropriate treatment and rehabilitation plan can be implemented.

DOCUMENTATION OF FINDINGS

The final phase of the injury evaluation format is the documentation of findings. The medicolegal climate of sports necessitates careful and systematic documentation of injuries. Of no less importance is the role documentation of injury plays in the establishment of a bonafide profession. An effective system of documentation should include gathering and recording of specific information about an injury with respect to subjective and objective information, clinician assessment, and plan of treatment (SOAP Notes).

SOAP Notes

Documentation of acute athletic injury can be effectively accomplished through a system designed to record both subjective and objective findings and to document the immediate and future treatment plan for the athlete. This method combines information provided by the athlete and the observations of the examiner.

The box on p. 275 presents a recommended injury report form that includes the components of documentation discussed above. This form also includes a provision to document findings arising from more definitive evaluation or from the examiner's subsequent day evaluation.

S (SUBJECTIVE). This component includes the sub-

jective statements provided by the injured athlete. History taking is designed to elicit the subjective impressions of the athlete relative to time, mechanism, and site of injury. The type and course of the pain and the degree of disability experienced by the athlete are also noteworthy.

O (OBJECTIVE). Objective findings result from the sports therapist's visual inspection, palpation, and assessment of active, passive, and resistive motion. Findings of special testing should also be noted here. Thus the objective report would include assessment of posture, presence of deformity or swelling, and location of point tenderness. Also, limitations of active motion and pain arising or disappearing during passive and resistive motion should be noted. Finally, the results of special tests relative to joint stability or apprehension are also included.

A (ASSESSMENT). Assessment of the injury is the sports therapist's professional judgment with regard to impression and nature of injury. Although the exact nature of the injury will not always be known initially, information pertaining to suspected site and anatomical structures involved is appropriate. A judgment of severity may be included but is not essential at the time of acute injury evaluation.

P (PLAN). The plan should include the first aid treatment rendered to the athlete and the sports therapist's intentions relative to disposition. Disposition may include referral for more definitive evaluation or simply application of splint, wrap, or crutches and a request to report for reevaluation the next day. If the injury is of a more chronic nature, the examiner's plan for treatment and therapeutic exercise would be appropriate.

INJURY REPORT FORM

ATHLETE'S NAME _____   DATE OF INJURY _____

INJURY SITE: R L _____   TODAY'S DATE _____

SPORT _____

Subjective findings (history):

Objective findings (inspection, palpation, mobility, and special tests):

Assessment (impression):

Plan (treatment administered and disposition):

Follow-up notes: Date _____

EVALUATED BY _____

RECORDED BY _____

SUMMARY

1. The components of the preparticipation examination include a medical history and evaluation of flexibility, strength, body composition, and fitness.
2. On-field evaluation requires the establishment of an emergency plan and early recognition of life-threatening injury.
3. Off-field evaluation permits a more detailed assessment of injury and may begin with upper- or lower-quarter screening.
4. The important components of off-field evaluation include history; inspection; palpation; assessment of active, passive, and resistive motion; and special tests.
5. The final phase of injury evaluation is effective recordkeeping, which includes documentation of subjective and objective findings, the evaluator's assessment, and the plan for injury management and treatment.

REFERENCES

1 Clarkson HM, Gilewich GB: *Musculoskeletal assessment: joint range of motion and manual muscle strength,* Baltimore, 1989, Williams & Wilkins.
2 Cooper KH: A means of assessing maximal oxygen intake, *J Am Med Assoc* 203:135-138, 1968.
3 Cyriax J: *Textbook of orthopaedic medicine: diagnosis of soft tissue lesions,* vol 1, London, 1982, Bailliere Tindall.
4 Daniels L, Worthingham C: *Muscle testing: techniques of manual examination,* Philadelphia, 1980, WB Saunders.
5 Denegar CR, Saliba EN: On the field management of the potentially cervical spine injured football player, *Athletic Training* 24:108-111, 1989.
6 Feinstein RA, Soileau EJ, Daniel WA: A national survey of preparticipation requirements, *Phys Sports Med* 16:51-59, 1988.
7 Feld F, Blanc R: Immobilizing the spine-injured football player, *J Emerg Med Serv* 12:38-40, 1988.
8 Jackson AS, Pollock ML: Practical assessment of body composition, *Phys Sports Med* 13:76-90, 1985.
9 Lephart SM, Perrin DH, Minger K, et al.: Sports specific functional tests for the anterior cruciate ligament insufficient athlete, *Athletic Training* 26:44-50, 1991.
10 National Collegiate Athletic Association: *NCAA Sports Medicine Handbook,* Mission, KS, 1987, NCAA.
11 Nockin CC, White JD: *Measurement of joint motion: a guide to goniometry,* Philadelphia, 1985, FA Davis.

12 Perrin DH: *Isokinetic exercise and assessment,* Champaign, Ill, 1993, Human Kinetics.

13 Powell J: 635,000 injuries annually in high school football, *Athletic Training* 22:19-22, 1987.

14 Ray RL, Feld FX: The team physician's medical bag in emergency treatment of the injured athlete, *Clin Sports Med* 8:139-146, 1989.

15 Slaughter MH, Lowman T, Blileau R, et al.: Skinfold equations for estimation of body fatness in children and youth, *Hum Biol* 60:709-723, 1988.

16 Vegso JJ, Bryant MH, Torg JS: Field evaluation of head and neck injuries. In Torg JS, editor: *Injuries to the head, neck, and face,* Philadelphia, 1982, Lea & Febiger.

17 Wilmore JH: *Training for sport and activity: the physiological basis of the conditioning process, ed 2,* Boston, 1982, Allyn and Bacon.

Back Rehabilitation

18

Dan Hooker

OBJECTIVES

After completion of this chapter, the student should be able to do the following:

- Discuss the importance of a thorough evaluation of the back before developing a rehabilitation plan.

- Describe the acute vs. reinjury vs. chronic stage model for treating low back pain.

- Explain the eclectic approach for rehabilitation of back pain in the athletic population.

- Discuss basic- and advanced-level training in the reinjury stage of treatment.

- Discuss the rehabilitation approach to specific conditions affecting the back.

Back pain has been a problem for all the ages. In most cases, low back pain in athletes does not have serious or long lasting pathology. It is generally accepted that the soft tissues (ligament, fascia, and muscle) can be the initial pain source. The athlete's response to the injury and to the provocative stresses of evaluation is usually proportional to the time since the injury and the magnitude of the physical trauma of the injury. The soft tissues of the lumbar region should react according to the biological process of healing, and the time lines for healing should be similar to other body parts. There is no substantiation that athletic injury to the low back should cause a pain syndrome whose symptoms last longer than 6 to 8 weeks.[8,27]

ACUTE VS. CHRONIC BACK PAIN

The low back pain that athletes most often experience is an acute, painful experience rarely lasting longer than 3 weeks. The athlete rarely misses a practice and even more rarely misses a game because of this type of back pain. As with many athletic injuries, sports therapists often go through exercise or treatment fads in trying to rehabilitate the athlete with low back pain. The latest fad might involve flexion exercise, extension exercise, joint mobilization, dynamic muscular stabilization, abdominal bracing, myofascial release, electrical stimulation protocols, and so on. To keep perspective, as sports therapists select exercise and modalities, they should keep in mind that 90% of people with back pain get resolution of the symptoms in 6 weeks regardless of the care administered.[27,38]

There are athletes who have pain persisting beyond 6 weeks. This group of athletes will generally have a history of reinjury or exacerbation of previous injury. They describe a low back pain that is similar to their previous back pain experience.

These athletes are experiencing an exacerbation or reinjury of previously injured tissues by continuing to apply stresses that may have created their original injury. This group of athletes needs a more specific and formal treatment and rehabilitation program.[8,27]

There are also people who have chronic low back pain. This is a very small percentage of the population suffering from low back pain and an even smaller percentage of the athletic low back pain subgroup. The difference between the athlete with an acute injury or reinjury and a person with chronic pain has been defined by Waddell. He states that "Chronic pain becomes a completely different clinical syndrome from acute pain."[38] Acute and chronic pain are not only different in time scale but are fundamentally different in kind. Acute and experimental pains bear a relatively straightforward relationship to peripheral stimulus, nociception, and tissue damage.

There may be some understandable anxiety about the meaning and consequences of the pain, but acute pain, disability, and illness behavior are generally proportionate to the physical findings. Pharmacological, physical, and even surgical treatments directed to the underlying physical disorder are generally highly effective in relieving acute pain. Chronic pain, disability, and illness behavior, in contrast, become increasingly dissociated from their original physical basis, and there may be little objective evidence of any remaining nociceptive stimulus. Instead, chronic pain and disability become increasingly associated with emotional distress, depression, failed treatment, and adoption of a sick role. Chronic pain progressively becomes a self-sustaining condition that is resistant to traditional medical management. Physical treatment directed to a supposed but unidentified and possibly nonexistent nociceptive source is not only understandably unsuccessful but may cause additional physical damage. Failed treatment may both reinforce and aggravate pain, distress, disability, and illness behavior.[38] This chapter will not attempt to deal with the evaluation or treatment of this type of patient but will concentrate on the acute injury and reinjury scenarios.

THE IMPORTANCE OF EVALUATION

In many instances after referral for medical evaluation, the athlete returns to the sports therapist with a diagnosis of low back pain. While this is a correct diagnosis, it does not offer the specificity needed to help direct the treatment planning. The sports therapist planning the treatment would be better served with a more specific diagnosis such as spondylolysis, disk herniation, quadratus lumborum strain, piriformis syndrome, or sacroiliac ligament sprain.

Regardless of the diagnosis or the specificity of the diagnosis, the importance of a thorough evaluation of the athlete's back pain is critical to good care. The sports therapist should become an expert on this individual athlete's back. Taking the time to perform a comprehensive evaluation will pay great rewards in the success of treatment and rehabilitation. The evaluation has six major purposes:

1. Clearly locates areas and tissues that might be part of the problem. The sports therapist should use this information to direct treatments and exercises.[21]

2. Establishes the baseline measurements used to assess progress and guide the treatment progression and helps the sports therapist make specific judgments on the progression of or changes in specific exercises. The improvement in these measurements also guides the return to practice and play and provides one measure of the success of the rehabilitation plan.[21]

3. Provides some provocative guidance to help the athlete probe the limits of their condition, help them better understand their problem, present limitations, and understand the management of their injury problem.[21]

4. Establishes confidence in the sports therapist and increases the placebo effect of the therapist-athlete interaction.[37,38]

5. Decreases the anxiety of the athlete, thereby increasing their comfort, which will increase their compliance with the rehabilitation plan; a more positive environment is created, and the therapist and patient avoid the "no one knows what is wrong with me" trap.[8]

6. Provides information for making judgments on pads, braces, and corsets.

The box provides a detailed scheme for evaluation of back pain.

ACUTE STAGE, REINJURY STAGE, CHRONIC STAGE MODEL

In discussing the treatment of the athlete with low back pain, the discussion can be much more specific and meaningful if treatment plans are lumped into two stages. Stage I (acute stage) treatment consists mainly of the modality treatment and pain relieving exercises. Stage II treatment involves treating athletes with a reinjury or exacerbation of a previous problem. The treatment plan in stage II goes beyond pain relief, strengthening, stretching, and mobilization to include trunk stabilization and movement training sequences and to provide a specific, guided program to return the athlete to the chosen sport.[27]

Stage I (Acute Stage) Treatment

INITIAL PAIN MANAGEMENT

Modulating pain should be the initial focus of the sports therapist. Progressing rapidly from pain man-

LUMBAR AND SACROILIAC JOINT OBJECTIVE EXAMINATION

A. Observation
B. Standing Position
  1. Posture—alignment
  2. Gait
    a. Patient's trunk frequently bent laterally or hips shifted to one side
    b. Walks with difficulty and limps
  3. Alignment and symmetry
    a. Level of malleoli
    b. Level of popliteal crease
    c. Trochanteric levels
    d. PSIS and ASIS positioning
    e. Levels of iliac crests
      1. If there is sacroiliac dysfunction the iliac crests will be unlevel; the ASIS and the PSIS will also be unlevel but in the opposite direction. Slight changes in leg length are probably insignificant. With shortening of ½ inch or more, there is a tendency for the pelvis to try and right the upper sacral surface. In the long leg, the ilium tends to move posterior or the short leg ilium moves anterior
  4. Standing forward bending of trunk—(standing flexion test)
    a. Note extent of cranial movement of the PSIS
      1. If one PSIS moves further cranially, a motion restriction is possibly present on that side of the inominates
      2. If the PSISs move at different times, the side that moves first is usually the side with restriction
  5. Lumbar spine active movements
    a. With sacroiliac dysfunction, the athlete will experience exacerbation of pain with side bending toward painful side
    b. Often a lumbar lesion is present along with sacroiliac dysfunction. Side bending toward sacroiliac joints will often aggravate this
  6. Single leg standing backward bending is a provocation test to produce pain from spondylolysis or spondylolisthesis
C. Sitting Position
  1. Sitting forward bending trunk test (sitting forward flexion test)
    a. Note extent of cranial movement of PSIS
      1. Involved PSIS moves more cranially
        a. Blocked joint moves solidly as one, while the sacrum on the painless side is free to move through its small range with the lumbar spine
  2. Rotation—Check lumbar spine
  3. Hip internal rotation
    a. Leg on the involved side may reproduce pain. This is thought to be a piriformis irritation pain and is reproduced as the muscle is stretched
    b. Range of motion
  4. Hip external rotation
    a. Range of motion
D. Supine Position
  1. Hip external rotation—piriformis contracture may cause exaggerated external rotation posture of involved hip.
  2. Palpation of symphysis pubis—for postural deviations and tenderness. Some sacroiliac joint problems create pain and tenderness in this area. Sometimes the presenting subjective symptoms mimic adductor or groin strain, but objective evaluation of muscle strength and tenderness are negative for strain of these groups
  3. Straight leg raising (SLR)
    a. Applies stress to sacroiliac joint—can indicate a unilateral torsional stress of the sacroiliac joint; however, could also be a coexisting lumbar problem
    b. Interpretation of SLR:
      1. 30 degrees—hip or very inflamed nerve
      2. 30 to 60 degrees—sciatic nerve involvement
      3. 70 to 90 degrees—sacroiliac joint
      4. Bilateral SLR—lumbar spine problem
      5. Neck flexion—exacerbates symptoms—disk or root irritation
      6. Ankle dorsiflexion or Lasègue sign—usually indicates sciatic nerve or root irritation
  4. Sacroiliac compression and distraction tests
    a. Tests useful in excluding joint irritability, hypermobility, and serious disease, usually negative unless classical pathology exists
  5. Patrick's test—flexion abduction external rotation (FABER)
    a. When pushed into extension may cause exacerbation of sacroiliac lesion—assess irritable motion
  6. Flexion adduction internal rotation (FADIR)—will give iliolumbar ligament stretch
  7. Bilateral knees to chest—will usually exacerbate lumbar spine symptoms as the sacroiliac joints move with the sacrum in this maneuver
  8. Single knee to chest—if pain is reported in the posterolateral thigh—indicates sacrotuberous irritation
  9. Single knee to opposite shoulder—if pain is reported in the PSIS area, this indicates sacroiliac ligament irritation
E. Sidelying—Each Side
  1. Anterior and posterior pelvic tilt—pain on movement indicates irritation of sacroiliac joint. Also gives direction of movement clues used in treatment
  2. Iliotibial band length—long standing sacroiliac joint problems sometimes create tightness of iliotibial band
F. Prone position
  1. Palpation

Continued.

LUMBAR AND SACROILIAC JOINT OBJECTIVE EXAMINATION—cont'd

a. Tenderness medial to or around PSIS that is well localized indicates sacroiliac problem

b. Gluteus maximus area—Sacrotuberous and sacrospinous ligaments are in this area, as well as piriformis and sciatic nerve. Changes in tension, tenderness, and springiness can occur from positional changes of ilium

c. Tenderness or alignment changes from S1 to T10 interspaces indicates lumbar problems

d. Anteroposterior or rotational stresses to lumbar spinous processes

e. Sacral provocation tests

  1. Do this series of tests only when applicable: If unable to reproduce signs and symptoms by now do not do if by previous tests the joint has been found to be hypermobile

    a. Anteroposterior pressure of sacrum at center of its base

    b. Anteroposterior pressure of sacrum on each side of sacrum just medial to PSIS

  2. Hip extension knee flexion stretch will provoke the L-3 nerve root. Pain similar to nerve pain down the anterolateral thigh would be a positive finding

G. Manual muscle test—if the lumbar spine or posterior hip muscle is strained, active movement against gravity or resistance should provoke the complaints of similar pain to pain under evaluation.

  1. Hip extension—isometric and isotonic

  2. Hip internal rotation

  3. Hip external rotation

  4. Arm and shoulder extension

  5. Arm, shoulder, and neck extension

  6. Resisted trunk extension

---

agement to specific rehabilitation should be a primary goal of the acute stage of the rehabilitation plan.

The most common treatment for pain relief in the acute stage is to use ice for analgesia. Rest, but not total bed rest, is used to allow the injured tissues to begin the healing process without the stresses that created the injury.[9] Along with rest, the athlete should be taught to increase comfort with favorable body positioning. They should also be taught to avoid positions and movements that increase any sharp, painful episodes. The limits of these movements and positions that provide comfort should be the initial focus of any exercises. Outside support, in the form of corsets and the use of props or pillows to enhance comfortable positions, also needs to be included in the initial pain management phase of treatment.[27,38]

POSITIONING AND PAIN RELIEVING EXERCISES

Most athletes with back pain have some fluctuation of their symptoms in response to certain postures and activities. The sports therapist logically treats this athlete by reinforcing pain reducing postures and motions and by starting specific exercises aimed at specific muscle groups or specific ranges of motion. A general rule to follow in making these decisions is as follows: any movement that causes the back pain to radiate or spread over a larger area should not be included during this phase of treatment. Movements that centralize or diminish the pain are correct movements to include at this time.[3,24]

Including some exercise in the initial pain management phase generally has a positive effect on the athlete. The exercise encourages them to be active in the rehabilitation plan and helps them to regain lumbar movement.[14,38]

When a patient relieves his pain through exercise and attention to proper postural control, he is much more likely to adopt these procedures into his daily routine. A patient who has his pain relieved via some other passive procedure, and then taught exercises will not be able to readily see the connection between relief and exercise.[3]

The types of exercises that may be included in the initial pain management phase include the following:

1. Lateral shift corrections
2. Extension exercises
3. Flexion exercises
4. Mobilization exercises
5. Myofascial stretching exercises

Lateral shift corrections and extension exercises

Lateral shift corrections and extension exercises should be discussed together because the indications for use are similar, and extension exercises will immediately follow the lateral shift corrections.

The indications for the use of lateral shift corrections are as follows:

1. Subjectively, the athlete complains of unilateral pain reference in the lumbar or hip area.

Keep hands high on iliac crest so you don't pull on sacral area.

2. The typical posture is scoliotic with a hip shift and reduced lumbar lordosis.
3. Walking and movements are very guarded and robotic.
4. Forward bending is extremely limited and increases the pain.
5. Backward bending is limited.
6. Side bending toward the painful side is minimal to impossible.
7. Side bending away from the painful side is usually reasonable to normal.
8. A test correction of the hip shift either reduces the pain or causes the pain to centralize.
9. The neurological examination may or may not elicit the following positive findings:
   a. Straight leg raising may be limited and painful, or it could be unaffected.
   b. Sensation may be dull, anesthetic, or unaffected.
   c. Manual muscle test may indicate unilateral weakness of specific movements, or the movements may be strong and painless.
   d. Reflexes may be diminished or unaffected.[3,24]

The athlete will be assisted by the sports therapist with the initial lateral shift correction. The athlete is then instructed in the techniques of self-correction. The lateral shift correction is designed to guide the athlete back to a more symmetrical posture. The sports therapist's pressure should be firm and steady and more guiding than forcing. The use of a mirror to provide visual feedback is recommended for both the therapist-assisted and self-corrected maneuvers. The specific technique guide for sports therapist-assisted lateral shift correction is as follows (Figure 18-1):

1. Preset the athlete by explaining the correction maneuver and the roles of the athlete and the sports therapist.
   a. The athlete is to keep the shoulders level and avoid the urge to side bend.
   b. The athlete should allow the hips to move under the trunk and should not resist the pressure from the sports therapist but allow the hips to shift with the pressure.
   c. The athlete should keep the sports therapist informed about the behavior of their back pain.
   d. The athlete should keep their feet stationary and not move after the hip shift correction until the standing extension part of the correction is completed.

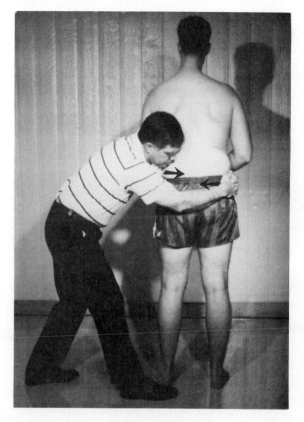

Fig. 18-1. Lateral shift correction position with assistance from the sports therapist.

   e. They should practice the standing extension exercise as part of this initial explanation.
2. The sports therapist should stand on the athlete's side that is opposite their hip shift. The athlete's feet should be a comfortable distance apart, and the sports therapist should have a comfortable stride stance aligned slightly behind the athlete.
3. Padding should be placed around the athlete's elbow, on the side next to the sports therapist, to provide comfortable contact between the athlete and the sports therapist.
4. The sports therapist should contact the athlete's elbow with their shoulder and chest with their head aligned along the athlete's back. Their arms should reach around the athlete's waist and apply pressure between the iliac crest and the greater trochanter.
5. The sports therapist should gradually pull the athlete's hips toward him or her. If the pain

increases, the sports therapist should ease the pressure and maintain a more comfortable posture for 10 to 20 seconds, then again pull gently. If the pain increases again, the sports therapist should again lessen the pull and allow comfort, then instruct the athlete to actively extend gently, pushing their back into and matching the resistance supplied by the therapist. The goal for this maneuver is an overcorrection of the scoliosis, reversing its direction.

6. Once the corrected or overcorrected posture is achieved, the sports therapist should maintain this posture for 1 to 2 minutes. This procedure may take 2 to 3 minutes to complete, and the first attempt may be less than a total success. Repeated efforts 3 to 4 minutes apart should be attempted during the first treatment effort before the sports therapist stops the treatment for that episode.

7. The sports therapist gradually releases pressure on the hip while the athlete does a standing extension movement. The athlete should complete approximately six repetitions of the standing extension movement, holding each 15 to 20 seconds.

8. Once the athlete moves their feet and walks even a short distance, the lateral hip shift usually will reoccur, but to a lesser degree. The athlete then should be taught the self-correction maneuver. The athlete should stand in front of a mirror and place one hand on the hip where the sports therapist's hands were and the other hand on the lower ribs where the therapist's shoulder was.

9. The athlete then pushes their hip under their trunk, watching the mirror to keep their shoulders level and trying to achieve a corrected or overcorrected posture. They should hold this posture for 30 to 45 seconds and then follow with several standing extension movements as described in step 7.[3,24]

Extension exercise

The indications for the use of extension exercise are as follows:

1. Subjectively, back pain is diminished with lying down and increased with sitting. The location of the pain may be unilateral, bilateral, or central, and there may or may not be radiating pain into either or both legs.

2. Forward bending is extremely limited and increases the pain, or the pain reference location enlarges as the athlete bends forward.

3. Backward bending can be limited, but the movement centralizes or diminishes the pain.

4. The neurological examination is the same as outlined for lateral shift correction.[3,25]

The efficacy of extension exercise is theorized to be from one or a combination of the following effects:

1. A reduction in the neural tension.

2. A reduction of the load on the disk, which in turn decreases disk pressure.

3. Increases in the strength and endurance of the extensor muscles.

4. Proprioceptive interference with pain perception as the exercises allow self-mobilization of the spinal joints.

Hip shift posture has previously been theoretically correlated to the anatomical location of the disk bulge or nucleus pulposus herniation. Creating a centralizing movement of the nucleus pulposus has been the theoretical emphasis of hip shift correction and extension exercise. This theory has good logic, but research on this phenomenon has not been supportive.[26] However, in explaining the exercises to the athlete, the use of this theory may help increase the athlete's motivation and compliance with the exercise plan.

End-range hyperextension exercise should be used cautiously when the athlete has facet joint degeneration or impingement of the vertebral foramen borders on neural structures. Also, spondylolysis and spondylolithesis problems should be approached cautiously with any end-range movement exercise using either flexion or hyperextension.

The following exercises are included as extension exercises. This list is not exhaustive but is representative of most of the exercises used clinically:

1. Prone on elbows (Figure 18-2)
2. Prone on hands (Figure 18-3)
3. Alternate arm and leg (Figure 18-4)
4. Standing extension (Figure 18-5)
5. Supine hip extension—butt lift or bridge (Figure 18-6)
   a. Double leg support
   b. Single leg support
6. Prone single leg hip extension (Figure 18-7)
   a. Knee flexed
   b. Knee extended
7. Prone double leg hip extension (Figure 18-8)
   a. Knees flexed

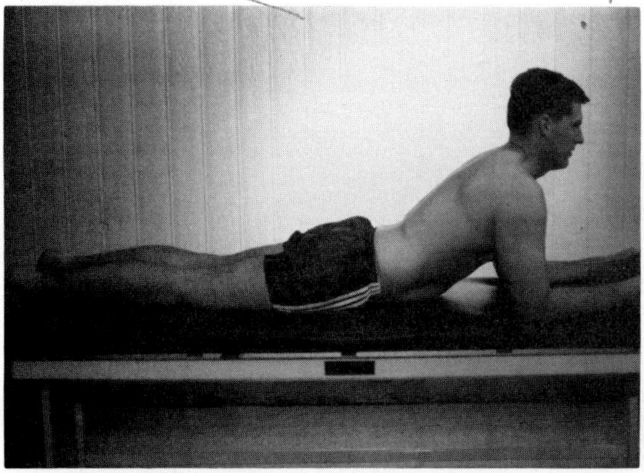

Fig. 18-2. Prone extension on elbows.

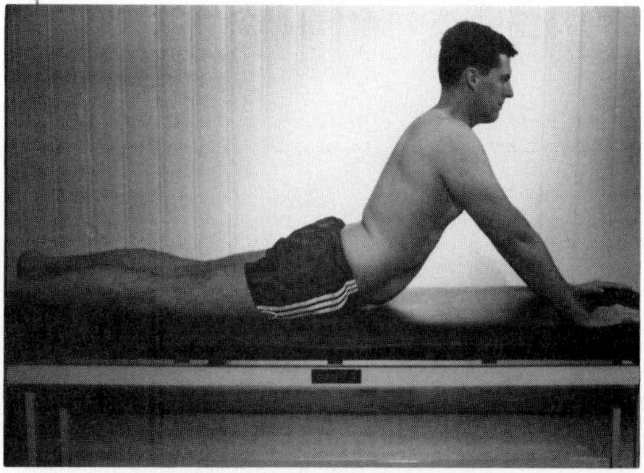

Fig. 18-3. Prone extension on hands.

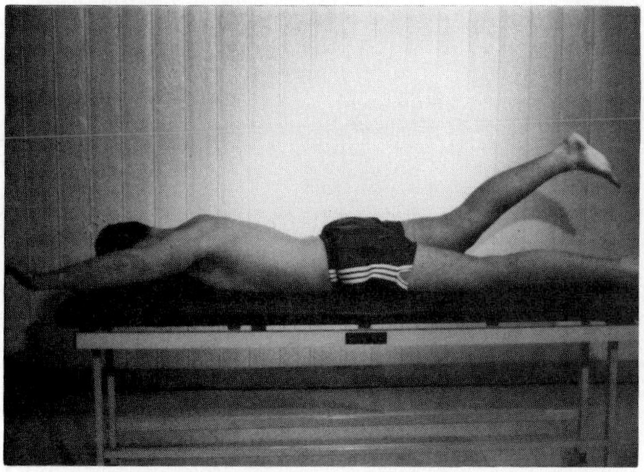

Fig. 18-4. Alternating arm and leg extension.

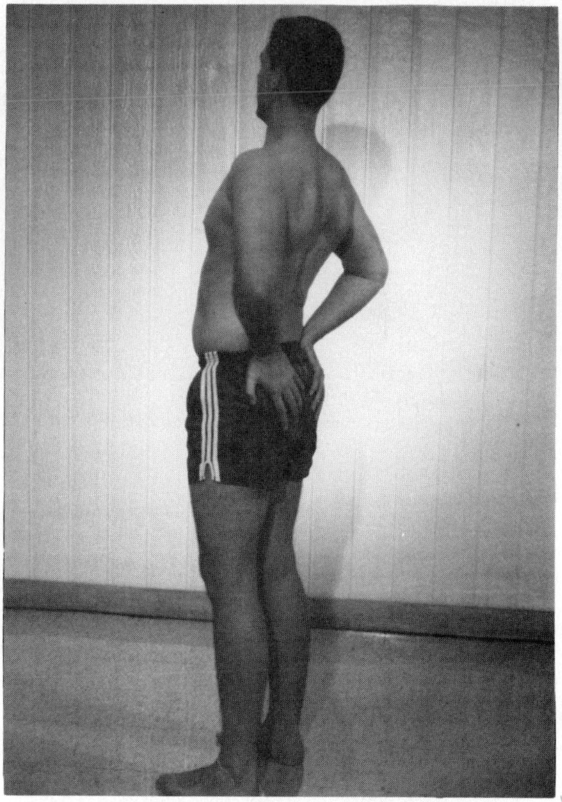

Fig. 18-5. Standing extension.

   b. Knees extended
8. Trunk extension—prone (Figure 18-9)
   a. Hands near head
   b. Arms extended—superman position

The order in which exercises are presented is not significant. Instead, each sports therapist should base the starting exercises on the evaluative findings. Jackson, in a review of back exercise, stated "... no support was found for the use of a preprogrammed flexion regimen that includes exercises of little value or potential harm and is not specific to the current needs of the patient, as determined by a thorough back evaluation." The review also included a report of Ken-

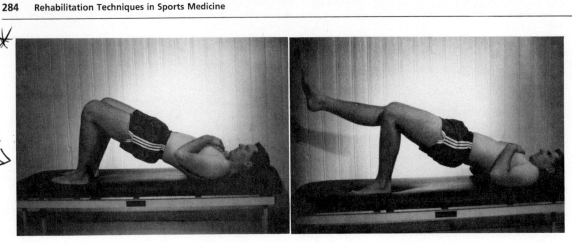

Fig. 18-6. Supine hip extension. A, Double leg support. **B,** Single leg support.

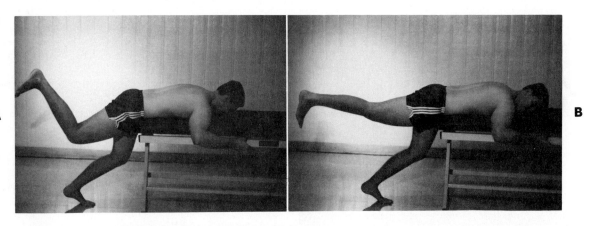

Fig. 18-7. Prone single leg hip extension. A, Knee flexed. **B,** Knee extended.

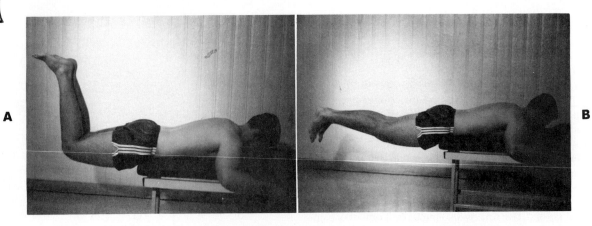

Fig. 18-8. Prone double leg hip extension. A, Knee flexed. **B,** Knee extended.

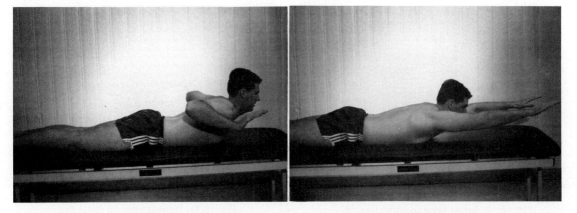

Fig. 18-9. Trunk extension. A, Hands near head. **B,** Superman position.

dall and Jenkins' study, which stated that one third of the patients for whom hyperextension exercises had been prescribed worsened.[17]

Flexion exercises

The indications for the use of flexion exercises are as follows:

1. Subjectively, back pain is diminished with sitting and increased with lying down or standing. Pain is also increased with walking.
2. Repeated or sustained forward bending eases the pain.
3. The athlete's lordotic curve does not reverse as they forward bend.
4. The end range of or sustained backward bending is painful or increases the pain.
5. Abdominal tone and strength are poor.

In his approach, Saal elaborates on the thought that, "No one should continue with one particular type of exercise regimen during the entire treatment program."[27] We concur with these thoughts and believe starting with one type of exercise should not preclude rapidly adding other exercises as the athlete's pain resolves and other movements become more comfortable.

The efficacy of flexion exercise is theorized to be from one or a combination of the following effects:

1. A reduction in the articular stresses on the facet joints.
2. Stretching to the dorsolumbar fascia and musculature.
3. Opening of the intervertebral foramen.
4. Relief of the stenosis of the spinal canal.
5. Improvement of the stabilizing effect of the abdominal musculature.

6. Increasing the intraabdominal pressure because of increased abdominal muscle strength and tone.
7. Proprioceptive interference with pain perception as the exercises allow self-mobilization of the spinal joints.[17]

Flexion exercises should be used cautiously or avoided in most cases of acute disk prolapse and when a laterally shifted posture is present. In patients recovering from disk related back pain, flexion exercise should not be commenced immediately after a flat lying rest interval longer than 30 minutes. The disk can become more hydrated in this amount of time, and the athlete would be more susceptible to pain with postures that increase disk pressures. Other less stressful exercises should be initiated first and flexion exercise done later in the exercise program.[3,25]

The following exercises are included as flexion exercises. Again this list is not exhaustive but is representative of the exercises used clinically.

1. Single knee to chest (Figure 18-10)
   a. Stretch holding 15 to 20 seconds
   b. Same as step 2
2. Double knee to chest (Figure 18-11)
   a. Stretching—holding posture 15 to 20 seconds
   b. Mobilizing—using a rhythmic rocking motion within a pain-free range of motion
3. Posterior pelvic tilt (Figure 18-12)
4. Partial sit-up (Figure 18-13)
5. Rotation partial sit-up (Figure 18-14)
6. Slump sit stretch position (Figure 18-15)
7. Flat footed squat stretch (Figure 18-16)
8. Hamstring stretch (Figure 18-17)
9. Hip flexor stretch (Figure 18-18)

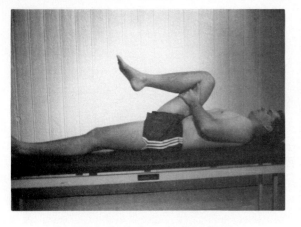

Fig. 18-10. Single knee to chest flexion.

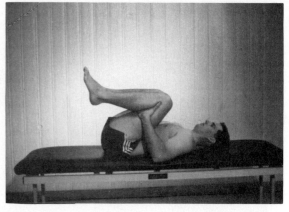

Fig. 18-11. Double knee to chest flexion.

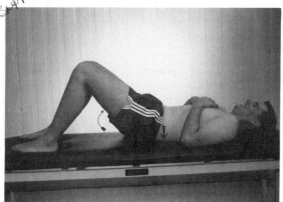

Fig. 18-12. Posterior pelvic tilt.

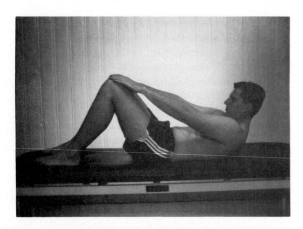

Fig. 18-13. Partial sit-up.

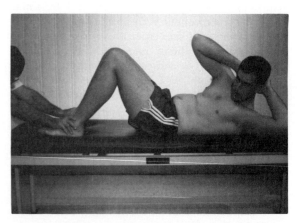

Fig. 18-14. Partial sit-up with rotation.

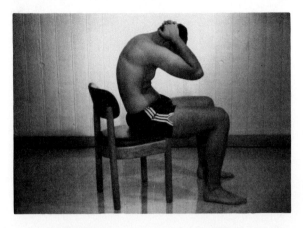

Fig. 18-15. Slump sit stretch position.

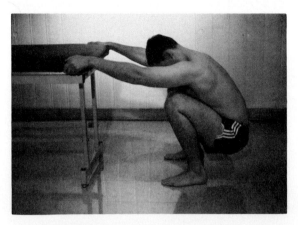

Fig. 18-16. Flat-footed squat stretch.

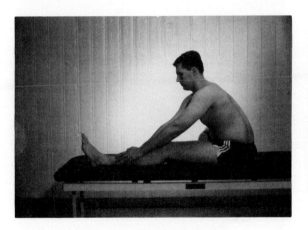

Fig. 18-17. Hamstring stretch.

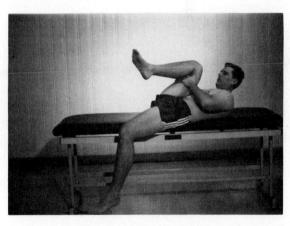

Fig. 18-18. Hip flexor stretch.

Joint mobilization

The indications for the use of a joint mobilizing exercise are as follows:

1. Subjectively, the athlete's pain is centered around a specific joint area and increases with activity and decreases with rest.
2. The accessory motion available at individual spinal segments is diminished.
3. Passive range of motion is diminished.
4. Active range of motion is diminished.
5. There may be muscular tightness or increased fascial tension in the area of the pain.
6. Back movements are asymmetrical when comparing right and left rotation or sidebending.
7. Forward and backward bending may steer away from the midline.

The efficacy of mobilization is theorized to be from one or a combination of the following effects:

1. Tight structures can be stretched to increase the range of motion.
2. The joint involved is stimulated by the movement to more normal mechanics, and irritation is reduced because of better nutrient waste exchange.
3. Proprioceptive interference occurs with pain perception as the joint movement stimulates normal neural firing whose perception supercedes nocioceptive perception.

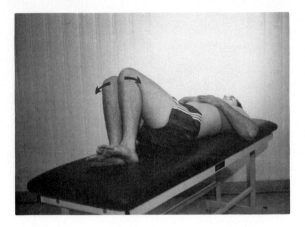

Fig. 18-19. Knee rocking side-to-side self-mobilization.

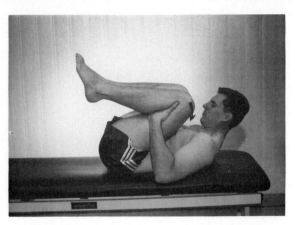

Fig. 18-20. Knees toward chest rocking self-mobilization.

Mobilization treatment is very multidimensional and is easily adapted to any back pain problem. The mobilizations can be active or passive or assisted by the sports therapist. All ranges (flexion, extension, sidebending, rotation, and accessory) can be incorporated within the exercise plan. The mobilizations can be carried out according to Maitland's grades of oscillation as discussed in Chapter 10. The magnitude of the forces applied can range from grade 1 to grade 4 depending on levels of pain. Because of the great variety in the motions mentioned above, we will limit our list to self-mobilization exercises. The theory, technique, and application of the sports therapist-assisted mobilizations are best gained through guided study with an expert practitioner.[21]

The following exercises are included as self mobilization exercises:

1. Knee rocking side to side (Figure 18-19)
2. Knees toward chest rock (Figure 18-20)
3. Supine hip lift-bridge-rock (Figure 18-21)
4. Pelvic tilt or pelvic rock butt out-tail tuck (Figure 18-22)
5. Kneeling—dog tail wags (Figure 18-23)
6. Sitting or standing rotation (Figure 18-24)
7. Sitting or standing side bending (Figure 18-25)
8. Standing hip shift side to side (Figure 18-26)
9. Standing pelvic rock butt out-tail tuck (Figure 18-27)
10. Various sidelying and backlying positions to both stretch and mobilize specific joint areas (Figure 18-28)

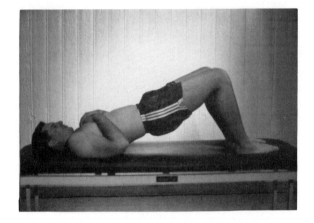

Fig. 18-21. Supine hip lift.

Myofascial stretching

The indications for treating low back pain with myofascial stretching and treatment techniques are as follows:

1. Subjectively, in athletes, early season muscle soreness and fatigue from repetitive motions are common antecedent mechanisms. Athletes are also susceptible later in their season as fatigue and stress overload specific muscle groups. There may be a history of sudden onset during or shortly after an acute overload stress, or there may be a gradual onset with repetitive or postural overload of the affected muscle. The pain may be an incapacitating event in

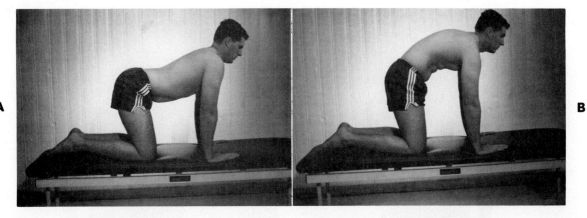

A   B

Fig. 18-22. Pelvic tilt or pelvic rock. **A,** Butt out (horse position). **B,** Tail tuck (cat position).

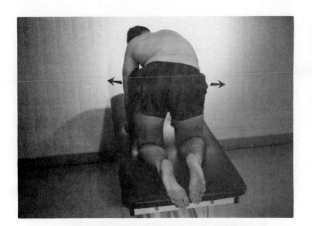

Fig. 18-23. Kneeling dog tail wags.

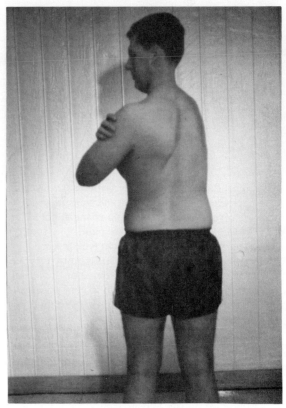

Fig. 18-24. Standing rotation.

the case of acute onset, but it may also be a nagging, aggravating type of pain with an intensity that varies from an awareness of discomfort to a severe unrelenting type of pain. The pain location is usually a referred pain area, and the actual myofascial trigger point is often remote to the pain area. These trigger points can be present but quiescent until they are activated by overload, fatigue, trauma, or chilling. These points are called *latent trigger points.* This deep, aching pain can be specifically localized, but the athlete is not sensitive to palpation in these areas. This pain can often be

*To decrease compression of discs you can have patient lay on their sides and bring both legs up.

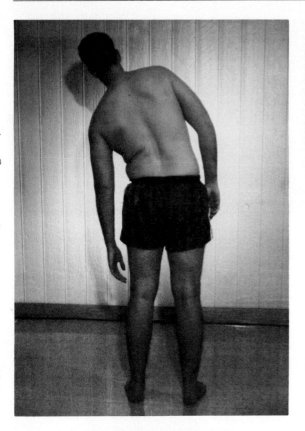

Fig. 18-25. Standing side bending.

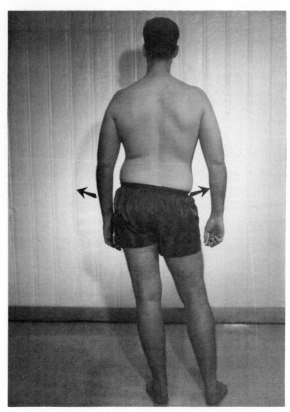

Fig. 18-26. Standing hip shift side-to-side.

reproduced by maintaining pressure on a hypersensitive myofascial trigger point.

2. Passive or active stretching of the affected myofascial structure increases pain.

3. The stretch range of muscle is restricted.

4. The pain is increased when the muscle is contracted against a fixed resistance or the muscle is allowed to contract into a very shortened range. The pain in this case is described as a muscle cramping pain.

5. The muscle may be slightly weak.

6. Trigger points may be located within a taut band of the muscle. If taut bands are found during palpation, explore them for local hypersensitive areas.

7. Pressure on the hypersensitive area will often cause a "jump sign"; as the sports therapist strums the sensitive area, the athlete's muscle involuntarily jumps in response.

8. 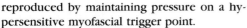The primary muscle groups that create low back pain in athletes are the quadratus lumborum and the piriformis muscles.[18,31,34,35]

Travell and Simons have devoted two volumes to the causes and treatment of various myofascial pains.[34,35] They have done a very thorough job of describing the symptoms and signs of each area of the body, and they give very specific guidance on exercises and positioning in their treatment protocols.

GENERAL RECOMMENDATIONS FOR STAGE I (ACUTE STAGE) TREATMENT

The athlete should be encouraged to move through this stage quickly and return to practice and play as soon as range, strength, and comfort will allow. The addition of a supportive corset for practice and play during this stage should be based mostly on the comfort of the athlete. We suggest using an eclectic approach to the selection of the exercises, mixing the

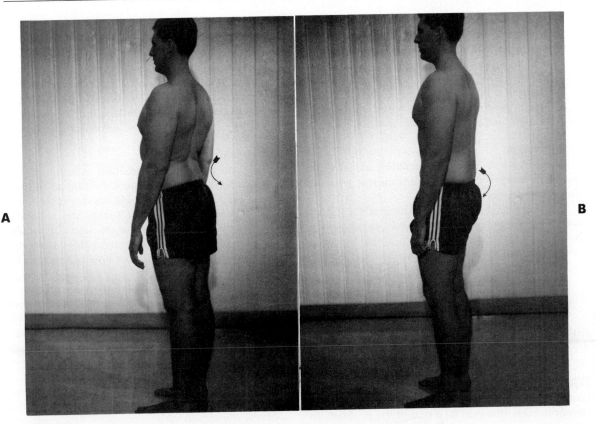

A   **B**

Fig. 18-27. Standing pelvic rock. A, Butt out. **B,** Tail tuck.

various protocols described according to the findings of the athlete's evaluation. Rarely will an athlete present with classic signs and symptoms that will dictate using one variety of exercise.

Stage II (Reinjury Stage) Treatment

In the reinjury or chronic stage of back rehabilitation, the goals of the treatment and training should again be based on a thorough evaluation of the athlete. Identifying the causes of the athlete's back problem and reoccurrences is very important in the management of their rehabilitation and prevention of reinjury. A goal for this stage of care is to make the athlete responsible for the management of their back problem. The sports therapist should identify specific problems and corrections that will help the athlete better understand the mechanisms and management of their problem.[27]

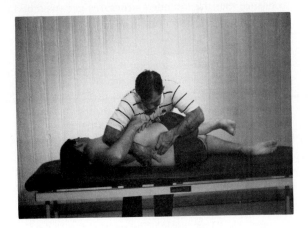

Fig. 18-28. Sidelying stretch. Sidelying position may be used to stretch specific joints.

Specific goals and exercises should be identified about the following:

1. Which structures to stretch
2. Which structures to strengthen
3. Incorporating dynamic stabilization into the athlete's daily life and exercise routine
4. Which movements need a motor learning approach to control faulty mechanics [27]

STRETCHING

Chapters 3 and 4 detail the stretching and strengthening exercises available for each muscle group of the trunk and hip.

In the sports therapist's evaluation of the athlete with back pain, the following muscle groups should be assessed for flexibility:

1. Hip flexors
2. Hamstrings
3. Low back extensors
4. Lumbar rotators
5. Lumbar lateral flexors
6. Hip adductors
7. Hip abductors
8. Hip rotators[10]

The sports therapist and the athlete need to plan specific exercises to stretch restricted groups, maintain flexibility in normal muscle groups, and identify hypermobility that may be a part of the problem. In planning, instructing, and monitoring each exercise, adequate thought and good instruction must be used to ensure that the intended structures get stretched and areas of hypermobility are protected from overstretching.[10,16]

Inadequate stabilization will lead to exercise movements that are so general that the exercise will encourage hyperflexibility at already hypermobile areas. Lack of proper stabilization during stretching may help perpetuate a structural problem that will continue to add to the athlete's back pain.

STRENGTHENING

There are numerous methods for strengthening the muscles of the trunk and hip. Muscles are perhaps best strengthened by using techniques of progressive overload to achieve specific adaptation to imposed demands (SAID principle). The overload can take the form of increased weight load, increased repetition load, or increased stretch load to accomplish physiological changes in muscle strength, muscle endurance, or flexibility of a body part.[10]

The treatment plan should call for an exercise that the athlete can easily accomplish successfully. Rapidly but gradually, the overload should push the athlete to challenge the muscle group needing strengthening. The sports therapist and the athlete should monitor continuously for increases in the athlete's pain or reoccurrences of previous symptoms. If those changes occur, the exercises should be modified, delayed, or eliminated from the rehabilitation plan.[17,27]

DYNAMIC STABILIZATION

Dynamic muscular stabilization, dynamic abdominal bracing, and finding neutral position all describe a technique used to increase the stability of the trunk. This increased stability will enable the athlete to maintain the spine and pelvis in the most comfortable and acceptable mechanical position that will control the forces of repetitive microtrauma and protect the structures of the back from further damage. Abdominal muscular control is one key to giving the athlete the ability to stabilize their trunk and control their posture. Abdominal strengthening routines are rigorous, and the athlete must complete them with vigor. However, in their functional activities, the athlete does not take advantage of abdominal strength to stabilize the trunk and protect the back.[16,22,29]

Kennedy's dynamic abdominal bracing exercises focus attention on the motor control of the external oblique muscles in various positions. Once this control is established, different positions and movements are added.[22] Saal describes this type of exercise as finding and maintaining the neutral position with muscle fusion. He specifically singles out the external oblique muscles as a major factor but describes a co-contraction of the abdominal and lumbar extensors, including the gluteus maximus, to maintain a corseting action on the lumbar spine. Adequate flexibility of hip muscles and other structures is also necessary to accomplish this muscle fusion concept.[27] The concept of increasing trunk stability with muscle contractions that support and limit the extremes of spinal movement is important, regardless of whether muscle fusion or dynamic abdominal bracing are the terms used to describe this action.

BASIC FUNCTIONAL TRAINING

Since strength and flexibility are not enough, the athlete must be committed to improving body mechanics and trunk control in all postures in both sport-related activities and in their activities of daily living. The sports therapist needs to evaluate the athlete's daily patterns and give them instruction, practice, and monitoring on the best and least stressful body mechanics for them in as many activities as possible.

The basic program follows the developmental sequence of posture control, starting with supine and prone extremity movement while actively stabilizing the trunk. The athlete is then progressed to all fours, kneeling, and standing. Emphasis on trunk control and stability is maintained as the athlete works through this exercise sequence.[16,23,27]

The most critical aspect for developing motor control is repetition of exercise. However, variability in positioning, speed of movement, and changes in movement patterns must also be incorporated. The variability of the exercise will allow the athlete to generalize their newly learned trunk control to the constant changes necessary in their sport. The basic exercise, including a trunk stabilizing contraction, is the key. Incorporating this stabilization contraction into various activities helps reinforce trunk stabilization and makes trunk control a subconscious automatic response.

The use of augmented feedback (EMG, palpation) of the trunk stabilizing contraction may be needed early in the exercise plan to help maximize the results of this exercise. The sports therapist should have the athlete internalize this feedback as quickly as possible to make the athlete apparatus-free and more functional. With augmented feedback, it is recommended that the patient be rapidly and progressively weaned from dependency on external feedback.

ADVANCED FUNCTIONAL TRAINING

Each activity that the athlete is involved in becomes part of the advanced exercise rehabilitation plan. The usual place to start is with the athlete's strength and conditioning program. Each step of the program is monitored and emphasis is placed on trunk stabilization for even the simple task of putting the weights on a bar or getting on and off of exercise equipment. Each exercise in their strength and conditioning program should be retaught, and the athlete is made aware of their best mechanical position and the proper stabilizing muscular contraction. The strength program is sport and athlete specific, attempting to strengthen weak areas and improve strength in muscle groups needed for better sports performance.[27]

Aerobic activities are also included in advanced programs. The same emphasis on technique and stabilization is used as the athlete begins aerobic conditioning activities. A functional progression should be used so that changes in symptoms can be controlled by working with lower-level exercises and then progressing to more difficult and stressful exercises.[27] Modification of normal aerobic conditioning for a particular sport may be an important part of eliminating some of the unnecessary stress from the athlete's overall program. Substituting an aquatic conditioning program for sprinting and running may keep the athlete participating effectively without increasing their back pain.

Using exercises designed to incorporate trunk control into specific skills is the next step in the exercise progression. Sport-specific skills should be tailored to the individual athlete. The sports therapist should work in concert with the coach and athlete to incorporate stabilization training with sports drills and postures. The sports therapist may not know the intricacies of pass blocking, but they can help coach and athlete identify good alignment and stabilization as the athlete performs each drill.[27]

The athlete should be taught to start their stabilizaton contraction before starting any movement. This presets the athlete's posture and stabilization awareness before their movement takes place. As the movement occurs, they will become less aware of the stabilization contraction as they attempt to accomplish the drill.

They may revert to old postures and habits, so feedback is important. The next step is to incorporate a firmer stabilization contraction during the power phase of the drill. The athlete is instructed to contract more firmly during initiation of a jump or push during change in direction. The drills should be constructed to have several changes in contraction strength planned as the athlete moves through the drill. Expect that the athlete may experience paralysis by analysis as they try to think through stabilizing contraction plus drill execution. Adequate practice time will be necessary before the athlete is ready to reenter a team practice. The athlete should find this stabilization control comfortable, efficient, and powerful.

Remember each athlete is different not only with their individual back problem but also with their abilities to gain motor skill. Each athlete will have differences in degree of control and in the speed at which they acquire these new skills of trunk stabilization.

Reducing stress to the back by using braces, orthotics, shoes, or comfortable supportive furniture (beds, desks, or chairs) is essential to help the athlete minimize chronic or overload stresses to their back. The stabilization exercise should be incorporated into their activities of daily living and sports activities.[30]

For most low back problems the stage I treatment and exercise programs will get the athlete back into their activities quickly. If the pain or dysfunction is pronounced or the problem becomes recurrent, an in-depth evaluation and treatment using stage I and stage II exercise protocols will be necessary. The team approach with athlete, doctor, sports therapist, and coach working together will provide the comprehensive approach needed to manage the athlete's back problem. Close attention to and emphasis on the athlete's progress will provide both the athlete and the sports therapist with the encouragement to continue this program.

REHABILITATION AND TREATMENT TECHNIQUES FOR SPECIFIC LOW BACK CONDITIONS

The following examples are included to illustrate the evaluation findings and the treatment techniques used for the more common low back problems found in the athletic population.

Muscular Strains

Evaluative findings include a history of sudden or chronic stress that initiates pain in a muscular area during the workout. There are three points on the physical examination that must be positive to indicate the muscle as the primary problem. There will be tenderness to palpation in the muscular area. The muscular pain will be provoked with contraction and with stretch of the involved muscle.

The treatment should include the standard protection, ice and compression. Ice may be applied in the form of ice massage or ice bags depending on the area involved. An elastic wrap or corset would protect and compress the back musculature. Additional modalities would include pulsed ultrasound as a biostimulative and electrical stimulation for pain relief and muscle reeducation. The exercises used in rehabilitation should make the involved muscle contract and stretch, starting with very mild exercise and progressively increasing the intensity and repetition loads. In general this would include active extension exercises such as hip lifts, alternate arm and leg, hip extension, trunk extension, and quadratus hip shift

exercises. A good series of abdominal strengthening and stabilization exercise would also be helpful. Stretching exercises might include the following: knee to chest, side lying leg hang, slump sitting, and knee rocking side to side.

When the athlete can perform functional activities on the same level as teammates, he or she may return to practice and competition. Initially, the athlete may wish to continue to use a brace or corset, but they should be encouraged to do away with the corset as their back strengthens and their performance returns to normal.[10,17]

Piriformis Muscle Myofascial Pain or Strain

The piriformis muscle refers pain to the posterior sacroiliac region, to the buttocks, and sometimes down the posterior or posterolateral thigh. The pain is usually described as a deep ache that can get more intense with exercise and with sitting with the hips flexed, adducted, and medially rotated. The pain gets sharper and more intense with activities that require decelerating medial hip and leg rotation during weight bearing.

Tenderness to palpation has a characteristic pattern with tenderness medial and proximal to the greater trochanter and just lateral to the posterosuperior iliac spine. Isometric abduction in the sitting position produces pain in the posterior hip buttock area, and the movement will be weak or hesitant. Passive hip internal rotation in the sitting position will also bring on posterior hip and buttock pain.

Rehabilitation exercises should include both strengthening and stretching. Examples of strengthening exercises are as follows:
1. Prone lying hip internal rotation with elastic resistance (Figure 18-29)
2. Hip lift bridges (Figure 18-30)
3. Hand knee position—fire hydrant exercise (Figure 18-31)
4. Sidelying hip abduction straight leg raises (Figure 18-32)
5. Prone hip extension exercise (Figure 18-33)
Examples of stretching exercise are as follows:
1. Long leg sitting with the involved hip and knee flexed and foot crossed over extended leg (Figure 18-34)
2. Backlying legs crossed hip adduction stretch (Figure 18-35)
3. Backlying with the involved leg crossed over the uninvolved leg, ankle to knee position, pull-

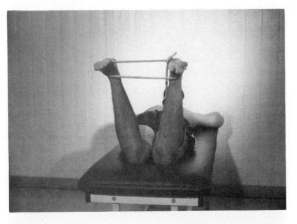

Fig. 18-29. Pronelying hip internal rotation with elastic resistance.

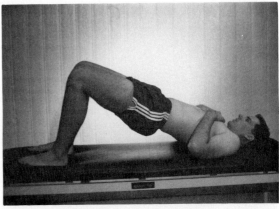

Fig. 18-30. Hip lift bridges.

Can flex knee & move front + back to get more muscles worked out. Do not arch back or roll forward.

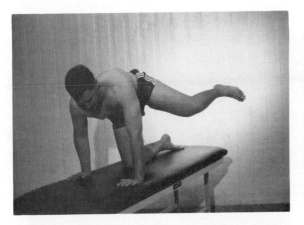

Fig. 18-31. Hand-knee position—fire hydrant exercise.

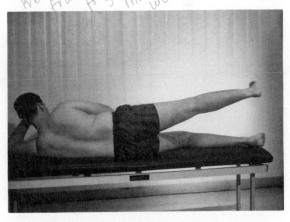

Fig. 18-32. Sidelying hip abduction straight leg raises.

If chip tilt will produce more tilt. Can use pillow on this.

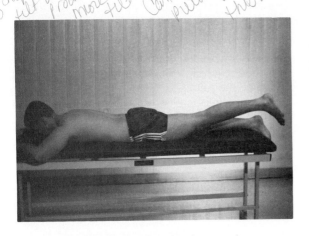

Fig. 18-33. Prone hip extension exercise.

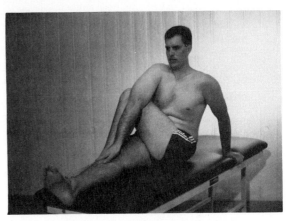

Fig. 18-34. Long leg sitting stretch.

older patients or other populations may not be able to get out of position

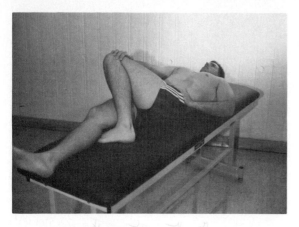

Fig. 18-35. Backlying legs crossed hip adduction stretch.

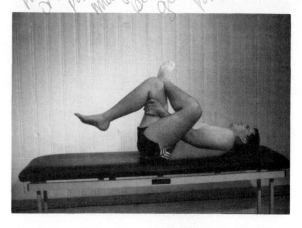

Fig. 18-36. Backlying legs crossed pulling uninvolved knee.

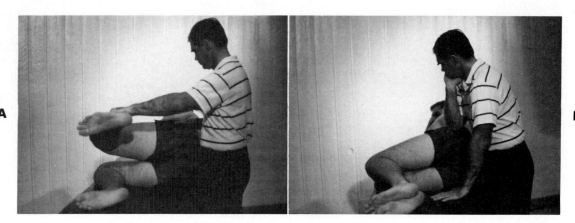

Fig. 18-37. Piriformis stretch using elbow pressure. **A,** Start-contract. **B,** Relaxation-stretch.

ing the uninvolved knee to the chest to create the stretch (Figure 18-36)
4. Contract-relax-stretch with elbow pressure to the muscle insertion during the relaxation phase (Figure 18-37)[18,31,34]

Quadratus Lumborum Myofascial Pain or Strain

Pain from the quadratus lumborum muscle is described as an aching, sharp pain located in the flank, lateral back area, and near the posterior sacroiliac region and upper buttocks. The athlete usually de-

scribes pain on moving from sitting to standing, standing for long periods, coughing, sneezing, and walking. Activities requiring trunk rotation or side bending aggravate the pain.

The muscle is tender to palpation near the origin along the lower ribs and along the insertion on the iliac crest. Pain will be aggravated on side bending, and the pain will usually be localized to one side. For example, with a right quadratus problem, side bending right and left would provoke only right sided pain. Supine hip hiking movements would also provoke the pain. Rehabilitation exercises should include both

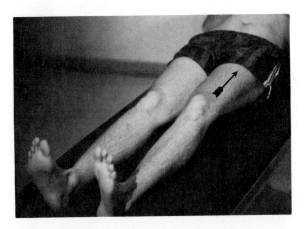

Fig. 18-38. Backlying—hip hike shifting.

strengthening and stretching. Examples of strengthening exercises are as follows:

1. Backlying—hip hike-shifting (Figure 18-38)
2. Standing with one leg on elevated surface and the other free to move below that level, hip hike the free side (Figure 18-39)
3. Backlying hip hike—resisted by pulling on the involved leg (Figure 18-40)

Examples of stretching exercises are as follows:

1. Sidelying over a pillow roll—leg hand stretch (Figure 18-41)
2. Supine self-stretch—legs crossed (Figure 18-42)
3. Hip hike exercise with hand pressure to increase stretch (Figure 18-43)
4. Standing one leg on a small book stretch (Figure 18-44)[34]

Treatment of Myofascial Pain and Trigger Points

The above examples of muscular oriented back pain could also have a myofascial origin. The major component in successfully changing myofascial pain is stretching the muscle back to a normal resting length. The muscle irritation and congestion that create the trigger points are relieved, and normal blood flow resumes, further reducing the irritants in the area. Stretching through a painful trigger point is difficult. A variety of comfort and counterirritant modalities can be used preliminary to, during, and after the stretching to enhance the effect of the exercise. Some of the methods used successfully are dry needling,

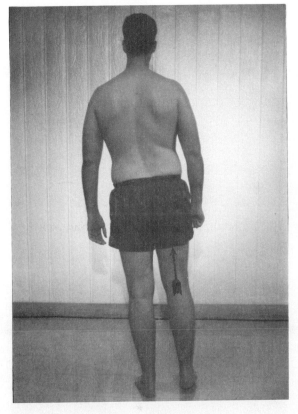

Fig. 18-39. Standing hip hike.

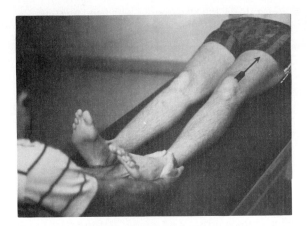

Fig. 18-40. Backlying—hip hike resisted.

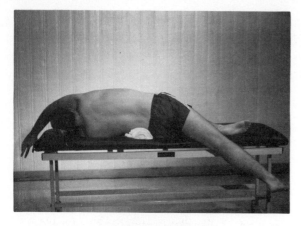

Fig. 18-41. Sidelying stretch over pillow roll.

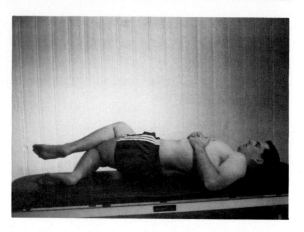

Fig. 18-42. Supine self-stretch—legs crossed.

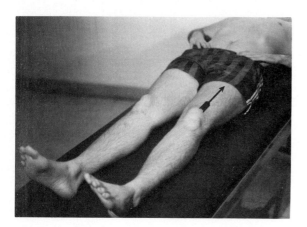

Fig. 18-43. Hip hike exercise with hand pressure.

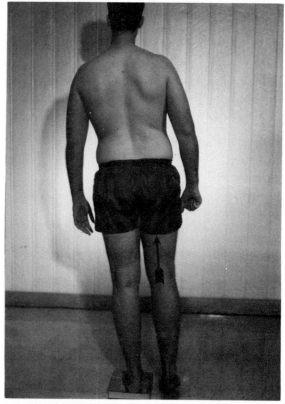

Fig. 18-44. Standing one leg up stretch.

local anesthetic injection, ice massage, friction massage, acupressure massage, ultrasound electrical stimulation, and cold sprays.

An example of a treatment plan is as follows:

1. Position the athlete comfortably but in a position that will lend itself to stretching the involved muscle group.
2. Caution the athlete to use mild progressive stretches rather than sudden, sharp, hard stretches.
3. Hot pack the area for 10 minutes, and follow with an ultrasound-electrical stimulation treatment over the affected muscle.

4. Use an ice cup, and use 2 to 3 slow strokes starting at the trigger point and moving in one direction toward their pain reference area and over the full length of the muscle.

5. Begin stretching well within the athlete's comfort. A stretch should be maintained a minimum of 15 seconds. The stretch should be released until the athlete is comfortable again. The next stretch repetition should then be progressively more intense if tolerated, and the position of the stretch should also be varied slightly. Repeat the stretch 4 to 6 times.

6. Hot pack the area, and have the athlete go through some active stretches of the muscle.

7. Refer to Travell and Simons' manual for specific references on other muscle groups.[18,34,35]

Lumbar Facet Joint Sprains

The athlete will report a sudden acute episode that caused the problem, or they will give a history of a chronic repetitive stress that caused the gradual onset of a pain that got progressively worse with continuing activity. The pain is local to the structure that has been injured, and the athlete can clearly localize the area. The pain is described as a sore pain that gets sharper in response to certain movements or postures. The pain is located centrally or just lateral to the spinous process areas and is deep.

Local symptoms will occur in response to movements, and the athlete will usually limit the movement in those ranges that are painful. When the vertebra is moved passively with a posteroanterior or rotational pressure through the spinous process the pain may be provoked. On palpation around the spinous process there will be local tenderness.

The treatment should include the standard protection, ice, and compression as mentioned previously. Both pulsed ultrasound and electrical stimulation could also be used similarly to the treatment of muscle strains but localized to the specific joint area.

The exercises used in the rehabilitation should involve joint mobilization to help reduce pain and increase joint nutrition. The athlete should be instructed in trunk stabilization exercises and in good postural control. Strengthening exercises for abdominals and back extensors should initially be limited to a pain-free range. Stretching in all ranges should start well within a comfort range and gradually increase until trunk movements reach normal ranges. Athletes should be supported with a corset or range limiting brace when they return to their competitive activity, which should be used only temporarily until normal strength, muscle control, and pain-free range are achieved.*

Hypermobility Syndromes (Spondylolysis/Spondylolisthesis)

The athlete usually has a relatively long history of feeling something go in their back. They complain of a low back pain described as a constant persistant ache across the back (belt type). This pain does not usually interfere with their workout performance but is usually worse when fatigued or after sitting in a slumped posture for an extended time. The athlete may also complain of a tired feeling in the low back. They describe the need to move frequently and get temporary relief of pain from self-manipulation. They often describe self-manipulative behavior more than 20 times a day. Their pain is relieved by rest, and they do not usually feel the pain during exercise. On physical examination, the athlete usually will have full and painless trunk movements, but there will be a wiggle or hesitation at the mid-range of forward bending. On backward bending their movement may appear to hinge at one spinal segment. When extremes of range are maintained for 15 to 30 seconds, the athlete feels a lumbosacral ache. On return from forward bending, the athlete will use thigh climbing to regain the neutral position. On palpation there may be tenderness localized to one spinal segment. Excessive movement may be noticed when applying posteroanterior pressure to the spinal segment. Athletes with this problem will fall into the reinjury stage of back pain and may require extensive treatment to regain stability of the trunk.

The athlete's pain should be treated symptomatically with the major focus for rehabilitation placed on exercises to strengthen, stabilize, and control the hypermobile segment. (See discussion of reinjury stage treatment.) The athlete should avoid manipulation and self-manipulation. Corsets and braces are beneficial if the athlete uses them only for support during higher-level activities and for short (1 to 2 hour) periods to help avoid fatigue.[16,27]

---

*References 10, 20, 21, 33, 36.

Disk Related Back Pain

The athlete will report a centrally located pain that radiates unilaterally or spreads across the back. They may describe a sudden or gradual onset after a workout that becomes particularly severe after they have rested and then tried to resume their activities. They may complain of tingling or numb feelings in a dermatomal pattern or sciatic radiation. Forward bending and sitting postures increase their pain. The athlete's symptoms are usually worse in the morning on first arising and get better through the day. Coughing and sneezing may increase their pain.

On physical examination, the athlete will have a hip shifted, forward bent posture. On active movements, side bending toward the hip shift is painful and limited. Side bending away from the shift is more mobile and does not provoke the pain. Forward bending is very limited and painful, and guarding is very apparent. On palpation there may be tenderness around the painful area. Posteroanterior pressure over the involved segment increases the pain. Passive straight leg raising will increase the back or leg pain during the first 30 degrees of hip flexion. Bilateral knee-to-chest movement will increase the back pain. Neurological testing (strength, sensory reflex) may be positive for differences between right and left.

The athlete should be treated with pain reducing modalities (ice, electrical stimulation) initially. The sports therapist should then use the lateral shift correction and extension exercise. This should be followed by self-correction instruction and gentle strengthening and mobilizing exercises. When pain and posture return to normal, abdominal and back extensor strengthening should be emphasized. This athlete may recover easily from the first episode, but if repeated episodes occur, then they should also start on the reinjury stage of back rehabilitation.*

Sacroiliac Joint Dysfunction

The athlete will relate a gradual onset of dull, achy back pain near or medial to the posterosuperior iliac spine (PSIS). The pain may radiate into the buttocks and posterolateral thigh. Athletic activities involving unilateral forceful movements, such as punting, hurdling, throwing, jumping, or trunk rotations with both feet fixed (swinging a club or bat), are the usual ac-

tivities associated with the onset of pain. There may also be a sudden onset usually associated with landing heavily on a single leg. The athlete may describe a heaviness or dullness or deadness in the leg or referred pain to the groin, adductor, or hamstring on the same side. Doing a hip flexion activity with the affected leg may increase the pain. The pain may be more noticeable during the stance phase of walking.

This problem is more common in females and younger, more flexible males. There may be a leg length difference, and the anterorsuperior iliac spine (ASIS) and PSIS are asymmetrical when compared to the opposite side.

On active movements in forward bending, there is a block to normal movement, and the PSIS on the affected side will move sooner than the normal side. Side bending toward the painful side will increase the pain. Straight leg raising will increase pain in the sacroiliac joint area after 45 degrees of motion. On palpation, there may be tenderness over the PSIS, medial to the PSIS, in the muscles of the buttocks, and anteriorly over the pubic symphysis. The back musculature will have increased tone on one side.

To treat this problem, the sports therapist should mobilize the sacroiliac joint to correct the postural asymmetry. This should be followed by a contract-relax stretch of the hip, again aimed at correcting the postural asymmetry. A bilateral hip lifting bridge exercise may be used to help stabilize the pelvis. Corsets or belts may also help to stabilize the pelvis during activities. Self-stretching to correct the postural asymmetry should also be taught to the athlete.*

SUMMARY

1. The low back pain that athletes most often experience is an acute, painful experience of relatively short duration that seldom causes significant time loss from practice or competition.
2. Regardless of the diagnosis or the specificity of the diagnosis, a thorough evaluation of the athlete's back pain is critical to good care.
3. Back rehabilitation may be classified as a two-stage approach. Stage I (acute stage) treatment consists mainly of the modality treatment and pain relieving exercises. Stage II treatment involves treating athletes with a reinjury or exacerbation of a previous problem.

*References 7, 10, 12, 14, 17, 29, 30, 32.

*References 4, 5, 11, 15, 39.

4. The types of exercises that may be included in the initial pain management phase include the following: lateral shift corrections, extension exercises, flexion exercises, mobilization exercises, and myofascial stretching exercises.

5. It is suggested that the sports therapist use an eclectic approach to the selection of exercises, mixing the various protocols described according to the findings of the athlete's evaluation.

6. Specific goals and exercises included in stage II should address which structures to stretch, which structures to strengthen, incorporating dynamic stabilization into the athlete's daily life and exercise routine, and which movements need a motor learning approach to control faulty mechanics.

7. The rehabilitation program should be based on functional training, which may be divided into basic and advanced phases.

8. Back pain can result from one or a combination of the following problems including muscle strain, piriformis muscle or quadratus lumborum myofascial pain or strain, myofascial trigger points, lumbar facet joint sprains, hypermobility syndromes, disk-related back problems, or sacroiliac joint dysfunction.

REFERENCES

1 Beattie P: The use of an eclectic approach for the treatment of low back pain: a case study, *Phys Ther* 72(12):923-928, 1992.

2 Binkley J, Finch E, Hall J, et al.: Diagnositic classification of patients with low back pain: report on a survey of physical therapy experts, *Phys Ther* 73(3):138-155, 1993.

3 Bittinger J: *Management of the lumbar pain syndromes*, Course Notes, 1980.

4 Cibulka M: The treatment of the sacroiliac joint component to low back pain: a case report, *Phys Ther* 72(12):917-922, 1992.

5 Cibulka M, Delitto A, Koldehoff R: Changes in innominate tilt after manipulation of the sacroiliac joint in patients wtih low back pain: an experimental study, *Phys Ther* 68(9):1359-1370, 1988.

6 Cibulka M, Rose S, Delitto A, et al.: Hamstring muscle strain treated by mobilizing the saroiliac joint, *Phys Ther* 66(8):1220-1223, 1986.

7 Crock H: Internal disk disruption: a challenge to disk-prolapse fifty years on. The Presidential address: ISSLS, *Spine* 11(6):650-653, 1986.

8 DeRosa C, Porterfield J: A physical therapy model for the treatment of low back pain, *Phys Ther* 72(4):261-272, 1992.

9 Deyo R, Diehl A, Rosenthal M: How many days of bed rest for acute low back pain?: a randomized clinical trial, *New Engl J Med* 315:1064-1070, 1986.

10 Donley P: Rehabilitation of low back pain in athletes: the 1976 Schering symposium on low back problems, *Athletic Training* 12(2), 1977.

11 Erhard R, Bowling R: The recognition and management of the pelvic component of lowback and sciatic pain, *APTA* 2(3):4-13, 1979.

12 Farfan H: Muscular mechanism of the lumbar spine and the position of power and efficiency, *Orthop Clin North Am* 6(1):135-144, 1975.

13 Friberg O: Clinical symptoms and biomechanics of lumbar spine and hip joint in leg length inequality, *Spine* 8(6):643-650, 1983.

14 Frymoyer J: Back pain and sciatica: medical progress, *New Engl J Med* 318(5):291-300, 1988.

15 Grieve G: The sacro-iliac joint, *Physiotherapy* 62:384-400, 1976.

16 Grieve G: Lumbar instability, Congress lecture, *Physiotherapy* 68(1):2-9, 1982.

17 Jackson C, Brown M: Analysis of current approaches and a practical guide to prescription of exercise, *Clin Orthop Rel Res* 179:46-54, 1983.

18 Lewit K, Simons D: Myofascial pain: relief by post-isometric relaxation, *Arch Phys Med Rehabil* 65(8):452-456, 1984.

19 Lindstrom I, Ohlund C, Eek C, et al.: The effect of graded activity on patients wtih subacute low back pain: a randomized prospective clinical study with an operant-conditioning behavioral approach, *Phys Ther* 72(4):279-290, 1992.

20 Maigne R: Low back pain of thoracolumbar origin, *Arch Phys Med Rehabil* 61(9):391-395, 1980.

21 Maitland G: *Vertebral manipulation*, ed 5, London, 1990, Butterworth and Company (Pub) Ltd.

22 Mapa B: An Australian programme for management of low back problems, *Physiotherapy* 66(4):108-111, 1980.

23 McGraw M: *The neuro-muscular maturation of the human infant*, New York, 1966, Hafner Publishing.

24 McKenzie R: Manual correction of sciatic scoliosis, *New Zealand Med J* 76(484):194-199, 1972.

25 McKenzie R: *The lumbar spine: mechanical diagnosis and therapy, spinal publications*, New Zealand, 1981, Lower Hutt.

26 Porter R, Miller C: Back pain and trunk list, *Spine* 11(6):596-600, 1986.

27 Saal J: I. Rehabilitation of football players with lumbar spine injury, *Phys Sports Med* 16(9):61-68, 1988.

28 Saal J: Rehabilitation of football players with lumbar spine injury, *Phys Sports Med* 16(10):117-125, 1988.

29 Saal J: Dynamic muscular stabilization in the nonoperative treatment of lumbar pain syndromes, *Orthop Rev* 19(8):691-700, 1990.

30 Saal J, Saal J: Nonoperative treatment of herniated lumbar intervertebral disk with radiculopathy: an outcome study, *Spine* 14(4):431-437, 1989.

31 Steiner C, Staubs C, Ganon M, et al.: Piriformis syndrome: pathogenesis, diagnosis, and treatment, *J AOA* 87(4):318-323, 1987.

32 Tenhula J, Rose S, Delitto A: Association between direction of lateral lumbar shift, movement tests, and side of symptoms in patients with low back pain syndrome, *Phys Ther* 70(8):480-486, 1990.

33 Threlkeld A: The effects of manual therapy on connective tissue, *Phys Ther* 72(12):893-902, 1992.

34 Travell J, Simons D: *Myofascial pain and dysfunction: the lower extremities*, Baltimore, 1992, Williams and Wilkins.

35 Travell J, Simons D: *Myofascial pain and dysfunction: the*

trigger point manual, Baltimore, 1992, Williams and Wilkins.

36 Twomey L: A rationale for treatment of back pain and joint pain by manual therapy, *Phys Ther* 72(12):885-892, 1992.

37 Waddell G: Clinical assessment of lumbar impairment, *Clin Orthop Rel Res* 221:110-120, 1987.

38 Waddell G: A new clinical model for the treatment of low-back pain, *Spine* 12(7):632-644, 1987.

39 Walker J: The sacroiliac joint: a critical review, *Phys Ther* 72(12):903-916, 1992.

Rehabilitation of Shoulder Injuries

19

Lori A. Thein

OBJECTIVES

After completion of this chapter, the student should be able to do the following:

- Discuss important rehabilitation concepts for treating shoulder injuries.

- Relate biomechanical principles to the rehabilitation of various shoulder injuries/pathologies.

- Discuss criteria for progression of the rehabilitation program for different shoulder injuries/pathologies.

- Discuss treatment of overuse problems, injuries to the joint structures and bones, and injuries involving the soft tissues of the shoulder.

- Describe and explain the rationale for various treatment techniques in the management of shoulder injuries.

- Describe the relationship between shoulder girdle biomechanics and the choice of exercise techniques.

- Outline a program of therapeutic exercise designed to manage various shoulder injuries.

- Describe how exercise techniques for a given injury would change for athletes in different positions or different sports.

INTRODUCTION

The shoulder girdle is a complex series of joints and articulations that function together in a intricate pattern of gliding, rolling, and rotating to produce coordinated motion. Although the glenohumeral joint is most apparent when considering the shoulder, the acromioclavicular and sternoclavicular joints and the scapulothoracic and costovertebral articulations are essential to normal shoulder motion and function. Additionally, the suprahumeral (or subacromial) space is considered an articulation by some and is of critical importance when considering rotator cuff pathology. Each area is prone to specific injuries in sports, and the sports therapist should be aware of the structures at risk in a given sport. This knowledge will aid in the evaluation process and supports the functional progression.

The glenohumeral joint trades stability for mobility so that the hand may be placed in a multitude of positions for a variety of tasks. Unlike the hip joint, which has stability via the bony articulation of the femoral head and the acetabulum, the glenohumeral joint has no intrinsic bony stability. The glenoid fossa is shallow and slightly curved, while the humeral head is a large, spherical structure (Figure 19-1). This joint can be likened to a large ball sitting on a shallow plate. As such, the stability must be provided by the

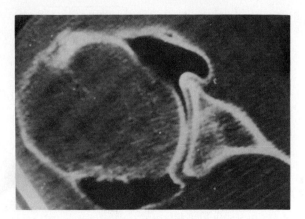

Fig. 19-1. CAT arthrogram of the glenohumeral joint.
The articular cartilage and the glenoid labrum provide
additional static support to the bony glenoid. This further
increases the stability of the glenohumeral joint.
(From Rockwood CA, Matsen FA:*The shoulder.* Philadelphia, 1990,
WB Saunders.)

surrounding soft tissues. This fact underscores the
importance of a thorough rehabilitation program.
Matsen et al. state

> In spite of this lack of coverage, the normal shoulder
> precisely constrains the humeral head to within 1
> millimeter of the center of the glenoid cavity throughout
> most of the arc of movement. It is amazing that this
> seemingly unstable joint is able to provide this precise
> centering, resist the gravitational pull on the arm hanging
> at the side for long periods, allow for the lifting of large
> loads, permit throwing a baseball at speeds approaching
> 100 mph, and hold together during the application of an
> almost infinite variety of forces of differing magnitude,
> direction, and abruptness.[26]

Because of the complexity of this series of joints
and articulations and the heavy reliance on soft tissues
to provide both static and dynamic stability, a thorough evaluation is essential. Often one or more problems coexist to produce the athlete's symptoms; the
key to shoulder evaluation is to determine which
problem is the primary underlying etiology and
which problems are secondary results. A good example is the relationship between impingement syndrome and instability. In the young athlete, instability
is often the underlying problem and impingement
syndrome a secondary problem. Failure to realize this
will result in treatment for the wrong problem and
an unsatisfactory outcome. The subjective examination must include open-ended questions to prevent

leading the athlete to a predetermined conclusion,
and a detailed physical examination will prevent overlooking a secondary problem. Comparisons must be
made to the uninvolved side, keeping in mind issues
of dominance and unilateral sports.

Evaluating the athlete's sport can provide clues to
the problem, as well as form the basis for a functional
progression. Many athletes fail to return to their previous level of activity because they cannot bridge the
gap between formal rehabilitative exercises and functional activity. Each athlete must complete a functional progression before returning fully to their
sport. However, early, controlled participation can
provide an outlet for activity, a team support system,
and a mark of short-term goal achievement. Decisions
about controlled return to activity must be made by
the individual rehabilitation expert, keeping in mind
the demands of the sport on the athlete's shoulder.
This chapter will provide basic information on the
pathomechanics and rehabilitation of shoulder complex injuries. It is beyond the scope of this or any
other text to provide precise rehabilitation activities
for every possible situation. The information is not
intended to be all-inclusive but rather to provide an
understanding of the relationships among anatomy,
biomechanics, and the rehabilitation process, as well
as supply examples of exercise techniques that might
be used in various situations.

COMMON ISSUES IN SHOULDER REHABILITATION

There are several basic tenets that underlie all shoulder rehabilitation procedures. Although some of
these are more critical in certain pathologies, these
principles should be considered when treating any
athlete with a shoulder problem.

Clearly, the shoulder must achieve full range of
motion and strength during the course of rehabilitation. The shoulder must also achieve normal proprioception. Like the relationship between a sore,
swollen knee and poor quadriceps strength, sore, inflamed subacromial soft tissues will produce supraspinatus dysfunction. The supraspinatus will fail to
stabilize and depress the humeral head, leading to
poorly controlled motion, functional impingement,
weakness, and pain. This starts a self-perpetuating cycle that must be broken with therapeutic intervention. The supraspinatus must be retrained to stabilize
and depress the humeral head to restore normal biomechanics. This can be accomplished with PNF tech-

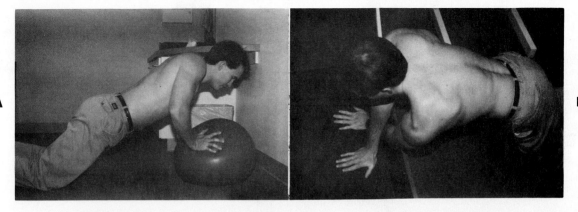

Fig. 19-2. Proprioceptive exercises for the shoulder. A, Push-ups on a gym ball. **B,** Walking on hands on the treadmill.

niques and various closed-kinetic chain exercises. These exercises include push-ups on a gym ball, using a Shuttle 2000-1* with the arms, walking on their hands on the treadmill, and various gym ball activities (Figure 19-2).[11,16]

Isokinetic strengthening is used in most shoulder rehabilitation programs. Training procedures typically include shoulder abduction/adduction, flexion/extension, and internal/external rotation. Reciprocal concentric contractions can be combined with concentric/eccentric contractions of a specific movement pattern depending on the problem. Velocity spectrum from 30 degrees/second to 450 degrees/second may be used with shoulder rehabilitation. Range-of-motion limits may be necessary in some cases (Figure 19-3). For example, in early rehabilitation after an anterior dislocation, full external rotation at 90 degrees abduction may require limitations. Patients with impingement syndrome may not tolerate elevation past 90 degrees.

There are many published studies providing information on the norms for shoulder strength.† These studies are specific to the population tested, isokinetic dynamometer choice, test speed, and test position. For example, shoulder rotation may be tested standing in slight abduction, sitting in 90 degrees

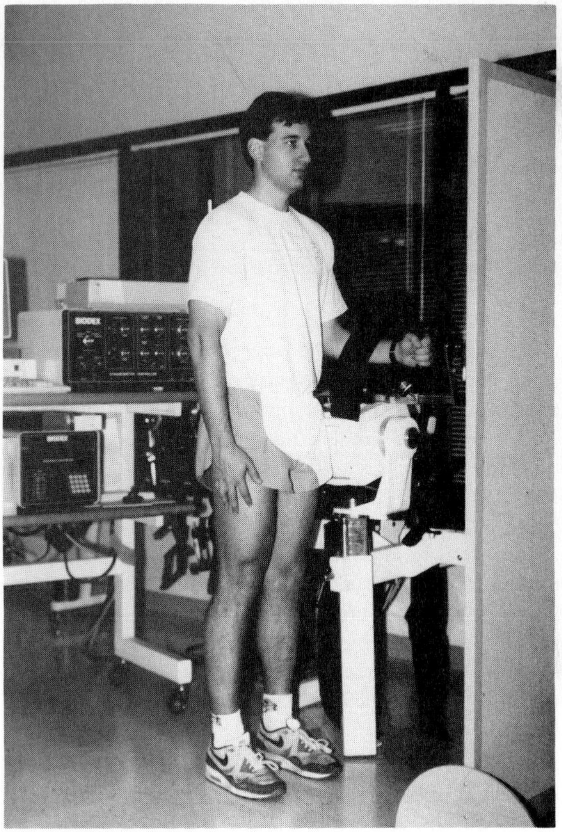

*Shuttle 2000-1, Glacier, WA.
†References 4, 12, 15, 19, 24, 33, 44, 46.

Fig. 19-3. Isokinetic exercise for the shoulder.

TABLE 19-1

Average Normal Values (ft-lbs) for Isokinetic Shoulder Strength as Measured on a Cybex II Dynamometer

Test Motion	Male 60 Deg/Sec (Mean ± SD)	Male 180 Deg/Sec (Mean ± SD)	Female 60 Deg/Sec (Mean ± SD)	Female 180 Deg/Sec (Mean ± SD)
Internal rotation	33.2 ± 11.8	30.2 ± 10.9	17.9 ± 2.9	16.0 ± 3.0
External rotation	21.8 ± 5.7	19.9 ± 6.0	13.0 ± 2.0	10.8 ± 2.1
Abduction	37.5 ± 11.4	28.4 ± 9.9	19.5 ± 5.9	13.9 ± 4.6
Adduction	61.0 ± 15.2	52.6 ± 16.7	34.2 ± 6.7	27.8 ± 4.2
Extension	53.9 ± 14.3	44.2 ± 12.8	28.4 ± 4.3	22.9 ± 5.0
Flexion	43.0 ± 9.3	34.1 ± 7.4	24.0 ± 4.5	18.6 ± 4.4

From Ivey et al.: *Arch Phys Med Rehab* 66:384-386, 1985.

TABLE 19-2

Ratios (Operated/Nonoperated) of the Averages of Peak Values × 100 for Each Group (± Standard Deviation)

	Abduction		External Rotation		Flexion	
	60 Deg/Sec	180 Deg/Sec	60 Deg/Sec	180 Deg/Sec	60 Deg/Sec	180 Deg/Sec
All 6 months	70 ± 30	55 ± 30	75 ± 30	65 ± 30	65 ± 20	65 ± 25
All 12 months	80 ± 25	80 ± 40	90 ± 30	90 ± 30	75 ± 25	75 ± 30
Small 6 months	80 ± 35	60 ± 35	80 ± 30	75 ± 35	80 ± 15	75 ± 20
Small 12 months	90 ± 20	90 ± 35	105 ± 25	100 ± 20	80 ± 25	80 ± 20
Large 6 months	65 ± 30	55 ± 30	70 ± 30	60 ± 30	55 ± 15	55 ± 20
Large 12 months	80 ± 30	80 ± 40	85 ± 35	80 ± 30	75 ± 20	75 ± 30

From Walker SW et al.: *J Bone Joint Surg* 69A (7):1041-1044, 1987.

abduction, supine in 90 degrees abduction, in the plane of the scapula, or in the prone position. As such, the values obtained are specific to that study. Table 19-1 presents normal values for shoulder testing at 60 and 180 degrees/second in a group of 18 men and 13 women 21 to 50 years of age. Table 19-2 presents the isokinetic strength of a group of patients at 6 and 12 months after repair of a small or a large rotator cuff tear. Falkel et al. found that swimmers produced more rotational torque when tested in the prone position, which more closely simulates their sport.[12] Subjects produced more torque when testing rotation in the plane of the scapula rather than in flexion.[13] Finally, Wilk et al. have extensively studied isokinetic shoulder strength testing and identified 15 guidelines for standardization of isokinetic shoulder testing. These guidelines should be incorporated to ensure reliable isokinetic values[46] (see the box).

Resistive tubing exercises should be avoided until the patient has formed a solid base of pain-free ex-

---

GUIDELINES FOR STANDARDIZATION OF ISOKINETIC SHOULDER TESTING

1. Planes of motion to evaluate
2. Testing position/stabilization
3. Axis of joint motion
4. Client education
5. Active warm-up
6. Gravity compensation
7. Rest intervals
8. Test collateral extremity first
9. Standardize verbal commands
10. Standardize visual feedback
11. Testing velocities used
12. Test repetitions
13. System calibration
14. System level/stabilized
15. Use of windowed data/semihard end stop

From Wilk KE, Arrigo CA, Andrews JR: Standardized isokinetic testing protocol for the throwing shoulder: the thrower's series, *Isokinetics Exer Sci* 1(2):63-71, 1991.

ercises and is free from recurrent exacerbations of pain. Resistive tubing provides the most resistance at the end of the range where strength is the least, resulting in patients overworking their shoulders. Sport-specific speeds, ranges, and repetitions can be achieved using tubing; however, these activities should be reserved for the latter stages of rehabilitation.

Patients respond best to high-repetition, low-resistance programs. It must be reinforced that the patient's goal is to complete the repetitions, even if this means decreasing the weight. If the patient is unable to complete a set of 30 repetitions with a given weight, they should decrease the weight and complete the set. Additionally, the more frequently during the day they can perform their exercises, the better. Too often, patients return home at the end of a long day and try performing too many exercises. Spacing exercise sets out over the course of the day tends to be better tolerated by the athlete with shoulder pain. The athlete should be counseled to expect only fatigue with their exercises. If they experience pain with any exercises, the sports therapist should be informed and the program modified. Too often, athletes and therapists have unreasonable expectations about the amount of weight that can be tolerated. A great deal of force must be produced by the supraspinatus during activities such as abduction, owing to its insertion close to the axis of rotation and the length of the arm (lever arm) being lifted.

The scapulothoracic joint is the base of support for the shoulder. The entire shoulder girdle must be considered, not just the tissues directly involved with the pathology. The rotator cuff needs a solid base of support from which to function. This is an example of mobility imposed upon stability. If the base is unstable, the extremity will be unstable, setting the stage for impingement, subluxations, or dislocations. Several exercises can be performed to strengthen the periscapular musculature. Simple protraction and retraction with weights or manual resistance can be used to strengthen and provide proprioceptive feedback (Figure 19-4). Moseley et al. performed EMG analysis of the scapular muscles during rehabilitation exercises and developed a core of four exercises that exercised the periscapular muscles. These muscles were identified as the upper, middle, and lower trapezius, levator scapula, rhomboids, pectoralis minor, and the middle and lower serratus anterior. These four exercises are as follows: 1) scaption in internal rotation (scapular plane elevation), 2) rowing, 3) push-ups with a plus, and 4) press-up (Figure 19-5).[27]

Scapular strengthening should be a part of every shoulder rehabilitation program.

Finally, the best outcome can be expected with interventions applied simultaneously rather than sequentially. Often patients try rest, then medications, then a cortisone injection, and then therapy. If controlled activity, appropriate medications, and rehabilitation are applied simultaneously, the chances of a successful outcome are enhanced.

IMPINGEMENT SYNDROME

The subacromial (or suprahumeral) space and the interposed soft tissues form the anatomical basis for impingement syndrome. The coracoacromial ligament spans the coracoid process to the acromion, forming an arch over the humeral head. Between this arch and the humeral head lie the articular cartilage, long head of the biceps and supraspinatus tendons, and the subacromial bursa (Figure 19-6). Impingement syndrome is often considered an overuse problem, but it frequently originates with an acute traumatic episode, such as a fall. Although there is no objective injury (for example, fracture or rotator cuff tear), the contusion to these soft tissues sets up a cycle of pain, biomechanical changes, and weakness that is self-perpetuating. Swelling in the subacromial bursa further compromises an already small space, thereby irritating the biceps and rotator cuff tendons. Patients with a type II or type III acromion injury may be more susceptible to impingement syndrome than those with a type I acromion injury because of these mechanical factors (Figure 19-7).

In athletes without a history of trauma, repetitive overhead motion is usually the causative factor. Tendon degeneration occurs with fatigue of the musculotendinous unit. This is particularly evident in activities requiring rapid eccentric contraction of the external rotators such as throwing and tennis serving. Nirschl describes a process of tendon degeneration that results in a dull, gray, edematous tissue. Tendon tissue resected from a site of chronic inflammation often reveals few inflammatory cells but instead changes more representative of a degenerative process.[31]

In addition to the mechanical aspects of impingement, the vascular supply adds another component to this problem. Rathbun and Macnab performed vascular studies of the supraspinatus and biceps tendons and discovered that each has an area of avascularity that is apparent when the humerus is adducted at the side. This area of avascularity extends from 1 centi-

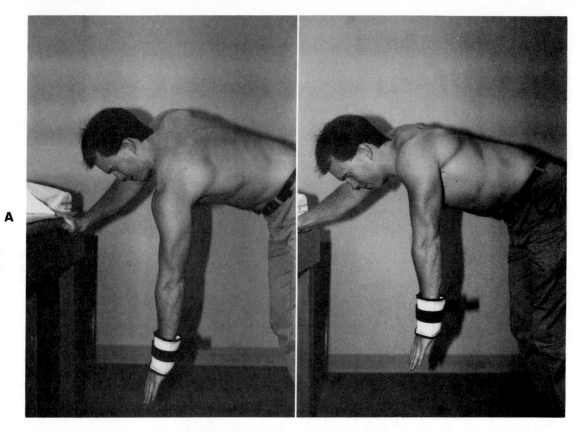

Fig. 19-4. Resisted scapular motion. A, Retraction.

meter proximal directly to the insertion on the greater tuberosity. The vascular supply returns when the arm is abducted 15 degrees and therefore has significant implications in rehabilitation exercise design.

Superimposed instability may confuse the typical impingement picture. When underlying instability is present, the rotator cuff may become overworked. The supraspinatus functions to compress the humeral head into the glenoid fossa and to depress the humeral head during abduction. If the supraspinatus is overworked trying to stabilize the humeral head, then it is unable to effectively function to depress the humeral head. The resultant upward movement decreases the subacromial space and irritates the subacromial soft tissues, thus perpetuating the impingement process.

Neer describes three stages of impingement. Stage I is characterized by edema and hemorrhage and is generally seen in athletes under age 25. However,

with increased sports participation in the later years and earlier intervention, stage I impingement may be seen at any age. Symptoms include the following: 1) painful arc between 60 and 120 degrees of elevation, 2) pain with overpressure to abduction (positive Neer's impingement sign), 3) pain with overpressure to internal rotation at 90 degrees foward flexion (positive Hawkins' impingement sign), and 4) pain with resisted supraspinatus testing (arm elevated to 90 degrees, horizontally adducted 30 degrees and fully internally rotated; pressure is applied downward while that patient resists upward) (Figure 19-8). Palpable tenderness over the greater tuberosity is often present, and the patient may complain of pain into the C5 dermatome.[29]

Stage II impingement is typically seen in patients between 25 and 40 years of age and is characterized by fibrosis and tendinitis. Hawkins and Abrams feel that age is variable and that duration of symptoms is of greater significance.[14] Stage II is a progression of

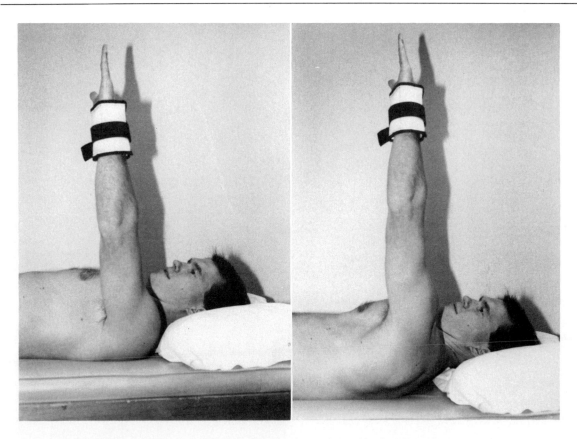

Fig. 19-4, cont'd. B, Protraction exercises may be performed with cuff weights or manual resistance.

stage I and includes all of the stage I symptoms but may additionally include night pain, activity limiting pain, crepitus, and a catching sensation at approximately 100 degrees of abduction. There may be early signs of adhesive capsulitis.

A prolonged history of chronic pain and tendinitis is the hallmark of stage III impingement. This patient typically averages 60 years of age and often presents with a frank rotator cuff tear. A small incident may extend a small partial tear into a complete tear. Night pain is a common complaint, and pain and loss of motion generally prohibit any athletic endeavors. Frequently, stage III impingement symptoms cannot be completely resolved conservatively. After failed conservative management, surgical intervention is considered. Surgical treatment usually includes a rotator cuff repair and subacromial decompression.

Medical management for stage I and II impingement includes oral nonsteroidal antiinflammatory medication and occasionally in stage II the judicious

use of a subacromial corticosteroid injection. The key to management and prevention of reoccurrence, however, is a thorough and complete rehabilitation program. Surgery to resect the coracoacromial ligament and the distal clavicle is generally not considered until the patient has failed 6 months to 1 year of appropriate conservative treatment and has a positive impingement test.[29,30] A subacromial injection of lidocaine that results in relief of the patient's pain is considered a positive impingement test and distinguishes the patient who is likely to improve with a subacromial decompression (see Figure 19-8).

Key Issues in Impingement Rehabilitation

There are several key issues that are essential to a good outcome when rehabilitating athletes with impingement syndrome. First, there must be adequate laxity in the inferior capsule to allow the humeral head to glide caudally during elevation. Biomechan-

Stage 3 - atrophy of muscles.

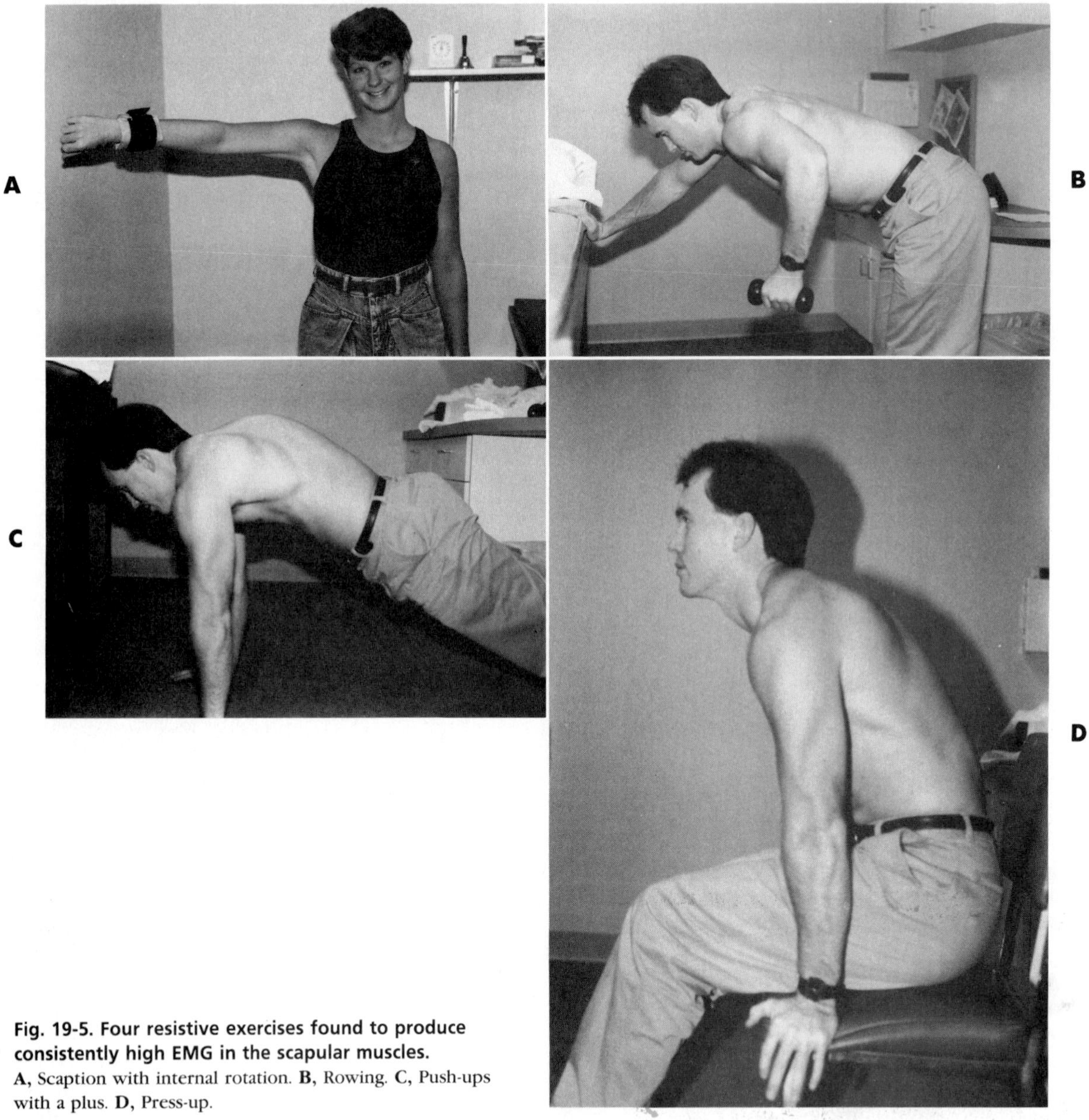

Fig. 19-5. Four resistive exercises found to produce consistently high EMG in the scapular muscles.
A, Scaption with internal rotation. B, Rowing. C, Push-ups with a plus. D, Press-up.

ically, the humeral head glides inferiorly on the glenoid during elevation. If there is inadequate capsule mobility, impingement will occur with elevation, regardless of rotator cuff strength and flexibility. If mobility is lacking, joint mobilization must be incorporated as part of the treatment plan.

Exercises should avoid the impingement zone. The impingement zone is traditionally considered to be forward elevation. However, this painful zone may occur in different ranges in certain athletes, depending on their sport and anatomy. As a rule, any abduction past 90 degrees should be performed in external rotation; any flexion past 90 degrees in neutral or external rotation, and "empty can" strengthening

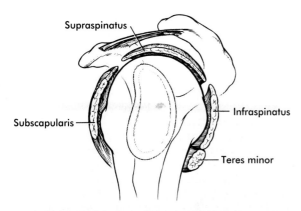

Fig. 19-6. Sagittal view of the normal shoulder. Note the close anatomical relationship between the coracoacromial arch and the underlying supraspinatus tendon. This forms the anatomical basis for impingement syndrome.
(From Rockwood CA, Matsen FA: *The shoulder,* Philadelphia, 1990, WB Saunders.)

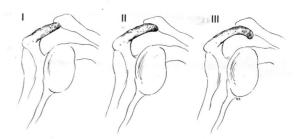

Fig. 19-7. Three types of acromion morphology defined by Bigliani and Morrison. They found type I, with its flat surface, to provide the least compromise of the supraspinatus outlet, whereas type IIIs sudden discontinuity or hood was associated with the highest rate of rotator cuff pathology in their cadaver study.
(From Rockwood CA, Matsen FA: *The shoulder,* Philadelphia, 1990, WB Saunders.)

(scaption in internal rotation) only to 90 degrees elevation.

Instability must be ruled out as a causative factor during the shoulder evaluation. Shoulder subluxation occurs in a high percentage of athletes presenting with stage I impingement. The symptoms are often very subtle and may go unnoticed by the athlete. A thorough history and detailed examination can identify those athletes with underlying instability. If instability is a component of the athlete's impingement syndrome, it must be treated concurrently. Treating only the symptoms will result in continued pain, while treating the instability (the cause) will produce a successful outcome. Overlooking this common association will lead to progression of the impingement lesion.

Finally, the long head of the biceps and supraspinatus tendons' positional avascularity must be incorporated into rehabilitation exercises. These muscles should be trained with the arm slightly abducted and not with the elbow held tightly against the side. This is in contrast to some published rehabilitation programs that demonstrate sidelying external rotation performed in humeral adduction.

Rehabilitation by Phase

EARLY PHASE. Although there will be many specific goals for the early phase of rehabilitation, the overall goals and criteria for progression to the intermediate

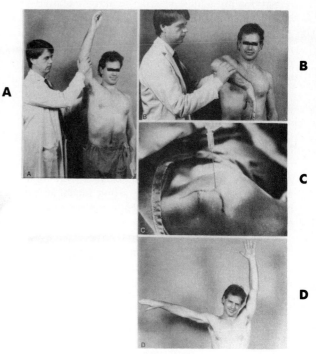

Fig. 19-8. Impingement signs and test. A, Neer's impingement sign. **B,** Hawkin's impingement sign. **C,** Impingement test. Ten milliliters of 1% lidocaine is injected into the subacromial space. A pain-free impingement sign after injection is considered a positive impingement test. **D,** Painful arc.
(From Rockwood CA, Matsen FA: *The shoulder,* Philadelphia, 1990, WB Saunders.)

phase include restoration of normal articular biomechanics (active and passive), establishment of a baseline of tolerable activity (including rehabilitation exercises and sports involvement), and control of pain. The key will be controlling the level and frequency of load on the rotator cuff, then gradually and systematically increasing this level and frequency.

Activity modification is a critical component of the treatment program. Only with some control over the activity level can a stable baseline of tolerated activity be established. Additionally, some patients with stage I impingement may recover completely with time and activity modification only.[29] Complete rest is necessary in stage II and III impingement only. Complete rest implies rest only from the aggravating activities, not immobilization. In most stage I cases, the sport can be modified to allow some participation. This may mean swimming with fins or only kicking for the swimmer or hitting only ground strokes at 50% intensity for the tennis player. The activity should be evaluated and participation allowed on a limited basis. Additionally, the athlete's sport must be evaluated to rule out technique faults that may underlie impingement syndrome. Some athlete's money would be better spent on coaching than on expensive equipment.

Upper extremity peripheral aerobics using an upper body ergometer or other upper extremity endurance activity should be incorporated to promote circulation through the area. Nirschl describes the benefits of this activity as increased oxygenation, nutrition, and collateral circulation, as well as enhancement of biochemical changes associated with endurance training.[31] Cross-country skiing machines and rowing ergometers make good alternatives to an upper body ergometer.

Stretching should be incorporated immediately in the early phase. Any muscle tightness found on evaluation should be treated with static stretches held for 2 to 3 minutes each. Four commonly used stretches specifically for the rotator cuff include: 1) internal rotation at 80 degrees abduction, 2)external rotation at 90 degrees abduction, 3) 135 degrees elevation, and 4) full overhead elevation with external rotation (Figure 19-9). Stretches should be performed with a cuff weight, baton, or cane to allow full relaxation of the shoulder girdle muscles. Avoid overstretching, particularly in the hypermobile athlete. The sports therapist should counsel the athlete to ensure full understanding of this concept.

Joint mobilization should be used in those patients who demonstrate decreases in joint mobility. Of particular importance is inferior humeral glide. This mobility is necessary for proper glenohumeral mechanics in overhead motion. Additionally, any patients with a component of adhesive capsulitis will require extensive joint mobilization. The specifics of mobilization are discussed in Chapter 10.

Biomechanical reeducation is necessary in all patients demonstrating loss of normal articular biomechanics. In those patients with late stage I and stage II impingement, pain may inhibit the supraspinatus, leading to shoulder hiking and substitution during elevation. This attempts to elevate the acromion because the supraspinatus is no longer depressing the humeral head. Patients often lose their normal scapulohumeral rhythm, and the scapula and humerus move as a single unit during elevation. The patient must learn to elevate the humerus while maintaining the scapula in retraction. A proprioceptive exercise to train this requires the patient to actively stabilize the scapula in retraction while actively abducting the upper arms. Performing this with the elbows flexed decreases the torque demands on the rotator cuff, allowing for better technique. A mirror can provide visual feedback to discourage shoulder hiking (Figure 19-10). Proprioceptive training to teach the supraspinatus to depress the humeral head is also essential to breaking the pain-impingement cycle and can be achieved using PNF techniques outlined in Chapter 11.

Supraspinatus strengthening will be the core of the shoulder strengthening program because of its role in impingement syndrome. Chandler et al. found strength imbalances between the internal and external rotator musculature and felt that exercises to strengthen the posterior cuff may prevent or lessen the severity of overuse injuries.[7] Exercises producing high EMG activity in the supraspinatus include the following: 1) scaption in internal rotation, 2) flexion, 3) scaption in external rotation, and 4) military press (Figure 19-11).[7]

In addition to specific supraspinatus strengthening, other shoulder strengthening exercises should be performed. Those supplemental exercises producing high EMG activity in the external rotators as a group include the following: 1) external rotation in sidelying position, 2) external rotation in prone position at 90 degrees abduction, and, 3) horizontal abduction in external rotation (Figure 19-12).[42] The long head of the biceps should be trained by performing elbow curls in a position of shoulder extension. The periscapular musculature must be strengthened to pro-

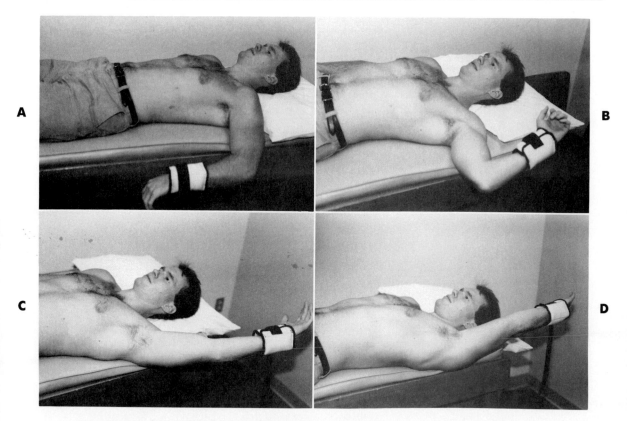

Fig. 19-9. Four basic shoulder stretching exercises. A, Internal rotation at 80 degrees abduction. **B,** External rotation at 90 degrees abduction. **C,** Overhead at 135 degrees abduction. **D,** Full overhead position in external rotation. Caution must be used with stretches **B** to **D** in athletes with anterior instability.

vide a solid base of support for the shoulder. The core scapular exercises outlined earlier should be incorporated. Occasionally, these exercises are too painful for the athlete early in the rehabilitation program. In this situation, simple scapular protraction and retraction should be included until the core exercises are tolerated (see Figure 19-4).

Finally, the patient must be reminded that ice should be used on a regular basis (two to three times daily) to control pain and inflammation.

INTERMEDIATE PHASE. The chief goal in the intermediate phase is to develop a solid strength base in the rotator cuff. This will provide the basis for sport-specific training in the next phase. This phase can be likened to the strength phase in a traditional strength-training program.[37] The baseline established in the early phase is the point of return if the athlete suffers a setback in their program.

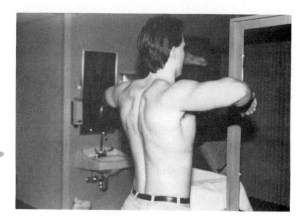

Fig. 19-10. Active shoulder abduction to 90 degrees while maintaining scapular retraction.

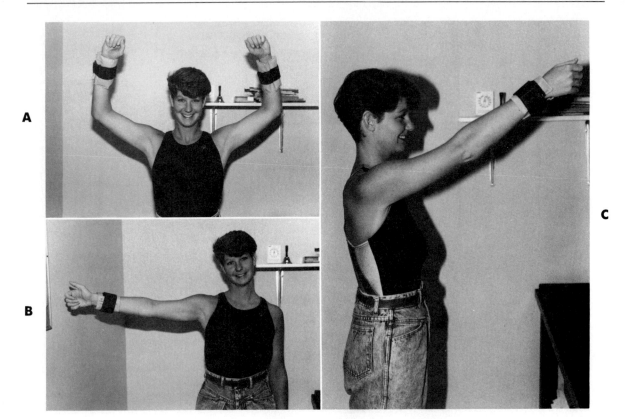

Fig. 19-11. Four resistive exercises found to produce consistently high EMG in the suspraspinatus. A, Military press. **B,** Flexion. **C,** Scaption in external rotation. **D,** Scaption in internal rotation (see Figure 19-5, A).

The stretching and upper extremity peripheral aerobics are simply a continuation of the early phase program. The athlete should be periodically reevaluated to ensure that the stretching is still appropriate and that he or she is not overstretching. Swimmers are notorious for a "more is better" attitude regarding their stretching. They often end up stretching their joint capsule after they have stretched the musculotendinous unit.

The strengthening program should be progressively increased in resistance and repetitions in an attempt to establish a strength and endurance base. The athlete should be progressed up to three sets of 30 repetitions on a daily basis. Resistive tubing exercises may be added as an adjunct to the free weight exercise program. Isokinetics may be added as an additional strengthening tool, keeping in mind issues regarding the impingement zone. Velocity spectrum training and concentric/eccentric training in various

positions are beneficial. However, free weight exercises train proprioception and balance in addition to strength; therefore tubing and isokinetics should not be a substitute for these exercises.

Exercises should gradually be moved from a single plane to sport-specific positions. This should be done as a transition technique to the late stage of rehabilitation. For example, throwing sport athletes should perform decelerations, and their rotation exercises may be moved to 90 degrees abduction, while swimmers may train their stroke on a Total Gym* (Figure 19-13). A tennis player may perform resistive pulleys or tubing exercises in a forehand or backhand pattern. An Inertial Exercise System† may be used to perform sport-specific high-speed repetitive acceleration and deceleration (see Figure 19-27).

---

*Total Gym, West Bend, WI.
†Impulse Inertial Exercise System, Newnan, GA.

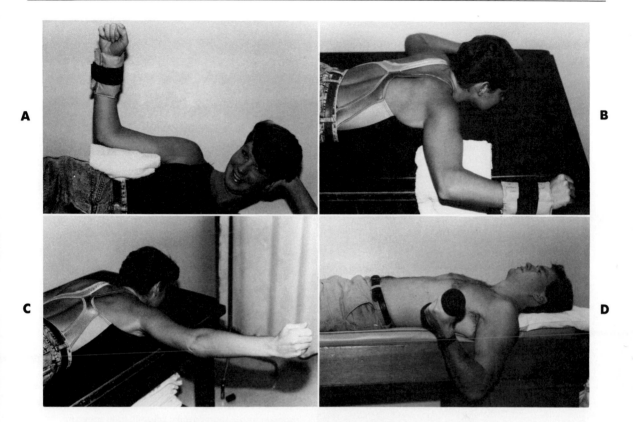

Fig. 19-12. Additional exercises to strengthen the external rotators and long head of the biceps. A, External rotation in sidelying position. **B,** External rotation in prone position. **C,** Horizontal abduction in external rotation. **D,** Biceps curls in shoulder extension.

LATE PHASE. The principal goal in the late phase is the conversion of the strength base formed in the intermediate phase into sport-specific training. This phase can be compared to the conversion phase in a traditional strength-training program.[37] Exercises should be modified to prepare the athlete for the final functional progression stage before full return to sport.

The athlete's exercise program should be modified to reflect the demands of the sport. Athletes involved in low-repetition, high-force activities should continue to increase the weight on their exercises while maintaining the number of repetitions. Swimmers and other athletes participating in high-repetition, low-resistance sports should continue to increase repetitions, progressing to sport-specific speeds, and maintain the resistance. Although most single-plane exercises should be modified to a multi-plane exercise reproducing the demands of the athlete's sport, a few

core exercises that isolate the supraspinatus should be continued on a maintenance basis. The four exercises producing the highest EMG in the supraspinatus should be maintained as a core exercise program, along with the four core scapular exercises (see Figures 19-5 and 19-9 to 19-11). The athlete should be fatigued after completing the exercise program but should not experience pain.

The stretching program should be done before and after exercising but for longer periods of time only if a flexibility deficit remains or if necessary because of the athlete's sport and position (such as, pitcher). Each treatment session should be concluded with ice.

FUNCTIONAL PROGRESSION PHASE. The goal of the functional progression phase is to prepare the athlete for return to their activity. A functional progression specifically stresses the healing tissues and provides neuromuscular coordination, activity-specific strength and endurance training, as well as confidence

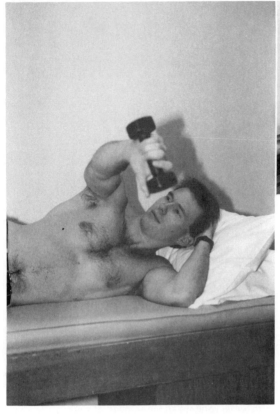

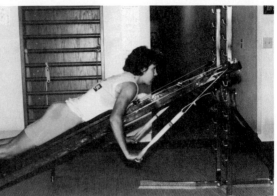

Fig. 19-13. Deceleration exercises. A, Deceleration exercises and **B,** total gym training can convert a strength program into a sport-specific rehabilitation program.

for the athlete returning to activity. It is a progression of the progressive resistive exercise program and prepares the athlete physically and psychologically for return to their sport. Initially, the sports therapist should control the many participation variables, including contact, intensity, duration, and specific drills/activities. As the athlete demonstrates readiness, the control of these variables is slowly passed on to the athlete.

It is imperative that the athlete complete a functional progression before fully returning to their sport. This includes a swimming program for the swimmer, a hitting program for the tennis player, or a throwing program for the baseball player.[1] Specificity of exercise is the underlying principle, and as such, the specific activity must be evaluated and the functional progression patterned after the activity. There are many standard programs for common sports, such as the throwing program. However, the gymnast recovering from impingement syndrome caused by

weight bearing on their hands will require a very different functional progression from that of the thrower. This requires a great deal of kinesiology-based creativity by the sports therapist.

Finally, the athlete should continue on a maintenance program of core exercises on a three times a day (TIW) basis, and ice should be used prophylactically after practice and games.

SUBACROMIAL DECOMPRESSION

In 1972, Neer described indications for performing an anterior acromioplasty in patients with longstanding impingement syndrome. Those indications were long-term disability from chronic bursitis or partial or complete supraspinatus tears.[28] Complete tears may be seen in middle-aged athletes who sustain a fall while skiing or other traumatic injury. Previously, lateral acromioplasty was performed as treatment, and Neer's study was the first documentation that the

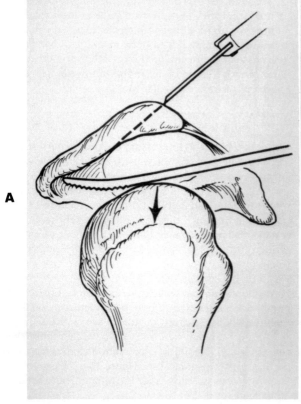
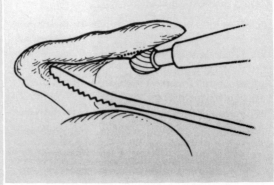

Fig. 19-14. Technique for subacromial decompression.
A, An osteotome is used to resect the anteroinferior surface of the acromion. **B,** Any irregularities are removed with a burr.
(From Rockwood CA, Matsen FA: *The shoulder,* Philadelphia, 1990, WB Saunders.)

impingement lesion was anterior rather than lateral. In a 1983 publication, Neer presented the following indications for anterior acromioplasty:

1. Positive arthrogram showing complete thickness rotator cuff tear.
2. Patients over 40 years of age with negative arthrograms but persistent disability for 1 year, despite appropriate conservative care and a positive impingement test.
3. Patients younger than 40 years of age with chronic stage II lesions and a prominent anterior acromion.
4. Patients undergoing other procedures where impingement is commonly associated (total shoulder replacement).[29]

Matsen and Arntz believe the good prognostic indicators for a successful subacromial decompression to be the following:

1. A well-motivated patient over 40 years of age.
2. Absence of posterior capsular stiffness.
3. Presence of subacromial crepitus.
4. Pain relieved by the subacromial injection of lidocaine.
5. A condition that is unrelated to the patient's occupation.[25]

There are several approaches to surgical decompression, both arthroscopic and open. The basic procedure involves resecting the anterior undersurface of the acromion and resecting the coracoacromial ligament (Figure 19-14). Additionally, any irregularities remaining on the undersurface of the acromion are smoothed off. Any inferiorly directed osteophytes are resected from the acromioclavicular joint, and the lateral 1.5 centimeters of the clavicle are resected if significant acromioclavicular pain is present. The shoulder is thoroughly irrigated to remove any bone fragments. Exploration and probing of the rotator cuff and appropriate debridement or repair are performed.[25]

Postoperative Rehabilitation

The rehabilitation program will vary with the degree and extent of rotator cuff repair and debridement. Variables include the following:

1. Arthroscopic vs. open procedure
2. Rotator cuff repair vs. debridement
3. Secondary pathology

The *progression* of activity is generally the same for both large and small rotator cuff tears; however, the program for large tears tends to lag 3 to 4 weeks behind that of the small tears because of additional soft tissue healing constraints. Some protection is necessary as the injured soft tissues heal. Sling immobilization for comfort is used for the first 2 weeks in small tears, and sling immobilization or an abduction brace is used for 5 weeks for large tears. During this time, elbow, hand, and wrist exercises should be performed to maintain their mobility. Strengthening exercises can be performed for the contralateral upper extremity and both lower extremities. Nonsteroidal antiinflammatory medication, TENS, and ice should be used to control pain and inflammation throughout all phases of rehabilitation. Cardiovascular training should consist of walking or stationary biking.

Early Phase

At 2 weeks, (small tears) or 5 weeks (large tears), the athlete may progress to the next (early) phase of rehabilitation. The goals of this phase are to restore mobility to the shoulder and maintain kinesthesia without disrupting the healing process. This requires primarily passive techniques. Codman's exercises, pulleys for shoulder mobility, shrugs, and passive stretching may be performed below 90 degrees elevation. Codman's exercises are performed to help restore mobility. Otherwise known as pendulum exercises, they are peformed passively, with the body providing momentum to swing the arm into flexion/extension, horizontal abduction/adduction, and circumduction. A cuff weight will add momentum and afford better relaxation than hand-held weights (Figure 19-15).

Passive range-of-motion exercises for flexion and abduction may be completed below 90 degrees elevation. Passive internal and external rotation at zero degrees abduction and external rotation at 90 degrees abduction are appropriate in this phase. These exercises can be performed by the sports therapist and taught to the athlete, who can carry out these exercises with a cane or other assistive equipment. No active abduction is allowed in this phase. However, gentle isometric strengthening for flexion, extension, adduction, abduction, and internal/external rotation is allowed. Proper kinesthetic awareness and firing patterns can be maintained by starting isometric exercises early. Grade I joint mobilization can decrease pain and maintain capsular mobility.

Intermediate Phase

Progression to the intermediate phase occurs at approximately 6 weeks for small tears and 8 weeks for large tears. The primary goals of the intermediate rehabilitation phase are the attainment of full range of motion and the application of specific stresses to affect the healing collagen. Codman's pendulum exercises and passive range-of-motion activities are continued in this phase. Active assisted range-of-motion techniques may be used by the therapist, using pain to guide the amount of assistance. Gentle progressive resistive exercises for flexion, extension, horizontal abduction, and rotation may be initiated, as well as gentle PNF D-1 pattern diagonals below 90 degrees elevation. Scapular stabilization procedures should be incorporated, including protraction and retraction with manual resistance (see Figure 19-4). Easy, active supraspinatus exercises may be initiated, but without resistance.

The pool is a good medium to achieve full motion in a supportive environment. Movements away from the bottom of the pool or parallel to the surface are active assisted, while movements toward the bottom are resistive. Simply allowing the arm to float up to the surface in chest-deep water is a good active-assisted abduction exercise. Gentle resistance can be applied to all shoulder muscle groups using the water as resistance (Figure 19-16).

Late Phase

At 9 weeks for small tears and 12 weeks for large tears, the athlete may progress to the late phase. During this rehabilitation phase, the surgical repair should be very stable, and the primary goal is to recondition the rotator cuff musculature. Passive stretching should be continued and joint mobilization techniques maintained as needed. Sport-specific stretching should be included to prepare the shoulder musculature for the demands of the athlete's sport. All phases occur along a continuum, and exercises should therefore become more sport specific toward the end of this phase. This specificity includes range

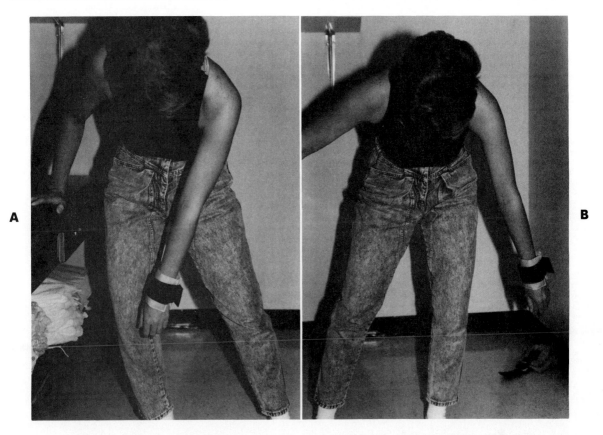

A   B

Fig. 19-15. Codman's exercises. Codman's exercises are performed passively, using body weight and momentum to swing the shoulder in various planes.

of motion, speed, repetitions, type of muscle contraction, open or closed chain, and muscle firing patterns.

Strengthening exercises for the rotator cuff should be performed with free weights and progressed to resisted tubing and isokinetics. Exercises that work the rotator cuff as a group rather than isolating the supraspinatus specifically are better tolerated by the athlete recovering from this surgery. Scaption in internal rotation and external rotation, flexion, and military press produce the highest EMG activity in the supraspinatus and as such should be progressed more slowly. Isokinetic exercise for shoulder internal and external rotation performed in 15 degrees abduction can be performed through a velocity spectrum. This activity should include both concentric and eccentric contractions.

Any exercises performed over 90 degrees elevation, such as the military press, should be initiated with caution. These exercises should be preceded by

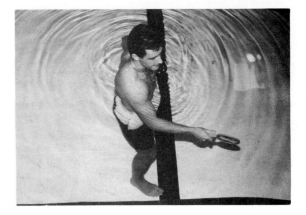

Fig. 19-16. Water for support or resistance. Water can be used as gentle support or resistance depending upon the relationship to the bottom of the pool and equipment used. In this case, equipment is used to increase the resistive surface area. The amount of resistance is relative to the speed of movement and surface area.

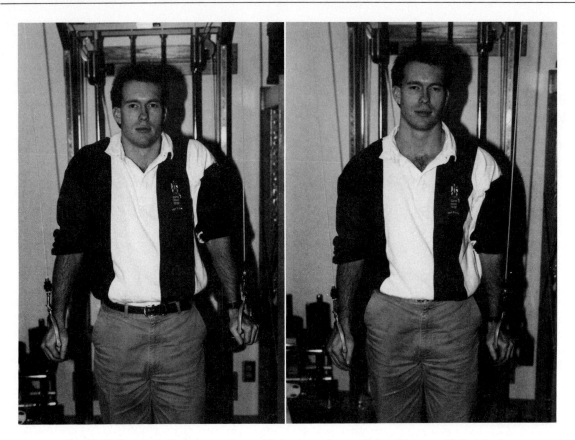

Fig. 19-17. Press-ups. Press-ups can be modified using pulleys until the athlete can lift their body weight.

PNF diagonal exercises above 90 degrees elevation. In this way, the amount of resistance at a given point in the range of motion can be modulated by the therapist. Additionally, it provides the therapist an opportunity to ensure proper muscle firing patterns.

The scapular stabilization exercise core should be progressed from the simple protraction and retraction exercises performed in the last phase to press-ups using pulleys and wall push-ups (Figure 19-17). These activities should be progressed to the core of scapular exercises outlined in the impingement section. Resistance and repetitions in all exercises should approximate the demands of the sport.

Functional Progression Phase

This phase should be minimally initiated at 14 weeks (small tears) or 18 weeks (large tears) or when full, pain-free range of motion and full measured strength are achieved. The goal in this phase is to specifically stress the healing tissue and train the musculature to tolerate the demands of a specific activity. A key element in making the transition from simple strengthening exercises to a functional progression is designing strength and endurance exercises to mimic the demands of the sport in as many aspects as possible. In this way, initiating activity, such as hitting a tennis ball, performing a back handspring, or throwing a softball, is both comfortable and familiar.

CLAVICLE FRACTURES

Clavicle fractures are a common injury in contact and collision sports. Fractures of the middle third are the most common and occur at the point where the cross-section changes from a prism to a flattened shape. It accounts for 80% of all clavicular fractures.[10] The mechanism of injury includes a fall on an outstretched arm, a direct blow to the clavicle (usually with a hockey or lacrosse stick), or most often, a fall directly on the shoulder.

The athlete with a clavicular fracture often splints the arm because of pain but may be able to elevate the arm up to 90 degrees. After this point, clavicular rotation is required to produce full elevation. There may be an obvious clinical deformity, and the proximal fragment may be displaced upward and backward.[10] Palpation reveals point tenderness and motion at the fracture site.

Treatment includes a figure-eight splint for 4 to 6 weeks if healing proceeds at a normal pace. Craig recommends a figure-eight splint for 6 weeks followed by a sling for an additional 3 to 4 weeks. Gentle mobilization and isometric exercises can be initiated at 6 weeks.[10] There are occasional cases of nonunion at this fracture site. Palpable tenderness and radiographic evidence determine when the splint can be removed. While the fracture is healing, the athlete must maintain cardiovascular conditioning and strength in the uninvolved extremities. Weight training, stationary biking, and stairstepping can be used as training techniques.

Early Phase

The primary goal in the early phase is to restore full range of motion and normal articular biomechanics to the shoulder girdle. This phase is initiated upon splint removal. Codman's exercises may be started immediately to help restore mobility. Active-assisted and passive mobility exercises for all restricted soft tissues in all planes can be introduced at this point.

Stretching should be initiated for any muscles demonstrating inflexibility. Keep in mind demands of specific sports. Cane exercises can be used as adjuncts for passive and active-assisted exercise. These exercises should be evaluated to ensure that the athlete is performing them using normal scapulothoracic biomechanics. Additionally, joint mobilization should be incorporated at the glenohumeral, sternoclavicular, or acromioclavicular joint based upon evaluation results.

PNF techniques can be used to restore strength and normal motor programming. Weight-bearing activities and other proprioceptive exercises described previously should be initiated in the early stage to ensure that the athlete learns proper technique from the beginning. Rehearsing motion patterns first in front of a mirror, then without a mirror, and finally

with the eyes closed will help retrain motor control. These motions should be incorporated into the strengthening program in the next phase with the use of tubing or other resistive equipment. They are also easily reproduced in a pool.

Isometric and isotonic strengthening exercises for all shoulder girdle muscles can be initiated when normal patterns of firing are demonstrated. These can be performed in the available range of motion.

Intermediate Phase

When full range of motion and normal articular biomechanics can be demonstrated, the athlete may be progressed to the intermediate phase. The chief goal in this phase is development of a strength base.

A full complement of shoulder strengthening exercises may be incorporated, including a rotator cuff program with free weights, resistive tubing, inertial exercise, isokinetics, and isotonic equipment. The proprioceptive benefits of free-weight exercise support its use through the entire rehabilitation program. There are essentially no exercises that are contraindicated at this point. However, pain should set the guidelines for exercise choices, resistance, and repetitions. Sport-specific strengthening should be initiated toward the end of the intermediate phase. Exercises should be progressed to ranges and patterns encountered in the athlete's sport (Figure 19-18).

Use of upper body ergometry or other upper body endurance equipment may be initiated at this point, and stretching exercises should be continued throughout this phase. A rowing ergometer can work both the upper and lower extremity, with particular focus on the scapular retraction musculature. The liberal use of ice is quite effective in controlling pain after exercise.

Late Phase

Athletes may be progressed to the late phase when they demonstrate a solid, pain-free strength base. The goal of this phase is to train the shoulder muscles for the specific strength, power, and endurance demands of their sport.

Strengthening exercises should be modified to reflect the demands of the sport. They should be performed with the range, pattern, speed, and muscle contraction type encountered in their sport as the basis. A full complement of upper extremity strengthening is indicated. Additional considerations include

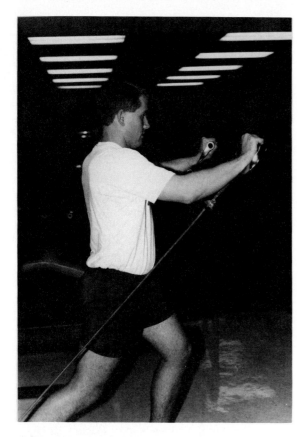

Fig. 19-18. Pulleys. Pulleys are versatile in their ability to replicate sport-specific activities.

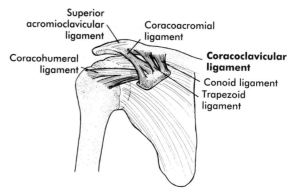

Fig. 19-19. Anatomy of the acromioclavicular joint and supporting ligaments.
(From Nicholas JA, Hershman EB, editors: *The upper extremity in sports medicine,* St Louis, 1990, Mosby.)

the cardiovascular demands of the sport, the number of repetitions in a typical contest, and the unilateral or bilateral nature of the sport. A core of key exercises should be continued on a maintenance basis for the duration of the season.

Functional Progression Phase

A functional progression must be completed before full return to sport. Preparation must include both physical and psychological readiness, particularly for athletes that sustained their fracture from contact in their sport. They must be fully prepared to encounter the same forces that caused their injury. A football player must get used to hitting a sled before he can feel ready to hit an opponent. A volleyball player must be ready to dive for a ball, and a gymnast must be prepared to take a fall without fear of reinjury. These activities must be initiated in a planned, progressive

manner. A functional progression is the only way to ensure the athlete's complete preparation to fully engage in their sport.

ACROMIOCLAVICULAR JOINT INJURIES
Anatomy

The acromioclavicular joint is a diarthrodial joint formed by the distal end of the clavicle and the acromion process of the scapula. The joint capsule is supported by the anterior, posterior, superior, and inferior acromioclavicular ligaments. The fibers of the superior ligament are reinforced by the muscle attachments of the trapezius and deltoid. The fibers of the coracoclavicular ligament run from the lateral inferior surface of the clavicle to the coracoid process of the scapula. It is comprised of two parts, the conoid and the trapezoid ligaments. These ligaments are the primary support for the acromioclavicular articulation and along with the sternoclavicular ligaments maintain the only connection of the upper extremity to the axial skeleton. Rockwood and Young feel that the acromioclavicular ligament provides horizontal stability, while the coracoclavicular ligaments provide vertical stability (Figure 19-19).[35] Approximately 45 degrees of upward clavicular rotation occurs during full overhead elevation.[35]

The mechanism of injury is usually a fall directly on the point of the shoulder with the arm at the side. This forces the acromion down, resulting in either a clavicular fracture or an acromioclavicular joint sprain. A fall on an outstretched arm is a second and less common mechanism of injury.

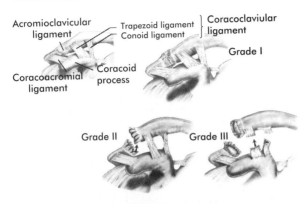

Acromioclavicular ligament — Trapezoid ligament — Coracoclaviular ligament — Conoid ligament

Coracoacromial ligament — Coracoid process

Grade I

Grade II   Grade III

Fig. 19-20. Acromioclavicular separations. In a grade I separation, damage occurs to the acromioclavicular ligament without displacement of the clavicle. Grade II separation implies subluxation from the additional injury to the coracoclavicular ligaments. In a grade III injury, both the acromioclavicular and coracoclavicular ligaments are torn, resulting in displacement of the clavicle.
(From Kulund DN: *The injured athlete,* ed 1, Philadelphia, 1982, JB Lippincott.)

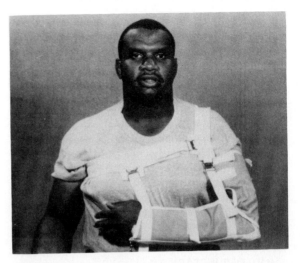

Fig. 19-21. Kenny-Howard sling. A Kenny-Howard sling may be used in the conservative treatment of grade III acromioclavicular sprains.
(From Nicholas JA, Hershman ED, editors: *The upper extremity in sports medicine,* St Louis, 1990, Mosby.)

Injuries are classified by severity and vary from author to author. Most categorize injuries into three grades of severity commonly seen by the sports therapist. Rockwood and Young have added an additional three classifications for severe and unusual cases of acromioclavicular injury. The type I injury involves a sprain of the acromioclavicular ligament and the joint capsule, with the coracoclavicular ligaments and deltoid and trapezius muscles intact. A type II injury includes disruption and widening of the acromioclavicular joint and coracoclavicular ligament sprains, with intact deltoid and trapezius muscles. The distal clavicle displacement is less than the full width of the clavicle.[9] A type III injury includes disruption of the acromioclavicular ligaments, with dislocation of the joint greater than the width of the clavicle and inferior displacement of the shoulder complex, disruption of the coracoclavicular ligaments with the coracoclavicular space increased more than 25% of the normal shoulder, and detachment of the deltoid and trapezius muscles from the distal clavicle (Figure 19-20).[35]

Treatment of Acromioclavicular Sprains

Most authors advocate conservative treatment for type I and II injuries, but there is some controversy over the treatment of type III injuries. Some prefer surgical repair in all or selected patients with type III injuries. However, most orthopedists working with athletes choose to treat this injury conservatively with a modified Kenny-Howard sling (Figure 19-21).[2] Use of this sling is controversial because some individuals experience severe skin problems. The athlete using the Kenny-Howard sling must be watched closely to avoid skin breakdown. Cox surveyed team physicians and chairpersons of orthopedic residency programs and found 86% of the team physicians and 72% of the chairpersons to favor conservative treatment of these injuries. He notes a trend from surgical to conservative care and from closed reduction to simple symptomatic treatment.[9] Tibone et al. evaluated isokinetic shoulder strength an average of 4.5 years after a type III injury and found no significant differences in strength between groups treated surgically and those treated conservatively.[41]

Type I injuries require only symptomatic treatment. The use of ice, antiinflammatory medications, and padding to protect the joint usually allows return to competition in 2 to 14 days. The athlete should have full, pain-free range of motion and symmetrical strength before returning to high-risk sports. Type II injuries often require some period of sling immobilization for comfort. The length of immobilization varies from author to author, but ranges from a few days for comfort to 3 to 6 weeks. Return to contact sports is typically in 8 to 10 weeks.[10] Immobilization length also varies in conservative treatment of type

III injuries. Bergfeld remarks that those who choose symptomatic treatment immobilize for 7 to 10 days for comfort only, and those electing aggressive treatment attempt to keep the joint reduced for 6 weeks. He notes that compliance with the sling drops off significantly at 3 weeks.[2] Craig feels that 6 to 8 weeks of upper extremity immobilization is unreasonable and impractical in a young, active person.[10]

The rehabilitation program for conservative management of acromioclavicular sprains is generally symptomatic. Isometric exercise, Codman's exercises, and mobility activities can be initiated when pain has subsided. The program can progress based upon the patient's symptoms and follows the same progression as those with impingement syndrome.

SHOULDER INSTABILITY

The unstable shoulder is one of the most common and difficult problems encountered in sports medicine. Instability occurs along a continuum, from subluxations producing secondary impingement syndrome to frank dislocations. Additionally, instability can occur in anterior, anteroinferior, posterior, or multiple directions. Each of these factors, along with the complex anatomy of the shoulder and demands by the athlete, make treatment of this problem quite challenging. As such, there are many differing ideas on both conservative and surgical treatment. The sports therapist must be aware as the philosophy and specific guidelines for instability treatment evolve.

Anatomy

The shoulder capsule is twice the surface area of the humeral head and is lined with synovium. It extends from the glenoid neck and labrum to the anatomical neck and proximal shaft of the humerus. Variations in the collagen type and orientation provide stability to the glenohumeral joint by changing function based on how and where they attach to the glenoid, labrum, and humerus.[32] Thickenings in the capsule form ligaments, termed the *superior, middle,* and *inferior glenohumeral ligaments* (Figure 19-22). Their function depends upon the collagen makeup, location of attachment, and the position of the arm.[32]

The superior glenohumeral ligament provides little static stability. It extends from the anterosuperior edge of the glenoid to the top of the lesser tuberosity. Selective cutting does not cause any significant translation anteriorly or posteriorly but does provide suspension to the humerus with the arm at the side.[38]

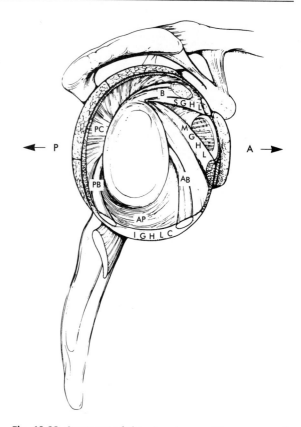

Fig. 19-22. Anatomy of the glenohumeral ligaments and inferior glenohumeral ligament complex *(IGHLC).*
P, Posterior; *A,* anterior; *SGHL,* superior glenohumeral ligament; *MGHL,* middle glenohumeral ligament.
(From Rockwood CA, Matsen FA: *The shoulder,* Philadelphia, 1990, WB Saunders.)

The middle glenohumeral ligament spans the supraglenoid tubercle to the base of the lesser tuberosity. It provides variable static stability to the shoulder and is absent or poorly defined in approximately 27% of the population.[32] This ligament limits external rotation at approximately 45 degrees abduction.

The inferior glenohumeral ligament is actually a ligament complex and plays the most important role in anteroinferior instability. It provides the primary restraint to external rotation between 45 and 90 degrees of abduction.[43] The inferior glenohumeral ligament extends from the anteroinferior labrum to the lesser tuberosity of the humerus. Turkel et al. distinguished three parts of this ligament and felt the superior band of the inferior glenohumeral ligament to be the major stabilizer.[43] Between this band and the

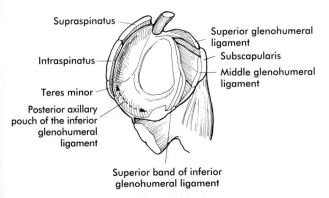

Fig. 19-23. Inferior aspect of glenohumeral ligament. The inferior aspect of the glenohumeral ligament is thinner than the middle portion and has been termed the *axillary pouch.* (From Nicholas JA, Hershman ED, editors: *The upper extremity in sports medicine,* St Louis, 1990, Mosby.)

posterior band of the inferior glenohumeral ligament lies the hammocklike structure termed the *axillary pouch* (Figure 19-23). This sling concept helps to explain why instability in one portion of the shoulder may affect the opposite side and has significant implications for treating instability.[32]

Factors Affecting Stability

There are multiple active and passive factors affecting glenohumeral stability. Passively, the size, shape, and tilt of the glenoid fossa may affect glenohumeral instability.[26] The glenoid is shaped like an inverted comma and may be either anteverted (75% of shoulders) or retroverted (25% of shoulders) relative to the scapular plane. Excessive retroversion has been correlated with posterior instability.[3,17] Hurley et al. concluded the following:

1. Rotator cuff strengthening should be the first course of treatment for posterior instability.
2. Soft tissue surgery has a high rate of recurrence.
3. The return to sports is variable.[17]

Fluid properties, such as joint volume and adhesion and cohesion, play a role in passive stability. The finite volume of joint fluid creates a situation where motion beyond a certain point is inhibited by a negative pressure, pulling the capsule inward.[26] This negative pressure (vacuum) is further enhanced by the normal negative intraarticular pressure. Adhesion and cohesion properties are best understood by visualizing two microscope slides with a drop of water in between. The slides may be easily slid back and forth

but are difficult to pull apart. This is a similar relationship to the humeral head in the glenoid fossa. The effectiveness of both of these fluid properties is diminished in a shoulder with increased capsular laxity. Additionally, introducing air into the joint significantly increased subluxation in all directions in one cadaver study.[26] This may be from the loss of the negative pressure in the joint.

Ligamentous and capsular restraints provide static stability to the glenohumeral joint. The superior, middle, and inferior glenohumeral ligaments have been discussed previously. These soft tissues provide stability in a small portion of the shoulder range, since they must be under tension to provide stability. The inferior glenohumeral ligament, with the posteroinferior capsule, provides the primary restraint to anterior translation, while the posteroinferior capsule alone provides the primary restraint to posterior translation.[26]

The glenoid labrum functions to deepen the glenoid fossa and provides additional stability (Figure 19-1). It serves as an attachment for the glenohumeral ligaments and the long head of the biceps tendon. The labrum frequently becomes detached during anterior dislocations (Bankart lesion) (Figure 19-24).

Dynamic muscular stability is of primary importance to the sports therapist. Selective contraction of the shoulder girdle muscles can provide significant stability to the glenohumeral joint. The rotator cuff and long head of the biceps function to secure the humeral head of the glenoid fossa and maintain its central position. Additionally, selective muscle contraction can adjust tension in the capsule, thus acting like dynamic ligaments. For example, contraction of the infraspinatus and teres minor produces tension in the inferior glenohumeral ligament at forces of external rotation greater than 20 pounds, thus reinforcing this ligament.[6] This dynamic muscular stability is the focus of the rehabilitation program.

Key Issues in Rehabilitation of the Unstable Shoulder

It is important to determine the direction of instability when establishing the rehabilitation program. Most instabilities are anterior and inferior but may be posterior or multidirectional. In the early and intermediate rehabilitation phases, many of the exercises will be the same, regardless of instability direction. This is because of the interrelationships within the capsular fibers. However, the program will be-

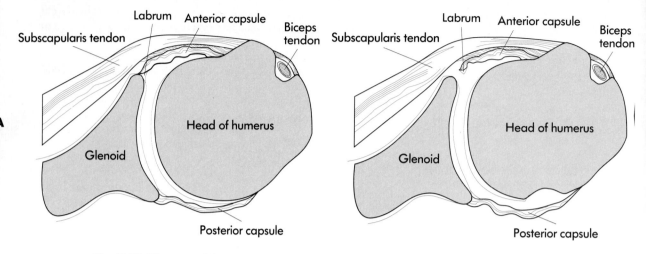

Fig. 19-24. Diagrams of the Bankart and Hill Sachs lesions. A, Normal glenohumeral joint and articulations. **B,** Bankart lesion where the labrum is pulled away from the anterior glenoid, along with a small piece of the glenoid. The Hill Sachs lesion is a compression fracture of the posterior humeral head.

come specialized as it approaches the late and functional progression phases.

The voluntary or involuntary nature of the dislocation/subluxation, the chronicity of the problem, age, and lifestyle will all play a role in program design. The athlete with a voluntary component or multiple dislocations will have difficulty fully recovering from this problem. The athlete who has sustained several dislocations will likely be immobilized for a shorter length of time and progress faster in the rehabilitation program than the athlete with a first-time dislocation. The backstroke swimmer with subluxations will require different rehabilitation than the wrestler who sustained an acute dislocation. In addition, the athlete with an unstable shoulder, with or without frank dislocation, will often present with impingement syndrome as well.

The acronyms TUBS and AMBRI have been used to guide treatment decisions. Those athletes with a *T*raumatic *U*nidirectional injury and a *B*ankart lesion often require *S*urgery, while those with *A*traumatic, *M*ultidirectional, *B*ilateral instability usually respond best to *R*ehabilitation; however, these athletes often progress to *I*nferior capsular shift procedures. The Bankart lesion is an avulsion of the capsulolabral complex from the anteroinferior neck of the glenoid (see Figure 19-24). A second defect frequently seen with anterior dislocations is the Hill-Sachs lesion. This is a posterior humeral head defect resulting from

compression of the humeral head on the anterior glenoid lip as is passes out anteriorly and rests against the glenoid fossa (see Figure 19-24). Burkhead and Rockwood evaluated the results of a conservative rehabilitation program on unstable shoulders and found a 16% good or excellent result in those with traumatic subluxations and an 80% good or excellent result in those with atraumatic subluxations.[5]

All stretching and joint mobilization activities must be approached with caution when dealing with instability. The underlying problem is excessive mobility and a resultant unstable shoulder. Overstretching the joint capsule will only compound the problem. Gentle stretching exercises should be incorporated where musculotendinous inflexibility is noted. The athlete should be cautioned that a "more is better" attitude applied to stretching can be detrimental in this situation. Training the athlete to feel levels of overstretch is the first step in proprioceptive training.

Proprioceptive training will be essential in the rehabilitation program. Smith and Brunolli demonstrated the loss of joint proprioception after anterior glenohumeral dislocation.[40] Because of the unstable shoulder's increased joint capsule laxity, mechanoreceptors are not excited until the humeral head is subluxed and the joint capsule stretched. The soft tissues about the shoulder must be retrained to fire before the humeral head has passed anatomical limits.

Rehabilitation of the Unstable Shoulder

Rehabilitation for both posterior and anteroinferior dislocations will be considered together. Specific differences between programs for anterior vs. posterior dislocations will be noted in each phase. Additionally, athletes experiencing subluxation should be initiated in their program with intermediate phase activities.

EARLY PHASE. The goal in the early rehabilitation phase is to protect the injured soft tissues during initiation of the healing process. Some period of immobilization may be required and will vary depending upon age, number of previous dislocations, and philosophy of the primary caregiver. Length of immobilization may vary from days (for comfort only) to 3 to 6 weeks. A number of studies demonstrates different outcomes based on immobilization length.[21,36,39] Matsen et al. conclude that the incidence of recurrence is not significantly affected by type and length of immobilization.[26] However, there is consensus that athletes under age 20 are at significant risk for reinjury from the high rate of avulsion of the capsulolabral complex from the anterior glenoid lip (Bankart lesion). Matsen et al. suggest immobilization from 2 to 5 weeks for young athletes and shorter periods for athletes over age 30.[26] Athletes with an acute posterior dislocation may be immobilized in neutral rotation rather than in a traditional sling in internal rotation. This will decrease the tension on the posterior structure while healing.

Exercises for the contralateral extremity and the lower extremities may be performed during this rehabilitation phase. An exercise bike or walking may be used as cardiovascular conditioning. The sling may be removed for elbow, wrist, and hand mobility activities. Strengthening exercises may be performed for the wrist and forearm as long as traction is not placed on the humerus in doing so. The liberal use of ice will reduce shoulder pain.

INTERMEDIATE PHASE. The goal in the intermediate phase is to achieve full active range of motion and a baseline of strength. This phase begins 2 to 5 weeks after injury for the athlete with an acute dislocation and as soon as pain subsides for the athlete with subluxation or a chronic instability. Those with a subluxating shoulder or chronic instability will likely have little or no loss of mobility, and therefore the exercise program should focus on strength.

Mobility activities should consist of Codman's pendulum exercises; active, passive, and active-assisted exercises; pulleys; and gentle stretching. Pain should be a guide for frequency and intensity of the exercise program. Overstretching the healing tissue will only delay return to sport. These mobility activities are similar, regardless of the dislocation direction.

The strengthening program should be initiated with isometric exercises performed in neutral position. This includes flexion, extension, abduction, adduction, internal, and external rotation. The athlete should be cautioned that this does not mean "all or none." The amount of force should stay below the level of pain and should gradually increase as healing occurs. These exercises should be performed hourly based on their daily schedule. Students are encouraged to perform 10 to 20 repetitions of each exercise every time they go into a new class.

When tolerated, these isometric exercises should be progressed to isotonic exercises through a range of motion. Performing exercises in the plane of the scapula will prevent undue strain on the anterior or posterior capsule. The exercises for the rotator cuff outlined in the impingement section may be used at this stage of rehabilitation. The compressive role of the rotator cuff makes it a key in rehabilitation of both the anterior and posterior dislocation and subluxations. The infraspinatus and teres minor should receive special attention because of their role in producing tension in the inferior glenohumeral ligament. Exercises should be performed in a controlled manner, focusing on normal movement patterns and control of the weight. As such, free weight exercises are optimal for retraining proprioception while strengthening. PNF techniques may be used to facilitate return of normal firing patterns. Scapular stabilizing exercises should be incorporated; particular attention should be paid to the posterior capsule stress when performing scapular protraction exercises in athletes with posterior dislocations (for example, any push-up activities).

Isokinetic exercise may be used to develop a solid baseline of strength. Exercises should again be performed in a controlled manner. Internal and external rotation should be performed in slight abduction, and high-speed exercise should be limited to 90 degrees of elevation. Slow, controlled motions may be performed past 90 degrees. The goal is to achieve a solid strength base to be converted to functional strength and endurance in the next phase. When the athlete has full, pain-free range of motion, full strength, and is free of symptom exacerbations, they may be progressed to the next phase.

LATE PHASE - PROVOCATIVE PROGRAM. The purpose

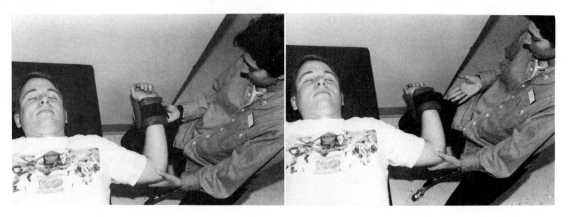

Fig. 19-25. Provocative exercise. The athlete is asked to "catch" the weight as the therapist drops it. The athlete must be relaxed and the therapist prepared to protect the athlete's shoulder.

of this phase is to convert the athlete's baseline strength into the appropriate power and endurance demands of their sport. A second goal is to prepare the athlete for forces encountered in their sport that put them at risk for reinjury. To this end, a provocative program is an essential component of the rehabilitation program.

Strengthening exercises should be advanced to overhead positions. Flexion should be performed through a full range of motion, and rotation exercises should be performed at 90 degrees abduction. Resistive tubing exercises may be added for endurance and should be progressed to high speeds to more closely simulate sport activities. These exercises may also be performed in an overhead position. The exercises should reproduce the demands of the sport in working range of motion, speed, repetitions, open vs. closed chain, and motor patterns. The athlete with shoulder subluxations will have a very different program from the athlete with a frank dislocation, in addition to program differences related to sport. Exercises should continue to focus on strengthening all muscles in the upper kinetic chain, with particular attention to the rotator cuff. However, instead of isolating the rotator cuff as in the intermediate phase, the rotator cuff is now asked to work in concert with other shoulder musculature. Latissimus pull-downs, military press, pectoral flys, and bench pressing may be used as tools to train glenohumeral stabilization while other muscle groups are working as primary movers.

A program to present controlled perturbations to the shoulder in provocative positions is a necessary

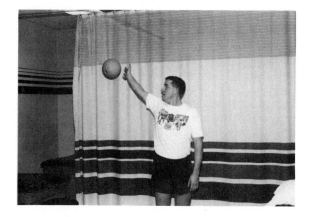

Fig. 19-26. Provocative plyometric ball activity. The athlete is required to catch the ball in progressively provocative positions at higher velocities.

precursor to the functional progression. This prepares the athlete both physically and psychologically and retrains the proprioceptive system to respond to a stimulus. Those athletes with anterior dislocations/subluxations should be stressed or "perturbed" in abduction and external rotation, while those with posterior instability should be stressed in a position of flexion, adduction, and internal rotation. A simple beginning exercise for anterior instability requires the athlete to lie on their back with their arm unsupported, in 90 degrees abduction and full external rotation. The athlete is asked to close their eyes and completely relax their shoulder, while the therapist supports a weight in their hand. The therapist must

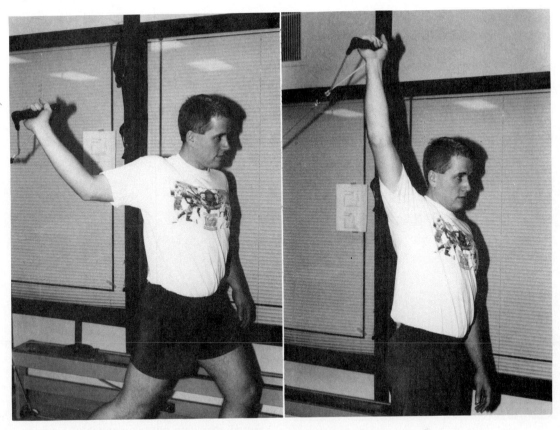

Fig. 19-27. Provocative training on the impulse inertial exercise system. High speed, low resistance movements in progressively provocative positions are used.

place their knee or other object just under the athlete's hand as a safeguard. When the athlete is completely relaxed, the therapist releases the athlete's hand, requiring the athlete to fire their rotator cuff to stabilize their shoulder (Figure 19-25). Activities like this can be progressed to catching a small plyometric ball in an overhead, externally rotated position at increasing velocities (Figure 19-26).

Exercises should be performed at the end range of motion for external rotation at various positions of abduction. The Inertial Exercise System* is a good piece of equipment for performing these exercises. Flexion, extension, abduction, and adduction can be performed in a full overhead position or at varying positions throughout the range of motion (Figure 19-

27). The athlete should be worked to fatigue in these positions, since they will encounter these situations when fatigued in a competitive setting. The therapist may also consider isokinetically testing athletes when they are fatigued, since this is the most critical time in a game situation.

Athletes who sustain a posterior dislocation may benefit from plyometric activities to perturb the shoulder. Because of the mechanism of injury (a posteriorly directed force along a flexed humerus), bench presses and wall push-ups should be progressed to plyometric wall-push-ups or push-ups using a Shuttle 2000-1* (Figure 19-28). This can be progressed to push-ups in the standard position, either using plyometrics for quick firing or repetition

---

*Impulse Inertial Exercise System, Newnan, GA.

*Shuttle 2000-1, Glacier, WA.

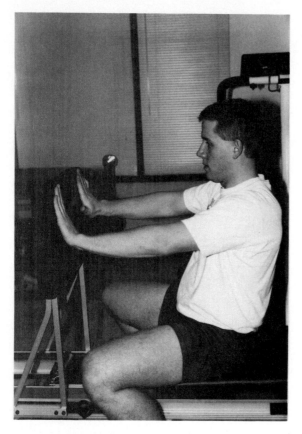

Fig. 19-28. Shuttle 2000-1. The Shuttle 2000-1 can be used for upper extremity proprioceptive exercises or plyometric activities.

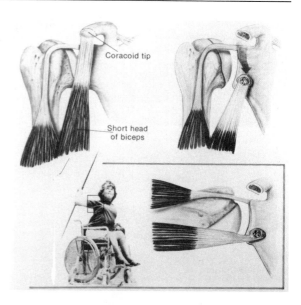

Fig. 19-29. The Bristow procedure. The coracoid along with the attached coracobrachialis and short head of the biceps is transferred to the anterior glenoid rim. (From Kuland DN: *The injured athlete*, ed 1, Philadelphia, 1982, JB Lippincott.)

for endurance. The athlete should demonstrate good control of the glenohumeral joint before placing it in any provocative situation.

FUNCTIONAL PROGRESSION PHASE. The functional progression phase is of particular importance in the athlete with an unstable shoulder. Simple strengthening alone will not prepare the neuromuscular system for the possibility of reinjury in a sports situation. The athlete must be confident in full use of their shoulder for all aspects of their sport. For the bicyclist with posterior instability, gradual controlled weight-bearing on both their hands and their elbows (aerobars) must be initiated for varying time periods and speeds. This should be progressed to training in this position when fatigued (for example, after rehabilitation exercises). The swimmer with multidirectional instability should be gradually returned to the pool,

with controls placed on stroke, speed, distance, and intensity. Gradually, the limitations should be decreased, changing only one variable at a time, until the previous level of activity is reached. This may take several weeks but is more acceptable than a reoccurrence and return to the early stage of rehabilitation.

The gymnast with subluxations or dislocation is a particular challenge to the sports therapist, and their rehabilitation and functional progression should mimic their particular event. One should expect a protracted course of rehabilitation and lengthy functional progression to fully return this athlete to their sport.

Surgical Stabilization Procedures

There are several stabilization procedures used to control anteroinferior dislocation. Each procedure has its benefits and drawbacks, and each surgeon has their own preference. Procedures are categorized by the mechanism of stabilization and generally include capsular procedures, coracoid transfer/bone blocks, and subscapularis transfers. The Bristow procedure is an example of a coracoid transfer. In this case, the

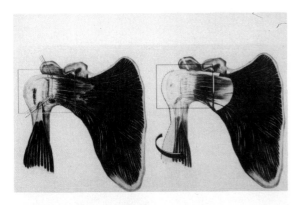

Fig. 19-30. The Magnusen Stack procedure. The subscapularis tendon and capsule are transferred to the lateral side of the bicipital groove, distal to the greater tuberosity.
(From Kuland DN: *The injured athlete,* ed 1, Philadelphia, 1982, JB Lippincott.)

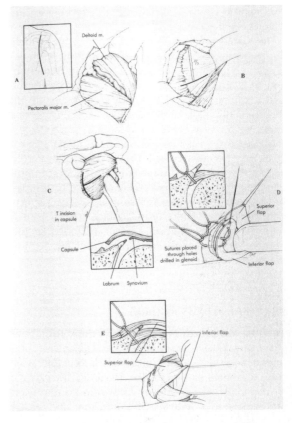

Fig. 19-31. The Bankart procedure and capsulolabral reconstruction. In a simple Bankart procedure, the detached glenoid labrum and anterior capsule are reattached to the anterior glenoid. To reconstruct the anterior capsule, a T-incision is made in the capsule, and the interior flap is pulled superiorly and attached to the anterior glenoid. The superior flap is sutured into place, reinforcing the anterior capsule.
(From Nicholas JA, Hershman ED, editors: *The upper extremity in sports medicine,* St Louis, 1990, Mosby.)

tip of the coracoid process, along with the short head of the biceps and coracobrachialis attachments, are detached and reattached at the anterior margin of the glenoid (Figure 19-29). One advantage of this procedure is the early rehabilitation because of the inherent stability provided by the bony block. However, the loss of 6 to 10 degrees or more of external rotation makes it an unacceptable procedure for a throwing athlete.[20] After a Bristow procedure, the athlete may begin stretching and range-of-motion exercises after the first week and resistive exercises at approximately 3 weeks. Exercises are the same as noted in the previous instability section.

The Putti-Platt procedure is an example of a subscapular muscle transfer procedure. Stability is provided by overlapping and shortening the subscapularis tendon by suturing the lateral portion to the anterior glenoid lip. The Magnuseon Stack procedure also transfers the subscapularis tendon. In this case, it is transferred from the lesser tuberosity to the greater tuberosity (Figure 19-30). However, both of these procedures usually result in a loss of external rotation motion, which may be unacceptable to some athletes. Passive and active-assisted range of motion may be initiated at 3 weeks after surgery and continued for 4 weeks. Gentle isometrics may be performed at this stage. At 6 weeks after surgery, resistive exercises may be added. Total rehabilitation will take 4 to 6 months. Jobe et al. feel that neither of these procedures are acceptable for the thrower because of significant external rotation loss.[20]

The Bankart operation and capsulolabral reconstruction are commonly used capsular procedures. The Bankart procedure directly addresses the Bankart lesion by reattaching the labrum to the glenoid rim via drill holes through the bone (Figure 19-31). This procedure results in little loss of external rotation, a key factor for throwing athletes. Capsulolabral procedures also address the Bankart lesion and additionally allow the surgeon to tighten the joint capsule if necessary. Because of the soft tissue nature of this reconstruction, the rehabilitation course may be longer than with bony procedures, and particular attention should be paid to performing exercises in the scapular plane.

Jobe et al. prefer to immobilize their athletes after a capsulolabral reconstruction in a position of 90 degrees abduction, 30 degrees horizontal adduction, and 45 degrees external rotation for 2 weeks.[20] The brace may be removed for gentle passive flexion, abduction, adduction, and external rotation. Isometric exercises for the shoulder and mobility exercises for the elbow may also be performed. Codman's exercises may be initiated at 2 to 3 weeks after surgery and more aggressive range-of-motion and strengthening exercises at 6 weeks. Isokinetic exercises may be initiated at 8 weeks. Return to noncontact sports is generally at 4 months and contact sports is at 6 months. In all procedures, the rehabilitation should follow the program outlined in the previous section once the appropriate stage of healing has been reached.

BRACHIAL PLEXUS INJURIES

The brachial plexus is formed from the ventral rami of C5 through T1. It passes between the anterior and middle scalene muscles, under the sternocleidomastoid, and behind the medial third of the clavicle to the axilla. It may be injured from compression (thoracic outlet syndrome), contusion, or traction injuries.

The typical picture of a brachial plexus injury in sports is that of a traction injury, usually the result of shoulder depression and lateral cervical flexion in the opposite direction. The point of contact on the shoulder is more medial that that of acromioclavicular joint injuries (Figure 19-32). This syndrome of brachial plexus stretch injuries is termed the *burner* or *stinger* syndrome. These injuries usually involve the C5 and C6 levels. The athlete will complain of a sharp, burning pain in the shoulder that radiates down the arm into the hand. Weakness in the muscles supplied by C5 to C6 (deltoid, biceps, supraspinatus, and infraspinatus) accompanies the pain. The weakness may last only a few minutes or indefinitely.

Clancy et al. have classified brachial plexus injuries into three categories.[8] A grade I injury results in a transient loss of motor and sensory function, which usually resolves completely within 2 weeks. Motor function usually returns within minutes. A grade II injury results in significant motor weakness and sensory loss that may last from 6 weeks to 4

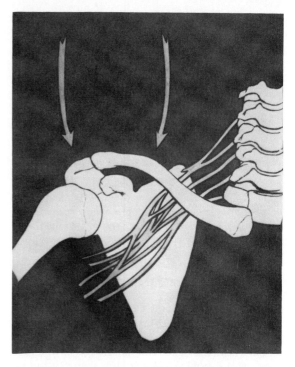

Fig. 19-32. Acromioclavicular joint injuries. The point of initial impact in acromioclavicular joint injuries is usually over the acromion, while in brachial plexus injuries, it is more medial.
(From Nicholas JA, Hershman EB, editors: *The upper extremity in sports medicine*, St Louis, 1990, Mosby.)

months.[45] EMG evaluation after 2 weeks will demonstrate abnormalities. Grade III lesions are characterized by motor and sensory loss for at least 1 year's duration.

Athletes are allowed to return to play when they have full, pain-free range of motion, full strength, and no prior episodes in that contest.[45] Additionally, football players should use a cervical neck roll. The goals of treatment are to restore normal mobility in the neck and upper extremity and to strengthen any weakened muscles and the cervical musculature.

Early Phase

The goal in this phase is to restore normal mobility to the neck and upper extremity. This phase should be initiated when the athlete's acute pain has subsided. Gentle passive stretching of the cervical muscles should be performed by the sports therapist who can control the degree of stretch. Stretches should focus on all cervical spine motions, and lateral flexion should be approached cautiously in the acute phase. Gentle isometric exercises for the cervical musculature and isotonic exercises for the upper extremity may be initiated. Strength training for all other extremities and cardiovascular conditioning may be continued. Ergometer rowing provides isometric resistance to all posterior spine stabilizing muscles while working both the upper and lower extremities. When full, pain-free range of motion of the cervical spine is achieved, the athlete may progress to the next phase.

Intermediate Phase

The goal in this phase is the restoration of strength in the neck and arm musculature. Cervical spine muscle strengthening may be performed through a range of motion. Isokinetic exercise for the shoulder will facilitate full return of strength. All muscle groups demonstrating weakness should be worked both concentrically and eccentrically and at a variety of speeds. Weakness may be undetectable by manual testing techniques because of an athlete's baseline of strength that is greater than that of a sedentary individual. The sports therapist should incorporate their knowledge of neuroanatomy to train the muscle groups innervated by the specific lesion level. Cardiovascular conditioning may be progressed to running, if this is a functional activity for the athlete's sport. When the athlete has achieved a solid baseline of strength, they may be progressed to the next phase. This may be only a matter of days in the athlete with a grade I injury.

Late Phase

The rehabilitation goal in the late phase is to convert the established strength into power or endurance as dictated by the demands of the sport. The strengthening program should become sport-specific, with emphasis on the speed, range of motion, repetitions, type of muscle contraction, open or closed chain, and motor programming required by the sport. Cervical strengthening should be continued and cardiovascular training advanced. The strength program should be maintained at least three times weekly for the duration of the season. When the athlete demon-

strates full strength, endurance, and power as demanded by their sport, they may begin a functional progression.

Functional Progression Phase

The athlete must complete a functional program before returning to their sport. The sports therapist must design a program of progressive return to activity to prepare the athlete for both the physical and psychological aspects of return to the activity that caused their injury. Because of the apprehension caused by neurological injuries, the psychological component may be even more critical for the athlete. The athlete with chronic burners should have their playing style evaluated, since they may be placing themselves at undue risk with their behavior. Additionally, football players should use a cervical roll as a mechanical block to excessive lateral flexion. As the athlete is progressed back into their sport, every attempt should be made to prevent a reoccurrence of the injury. This includes evaluation of playing style and physical and psychological readiness.

THORACIC OUTLET SYNDROME

Thoracic outlet syndrome is a collection of signs and symptoms resulting from compression of the subclavian artery, vein, and brachial plexus. The symptoms are typically complaints of pain, paresthesia, and paresis of the neck, upper extremity, and hand. This generally follows activities involving overhead use of the arm or carrying heavy objects in the hand or across the shoulder. There are two common patterns, an upper root pattern (C5 to C7) and a lower root pattern (C8 to T1).[16] The lower roots, and specifically the ulnar nerve, are more commonly involved because of the anatomical position of the medial cord.[23] The cause of neurovascular bundle compression may be soft tissue or bony. The compressing structures include, but are not limited to, a cervical rib, the scalene musculature, or the costoclavicular joint (Figure 19-33).[16,23] Sleeping in a hyperabducted position may also initiate symptoms.

Evaluation procedures attempt to reproduce symptoms via provocative tests. These include Adson's maneuver, Halstead's maneuver, and the costoclavicular, hyperabduction, and 3-minute elevated arm tests.[23] Although the symptoms in the majority of patients are neurological, these tests evaluate the

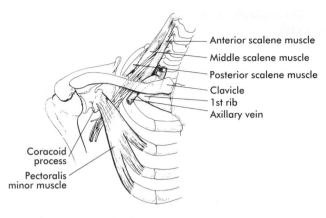

Fig. 19-33. Pertinent anatomy in thoracic outlet syndrome.
(From Mascaro D, Pratt NE: *Clinical musculoskeletal anatomy,* Philadelphia, 1991, JB Lippincott.)

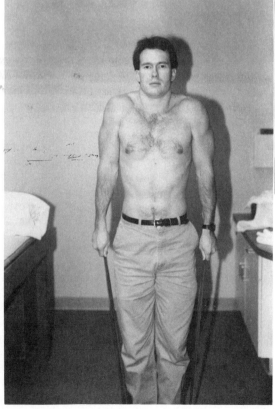

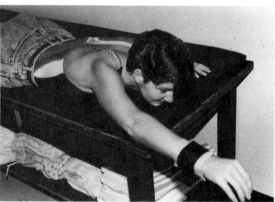

Fig. 19-34. Exercises used in the treatment of thoracic outlet syndrome. A, Upper trapezius strengthening. **B,** Lower trapezius strengthening.

C 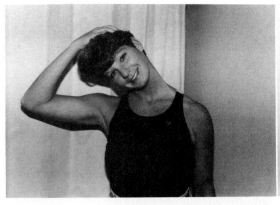   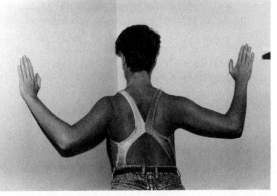 D

Fig. 19-34, cont'd. C, Lateral neck flexor stretch. **D,** Pectoral stretching.

vascular component by assessing pulse changes with arm and head position changes.

Treatment of Thoracic Outlet Syndrome

Conservative management of thoracic outlet syndrome results in 50% to 90% recovery rate and is therefore the first course of treatment. Postural exercises should be the focus of the exercise program.[16,22,23] Leffert emphasizes the importance of evaluating the patient's lifestyle and work habits to identify where postural problems lie.[22] The athlete's sport must be assessed if they are experiencing symptoms during participation. The importance of maintaining good posture throughout the day must be emphasized to the athlete.

Therapeutic exercises should focus on the strengthening and stretching of specific soft tissues. Lutz and Gieck emphasize stretching the scalenes, lateral neck flexors, and pectoral muscles while strengthening the upper, middle, and lower trapezius; serratus anterior; erector of spine; and deltoid muscles (Figure 19-34).[23] Proper breathing technique is also important in the prevention and treatment of scalene syndrome. The scalenes are accessory breathing muscles, and improper breathing techniques will cause tightening of these muscles and exacerbation of their symptoms. Proper abdominal breathing techniques should be taught, and athletes should be aware of their breathing style.

Failure to respond to appropriate, supervised physical therapy may necessitate surgical intervention. Leffert reports the indications for surgery to be the following:

1. Failure to respond to physical therapy.
2. Functionally significant muscle weakness or sensory loss in the hand.
3. Intractable pain.
4. Impending vascular catastrophe.[22]

The surgical procedure will vary depending upon the anatomical basis for the patient's symptoms.

SUMMARY

1. The shoulder girdle is a series of joints and articulations that function together to provide smooth, coordinated movement. The importance of the scapula and scapular muscles must be acknowledged.
2. Evaluation of the athlete's position and sport, in addition to evaluation of their shoulder girdle, will provide important information about their injury and rehabilitation needs.
3. Isokinetic exercise is a valuable tool in the rehabilitation of shoulder injuries. The sport therapist should make decisions about position, speed, and intensity based on their understanding of the pathology and healing process.
4. Proprioceptive exercises should be initiated early in the rehabilitation process and form the basis for subsequent exercises. Free weight exercises are a good way to carry proprioceptive activities into the intermediate and late rehabilitation phases.
5. The rotator cuff plays a primary role in the treatment of many shoulder problems. The importance of the rotator cuff in dynamic stability makes rotator cuff strengthening exercises the

core program when treating anterior or posterior instability.

6. The scapula is the support base for the glenohumeral joint. Scapular strengthening and stabilizing exercises should be a part of every shoulder rehabilitation program.

7. A functional progression prepares the athlete both physically and psychologically for return to their sport. The functional progression is an extension of the progressive resistive exercise program and progressively increases the athlete's participation in their sport. This should be tailored specifically to the needs of each individual athlete.

8. An understanding of the anatomy, pathology, biomechanics, and healing process of a particular injury or surgical procedure provides the best basis for determining the appropriateness of any given exercise. The sports therapist should be familiar with these aspects of shoulder care in the athlete.

9. Rehabilitation techniques change based on new research findings and new surgical procedures. The sports therapist must remain abreast of these changes and update their programs based on these findings and their experience.

10. Reevaluation throughout the rehabilitation process will provide data on its effectiveness. The programs included in this chapter are not absolute, but interactive, and require positive feedback from outcome-based evaluations.

REFERENCES

1 Axe MJ, Konin J: Distance based criteria interval throwing program, *J Sport Rehab* 1(4):326-336, 1992.

2 Bergfeld JA: Acromioclavicular complex. In Nicholas JA, Hershman EB, editors: *The upper extremity in sports medicine,* St Louis, 1990, Mosby.

3 Brewer BJ, Wubben RC, Carrera GF: Excessive retroversion of the glenoid cavity. A cause of nontraumatic posterior instability of the shoulder, *J Bone Joint Surg* 68(5):724-731, 1986.

4 Brown L, Niehues S, Harrah A, et al.: Upper extremity range of motion and isokinetic strength of the internal and external shoulder rotators in major league baseball players, *Am J Sports Med* 16:577-585, 1988.

5 Burkhead WZ, Rockwood CA: Treatment of instability of the shoulder with an exercise program, *J Bone Joint Surg* 74[A](6):890-896, 1992.

6 Cain PR, Mutschler TA, Fu FH, et al.: Anterior stability of the glenohumeral joint: a dynamic model, *Am J Sports Med* 15(2):144-148, 1987.

7 Chandler TJ, Kibler WB, Stracener EC, et al.: Shoulder strength, power, and endurance in college tennis players, *Am J Sports Med* 20(4):455-458, 1992.

8 Clancy WG, Brand RL, Bergfeld JA: Upper trunk brachial plexus injuries in contact sports, *Am J Sports Med* 5:209, 1977.

9 Cox JS: Current method of treatment of acromioclavicular joint dislocations, *Orthopaedics* 15(9):1041-1044, 1992.

10 Craig EV: Fractures of the clavicle. In Rockwood CA, Matsen FA, editors: *The shoulder,* Philadelphia, 1990, WB Saunders.

11 Dickoff-Hoffman S: *Post-operative elbow rehabilitation.* Presented at the HealthSouth Sports Medicine Seminar: The Shoulder, Dallas, TX, 1992.

12 Falkel J, Murphy T, Murray T: Prone positioning for testing shoulder internal and external rotation on the Cybex II isokinetic dynamometer, *J Orthop Sports Phys Ther* 8:368-370, 1987.

13 Greenfield BH, Donatelli R, Wooden MJ, et al.: Isokinetic evaluation of shoulder rotational strength between the plane of scapula and the frontal plane, *Am J Sports Med* 18(2):124-128, 1990.

14 Hawkins RJ, Abrams JS: Impingement syndrome in the absence of rotator cuff tear, *Orthop Clin North Am* 18(3):373-382, 1987.

15 Hinton RY: Isokinetic evaluation of shoulder rotational strength in high school baseball pitchers, *Am J Sports Med* 16(3):274-279, 1988.

16 Howell JW: Evaluation and management of thoracic outlet syndrome. In Donatelli R, editor: *Physical therapy of the shoulder,* New York, 1987, Churchill Livingstone.

17 Hurley JA, Anderson TE, Dear W, et al.: Posterior shoulder instability: surgical versus conservative results with evaluation of glenoid version, *Am J Sports Med* 20(4):396-400, 1992.

18 Irrgang JJ, Whitney SL, Harner CD: Nonoperative treatment of rotator cuff injuries in throwing athletes, *J Sports Rehab* (1)3:197-222, 1992.

19 Ivey F, Cahlhoun J, Rusche K, et al.: Normal values for isokinetic testing of shoulder strength, *Arch Phys Med Rehabil* 66:384-386, 1985.

20 Jobe FW, Tibone JE, Jobe CM, et al.: The shoulder in sports. In Rockwood CA, Matsen FA, editors: *The shoulder,* Philadelphia, 1990, WB Saunders.

21 Kiviluoto O, Pasila M, Jaroma H, et al.: Immobilization after primary dislocation of the shoulder, *Acta Orthop Scand* 51:915-919, 1980.

22 Leffert RD: Neurological problems. In Rockwood CA, Matsen FA, editors: *The shoulder,* Philadelphia, 1990, WB Saunders.

23 Lutz FR, Gieck JH: Thoracic outlet compression syndrome, *Athletic Training* 21(4):302-311, 1986.

24 Maddux REC, Kibler WB, Uhl T: Isokinetic peak torque and work values for the shoulder, *J Orthop Sports Phys Ther* 10(7):264-269, 1989.

25 Matsen FA, Arntz CT: Subacromial impingement. In Rockwood CA, Matsen FA, editors: *The shoulder,* Philadelphia, 1990, WB Saunders.

26 Matsen FA, Thomas SC, Rockwood CA: Anterior glenohumeral instability. In Rockwood CA, Matsen FA, editors: *The shoulder,* Philadelphia, 1990, WB Saunders.

27 Moseley JB, Jobe FW, Pink M, et al.: EMG analysis of the scapular muscles during a shoulder rehabilitation program, *Am J Sports Med* 20(2):128-134, 1992.

28 Neer CS: Anterior acromioplasty for the chronic impingement syndrome in the shoulder, *J Bone Joint Surg* 54[A](1):41-50, 1972.

29 Neer CS: Impingement lesions, *Clin Orthop* 173:70-77, 1983.

30 Neviaser RJ: Lesions of the biceps and tendinitis of the shoulder, *Orthop Clin North Am* 11(2):343-348, 1980.

31 Nirschl RP: Soft-tissue injuries about the elbow, *Clin Sports Med* 5(4):637-652, 1985.

32 O'Brien SJ, Arnoczky SP, Warren RF, et al.: Developmental anatomy of the shoulder and anatomy of the glenohumeral joint. In Rockwood CA, Matsen FA, editors: *The shoulder,* Philadelphia, 1990, WB Saunders.

33 Pawlowski D, Perrin D: Relationship between shoulder and elbow isokinetic peak torque, torque acceleration energy, average power, and total work and throwing velocity in intercollegiate pitchers, *Athletic Training* 24(2):129-132, 1989.

34 Pianka G, Hershman EB: Neurovascular injuries. In Nicholas JA, Hershman EB, editors: *The upper extremity in sports medicine,* St Louis, 1990, Mosby.

35 Rockwood CA, Young DC: Disorders of the acromioclavicular joint. In Rockwood CA, Matsen FA, editors: *The shoulder,* Philadelphia, 1990, WB Saunders.

36 Rowe CR: Acute and recurrent anterior dislocations of the shoulder, *Orthop Clin North Am* 11:253-269, 1980.

37 Sanders MT: Weight training and conditioning. In Sanders B, editor: *Sports physical therapy,* Norwalk, CT, 1990, Appleton & Lange.

38 Schwartz RE, O'Brien SJ, Warren RF, et al.: Capsular restraints to anterior-posterior motion of the abducted shoulder: a biomechanical study, *Ortho Trans* 12(3):727, 1988.

39 Simonet WT, Cofield RH: Prognosis in anterior shoulder dislocation, *Am J Sports Med* 12:19-24, 1984.

40 Smith FL, Brunolli J: Shoulder kinesthesia after anterior glenohumeral dislocation, *Phys Ther* 69:106-112, 1989.

41 Tibone J, Sellers R, Tonino P: Strength testing after third-degree acromioclavicular dislocations, *Am J Sports Med* 220(3):328-331, 1992.

42 Townsend H, Jobe FW, Pink M, et al.: Electromyographic analysis of the glenohumeral muscles during a baseball rehabilitation program, *Am J Sports Med* 19(3):264-275, 1991.

43 Turkel SJ, Panio MW, Marshall JL, et al.: Stabilizing mechanisms preventing anterior dislocation of the glenohumeral joint, *J Bone Joint Surg* 63[A]:1208-1217, 1981.

44 Walker SW, Couch W, Boester G, et al.: Isokinetic strength of the shoulder after repair of a torn rotator cuff, *J Bone Joint Surg* 69[A](7):1041-1044, 1987.

45 Warren RF: Neurological injuries in football. In Jordan BD, Tsairis P, Warren RF, editors: *Sports neurology,* Rockville, MD, 1989, Aspen Publications.

46 Wilk KE, Arrigo CA, Andrews JR: Standardized isokinetic testing protocol for the throwing shoulder: the thrower's series, *Isokin Exer Sci* 1(2):63-71, 1991.

Rehabilitation of Elbow Injuries

Steven Dickoff-Hoffman and Danny Foster

OBJECTIVES

After completion of this chapter, the student should be able to do the following:

- Discuss important rehabilitation concepts for treating injuries to the elbow.

- Discuss treatment of acute inflammation, injuries involving the joint structures, and injuries involving the musculotendinous units of the elbow.

- Discuss various exercise techniques in the management of elbow soft tissue recovery.

- Recognize and explain the differences between rehabilitation procedures for elbow joint restrictions and joint laxities.

- Outline a plan of therapeutic exercise designed to manage common elbow trauma.

Rehabilitation of elbow injuries in sports requires a complete understanding of the stresses imposed on the elbow during various athletic activities. In sports activities, the upper extremity usually functions in an open kinetic chain. However, there are sports, such as gymnastics and wrestling, that require the upper extremity to function in a closed-chain fashion. Both open- and closed-chain athletic activities can result in injury, which would necessitate the development of specific rehabilitation programs aimed at complete functional restoration, thereby allowing the athlete to resume activity without risk of reinjury.

The elbow is a hinged joint that is capable of 145 degrees of flexion from a fully extended position. In some cases of joint hyperelasticity, the joint may hyperextend a few degrees beyond neutral.

The elbow consists of the humeroulnar, humeroradial, and radioulnar articulations (Figure 20-1). The concave radial head articulates with the convex surface of the capitellum of the distal humerus and is connected to the proximal ulna via the annular ligament. The proximal radioulnar joint constitutes the forearm, which when working in conjunction with

the elbow joint permits approximately 90 degrees of pronation and 80 degrees of supination.

In athletic activity, the elbow must perform several functions. In throwing sports, the elbow helps to propel an object at a rapid velocity with accuracy. In power sports, such as hitting, the elbow must possess static stability and adequate dynamic strength to be able to transfer force to a hitting implement. In swimming, the elbow must be able to produce power and stability to propel the swimmer through the water. In gymnastics, the elbow functions in a closed-chain fashion in both static and dynamic modes to provide stability and propulsive power.

Regardless of the injured anatomical structure within the elbow joint, the rehabilitation program must be designed to address inflammation, restricted mobility, pain, weakness, and functional disability. The ultimate goal of any rehabilitation program is to permit the athlete to be able to resume athletic competition with minimal functional disability and risk of reinjury. The goals of elbow rehabilitation may be simply categorized as follows:

1. Diminish pain and inflammation.

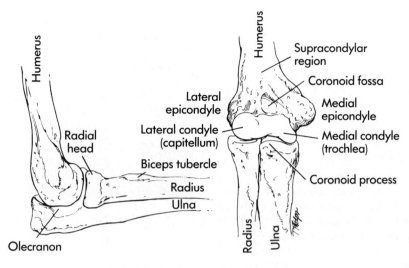

Fig. 20-1. Anatomy of the elbow joint.

2. Regain normal joint arthrokinematics.
3. Regain strength, power, and endurance of the forearm and elbow complex.
4. Retrain the elbow to perform functionally.
5. Minimize the risk of reinjury.

TECHNIQUES FOR MANAGING ACUTE INFLAMMATIONS

Soft tissue that has been irritated undergoes a cellular response that creates inflammation. The physiology of the healing process and a thorough discussion of the phases of inflammation and healing were detailed in Chapter 1. Of prime concern is the control and reduction of joint effusion, which can cause articular cartilage degradation and an early onset of osteoarthritis.[21,22] Enhancing circulation of synovial fluid and resorption of synovial effusion are important goals in the early stages of joint inflammation, not only because articular cartilage nutrition is enhanced but also because arthrofibrosis and restricted mobility are prevented.

Common initial techniques designed to reduce inflammation to injured tissue are (1) cryotherapy, (2) local compression, and (3) the use of nonsteroidal antiinflammatory drugs (NSAIDs). Although any injury, to some extent, becomes acutely inflamed, those resulting from acute, excessive mechanical trauma are subluxations and dislocations of the humeroulnar joint (medial elbow), strains of the wrist flexor mass, and strains of the elbow flexor group. Most elbow dislocations are posterior and involve disruption of many soft tissue structures surrounding the joint. Less commonly, fractures of the distal humerus, olecranon, midradius or ulna, and radial head elicit obvious deformity and weakness. Usually there is reduced range of motion and acute localized swelling at the site of the fracture. Pain under these circumstances may not indicate specific pathology, but usually a history and patient perception are good early indicators. Acute inflammation from repetitive forces at or through the elbow generally indicates significant degenerative pathology. In a young athlete, such inflammation represents difficult management. Among this category of trauma, the sports therapist commonly sees medial epicondylitis (little league elbow, golfer's elbow, racquetball elbow), lateral epicondylitis (tennis elbow, epicondylagia lateralis, tendinitis of the short radial extensor muscle of wrist), radial head degeneration, traction spurs, olecranon fossitis, and triceps tendinitis.

Cryotherapy

Cryotherapy in elbow rehabilitation is a common modality universally applied in acute trauma management; however, the sports therapist must be aware of the physiological and psychological responses to cold in the elbow region. Circulation here is usually very good, while limb density is low. These factors must be considered in modifying the time or temperature of the cooling agent when treating the elbow. Tolerable but vigorous local ice is commonly applied for 15 to 30 minutes as soon after an initial evaluation as possible, preferably within the hour. Some clinical practices expand the treatment time considerably, but the sports therapist should be concerned about the effective skin temperature and the depth of tissue damage. Adjustments of the effective skin temperature can be made with wet or dry toweling or cloth. Some sports therapists have used glycerol or skin protectants in this area, especially for sensitive patients. Unless open wounds are present, acute applications of ice or cold should be combined with external compression and elevation of the limb. After the initial cold treatment, icing throughout the inflammatory period is standard procedure. Cold can be applied periodically after the onset of injury, over the wrapping, as often as is feasible. Each session may last from 15 to 30 minutes once the perception of cold is felt.

If the temperature of the skin and cooling agent is close to 85°F, then extended cooling is usually tolerated well, as well as vigorous cooling through a wet wrapping. If the effective skin temperature is closer to 60°F, then the 15- to 30-minute time limit appears prudent to prevent superficial tissue damage. A possible guide might be one treatment every 2 waking hours during the acute stage (1 to 7 days, usually) so that if some hours are missed, the maximum expected benefit would still be achieved. Optimal directed care is, practically, three to four times daily. Adjunctive care with cold during immediate care or shortly thereafter is frequently used to enhance antiswelling and antipain effects. Some of these adjunctive therapies for the elbow region, as reported in the literature and used in clinical practice, are galvanic stimulation (high voltages, interferential or standard), microcurrent stimulation, and cold pressure or other pressure devices (Figure 20-2). Because the effectiveness of these adjunctive approaches is still a matter of clinical judgment, the sports therapist is directed to texts on therapeutic modalities for further discussion.

Local Compression

Circulation is definitely diminished by elbow flexion above 90 degrees because of soft tissue compression. The effect is even more pronounced in the well-developed athlete. That type of compression may be

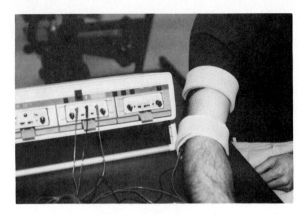

Fig. 20-2. Galvanic stimulation.

effective immediately after an injury but loses its cost-benefit ratio with many bony and soft tissue injuries. External compression with an Ace-type elastic wrap, elastic stockinette, or full-arm mesh sleeve may be applied to the elbow, either singly or in combination with elbow flexion. When applying Ace-type wraps to this area, attempt to place the elbow in the resting position before application because moving to this position once the wrap is applied usually results in increased compression at the proximal forearm and elbow and then distal arm stasis, swelling, or numbness. Full elbow flexion, used as compression, should be avoided after dislocations, fractures, and joint compression injuries.

Instructions to the athlete concerning skin color, feelings of numbness and tingling, throbbing, and other signs of circulatory distress should be made clear. Some practical instructions for a variety of problems for which the above symptoms may develop during treatment by compression include the following: (1) first, elevate the hand, and if this is not helpful in 2 to 3 minutes, lie down and elevate the entire arm with pillows; (2) if not relieved within 5 minutes, apply ice to the wrapped area; (3) again, if not relieved within 5 minutes, loosen the wrap or compression; and (4), should none of this work to relieve the signs of excessive compression, use a referral protocol.

Medications

NSAIDs and certainly steroidal antiinflammatories have their greatest effect in the long term by early administration, less than 4 hours after an injury. However, tissue healing responses (as measured by tissue strength) may be diminished during a window period early in recovery. This effect holds the sports therapist to a steady progression in rehabilitation, even in the face of significant pain relief and apparent full function.

Despite the recent and widespread use of NSAIDs, research evidence is not clear whether blocking cyclooxygenase activity with NSAIDs or blocking arachidonic acid synthesis by the use of steroids results in enhanced or diminished healing rates. Until this issue is resolved, the dramatic results often seen with NSAIDs need to be assessed in light of a false confidence factor, denoted in the terminology "combating inflammation".

MANAGING RESTRICTED MOTION AT THE ELBOW

Limited ranges of motion after surgery, long-term immobility, and trauma represent subacute or chronic complications of many elbow pathologies. They may be produced by soft tissue dysfunction and related to underlying contractures, adhesions, and muscle spasm. An inflamed or swollen joint results in capsular distention, which can create reflex muscle spasm resulting in restricted mobility of the contractile and noncontractile tissue elements.[1,21,22] Muscle weakness may also be a factor in the limitation of range of motion but is not considered in this discussion until the section of strengthening. Clinically, the athlete may present with flexion limitation more often than extension and with supination as equally limited as pronation. Progressive stages of medical collateral ligament tears in pitchers, fractures, and dislocations are common examples of injuries that develop motion restrictions.

The dangers of joint immobilization, arthrofibrosis, and adhesive capsulitis have been well documented.[6,10,21,22] Changes in collagen structure and a decrease in water content result in degeneration of articular cartilage.[17] Collagen fibrils composing the joint capsule become more disorganized and less able to stretch, thereby restricting the normal arthrokinematics of the elbow. Contractile tissues (muscle and tendon) experience reflex spasm, and if they remain in a shortened position, they will ultimately adapt to this shortened position.[17,44]

It is therefore imperative that early range-of-motion exercises be initiated to minimize the degenerative and deleterious effects of immobility. It is extremely important for the sports therapist to understand soft tissue healing constraints. Range-of-motion exercises to reverse motion restrictions should never exceed soft tissue healing limitations. The sports therapist must help to facilitate biological scar formation without compromising mobility. Common motion goals may involve maintaining available motion or retarding progressive mechanical restrictions, stimulating neurophysiological mechanoreceptors, inhibiting nociceptive stimuli, encouraging synovial fluid motion, maintaining nutrient exchange, and elongating hypomobile structures. This can be accomplished through the use of several treatment modalities including the use of continuous passive motion within a protective range to improve articular nutrition and prevent the onset of arthrofibrosis[12,14,31,34]; slow passive stretching (low force/long duration) to improve collagen flexibility and prevent the onset of adhesive capsulitis; and specific joint mobilization techniques to restore component mobility.

Passive Stretching

Stretching of noncontractile and contractile tissue can be implemented by the sports therapist and also taught to the athlete. These techniques may require a partner or the use of some apparatus. Athletes must have the techniques explained, the techniques must be observed, and the athlete must be given feedback early and regularly to avoid ineffective, overzealous, and sometimes disastrous results. Partner techniques can be used to obtain the most desirable results and are generally used early in the progression of rehabilitation.

Stretching techniques have been discussed in detail in Chapter 3. Recent literature is more supportive of using graded passive stretching or static stretching in which the stress is applied for a sustained period (20 to 30 seconds) to facilitate elongation of the tissues with long-term deformation.[20,23] PNF stretching techniques use a neurophysiological phenomenon that results in inhibition and relaxation of the antagonist muscle, thereby permitting a transient increase in range of motion.

For stretching the medial and lateral heads of the triceps and the anconeus, the athlete should be supine, arm slightly abducted, with the elbow flexed and slightly supinated (Figure 20-3). Facing the head of the athlete at the side, the sports therapist's hand farthest from the athlete should grasp the dorsal fore-

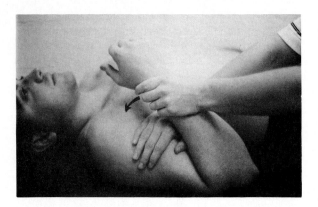

Fig. 20-3. Partner stretching of triceps (medial and lateral head) and anconeus.

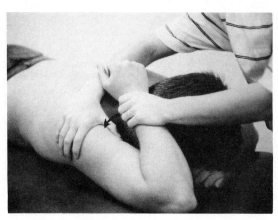

Fig. 20-4. Partner stretching of triceps, long head.

arm just proximal to the wrist; the other hand should stabilize the proximal humerus.

Gradual flexion is pursued in an arclike motion in an attempt to reach the athlete's fingers to the shoulder. Flexion agonist action can be resisted to facilitate triceps relaxation. The long head of the triceps may be ideally stretched with the athlete lying prone, shoulder fully flexed, and the pillow or table situated for full shoulder adduction (Figure 20-4). The sports therapist faces the athlete at the head and grips the forearm just proximal to the wrist with the hand closest to the head and stabilizes the athlete's shoulder posteriorly with the other hand. From a flexed and slightly supinated position, the forearm is moved gradually to full flexion.

Stretching into supination primarily involves the pronators and flexors of the wrist and hand, whereas stretching into pronation involves the supinator and extensors of the wrist and hand (Figure 20-5). Only the supinator and pronators (teres and quadratus) are presented here. For supination, the athlete lies supine with the arm flexed to about 90 degrees and fully medially rotated; the forearm is slightly flexed and fully pronated. The sports therapist should face the athlete, standing at the side and gripping the distal arm dorsally with the hand closest to the athlete, while the other hand stabilizes the upper arm dorsally just proximal to the elbow. The sports therapist gradually and fully extends the elbow and simultaneously draws the forearm farther ulnad.

The pronator teres may be stretched by two methods: one primarily for the humeral head and one pri-

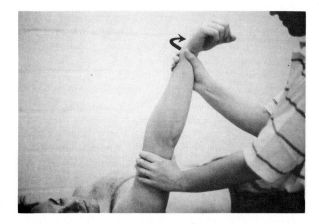

Fig. 20-5. Partner stretching of supinator.

marily for the ulnar head with the pronator quadratus. Humeral head stretching of the pronator is performed with the athlete supine, arm flexed to about 90 degrees and fully laterally rotated (Figure 20-6). The ulnar head and pronator quadratus are also stretched in this position. Additionally, the forearm is slightly flexed and fully supinated for the starting position. The sports therapist should sit at the athlete's side, holding the forearm in the lap and facing the hand. The sports therapist should then grip the dorsal and distal forearm with the hand toward the head and stabilize the upper ventral arm, proximal to the elbow, with the other hand. Gradually and fully extend the elbow while drawing the forearm maximally ul-

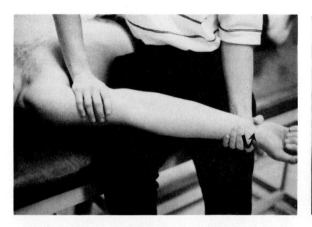

Fig. 20-6. Partner stretching of pronator teres and quadratus.

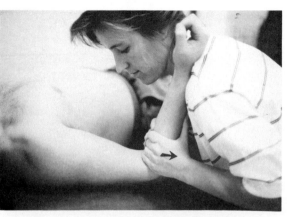

Fig. 20-7. Position for humeroulnar joint traction.

nad. The second stretching maneuver involves the same flexed starting position; however, the forearm remains in neutral position. The therapist this time retains a flexed elbow and draws the forearm maximally ulnad.

Each of the stretching maneuvers can be modified to use wands, poles, walls, tables, and changes in body position. The stretch should not be painful and should be sustained statically for at least 30 seconds, whether in continuous or intermittent time periods. The available evidence suggests that stretches lasting less than 30 seconds diminish the potential elongation gains, and stretches lasting greater than 30 seconds add no additional benefit to stress resistance.[20,23] Because the stretch is directed at tendinous and collagen-rich fascial components, damping of these tissues occurs over a matter of hours, and stretching once per day appears to be sufficient; any gains in motion should be followed by active shortening of the antagonistic muscle groups. This follow-up, active resistance exercising is designed to retain control and motion through subsequent treatment times.

Joint Mobilization

For the elbow to function normally during athletic activity, it is imperative that joint arthrokinematics and physiological component mobility be restored. Joint mobilization techniques using a graded system of oscillations and distraction as proposed in Chapter 10 should be incorporated to combat joint restrictions but must follow detailed evaluations and con-

stitute skilled technical performance. Otherwise, the neurophysiological and mechanical effects promoted with these techniques may be nullified by resulting joint trauma and hypermobility. This technique can be relatively safe if basic principles are followed. Although joint mobilization requires potentially extensive one-on-one time, it is definitely an effective treatment technique that can be used by the sports therapist.

To increase flexion of the humeroulnar joint, sustained or early oscillatory traction commonly precedes other accessory motions. For traction of the humeroulnar joint, the athlete lies supine with the wrist resting against the sports therapist's outside shoulder to allow the elbow to be in the resting position. The sports therapist uses the medial aspect of the inside hand over the proximal ulna on the volar surface and then reinforces this placement with the outside hand. Force through the hand is directed against the proximal ulna at a 45-degree angle to the ulnar shaft, which is parallel to the angulation of the joint surfaces (Figure 20-7).

Mobilization in this manner can begin at physiological elbow flexion angles less than the resting angle of 70 degrees but should progress by taking up the end of the available range and always applying a 45-degree direction to the pull along the shaft of the ulna. A distal glide also assists humeroulnar joint flexion, during which the traction position and maneuver is started, and then a pull is directed along the long axis of the ulna. The sustained or oscillatory mobilization grades range in their length of application;

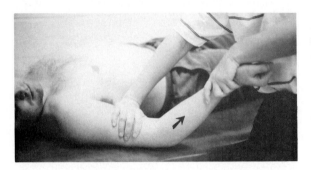

Fig. 20-8. Traction of the radiohumeral joint.

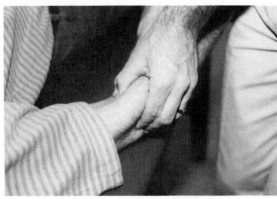

Fig. 20-9. Position for dorsal and volar radioulnar glides.

however, sustained pulls of over 1 minute without results indicate that another maneuver or technical adjustment may be more effective. Some experience is needed to gain an appreciation of tissue end feel, but the end result is objectively measured by gains in flexion range of motion.

Radiohumeral joint restrictions infrequently limit flexion or extension but may be involved with rotation restrictions. Traction of the radiohumeral joint proceeds axially along the radial shaft, and distraction glides are applied perpendicular to the head of the radius, either in a volar direction for flexion or a dorsal direction for extension (Figure 20-8). Likewise, to increase pronation and supination, the proximal radius is mobilized dorsally to increase pronation and volarly to increase supination (Figure 20-9). The resting position of the supported forearm is 70 degrees of flexion and about 35 degrees of supination. The treatment hand may rest on a table or plinth, with this position being maintained by the palm of the other hand. The direction of motion is in the plane of the radial notch of the ulna, parallel to the long axis of the ulna. The sports therapist needs to stabilize the humerus and proximal ulna medially with a hand coming from underneath the arm. The other hand is placed around the head of the radius with the fingers on the volar surface and the palm on the dorsal surface. Volar forces are accomplished by pushing through the palm and dorsal forces by pulling through the fingers.

Joint restrictions may occur from a variety of elbow traumas. Early attention to acute inflammatory treatment and subsequently early, active, pain-free range of motion may produce full and optimal results.

Subacute use of soft tissue mobilization and stretching is frequently effective for motion restrictions involving capsular or ligamentous adhesions and muscle spasm. In any case, gains in range of motion should be followed by exercises that address strengthening and neuromuscular control to provide neural feedback for the controlled muscular pattern that will be needed for the athlete to progress back to normal function.

MANAGING JOINT LAXITY OF THE ELBOW

In situations where the elbow joint exhibits excessive hypermobility secondary to joint laxity, efforts of the sports therapist should be directed toward increasing the stability of the joint. Thus the major goals for treating joint laxity become (1) to maintain a shortened physiological position of ligamentous tissue, (2) to increase tissue stress progressively without abnormal mechanical strain, (3) to strengthen the secondary muscular stabilizers, and (4) to retrain automatic reflex joint control. For chronic laxity, surgical treatment is frequently proposed. Conservative treatment concentrates primarily on strengthening activities.

Strengthening Activities

Regardless of whether the sports therapist is treating inflammation and restricted mobility or joint laxity, the athlete must begin to develop strength and power in preparation to resume competitive athletic activity. It is imperative that the athlete does not train through pain; however, the initiation of muscle ac-

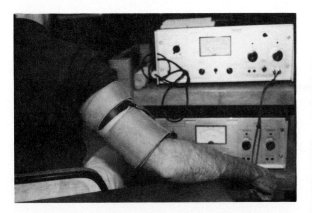

Fig. 20-10. Electrical stimulation of the triceps.

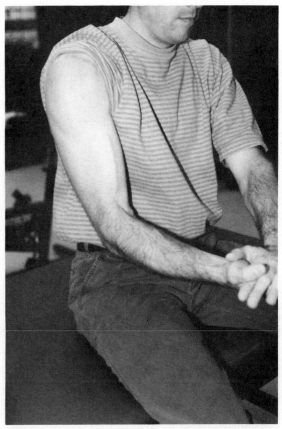

Fig. 20-11. Manually resisted isometrics to the elbow flexors.

tivity early in the rehabilitation phase is important to prevent muscle atrophy, initiate muscle reeducation, and facilitate effusion absorption.

ISOMETRIC EXERCISE. Electrical stimulation to facilitate muscle activity is an excellent way of initiating isometric muscle strength (Figure 20-10). Electrical stimulation can enhance isometric muscle strength and facilitate muscle contractions approximately 60% greater than what one can exhibit volitionally.[15,35] Progressing from electrical stimulation, the athlete can initiate a multiple angle isometric program, which, when performed at varying angles, facilitates a strengthening effect at ± 5 to 10 degrees above and below the angle at which the joint is exercised. Simply stated, a strengthening effect can be realized through a full range of motion as long as the athlete exercises isometrically at varying angles. Angles that are painful can be avoided. The following pictures demonstrate methods by which an athlete can exercise isometrically at varying positions (Figures 20-11 and 20-12).[1]

Early strengthening exercise is often restricted to the resting position at 70 degrees of elbow flexion with slight supination. In this position, isometric tension can be directed toward flexion and extension. Also in this position, shoulder and wrist exercises are encouraged. Maintaining forearm position has been promoted to impart stress to the surrounding musculature and joint structures without producing elongation or tension mechanical strain within the medial collateral ligament. Progression of these exercises usually follows a lack of symptoms during or after each session of exercise.

Endurance-type exercise intensity, frequency, and

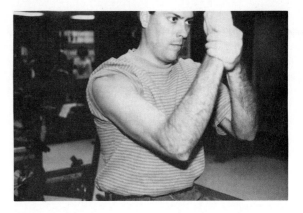

Fig. 20-12. Manually resisted isometrics to the elbow extensors.

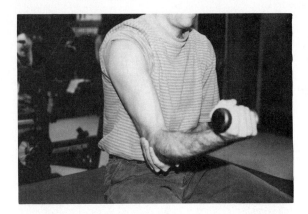

Fig. 20-13. Free weight resistance to the elbow flexors.

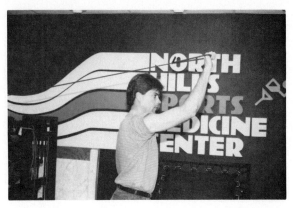

Fig. 20-14. Surgical tubing resistance to the elbow extensors.

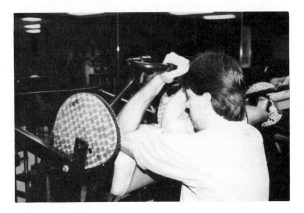

Fig. 20-15. Nautilus (R) multi-bicep machine.

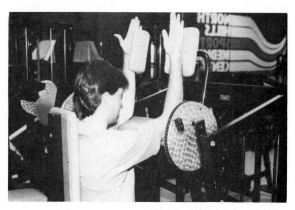

Fig. 20-16. Nautilus (R) tricep machine.

duration appear to enhance the metabolical functions in healing ligaments. Isometric exercises that progress in 10- to 20-degree positions from resting are promoted as early as tolerated; submaximal isometric tension is tolerated earlier than maximal. As long as prestress and poststress testing reveal no comparable change in valgus laxity, full supination and pronation appear to progress to full range before progression to full flexion and extension ranges. Usually, limits of strengthening exercises fall within 10 to 90 degrees of elbow flexion because this range provides the least valgus deformity and tension on the medial collateral ligament.

ISOTONIC EXERCISE. Isotonic exercise can be initiated after isometric training when the athlete exhibits

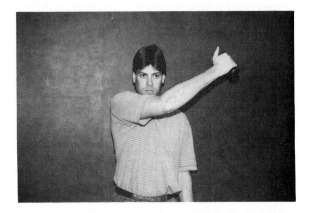

Fig. 20-17. D1 flexion pattern.

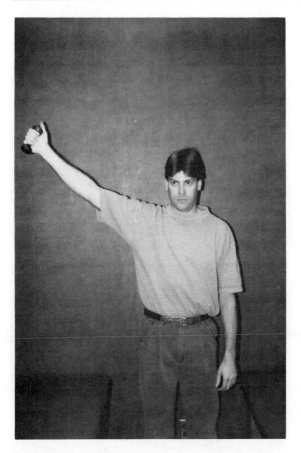

Fig. 20-18. D2 flexion pattern.

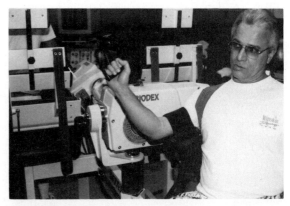

Fig. 20-19. Isokinetic resistance of the elbow on the biodex.

ISOKINETIC EXERCISE. Isokinetic exercise has the advantages of controlling speed and range of motion, providing biofeedback to the athlete, and using concentric and eccentric, work, power, and endurance training to exercise muscle (Figure 20-19). An isokinetic routine should be initiated when the athlete has full range of motion; normal arthrokinematics; and no pain, swelling, or instability. Isokinetic exercise should be performed through a velocity spectrum, which permits the athlete to exercise at slow speeds to improve strength, increase speeds for power, and over an extended period of time improve muscle endurance. The sports therapist should perform a biomechanical analysis of the specific athletic activities so that the isokinetic routine can include concentric and eccentric training that would be sport specific.

One of the advantages of isokinetic training is that it is accommodative, and resistance automatically adapts to muscle output, which would be related to either muscle weakness or pain. Isokinetic training should be used as a precursor to functional retraining and is a means by which objective comparative values can be obtained to notify the therapist and athlete of the differences between involved and uninvolved extremities, as well as antagonistic muscle groups.

CLOSED-KINETIC CHAIN EXERCISE. As stated previously, the elbow joint is primarily involved in athletic activities that occur in an open kinetic chain. For example, throwing activities create tremendous distraction forces on the elbow, which can create significant soft tissue strain.[13,24,25] There have been reports of joint instability resulting from continued distraction forces, as well as strain placed on static

pain-free range of motion. Many methods exist by which an athlete can exercise isotonically. Initially, the program should start with manual resistance so that the sports therapist can gain appreciation for areas of weakness and pain. These exercises can be performed in a cardinal plane and eventually progress to diagonal or functional patterns. Advantages of manual resistance include the emphasis on the area of weakness by imparting graded resistance, functional stabilization, and neurological facilitation.

Other methods of isotonic resistance include free weights, surgical tubing, and mechanical isotonic machinery (Figures 20-13 through 20-16). The athlete should exercise through available, pain-free motion at a controlled rate to fatigue. He or she should progress from a sequence exercising in cardinal planes to diagonal/functional patterns (Figures 20-17 and 20-18).

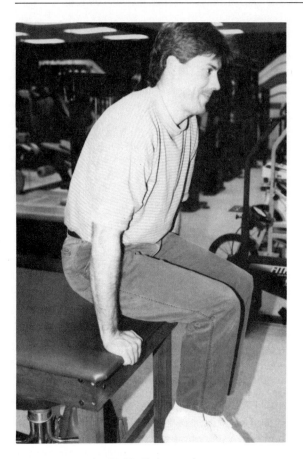

Fig. 20-20. Sitting push-up.

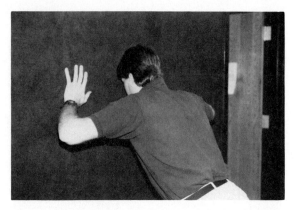

Fig. 20-21. Wall push-up.

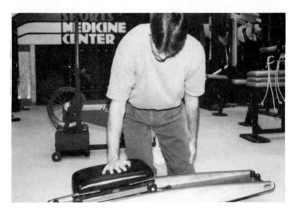

Fig. 20-22. Closed chain strengthening on the pro-fitter (R).

restraining structures.[3,36,42] In addition, other athletic activities, such as gymnastics and wrestling, involve placing the elbow and upper extremity in a close-packed position, which facilitates joint compressive forces and places extreme demands on the dynamic stabilizers of the elbow. Although the elbow is intrinsically stable because of its anatomical geometry, muscles and ligaments play a crucial role in providing additional static and dynamic control. Joint proprioceptors within the capsule provide a feedback mechanism whereby muscles contract in responses to various stresses, either compressive or distractive. An important component of elbow rehabilitation is improving static and dynamic stability of the elbow via closed-kinetic chain proprioceptive conditioning. These exercises help to facilitate joint stability and kinesthetic position sense.

Joint compression facilitates proprioceptors to en-

hance joint stability.[4] Intuitively, it makes sense that the initiation of an exercise program to facilitate joint stability would help minimize the incidence of hypermobility. The following exercises help to illustrate methods by which joint stability and co-contraction can be facilitated via closed-chain exercise (Figures 20-20 through 20-22). These activities not only increase static/dynamic control of the elbow, they help to exercise stabilizing muscles in isometric, concentric, and eccentric modes.

FUNCTIONAL RETRAINING. An analysis of the athletic activity that the athlete is returning to is important so that functional skills can be rehearsed and practiced in a controlled clinical environment before the athlete resumes competitive activity. Once the athlete has demonstrated full mobility, no swelling, no

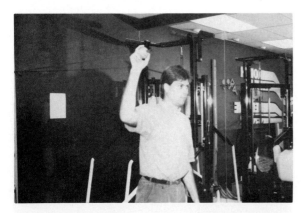

Fig. 20-23. Surgical tubing resistance to mimic throwing.

pain, "optimal" isokinetic strength parameters, and has completed an isometric/isokinetic/isotonic/ closed-chain strengthening routine, he or she can initiate a functional retraining program.

Skill training can only be enhanced through repetition. It is important that specific skills that the athlete must be able to perform in a competitive situation be demonstrated to the sports therapist so that he or she is certain that the athlete is not experiencing any disability. Examples of these activities would be swinging a racquet, throwing a ball, swinging a bat, or performing a handstand. All of these skills must be performed without pain or joint dysfunction. In addition to helping to "train" the athlete musculoskeletally, the performance of functional progressions helps to provide psychological confirmation that the athlete is able to perform these skills outside of the clinical environment. The following pictures demonstrate examples of functional activity (Figures 20-23 through 20-26).

Functional progressions have been discussed in detail in Chapter 12. Functional progression can be implemented by following these guidelines:

1. Open chain through controlled range of motion.
2. Open chain through pain-free range of motion.
3. Closed chain for stability and neuromuscular control.
4. Plyometrics.
5. Mimic functional activity.
6. Permission to compete when above objective criteria have been met.

PLYOMETRIC TRAINING. Plyometric training activities involve rapid muscle response using the myotatic

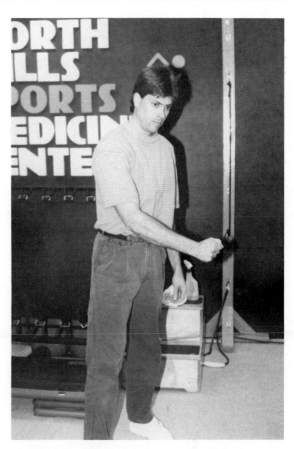

Fig. 20-24. Surgical tubing resistance to mimic tennis swing.

stretch reflex.[7,9,23,43] Plyometric activity involves rapid eccentric/concentric muscle activity aimed at improving power and neuromuscular control. These activities are highly specific and functional. Muscles need to be stressed in a rapid and repetitive fashion to improve power and endurance. Examples of plyometric activity include a resistive wall push-up (Figure 20-27), rapid flexion/extension with surgical tubing (Figure 20-28), and a ball toss with a weighted ball (Figure 20-29).

Preventing Recurrence

Of prime importance after a rehabilitation program is educating the athlete on how to maintain proper conditioning, biomechanics, and functional strength to prevent the recurrence of injury. Using the basic

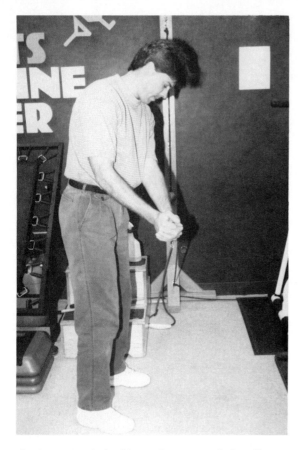

Fig. 20-25. Surgical tubing resistance to mimic golf swing.

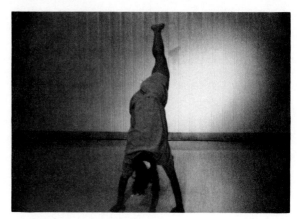

Fig. 20-26. Performance of gymnastic skills in clinical environment.

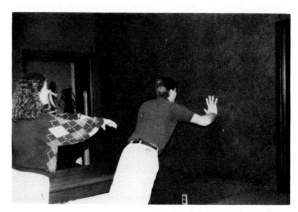

Fig. 20-27. Plyometric push-up.

components of rehabilitation, the athlete can then "fine tune" his or her program to prevent future injury.

Initially the activity must be analyzed from a biomechanical perspective. The stresses placed on the elbow joint must be understood so that muscle forces can be replicated in a training program. Strength, power, and endurance training using isotonic weights, surgical tubing, manual resistance, and functional repetition should take place. Proper biomechanics in sport are essential and should be reviewed with a competent coach or instructor. Joint flexibility is a key, especially in activities that require hyperelasticity of contractile and noncontractile tissue structures. Maintenance of proper body conditioning is important to reduce excessive strain on the elbow. Since virtually all athletic activity depends on coor-

dination and efficiency of all body parts, general body conditioning is paramount. Finally, and probably most important, the athlete must understand when to seek medical attention and not to delay obtaining advice from a sports therapist or physician when he or she is hurt. Many athletes attempt to play with pain and often develop injuries that could have been avoided if early advice had been sought.

Many "overuse" injuries result from inadequate rest; therefore an appreciation for training modification is quite important. This will allow the athlete to be treated and obtain appropriate advice for an early and safe return to athletic activity.

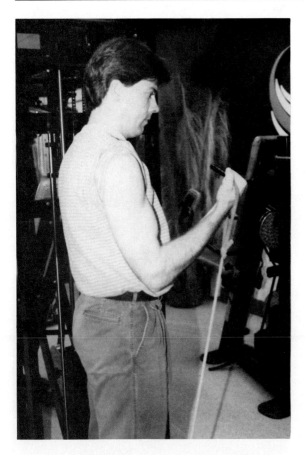

Fig. 20-28. Plyometrics with surgical tubing.

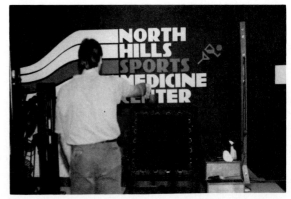

Fig. 20-29. Plyometrics with a weighted ball throwing into a plyoback (R).

TYPES OF INJURIES

The elbow is subjected to many stresses that may cause injury. These injuries can be inflammatory or traumatic and require appropriate intervention for a safe and expeditious return to athletic competition. This section will review common elbow injuries followed by rehabilitation guidelines for each problem.

Lateral Epicondylitis

Lateral epicondylitis is a tendinitis of the extensor tendon mechanism. Previous research has implicated the short radial extensor muscle of the wrist as the prime muscle involved, however, other authors have demonstrated that the entire extensor wad can be inflamed.[3,5,28] Lateral epicondylitis or "tennis elbow"

is a malady that is not only experienced by tennis or racquet sport players. Individuals who perform repetitive lifting or rotational movements with their forearm are prone to this problem. When rehabilitating lateral epicondylitis, it has been emphasized that strength and flexibility have to be restored to the forearm musculature.[29,30] Figures 20-30 through 20-33 demonstrate methods by which flexibility of the forearm pronators and supinators and wrist flexors and extensors can be obtained.

Static stretching is important to obtain mechanical deformation of inflexible tissue. Passive stretching of these muscle groups should be performed at least 5 to 6 times per day and the stretch held for 15 to 20 seconds.

STRENGTHENING. Strengthening in an iostonic, isokinetic, and plyometric mode can be applied in a variety of ways. Of prime importance is developing muscle endurance, which is obtained by having the athlete exercise with low loads (1 to 3 pounds) for extended periods until fatigued. Figures 20-34 through 20-36 demonstrate techniques of isotonic, isokinetic, and plyometric resistance to the forearm musculature. In addition, eccentric weakness of the wrist extensor muscles plays a role in the incidence of lateral epicondylitis; therefore this mode of training should be incorporated into the forearm conditioning program.[37,38] The athlete with tennis elbow must emphasize both concentric and eccentric conditioning to minimize risk of reinjury.

COUNTERFORCE BRACING. Counterforce bracing has been advocated by Nirschl and others.[29,30] The purpose of the counterforce brace is to redistribute com-

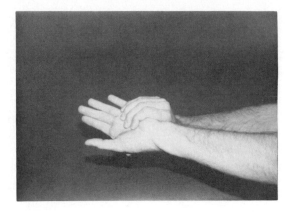

Fig. 20-30. Stretching the forearm pronators.

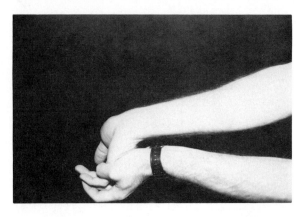

Fig. 20-31. Stretching the forearm supinators.

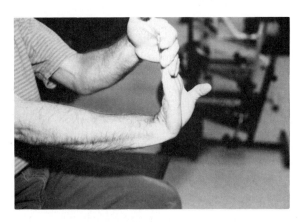

Fig. 20-32. Stretching the wrist flexors.

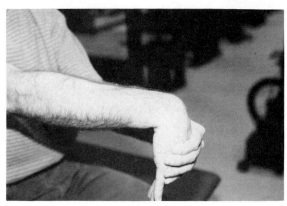

Fig. 20-33. Stretching the wrist flexors.

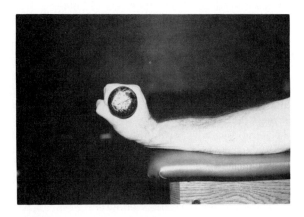

Fig. 20-34. Isotonic strengthening of the wrist extensors.

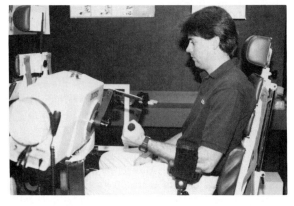

Fig. 20-35. Isokinetic strengthening of the forearm pronators/supinators.

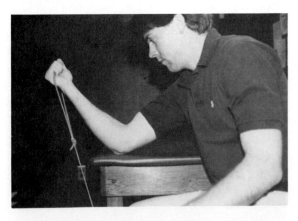

Fig. 20-36. Plyometrics of the forearm with tubing.

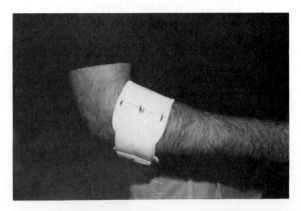

Fig. 20-37. Counterforce brace for lateral epicondylitis.

pressive forces on the extensor mechanism, thereby minimizing friction and stress and increasing the efficiency of force production. Studies have demonstrated that EMG activity of the wrist extensor muscles is enhanced after the application of a counterforce brace.[19,30] These braces can be used during the rehabilitation period, as well as when the athlete resumes competitive activity (Figure 20-37).

OTHER CONSIDERATIONS. Lateral epicondylitis is easier to prevent than it is to treat. The athlete should be on a vigorous flexibility and strength maintenance program emphasizing endurance and eccentric strength of the wrist extensor and flexor muscles. Proper technique in athletic activity is also important. Therefore the athlete should be observed by a coach or instructor who understands the biomechanical forces that the forearm undergoes during athletics. It is also important that if the athlete is a racquet sport participant, he or she chooses a racquet that is appropriate for hand size, grip, and competitive level. Measurement of appropriate grip width can be obtained by taking the length of the second palmar crease to the distal tip of the ring finger along the radial side (Figure 20-38). Racquet tension should not exceed 50 pounds for the recreational player.

Lateral epicondylitis may be recognized when the elbow is extended by extensor tendon pain, especially on isolated middle finger extension. Assuming other entities have been ruled out, this condition arising from playing tennis may be treated effectively through stretching, deep friction massage, or mobilization at the proximal attachment of the short radial extensor muscle of the wrist. Other wrist extensors

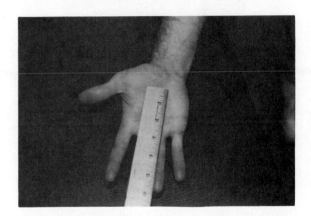

Fig. 20-38. Measurement of grip width.

have been implicated in this general syndrome. A host of preventive measures can be applied to prevent recurrences.

1. Players should receive advice about or pay attention to excessively tight strings, wet balls, and excessively small grip size.
2. Adequate conditioning decreases the chances of general body fatigue setting up poor stroke technique from poor positioning for the stroke.
3. Players should assess their stroke technique for errors.
4. Strengthening the grip and wrist extensors is paramount.
5. Periodic stretching of the extensors is important.

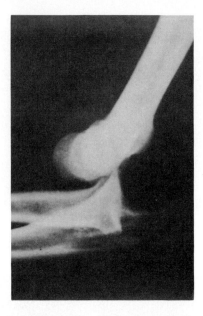

Fig. 20-39. Hyperextension of the elbow leading to posterior dislocation.

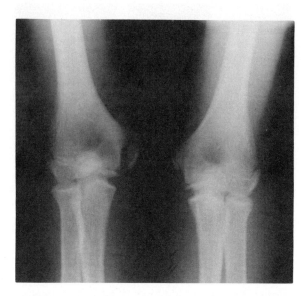

Fig. 20-40. Disruption of the medial humeral epiphysis in valgus stress overload.

6. Especially when hitting a lot of backhands, follow the workout with ice for 15 to 30 minutes.

Elbow Dislocations

The most common type of elbow dislocation is posterior. This typically occurs with a violent hyperextension force and is relatively common in contact sports and closed chain weight-bearing events (Figure 20-39). After immobilization, emphasis is placed on restoration of active and passive range of motion using passive stretching, inhibitory stretching, joint mobilization, and long axis distraction. Strengthening exercises for the biceps and triceps can be implemented using isotonics, manual resistance, free weights/surgical tubing, and isokinetics. Emphasis should be placed on eccentric strengthening of the biceps and supinators to minimize hyperextension forces. It takes approximately 8 to 10 weeks for the elbow joint capsule to totally heal after dislocation. Therefore a functional athletic progression routine is not implemented until that time. Before resumption of athletic activity, the athlete must have equal strength and flexibility, full range of motion, no sense of static or dynamic laxity, and the ability to perform his or her athletic activity without dysfunction.

Valgus Stress Overload

In the athlete, repetitive valgus stress overload can result in strain to the ulnar collateral ligament. In the adolescent athlete, this stress can also create traction on the epiphysis of the medial humeral epicondyle. Therefore growth plane injuries are quite common in adolescents who exhibit valgus stress overload (Figure 20-40). When the athlete is experiencing medial elbow pain, it is important that he or she rest the extremity and the soft tissues be treated with antiinflammatory modalities. During this time, the athlete can work on isotonic and plyometric strengthening of the elbow, wrist, and forearm. In addition, it is important to obtain flexibility of the shoulder internal and external rotators and work on proper body mechanics and form. Typically, valgus extension overload injuries occur in throwers who exhibit weakness of the scapular stabilizers and tightness of the shoulder internal rotators. This results in the thrower "opening up too early" when the elbow lags behind the shoulder during acceleration and the elbow is in a low position during acceleration and ball release.

Proper coaching is extremely important to emphasize 90 degrees of shoulder elevation and appropriate weight transference through the trunk to minimize valgus strain of the elbow during throwing. Even if the athlete has adequate strength of the forearm and elbow muscles, inappropriate form can perpetuate medial elbow symptoms. In extreme cases, rupture of the ulnar or medial collateral ligament can occur, which may require surgical correction.

If surgical intervention is necessary the sports therapist should use the following rehabilitation guidelines:

WEEKS 0-2

1. Functional brace 30 to 100 degrees.
2. Effusion/pain management.
3. Maintain range of motion of wrist/shoulder.
4. Strengthening of wrist—putty, spring loaded hand grip, isometrics.
5. Constant passive motion (CPM) of elbow within range of motion constraints.
6. Grade I-II mobilization—long axis distraction.

WEEK 3

1. Range of motion goal: 20 to 110 degrees.
2. Isotonic wrist strength—cuffs/reverse curls, etc.
3. Continuous passive motion.
4. Shoulder strength/flexibility, avoid external rotation stretch (valgus stress on elbow).
5. Joint mobilization to maintain range of motion.
6. Dynasplint if range of motion is not attained—low force/long duration.
7. Same exercises in Number 1 above.

WEEKS 4-6:

1. Increase range of motion to full extension to 130 degrees.
2. Aggressive joint mobilization if above not achieved.
3. Isotonic and active/assisted isokinetic resistance through full available range of motion.
4. Pronation, supination, broomstick wall up.
5. Discontinue functional brace at 6 weeks.

WEEKS 6-8:

1. Increase isotonic resistance to elbow.
2. As above, 1 through 3.

WEEK 8-4 MONTHS:

1. Isokinetic velocity spectrum training, power/endurance, eccentric.
2. Should be asymptomatic—treat symptoms with modalities.
3. Full flexibility and strengthening program for shoulder.

4 MONTHS-6 MONTHS:

1. Functional conditioning.
   a. Ball toss.

b. Closed-chain exercises.
c. Throwing progression when isokinetic ratio is within 80%.

2. Permission to resume athletic activity when the following occur:
   a. 100% strength.
   b. No pain.
   c. Full range of motion.
   d. No static or dynamic instability.
   e. Complete maturity of scar.

THROWING PROTOCOLS AFTER SURGERY

This program may be instituted for throwers after a recovery period from surgery, injection, or acute inflammation. Typical resting periods for the above conditions may be 2 weeks to 18 months. The athlete should have full, pain-free range of motion and comparable strength to the uninvolved side for the shoulder, elbow, and wrist. Stretching and upper extremity warm-up should be performed before the routine. Icing should be routine after each workout. Progression is based on 24-hour symptoms, but, particularly in postsurgical cases where circulation may not be optimal, forced rest for 48 hours may be needed to establish a tissue stress response. Throwing occurs every other day and conditioning with weight training on off days. The early routine consists of both short and long tosses.

For the short toss, start tossing the ball for 30 feet for 10 repetitions so that control feedback and technique can be gauged. The toss should be a three-quarter overhead style.

Increase every other day by 10 repetitions until 30 repetitions are reached. Then move up to half speed. Next increase to 40 feet, but drop back to 20 repetitions at half speed. Move progressively to 30 repetitions as tolerated. Finally move to 60 feet, starting back at 20 repetitions. Once reaching 30 repetitions with comfort, move to three-quarter speed.

For the long toss, start at 50 feet and 10 repetitions. Use the same gauge as in the short toss, and increase every other day if no symptoms occur. Use an overhead high toss only. Once reaching 30 repetitions at 50 feet, move to 70 feet and 20 repetitions and progress to 30 repetitions. Move from 70 feet to 100 feet and then to 130 feet as above. Optimal progression is 2 to 3 weeks.

The late routine also consists of short and long tosses. For the short toss, progress up to three-quarter speed. When comfortable, go to the mound. Then progress to the half-speed breaking ball. At three-quarter to full-speed, fast and breaking balls can be worked into games so that no more than 50 balls are thrown.

For the long toss, pitchers may want to stay with the early routine, whereas fielders may add more distance.

Ulnar Nerve Transposition

In throwing athletes, valgus stress can create strain on the ulnar nerve and cause it to periodically sublux. When the nerve subluxes, the athlete experiences paresthesia and pain along the ulnar nerve distribution. If chronic, muscle weakness of the contractile structures supplied by the ulnar nerve can result. It is sometimes necessary for the ulnar nerve to be transposed and surgically stabilized. After this technique, the athlete is typically in a posterior splint for approximately 1 week. He or she can perform finger and hand exercises when in the splint. After 1 week the splint is removed, and passive range of motion is initiated emphasizing full flexion and extension to 20 degrees. At approximately 21 days postsurgery, the athlete should be able to fully extend his or her elbow, exhibit full forearm pronation/supination, and initiate a vigorous isotonic and isokinetic elbow and forearm strengthening program. Emphasis is placed on biceps strength, particularly in an eccentric mode, to minimize hyperextension forces. As previously described with valgus stress overload, it is also important to emphasize proper form and elbow position, especially in throwing athletes so that the elbow does not lag behind the shoulder, and valgus strain is minimized.

SUMMARY

1. This chapter reviews the basic components of a rehabilitation program for the elbow.
2. The three joints of the elbow complex act independently between flexion and extension and supination and pronation, both in joint surface movement and in muscular activity; therefore application of this information aids in the use and positioning of the elbow segments in rehabilitation.
3. Prime considerations are a thorough understanding of the athletic activity that the athlete is considering returning to so that the rehabilitation program can be specifically designed for that purpose.
4. Adequate control of inflammation, pain, and joint

swelling are important to reduce muscle inhibition and minimize the possibility of joint contractures.
5. Early initiation of muscle activity and progression of resistive activities to improve strength, power, and endurance should follow. Many methods and techniques are available, however, all should be modified in accordance with the athlete's symptoms, specific diagnosis, and ultimately with regard to the biomechanical stresses imposed on the elbow during athletic activity.
6. Functional retraining and progression should follow, with activities designed to mimic the specific stresses that are going to be experienced on the athletic field.
7. The athlete needs to understand the importance of prevention. This includes maintenance of strength, flexibility, power, endurance, and overall body conditioning. He or she must know when to seek medical attention and modify competitive intensity to minimize the chance of an injury getting worse.

REFERENCES

1 Akeson W, Amiel D, LaVioletee D, et al.: The connective tissue response to immobility: an accelerated aging response, *Exp Gerontol* 3:298-301, 1968.
2 Andrews JR, McCluskey GM, McLeond WD: *Musculotendinous injuries of the shoulder and elbow in athletes,* Scherring Symposium presented at National Athletic Trainers Association Symposium, Summer 1976.
3 Arnheim D, Prentice W: *Principles of athletic training,* St Louis, 1993, Mosby.
4 Baratta R, Solomonow M, Zhou B, et al.: Muscular coactivation: the role of the antagonist musculature in maintaining knee stability, *Am J Sports Med* 16:113, 1988.
5 Berhang A: The many causes of tennis elbow, *N Y State J Med* 79:1363-1366, 1979.
6 Booth F: Physiological and biochemical effects of immobilization on muscle, *Clin Orthop* 219:15-20, 1987.
7 Bosco C, Komi P: Prestretch potentiation of human skeletal muscle during ballistic movement, *Acta Physiol Scand* 111:135, 1981.
8 Brodgen B, Crow M: Little Leaguer's elbow, *Am J Roentgenol* 83:671, 1980.
9 Chu D, Plummer L: The language of plyometrics, *NSCA Journal* 6:30, 1984.
10 Cooper R: Alterations during immobilization and regeneration of skeletal muscle in cats, *J Bone Joint Surg* 51(A):919-953, 1972.
11 Courson R: Rehabilitation of the throwers elbow, *Sportsmed Update,* Birmingham, Alabama, Spring 1989.
12 Coutts R (Moderator): Symposium: The use of continuous passive motion in the rehabilitation of orthopedic problems, *Contemp Orthop* 16(3):75-111, 1988.

13 DeHaven KE, Evarts CM: Throwing injuries of the elbow in athletes, *Orthop Clin North Am* 4:801-808, 1973.

14 Dehne E, Torp R: Treatment of joint injuries by immediate mobilization, *Clin Orthop* 77:218-232, 1971.

15 Delito A, Rose S, Lehman R, et al.: Electrical stimulation versus voluntary strengthening of the thigh after anterior cruciate ligament surgery, *Phys Ther* 68:660-663, 1988.

16 Del Pizzo W, Jobe F, Norwood L: Ulnar nerve entrapment syndrome in baseball players, *Am J Sports Med* 5(5):182-185, 1977.

17 Donatelli R, Owens-Burkhart H: Effects of immobilization on the extensibility of periarticular connective tissue, *J Orthop Sports Phys Ther* 3(2):67-72, 1981.

18 Grana W, Rahskin A: Pitcher's elbow in adolescents, *Am J Sports Med* 8:333, 1980.

19 Gruchow H, Pelltier D: An epidemiologic study of tennis elbow: incidence, recurrence, and effectiveness of prevention strategies, *Am J Sports Med* 7:234-238, 1979.

20 Hepburn G, Crivelli R: Use of elbow dynasplint for reduction of elbow flexion contracture: a case study, *J Orthop Sports Phys Ther* 5(5):269-274, 1984.

21 Hettinga D: Normal joint structures and their reaction to injury. I, *J Orthop Sports Phys Ther* 1(2):16-21, 1979.

22 Hettinga D: Normal joint structures and their reaction to injury. II, *J Orthop Sports Phys Ther* 1(3):83-87, 1979.

23 Ihara H, Nakiayama A: Dynamic joint control training for knee ligament injuries, *Am J Sports Med* 14:309-315, 1986.

24 Jobe F, Nuber G: Throwing injuries of the elbow, *Clin Sportsmed* 5(4):621-636, 1986.

25 King J, Breisford H, Tullos H: Analysis of the pitching arm of the professional baseball pitcher, *Clin Orthop* 67:116, 1969.

26 Knott M, Voss D: *Proprioceptive neuromuscular facilitation: patterns and techniques,* New York, 1968, Harper and Row.

27 Maitland G: *Extremity manipulation,* London, 1977, Butterworth Publishers.

28 Nirschl R: The etiology and treatment of tennis elbow, *J Sports Med* 2:308, 1974.

29 Nirschl R: Conservative treatment of tennis elbow, *Phys Sportsmed* 9:42-54, 1981.

30 Nirschl R: Soft tissue injuries about the elbow, *Clin Sport Med* 5:637-652, 1986.

31 Noyes F, Mangine R, Barber S: Early knee motion after open and arthroscopic anterior cruciate ligament reconstruction, *Am J Sports Med* 15(2):149-160, 1987.

32 Pappas A: Elbow problems associated with baseball during childhood and adolescence, *Clin Orthop* 164:30-41, 1982.

33 Richmond J, Southmayd W: Superficial anterior transposition of the ulnar nerve at the elbow for ulnar meuritis, *Clin Orthop* 16:42-44, 1982.

34 Salter B, Hamilton H, Wedge J, et al.: Clinical application of basic research on continuous passive motion for disorders and injuries of synovial joints: a preliminary report of a feasibility study, *J Orthop Res* 1(3):325-341, 1984.

35 Selkowitz D: Improvement in isometric strength of the quadriceps femoris as a result of electrical stimulation, *Phys Ther* 65:186-196, 1985.

36 Smith R, Brunolli J: Shoulder kinesthesia after glenohumeral joint dislocation, *Phys Ther* 69:106-112, 1989.

37 Stanish W, Rubinovich R, Curwin S: Eccentric exercise in chronic tendinitis, *Clin Orthop* 208:65-68, 1986.

38 Stauber W: Eccentric action of muscles: physiology, injury and adaptation, *Exerc Sport Sci Rev* 129:157, 1989.

39 Threlkeld A: The effects of manual therapy on connective tissue, *Phys Ther* 72(12):893-902, 1992.

40 Warren C, Lehman J, Koblanski J: Heat and stretch procedures: an evaluation using rat tail tendon, *J Musculoskel Med* 17-34, 1989.

41 Whiteside J, Andrews J: Common elbow problems in the recreational athlete, *Arch Phys Med Rehab* 50:122-126, 1976.

42 Wilson F, Andrews J, McClusky G: Valgus extension overload in the pitching elbow, *Am J Sports Med* 11(2):83-87, 1983.

43 Wilt F: Plyometrics—what it is and how it works, *Athletic Journal* 55b:76, 1975.

44 Woo S, Mathews J, Akeson W, et al.: Connective tissues' response to immobility: correlative study of biomechanical measurements of normal and immobilized rabbit knees, *Arthritis Rheum* 18:257, 1975.

Injuries to the Hand and Wrist

21

Scott Lephart

OBJECTIVES

After completion of this chapter, the student should be able to do the following:

- Describe common sports-related injuries of the wrist and hand.

- Describe the mechanism and pathology associated with hand and wrist injuries.

- Recognize and implement management protocols for the injuries.

- Describe rehabilitation objectives including flexibility and strength goals.

- Implement appropriate rehabilitation protocols for the various injuries.

- Apply appropriate protective devices to decrease incidence of recurrent injury to hand and wrist conditions.

The wrist and hand are exceedingly susceptible to injury in most sports. Sports requiring throwing, catching, grabbing, and falling constantly place the athlete's wrist and hand in positions that can result in injury. Injuries to the wrist and hand vary in degree of severity and range from soft tissue contusions to injuries requiring prolonged immobilization. Furthermore, the debilitation of an injury to the wrist and hand can vary from athlete to athlete and often depends on the athlete's position and reliance on the function of the wrist and hand for performance.

This chapter will outline the commonly encountered wrist and hand injuries in sports. The purpose of the chapter is to provide management and rehabilitation guidelines to appropriately protect, rehabilitate, and prevent recurrent injury to the region. It is important to keep in mind that the function of the hand is essential to daily activities outside athletic participation, and the functional integrity of the hand must never be compromised during care of these injuries.

WRIST INJURIES
Tendon Injuries of the Wrist

Repetitive use of the forearm, wrist, and hand in sports activity can result in tendinitis injuries, most of which can be classified as overuse inflammatory conditions. Tendon injuries are most prevalent in those sports in which throwing or a racket are used. Tendinitis and stenosing tenosynovitis are the most common sports-related tendon conditions of the wrist.[20] Both the flexor and extensor mechanisms can be involved, depending on the mechanism inducing the stress.

As is true with all overuse type injuries, acute management must include both the discontinuance of the activity responsible for the inflammatory condition and the use of conservative measures to reduce inflammation. In severe cases, splinting may be indicated to further reduce irritation to the involved tendons. Once the inflammatory condition is stabilized, the next step in the rehabilitation program is to restore flexibility. This is essential to prevent the formation of tendon adhesions, which can result in further inflexibility and the recurrence of the tendinitis upon return to sports activity. Once a sound flexibility program has been implemented, a resistive exercise program should be used emphasizing the development of strength and endurance of the involved musculature. Additionally, in sports such as tennis and racquetball, stroke mechanics must be analyzed to determine whether improper mechanics may have been responsible for producing the tendinitis.

DE QUERVAIN'S TENOSYNOVITIS. The most common stenosing tenosynovitis reported is de Quervain's, which is a result of repetitive ulnar deviation of the wrist.[15,17,18,20] De Quervain's stenosing tenosynovitis occurs at the radial styloid process where the long abductor of thumb and the short extensor of thumb pass through a fibroosseous canal.[20] Chronic irritation caused by ulnar deviation during tennis and golf swings produces the tenosynovitis within the fibroosseous canal. The condition presents pain with thumb use and gripping, inflammation at the radial styloid process, and crepitation when the wrist is extended and radially deviated.[19]

Most cases of de Quervain's tenosynovitis can be managed successfully with conservative measures including ice, antiinflammatory agents, and in severe cases immobilization until the acute pain subsequent to the inflammation subsides. The use of electrical modalities may also be indicated in cases where the inflammation is chronic. Phonophoresis, as described in an earlier chapter, may be beneficial by permitting antiinflammatory medications to be delivered to the injury site. Additionally, microamperage electrical nerve stimulation (MENS) therapy has been suggested to increase enkephalin production resulting in pain reduction.

A flexibility and strengthening protocol for the long abductor of thumb and the short extensor of thumb should be implemented once the pain and inflammation have subsided. Additionally, a thumb spica can be applied when returning the athlete to activity to prevent extreme ranges of thumb opposition and wrist ulnar deviation (Figure 21-1).

EXTENSOR MECHANISM TENOSYNOVITIS. The most common overuse injuries of the extensor mechanism occur in the radial extensor tendons of the wrist and the long and short radial extensors of wrist.[12,20] Athletes who perform wrist extension/radial deviation maneuvers including tennis and racquetball players, weight lifters, and rowers, are particularly susceptible

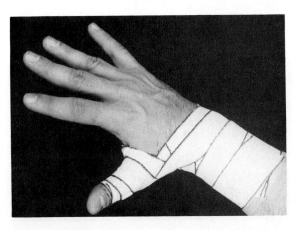

Fig. 21-1. Thumb spica taping. Thumb spica taping for de Quervain's tenosynovitis to prevent extreme ranges of thumb opposition and wrist ulnar deviation.

to developing insertional tenosynovitis. These tendons are also susceptible to overstretching during the deceleration phase of wrist flexion in golf, shotputting, and other throwing activities.[12] Clinically, pain is reproduced with passive flexion and active extension/radial deviation of the wrist and with direct palpation of the tendon insertion into the radial carpals.

The ulnar extensor of wrist is housed within a separate fibroosseous tunnel and is more superficial than the radial extensors of the wrist.[12] Furthermore, it is common to see fluid accumulation within the tendinous sheath, which is a common site of tenosynovitis for golfers and tennis players resulting from overuse.[3,9,20] Because of the tendon's superficial proximity, the thickened synovial sheath and tendon can be seen and palpated during forearm rotation.

Like most overuse inflammatory conditions, extensor tenosynovitis is acutely managed with rest and antiinflammatory measures. Immobilization may be indicated in severe cases, thus removing the stressful mechanism of chronic extension or overstretching from chronic flexion of the wrist (Figure 21-2). Strength and flexibility measures can be implemented for the extensor tendons once the acute inflammation has subsided.

FLEXOR MECHANISM TENDINITIS. Sports requiring sudden or chronic wrist flexion maneuvers can lead to flexor carpi ulnaris (FCU) irritation. The tendon insertion of the FCU includes the pisiform bone and the hypothenar fascia.[12] Irritation to the FCU tendon results in pain and strength deficits with gripping and

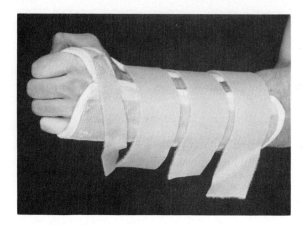

Fig. 21-2. Wrist immobilizer to prevent wrist flexion and extension.

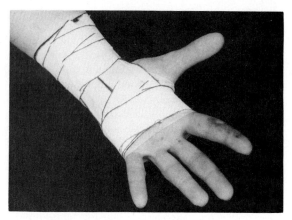

Fig. 21-3. Palmar checkrein taping to prevent wrist hyperextension.

flexion of the wrist caused by inflammation within the tendon. The FCU dominates wrist flexion activity. Maneuvers, such as curling dumbbells, releasing a ball during throwing, and swinging a golf club, commonly induce tendinitis. Pain is normally dispersed throughout the ulnar aspect of the wrist because of the broad tendinous insertion, although pain can usually be elicited upon palpation of the pisiform when inflamed.[12] Immobilization is usually suggested with FCU tendinitis because of the frequent use of the wrist flexor muscles in normal daily activities. In addition to immobilization, antiinflammatory measures are indicated until pain and swelling subside. Wrist flexion flexibility and strengthening exercises should be implemented once the acute symptoms have subsided.

CARPAL TUNNEL SYNDROME. Carpal tunnel syndrome is one of the most common wrist conditions associated with sports.[17,21,26] The condition is usually subsequent to an overuse wrist flexion activity, such as golf or tennis, which results in a flexor tenosynovitis. Swelling of the flexor tendons within the enclosed carpal tunnel space compresses the median nerve, resulting in pain or paresthesia in the radial aspect of the hand. Chronic carpal tunnel syndrome can result in thenar muscular atrophy because of the deinnervation caused by compression of the median nerve.

Conservative management includes immobilization and antiinflammatory measures in an attempt to relieve compression on the median nerve. In severe cases the decompression is performed surgically by releasing the transverse carpal ligament, which bounds the anterior aspect of the tunnel.[19]

TRIANGULAR FIBROCARTILAGE COMPLEX INJURIES. Sprains and fractures about the wrist and distal portions of the forearm may elicit symptoms of injury to the triangular fibrocartilage complex lying between the ulna and proximal row of carpal bones. The symptoms are usually reproduced by lateral motion of the wrist, either by impingement as the wrist is deviated ulnad or by distraction as the wrist is radially deviated.

Treatment of this condition ordinarily involves immobilization until healing has occurred. A complete tear of the complex, however, may indicate repair with or without augmentation to preserve its function in wrist stability. If locking and catching occur and persist, surgical excision is generally performed.[15]

Ligament Injuries of the Wrist

The major stabilizing ligaments of the wrist are the palmar intracapsular ligaments on the volar aspect of the wrist.[5] These intracapsular ligaments extend from their radial or ulnar origin to insert into their respective proximal row of carpal bones. The ligaments are sprained when the wrist is hyperextended and deviated, usually a result of falling when the hand attempts to break the athlete's fall.

Conservative management of wrist sprains involves antiinflammatory measures and supporting the wrist acutely for comfort. Surgery is usually only indicated in severe ligamentous injury resulting in instabilities of the carpal bones.[5] Rehabilitation of the overlying tendons is indicated to enhance dynamic stability in the region. Supportive taping is usually required when the athlete returns to activity to prevent hyperextension and terminal ranges of ulnar and radial deviation (Figure 21-3).

Fractures

SCAPHOID. The scaphoid is located in the lateral-distal carpal row. The lateral aspect of the scaphoid possesses a shallow waist, which is directly impinged by the distal radius when the wrist is extended and radially deviated. The most common mechanism of fracture of the scaphoid is falling on the outstretched arm while the wrist is extended. The force of the fall impinges the radius into the scaphoid and can fracture the bone at its narrow waist.

Differentiation between a scaphoid fracture and a soft tissue injury is often difficult. Therefore a radiographic evaluation is usually warranted when there is tenderness over the anatomical snuff box and when grip power is diminished.[15,17,18] Caution must be taken, however, not to dismiss the potential for a fracture existing should the initial radiographic evaluation prove negative, as is often the case. The continued presence of symptoms should guide the clinician toward subsequent reexamination of the wrist, either radiographically or by use of more sensitive procedures such as a bone scan or MRI. With early diagnosis, most scaphoid fractures can be managed with immobilization for approximately 3 months.[26] Immobilization usually consists of a short arm cast positioning the wrist in slight flexion with the thumb immobilized in abduction and opposition. The rules of sports, such as intercollegiate football, allow the athlete to wear an unyielding splint, thus allowing the athlete to return to competition while the scaphoid is healing. A protective silicone rubber short arm thumb spica splint can be simply devised, which immobilizes the fracture during sports activity.[27] The silicone splint should be removed, and the plaster cast should be reapplied immediately after the athletic event. Mobilization of the wrist is usually not warranted until complete fracture healing has occurred. Therefore flexibility and strengthening must include the entire hand and wrist region once the fracture has healed because of the prolonged period of immobilization.

HAMATE. The hamate is located in the medial-dorsal aspect of the wrist. The hamate possesses a hook-like projection that protrudes into the base of the hypothenar eminence. This protrusion can be fractured when a clublike device is in the palm of the hand and the wrist is deviated ulnad during swinging.[27] Golf, tennis, baseball, and squash may elicit the mechanism of a hamate fracture.[25,27] Normal wrist functions are unaffected by the fracture, and possibly the only signs of fracture may include tenderness to palpation and forceful ulnar deviation.

If the fracture is not displaced, a short arm cast is applied that extends to the little finger.[15,17,18] If the fracture is displaced, surgical excision of the fractured hook seems to be the most efficient management of hamate fractures in athletes.[27] After surgery the wrist is immobilized for 3 weeks. After the 3 weeks of immobilization, active motion can begin if pain is not present. The athlete can usually return to activity 6 weeks after surgery with protective taping.[27]

Rehabilitation of Wrist Injuries

The basic goals of rehabilitation of the wrist, which include arresting inflammation and restoring and enhancing flexibility and strength, are the same for both soft tissue injuries and fractures. Modifications and precautions may be indicated depending on the particular pathology of the injury, but the protocols tend to be similar.

Rehabilitation after fracture and immobilization of the wrist must initially focus on regaining active range of motion and then progress to restoring muscular strength, power, and endurance. Precaution should be taken to protect the fracture when the athlete returns to activity, and protective support is necessary after removal of the cast.

Most tendon inflammatory conditions of the wrist are a result of chronic irritation and can be classified as overuse injuries. To address the consequences of overuse, it is paramount to discontinue the activities responsible for the inflammatory condition. In addition to rest, the conservative measures of ice, antiinflammatory agents, and in severe cases, immobilization are necessary. The following outlines the treatment and rehabilitation protocol.

Treatment and Rehabilitation of Wrist Injuries
PHASE I: *Acute*
1. Rest/immobilization (Figure 21-2).
2. Ice (submersion or packs).
3. Oral antiinflammatory.

PHASE II: *Inflammation stabilized*
1. Cryokinetic techniques.
2. Active/active-assisted flexibility (Figure 21-4).
3. Active range of motion.

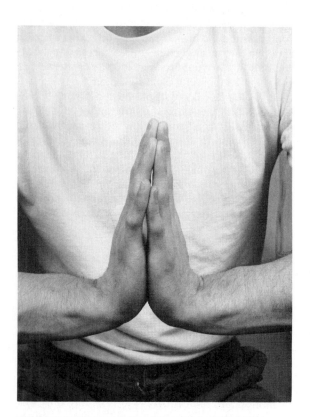

Fig. 21-4. Active-assisted wrist extension stretching.
Active-assisted wrist extension stretching with the athlete
using the uninvolved hand to assist stretching the involved
wrist to terminal extension.

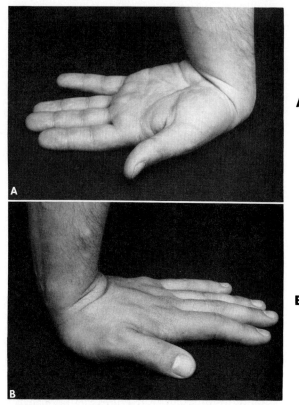

Fig. 21-5. Static stretching. Static stretching using a table to
assist terminal **A,** flexion, **B,** extension.

PHASE III: *Painfree range of motion*
1. Warm whirlpool/active range of motion.
2. Ultrasound.
3. Active/active-assisted flexibility.
4. Progressive resistance flexion, extension, supination, pronation, and deviation exercises
   (dumbell, elastic tubing, etc.) (Figures 21-6,
   21-7, and 21-8).

PHASE IV: *Near normal strength and range of motion*
1. Warm whirlpool/range of motion.
2. Active/active-assisted flexibility.
3. Progessive resistance exercises.
4. Sport-specific exercises (Figure 21-9).

Inherent in the process of rehabilitation of all injuries, including those to the wrist and hand, is the
importance of maintaining cardiovascular conditioning. Often, with injuries to the hand and wrist, the
athlete can continue to train aerobically specific to
his or her sport. In those cases where aerobic training
cannot be sport-specific, such as swimming, a form
of cross-training should be used, such as running or
biking. In addition, shoulder and elbow strengthening
should accompany hand and wrist rehabilitation to
enhance the overall function of the extremity.

FLEXIBILITY. Fractures and soft tissue overuse injuries of the wrist require rest and often prolonged
immobilization. After this period of rest or immobilization, restoring and enhancing flexibility of the
wrist flexor and extensors are necessary. The mechanism of wrist tendon involvement can be either eccentrically or concentrically induced, thus it is necessary to incorporate both flexion and extension exercises in the rehabilitation protocol, regardless of

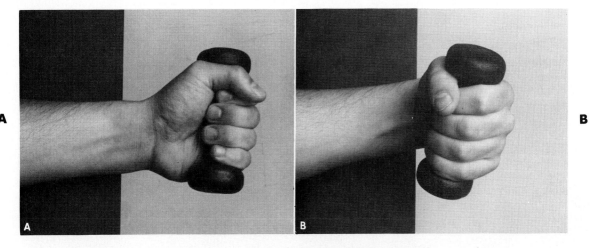

Fig. 21-6. Wrist flexion dumbell strengthening exercises.

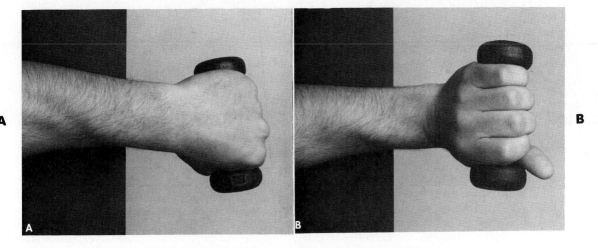

Fig. 21-7. Wrist extension dumbell strengthening exercises.

the specific condition. The use of a warm whirlpool with the athlete performing active motion while in the whirlpool will facilitate the goal of increased flexibility by increasing tissue temperature and elasticity.[21] Since the terminal ranges of flexion or extension may elicit pain at a fracture sight upon removal of the casting, the athlete should be encouraged to exercise within his or her pain-free ranges of motion.

The flexibility program should include both active and active-assisted stretching exercises. The stretching exercises should be performed actively to the

pain-free terminal range of motion. Upon reaching the terminal range of active motion, the athlete should perform an active-assisted stretch using the uninvolved hand (Figure 21-4). The terminal range of the active-assisted stretch should be held statically for 3 to 5 seconds (Figure 21-5). In addition to wrist flexion and extension, ulnar and radial deviation stretching should be integrated into the rehabilitation program.

STRENGTHENING. Rehabilitation of wrist tendon injuries must be monitored closely by the athletic

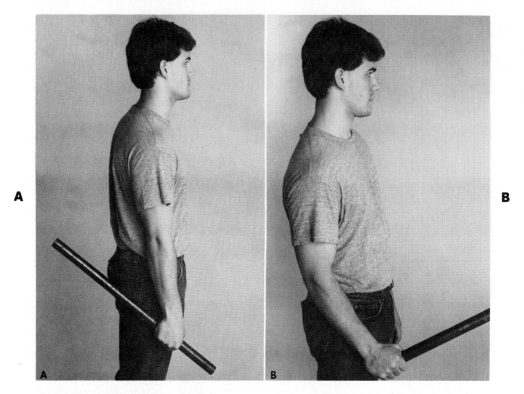

Fig. 21-8. Wrist deviation strengthening exercises. A, Wrist ulnar deviation strengthening exercise. **B,** Wrist radial deviation strengthening exercise.

trainer/therapist to prevent recurrence of the inflammation. The exercise program must develop both strength and endurance without inducing excessive irritation to the tendon. This can only be achieved if the athlete is willing to modify the exercises so that pain is not induced during the rehabilitation exercises. A protocol of progressive resistance exercise[13] using dumbell weights, elastic tubing, or other modalities is recommended to provide resistance to the exercising muscle. Three to four sets of 10 repetitions are generally recommended with increasing resistance incrementally from set to set or from session to session.

Wrist flexion and extension exercises should be performed with the elbow and forearm stabilized (Figure 21-6). This can easily be achieved with the elbow flexed to 90 degrees and positioning the forearm on a table with the hand and wrist extending beyond the table's end. Stabilization can also be achieved by securing the elbow tightly to the side while performing the exercises. All exercise should be performed throughout the entire range of motion and should be performed without pain in the involved tendon or bone (Figure 21-7). Ulnar and radial deviation and pronation/supination exercises should also be performed. Deviation exercises are easily performed using steel bar or hammerlike devices (Figure 21-8). Resistance can be modified by hand position. Rubber tubing can also be easily devised to exercise the pronator and supinator muscles and tendons.

The final stage of rehabilitation should include strengthening the musculature in patterns that are required upon return to sports activity. With creativity the athletic trainer/therapist can devise strengthening programs for the wrist and hand that are sport specific, thus decreasing the potential for recurrent injury upon return to competition. Examples of sport-specific exercises include releasing a baseball (Figure 21-9, A and B), the acceleration phase of a golf swing (Figure 21-9, C and D), and releasing a football.

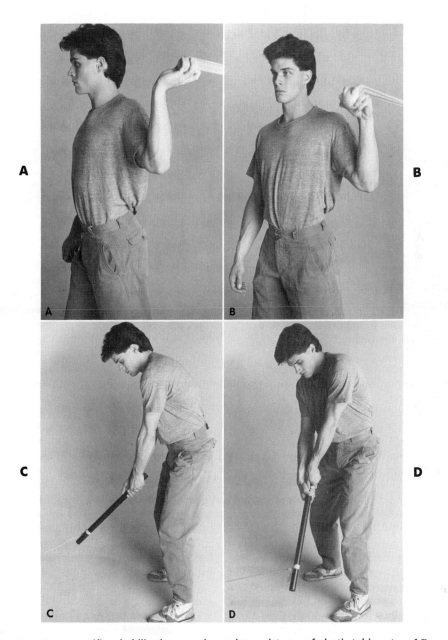

Fig. 21-9. Sport-specific rehabilitation exercises using resistance of elastic tubing. A and B, Wrist flexion during baseball throwing. **C and D,** Wrist flexion, extension, and deviation during a golf swing.

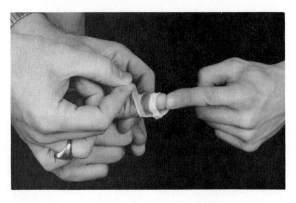

Fig. 21-10. Splint application of mallet finger. The athlete maintains slight DIP hyperextension while the splint is positioned on the volar aspect of the mallet finger.

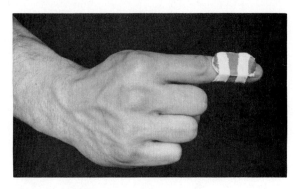

Fig. 21-11. Mallet finger splinting—dorsal aspect. Mallet finger splinting on the dorsal aspect of the finger for athletic participation.

HAND INJURIES
Tendon Injuries

EXTENSOR MECHANISM. Injuries to the extensor mechanism are common in sports that require catching a ball. Commonly, football receivers, baseball, basketball, and volleyball players are susceptible to having the ball hit the extended distal phalanx and forcefully flex the distal interphalangeal joint (DIP) or the proximal interphalangeal joint (PIP).[18]

One of the most common athletic injuries to the extensor mechanism is a rupture of the insertion of the extensor digitorum tendon from the distal phalanx resulting in a **mallet finger** or **drop finger**.[16] The athlete with a mallet finger is unable to actively extend the flexed DIP. The DIP is in a flexed position as a result of the flexor digitorum profundus tendon being unopposed when the extensor tendon has ruptured.

The exact involvement of a mallet finger can vary from stretching or rupturing the tendon to the tendon avulsing a piece of the distal phalanx.[16] Conservative management of the mallet finger involves immediate splinting of the DIP into a slightly hyperextended position to allow healing. It is not necessary to splint the PIP along with the DIP, which would result in stiffness to the PIP. McCue and others suggest 8 to 10 weeks of immobilization after injury and encourage the athlete to wear the splint during athletic activities for an additional 6 to 8 weeks to prevent reinjury.[16,17,18]

It is important that the splint is regularly alternated

from the dorsal to the volar surface of the finger. When the splint is moved, the athlete must stabilize the DIP, maintaining the hyperextended position while the splint is being reapplied (Figure 21-10). Cases of full-thickness skin necrosis have been reported as a result of impeded blood supply when the splint has been positioned on the dorsal surface of the finger for prolonged periods.[23] During athletic participation the splint should be positioned on the dorsal aspect of the finger if the athlete needs to catch or grasp during the event (Figure 21-11).

The **boutonniere deformity** is also a common injury to the hand in athletics. As with the mallet finger, a boutonniere deformity usually is the result of forceful flexion of the finger while the hand is extended. Forced flexion of the finger with the DIP extended results in flexion of the PIP and can rupture to the central slip of the extensor digitorum communis. The lateral bands of the flexor digitorum communis slide to the volar surface of the PIP, causing flexion of the interphalangeal joint (15 to 30 degrees) and extension of the DIP.[18] Rupture of the central slip renders the athlete unable to extend the PIP, thus resulting in the boutonniere deformity.

Management of the boutonniere deformity includes splinting of the PIP joint in an extended position for 6 to 8 weeks. The splint does not need to immobilize the metacarpal phalangeal joint (MCP) or the DIP. Additional splinting should occur for 6 to 8 weeks during athletic competition.[18]

FLEXOR MECHANISM INJURIES. Although injury to the flexor mechanism is not as common as injury to the extensor mechanism in the athletic population, forced extension of the finger can strain or rupture the flexor digitorum profundus (FDP) tendon. The most common mechanism of FDP rupture occurs when an athlete is grabbing an opponent's jersey and forcefully extends the finger, resulting in a **jersey finger.**[20] It is often difficult for the clinician to differentiate between a strain and complete rupture because of the mass of soft tissue and swelling in the volar aspect of the finger.

Management of the ruptured flexor tendon will depend on the exact pathology involved. Tendon ruptures will vary in degree of tendon retraction, volar plate involvement, and vinculum involvement. In most cases the tendon must be surgically repaired and the finger immobilized with the MCP flexed to 30 degrees and the interphalangeal joints flexed to 10 degrees for a minimum of 3 weeks.[18] Active motion is started at approximately the third week, with the protective splint reapplied immediately after the exercise. The splint is worn protectively up to 12 weeks after surgery but can be replaced with a mitten-type splint for some athletic competition if active gripping is not essential for performance.[18]

Ligament Injuries to the Hand

Capsular and ligamentous sprains of the fingers are frequent injuries in sports. The fingers are vulnerable whenever they are hyperextended or have axial, lateral, or rotary forces applied. Athletes refer to the hyperextension and axial compression injuries as *stoved* or *jammed* fingers. This type of injury usually results in a hemarthrosis to the proximal interphalangeal joint.

A lateral force of the finger can result in a collateral ligament sprain, compromising joint stability. However, a significant amount of laxity may not be evident if swelling is present, which stabilizes the joint. Conservative management of collateral sprains and severe capsular sprains includes splinting the finger in 30 degrees of flexion for 3 to 4 weeks. Active motion can begin 10 to 14 days after injury, and a protective splint should be worn for 4 to 6 weeks after injury during athletic competition.[11,15]

Injury to the ulnar collateral ligament (UCL) of the thumb, also referred to as **gamekeepers thumb** or **skiers thumb,** is a common athletic injury that results from the thumb being forcefully extended and abducted.[4,6,7,24] The pole of a skier extending the skier's thumb while falling or an opponent's jersey

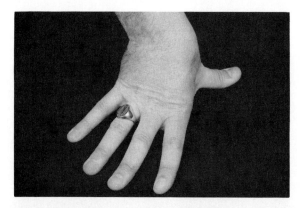

Fig. 21-12. Extension-abduction mechanism of gamekeeper's thumb.

forcefully extending an athlete's thumb are frequent mechanisms resulting in a sprain or rupture of the UCL at the level of the proximal phalanx of the thumb (Figure 21-12).

Gamekeepers thumb generally presents as a sprain or partial rupture to the UCL combined with a mild-to-moderate strain of the thumb flexor and adductor muscles. Diminished strength, swelling, and pain are associated with the injury, although instability is difficult to assess unless a complete rupture of the UCL has occurred. The potential for long-term functional loss and significant disability caused by inadequate treatment of this injury sets it apart from many other ligament injuries of the hand. Therefore considerable attention should be paid to designing a treatment and rehabilitation regimen that allows for adequate healing and logical progression back to optimal functional capability. The condition is managed conservatively with a thumb spica to support and protect the injury.[15,17] The spica is applied with the thumb adducted and slightly opposed for protection in athletic activities. In severe sprains or when the thumb is minimally used during the activity, further stabilization can be achieved by taping the thumb to the index finger (Figure 21-13).[15]

Fractures and Dislocations of the Hand

FRACTURES. The metacarpals of the hand are vulnerable to fracture any time a substantial force is applied to the bone in an axial loading fashion while the MCP is flexed. Typically boxers sustain metacarpal neck fractures known as a **boxer's** fracture.[2] In

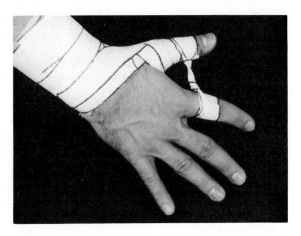

Fig. 21-13. Thumb spica with checkrein. Thumb spica with checkrein prevents extension and abduction of the thumb during athletic participation.

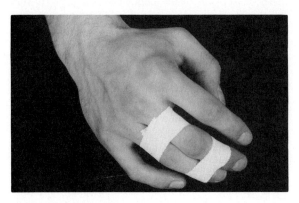

Fig. 21-14. Finger splinting. Finger splinting to the adjacent finger for athletic participation.

most cases, metacarpal fractures are treated with closed reduction and immobilization using a short arm cast for 4 to 6 weeks, which does not include immobilization of the PIP and DIP.[15]

Proximal phalanx fractures are commonly the result of a hyperextension mechanism. Improper reduction of this fracture can result in significant adhesions of the extrinsic tendons in this region.[15] The adhesions can severely restrict active motion at the PIP and DIP, which can be devastating to an athlete. Management involves closed reduction in most cases. The PIP is immobilized in 30 degrees of flexion, which tends to relax the extrinsic tendons and prevent significant tension adhesions. The collateral ligaments assist in stabilizing the MCP, thus maintaining control of the fractured proximal portion of the phalanx.[15]

Active motion can begin approximately 3 weeks after injury; sports activity can also begin at this time if significant healing has occurred. Wearing the splint can be discontinued for athletic participation at approximately 9 weeks and replaced by taping the finger to an adjacent finger for stabilization of the fracture (Figure 21-14).[15]

Oblique and transverse fractures through the cortical bone in the waist of the shaft of the middle phalanx are characteristic of sports-related finger injuries.[2,15] The dorsal insertion of the central slip of the extensor tendon into the base of the phalanx of the two slips of the flexor digitorum sublimis makes

these fractures anatomically susceptible to deformity.[2] Longitudinal traction, applied with or without flexion depending on the site of injury, is used to reduce these fractures. The fractures usually respond slowly to healing, thus traditionally they are splinted until completely healed. Stable fractures are splinted for 3 weeks before exercises are initiated. Unstable fractures may require percutaneous fixation with K wires and protection.[2,15]

DISLOCATIONS. The most common finger dislocation involves the PIP joint because of a hyperextension mechanism resulting in a dorsal dislocation.[2,15] This dislocation is easily reduced. The athlete will often reduce the dislocation on the field. Once reduced and fracture and volar plate involvement have been ruled out, the joint should be immobilized in 20 to 30 degrees of flexion for 3 weeks.[15] The athlete can generally return to competition at approximately 3 weeks, although the finger should be splinted by taping it to an adjacent finger for an additional 2 weeks. Active motion should be encouraged at 2 to 3 weeks after injury.

Rehabilitation of the Hand

The primary goal during rehabilitation of the hand is to restore active range of motion. Immobilization typically results in stiffness of the joints of the fingers, which then results in a lack of terminal ranges of flexion and extension. A thorough understanding of

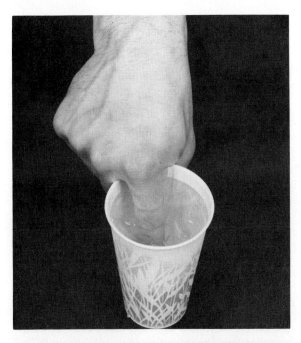

Fig. 21-15. Finger cryotherapy before exercise.

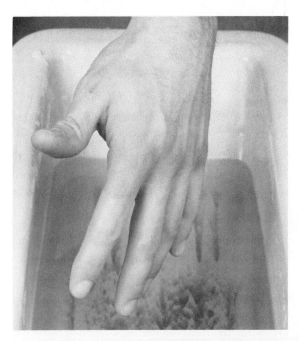

Fig. 21-16. Hand being dipped in paraffin.

the unique action of the hand musculature is necessary to isolate joint movements and enhance motion in all of the involved joints.

During the acute stage of rehabilitation of those conditions allowing for early mobilization of the joints, such as capsular sprains, active motion can be enhanced using the cryokinetic techniques.[14] Cryotherapy will assist in controlling the inflammation subsequent to the hand trauma and will reduce pain, thus facilitating active exercise (Figure 21-15).[10] Once the inflammation has been stabilized, heating modalities, such as warm whirlpools and paraffin, should be implemented to enhance tissue elasticity and assist with the restoration of active motion.[22] Paraffin has also proven to be effective in reducing chronic edema and hemarthrosis in the interphalangeal regions of the hand (Figure 21-16). The treatment and rehabilitation protocol are outlined below and in Table 21-1.

Treatment and Rehabilitation of Hand Injuries

PHASE I: *Acute*

1. Immobilization (dependent upon pathology; Table 21-1).

2. Ice packs; retain immobilization and keep splint dry.
3. Oral antiinflammatory.

PHASE II: *Begin Motion* (Table 21-1)

1. Warm whirlpool/active range of motion.
2. Isolated joint passive and active motion.
3. Reapply splint.

PHASE III: *Removal of Splint* (Table 21-1)

1. Warm whirlpool/active range of motion or paraffin followed by active range of motion.
2. Gripping strength exercises (Figure 21-18).
3. Isolated resistance exercises (Figures 21-19 and 21-20).
4. Dexterity exercises (Figure 21-21).

FLEXIBILITY OF THE HAND. Active motion exercises for the hand must include both gross motor exercises and isolated joint motion. All exercises of the hand should be performed gently and must be performed pain free. Gross motor exercises should be performed during a warm whirlpool or immediately after paraffin or cold application, as indicated. Both flexion and extension exercise are encouraged, regardless of the particular pathology. Generally the arm should be positioned in 90 degrees flexion and stabilized against

TABLE 21-1

Treatment and Immobilization of Finger Injuries

Injury	Constant Splinting (Weeks)	Begin Motion (Weeks)	Additional Splinting for Competition (Weeks)	Joint Position
Mallet finger	6–8	6–8	6–8	Slight DIP hyperextension
Collateral ligament sprains	3	2	4–6	30 degrees flexion
DIP and PIP dislocations	3	3	3	30 degrees flexion
Boutonniere deformity	6–8	6–8	6–8	PIP in extension; DIP, MCP not included
DIP, PIP fractures	9–11	3	3	30 degrees flexion
MCP fractures	3	3	4–6	30 degrees flexion
FDP repair	3–5	3	3–5	Depends on repair

Modified from Gieck JH, McCue FC III: Splinting of finger injuries, *Ath Train* 17:215, 1982.

the athlete's torso or on a table. Active motion protocols for the hand should be consistent with the principles of rehabilitation with regard to technique and duration. All exercises should be performed throughout the entire range of active motion, 3 to 4 sets of 8 to 10 repetitions. Pain, other than that induced by muscle fatigue, should terminate the exercise session. Flexion and extension exercises of the entire hand should be performed, followed by exercising each involved finger and isolating each involved joint.

Isolating each involved finger and each involved joint motion is necessary, particularly when the FDP and flexor digitor superficialis (FDS) tendons are involved. The FDP tendon inserts into the distal phalanx, while the tendon of the FDS inserts into the middle phalanx. To exercise the FDP, the DIP must be flexed while the MCP and PIP are stabilized (Figure 21-17).

After a period of immobilization, the hand's intrinsic muscles must also be reconditioned. The palmar and dorsal interosseous and the lumbrical muscle assist in flexion of the MCP and extension of the PIP joints, while the interosseous muscles are primarily responsible for abduction and adduction of the fingers. Active abduction and adduction exercises should be performed similar to flexion and extension exercises, beginning with exercising the hand as a whole followed by isolating each finger.

STRENGTHENING AND DEXTERITY EXERCISES FOR THE HAND. Active range-of-motion exercises initiate strengthening of the hand musculature but are not sufficient to regain both dexterity and power in the selected tendons and hand intrinsic muscles after immobilization. The principles of muscle strengthening in the injured hand are consistent with rehabilitation protocols for any injury. However, as compared to the technology available to rehabilitate other injuries, there are limited resistance modalities that exist specifically for the purpose of hand strengthening. Grip strength can be regained gripping a rubber ball or using gripping putty and hand grip coils. A hand dynamometer can be used to measure isometric grip strength (Figure 21-18). Gripping exercises should consist of a maximal and sustained voluntary contraction for 3 to 5 seconds in sets of 10 repetitions. Graded resistance protocols are difficult to achieve with gripping exercises, thus repetitions are usually increased as strength increases.

The strengthening needs of the thumb are unique because of the variety of thumb intrinsic muscles that need to be exercised. Active motion of the thumb must include adduction, abduction, flexion, extension, opposition, and circumduction. Once active range of motion is achieved, manual resistance exercises can easily be implemented. Manual resistance can either be performed by the athletic trainer/therapist or by the athlete (Figure 21-19). In addition to manual resistance, rubber bands can be used as a mode of progressive resistance (Figure 21-20). Strengthening of the finger's intrinsic muscles and tendons similarly can be achieved via manual resistance or using rubber bands for resistance.

Lastly, dexterity exercises should include pinch-

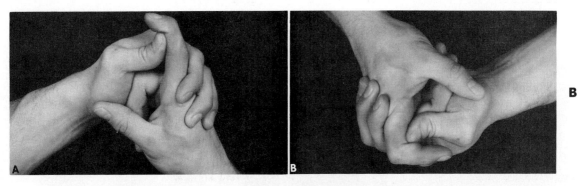

Fig. 21-17. Isolating joints for active range of motion for exercises. A, Stabilizing the MCP and PIP to exercise the DIP. **B,** Stabilizing the MCP to exercise the PIP.

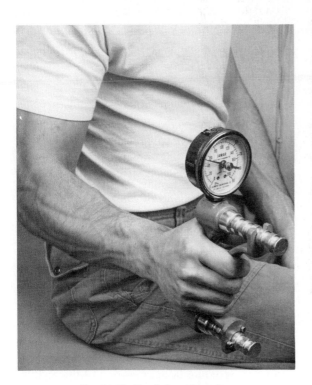

Fig. 21-18. Hand dynamometer.

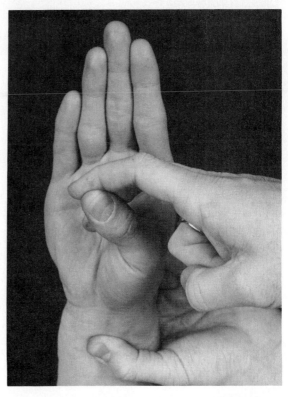

Fig. 21-19. Manual resistance for thumb opposition exercises.

ing, tearing, and other activities that are essential for not only athletics but for daily activities. Such activities include picking up coins, tearing tape, and gripping clubs, balls, or other objects requiring dexterity and tactile senses (Figure 21-21).

SUPPORT AND PROTECTION FOR RETURN TO SPORTS. Often the athlete can return to activity before complete healing of hand injuries. It is essential that the injuries are supported and protected during this period to prevent recurrent injury to the hand. Finger

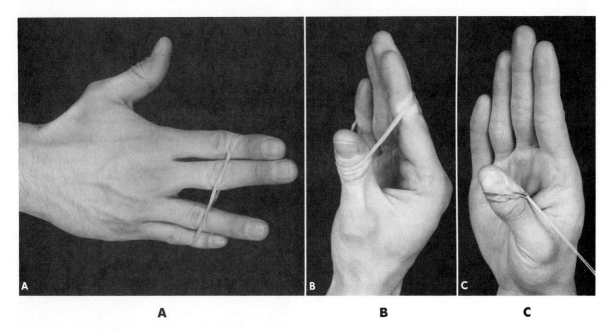

Fig. 21-20. Resistance exercises using rubber bands. A, Finger abduction exercise. **B,** Thumb abduction exercise. **C,** Thumb opposition exercise.

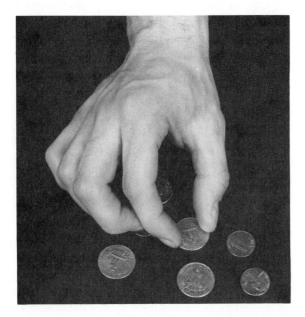

Fig. 21-21. Dexterity exercises for the hand.

splints can be modified to allow for gripping by moving the splint to the dorsal surface of the hand or in some cases using a flexible type of support device. Fingers with joint instability can be splinted to adjacent fingers for support or can be splinted to prevent unwanted motion. Finally, the thumb can be supported to prevent any or all motions depending on the needs of the particular athlete.

SUMMARY

1. Injuries to the wrist and hand are common in sports requiring the athlete to throw, catch, or grab or when the hand is involved in breaking the athlete's fall.
2. Wrist injuries are often subsequent to overuse activities, resulting in inflammation of the tendons in the region. Thus management of wrist inflammatory conditions must include rest from the sport for a period of time and in some cases immobilization.
3. Rehabilitation objectives after wrist injuries must initially focus on regaining active range of motion and then progress to restoring muscular strength, power, and endurance.

4. Hand injuries are generally a result of trauma induced by a ball, an opponent's jersey, or falling. These injuries include tendon and ligament disruptions, fractures, and dislocations.

5. The hands are relied on for dexterity during most daily activities, as well as for athletics. Therefore it is paramount that normal motion and function are reestablished after injury. Active motion exercises seem to be the most successful modality to rehabilitate the hand from such injuries.

6. The hand and wrist must be protected upon returning to athletic competition once rehabilitation is complete. Many taping, bracing, and supportive devices are available to decrease the incidence of recurrent injury upon return to sport participation.

The author would like to thank Kevin Conley, M.S., A.T.C., for his assistance with the preparation of this chapter.

REFERENCES

1 Bassett FH, Malone T, Gilchrist R, et al.: A protective splint of silicone rubber, *Am J Sports Med* 7(6):358-360, 1979.

2 Brunet ME, Haddad RJ: Fractures and dislocations of the metacarpals and phalanges, *Clin Sports Med* 5(4):773-781, 1986.

3 Burkhart SS, Wood MB, Linscheid RL: Post-traumatic recurrent subluxation of the extensor carpi ulnaris tendon, *J Hand Surg* 11[A]:519, 1986.

4 Commandre F, Viani JL: The football keeper's thumb, *J Sport Med Phys Fitness* 1(6):121-122, 1976.

5 Culver JE: Instabilities of the wrist, *Clin Sports Med* 5(4):725-740, 1986.

6 Curtin J, Kay NR: Hand injuries due to soccer, *Hand* 8:93-95, 1976.

7 Ganel A, Anronson Z, Engel J, et al.: Gamekeeper's thumb: injuries of the ulnar collateral ligament of the metacarpophalangeal joint, *Br J Sports Med* 14(2-3):92, 1980.

8 Gieck JH, McCue FC: Splinting of finger injuries, *Ath Train* 7:215, 1982.

9 Hajj AA, Wood MB: Stenosing tenosynovitis of the extensor carpi ulnaris, *J Hand Surg* 11[A]:519, 1986.

10 Hocatt JE, Jaffe R, Rylander C, et al.: Cryotherapy in ankle sprains, *Am J Sports Med* 10(5):316-319, 1982.

11 Isani A, Melone CP: Ligament injuries of the hand in athletics, *Clin Sports Med* 5(4):757-772, 1986.

12 Johnson RK: Soft tissue injuries of the forearm and hand, *Clin Sports Med* 7(2):329-348, 1988.

13 Kisner C, Colby LA: *Therapeutic exercises: foundations and techniques,* Philadelphia, 1985, FA Davis.

14 Knight KL: *Cryotherapy in sports medicine.* In Schubner K, Burke EJ, editors: *Relevant topics in athletic training,* New York, 1978, Movement Publications.

15 Kuland DN: *The injured athlete,* ed 2, Philadelphia, 1988, JB Lippincott.

16 McCue FC, Abbott JL: The treatment of mallet finger and boutonniere deformities, *Va Med Mon* 94:623, 1966.

17 McCue FC, Baugher H, Kuland D, et al.: Hand and wrist injuries in the athlete, *Am J Sports Med* 7(5):275-286, 1979.

18 McCue FC, Wooten SL: Closed tendon injuries of the hand in athletics, *Clin Sports Med* 5(4):741-755, 1986.

19 O'Donoghue DW: *Treatment of injuries to athletes,* ed 4, Philadelphia, 1984, WB Saunders.

20 Osterman LE, Moskow L, Low DW: Soft tissue injuries of the hand and wrist in racquet sports, *Clin Sports Med* 7(2):329-348, 1988.

21 Phalen GS: The carpal-tunnel syndrome: seventeen years experience in diagnosis and treatment of six hundred fifty-four hands, *J Bone Joint Surg* 48[A]:211, 1966.

22 Prentice WE: *Therapeutic modalities in sports medicine,* St Louis, 1990, Mosby.

23 Rayan GM, Mullins PT: Skin necrosis complicating mallet finger splinting and vascularity of the distal interphalangeal joint overlying skin, *J Hand Surg* 12[A](4):548-551, 1987.

24 Rovere GD: Treatment of "gamekeeper's thumb" in hockey players, *Am J Sports Med* 3:147-151, 1985.

25 Stark HH: Fracture of the hook of the hamate in athletics, *J Bone Joint Surg* 59[A]:575-582, 1977.

26 Woods MB, Dobyns JH: Sport-related extraarticular wrist syndromes, *Clin Orthop* 202:95-101, 1986.

27 Zemel NP, Stark HH: Fractures and dislocations of the carpal bones, *Clin Sports Med* 5(4):709-724, 1986.

Rehabilitation of Hip and Thigh Injuries

Bernard DePalma

OBJECTIVES

After completion of this chapter, the student should be able to do the following:

- Describe the functional anatomy of the hip and thigh.

- Discuss athletic injuries to the hip and thigh.

- Describe functional injury evaluation of the hip and thigh.

- Recognize abnormal gait cycles as they relate to hip and thigh injuries.

- Explain the behavioral approach to rehabilitation of the hip and thigh including short-term goals and rehabilitation timetables.

- Discuss the role of functional evaluation in determining when to return an athlete to competition, based on rehabilitation timetables.

This chapter describes functional rehabilitation programs that follow hip and thigh injuries. The behavioral approach, which uses short-term goal setting and rehabilitation timetables, characterizes these rehabilitation programs. The sports therapist and athlete together should develop the rehabilitation program with an emphasis on the sports therapist's functional evaluation and clinical findings. Each exercise program in this chapter should be presented to the athlete in terms of short-term goals. One objective for the sports therapist is to make the rehabilitation experience challenging for the athlete to promote adherence to the rehabilitation program. No matter how good the rehabilitation program is, it will not be effective if the athlete does not follow through.

The chapter presents a comprehensive review of injuries that commonly occur to the hip and thigh. Discussion of each injury includes a brief review of the literature, the functional evaluation and clinical findings pertinent to that injury, and a specific treatment and rehabilitation program. Keep in mind that the time sequences for programs presented in this chapter are approximations; shortening or lengthening the time sequences may be necessary depending upon the degree of injury.

HIP POINTER

A **hip pointer** can best be described as a subcutaneous contusion caused by a direct blow to the iliac crest or the anterosuperior iliac spine. In most cases, the contusion can cause separation or tearing of the origins or insertions of the muscles that attach to these two prominent bony sites.[12] Usually the athlete has no immediate concern, but within an hour of the injury, bleeding, swelling, and pain can severely limit the athlete's movement. In rare cases, a fracture of the crest may occur.[21] An x-ray film should be taken to rule out iliac crest fractures or avulsion fractures, especially in younger athletes.[12] If the hip pointer is not treated early, within approximately 2 to 4 hours, the athlete may experience severe pain and limited range of motion of the trunk because of the muscle attachments involved.

More serious injuries must also be ruled out. One athlete who reported the signs and symptoms of a hip pointer on the field later was determined to have a ruptured spleen.

A strain of the abdominal muscles at their attachment to the anterior and inferior iliac crest can easily be differentiated from a contusion by obtaining a good history of the mechanism of injury at the time it occurs. A forceful contraction of the abdominal muscles while the trunk is being passively forced to the opposite side may cause a strain of the muscles at their insertion to the iliac bone.[19]

Grade I Hip Pointer

EVALUATION AND CLINICAL FINDINGS. An athlete with a grade I hip pointer may have both normal gait cycle and normal posture. The athlete may complain of slight pain on palpation with little or no swelling. This athlete may also present with full range of motion of the trunk, especially lateral side bending to the opposite side of the injury. A grade I hip pointer usually does not prevent competition.

Grade II Hip Pointer

EVALUATION AND CLINICAL FINDINGS. An athlete with a grade II hip pointer may have moderate-to-severe pain on palpation, noticeable swelling, and an abnormal gait cycle. The gait cycle may be changed because of a short swing-through phase on the affected side; the athlete may take a short step and be reluctant to keep the foot off the ground. The athlete's posture may be slightly tilted to the side of the injury. Active hip and trunk flexion may cause pain, especially if the anterosuperior iliac spine is involved, because of the insertion of the sartorius muscle. Range of motion may be limited, especially lateral side bending to the opposite side of the injury and trunk rotation in both directions. This athlete could miss 5 to 14 days of competition.

Grade III Hip Pointer

EVALUATION AND CLINICAL FINDINGS. An athlete with a grade III hip pointer may have severe pain on palpation, noticeable swelling, and possible discoloration. The athlete's gait cycle could be abnormal, with very slow, deliberate ambulation and extremely short stride length and swing-through phase. The athlete's posture may present a severe lateral tilt to the

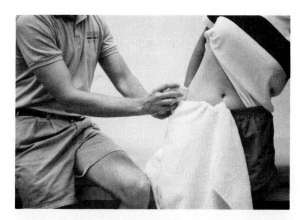

Fig. 22-1. Ice massage. Ice massage to hip pointer with side bending to opposite side.

affected side. Trunk range of motion may be limited in all directions. Active hip and trunk flexion may reproduce pain. This athlete could miss 14 to 21 days of competition.

TREATMENT AND REHABILITATION. Ice, compression, and rest should be started immediately. Subcutaneous steroid injection has decreased inflammation and enabled early range-of-motion exercises. Oral antiinflammatory medication is also beneficial in the early stages to reduce pain and inflammation. Transcutaneous electrical nerve stimulation (TNS) may be helpful on the day of injury to decrease pain and enable range-of-motion exercises.

To speed recovery, use ice massage for 10 minutes, followed by pain-free trunk active range-of-motion exercises. Concentrate on lateral side bending to the opposite side of the injury (Figure 22-1). When active swelling and inflammation stop, on approximately the second or third day, ultrasound is very beneficial for gaining range of motion after ice massage. Pain-free active range-of-motion exercises are vital to the recovery process. Active motion, usually started on the second day, helps promote healing and decreases the time the athlete is prohibited from practice and competition. On approximately days 3 to 5, hip abduction, flexion, and extension progressive resistive strengthening exercises (using an ankle cuff or weight boot) may be performed, as long as this activity does not cause pain (Figures 22-2 through 22-7). Trunk strengthening exercises may also be added. Compression should be maintained throughout the period with practice or competition. On returning to com-

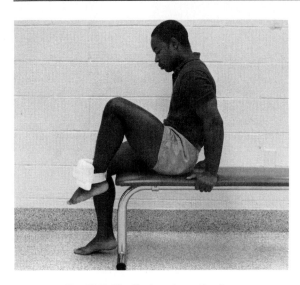

Fig. 22-2. Hip flexion strengthening.

petition, the athlete should wear custom-made protective doughnut padding.

Treatment of hip pointers

PHASE I: *Days 1-2*
1. Ice (massage).
2. Rest.
3. Compression.
4. Subcutaneous steroid injection.
5. Oral antiinflammatory medication.
6. TNS.

PHASE II: *Days 2-3*
7. Ultrasound.
8. Pain-free hip and trunk active range-of-motion exercises (concentrate on lateral side bending to the opposite side). Slow stretch held for 15 to 30 seconds times 3 to 5 sets daily.

PHASE III: *Days 3-5*
9. Pain-free hip abduction progressive resistive strengthening exercises: 3 sets of 10-15 repetitions daily.
10. Pain-free hip flexion progressive resistive strengthening exercises: 3 sets of 10-15 repetitions daily.
11. Pain-free hip extension progressive resistive strengthening exercises: 3 sets of 10-15 repetitions daily.
12. Pain-free active trunk flexion and extension strengthening exercises: 3 sets of 10-15 repetitions daily.

PHASE IV: *Day 5*
13. Functional sport-specific activities.
14. Custom-made, protective doughnut pad.

INJURY TO THE ILIAC SPINE
Anterosuperior Iliac Spine

The anterosuperior iliac spine serves as an attachment for the sartorius muscle. Pain at this site may indicate apophysitis, an inflammatory response to overuse.[1]

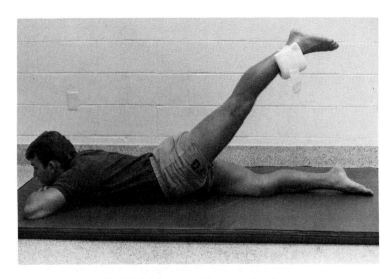

Fig. 22-3. Hip extension strengthening.

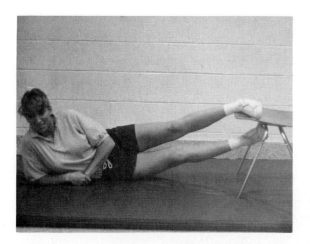

Fig. 22-4. Hip adduction strengthening.

Severe pain associated with disability requires an x-ray film to rule out an avulsion fracture.[1] Apophysitis or a contusion to the anterosuperior iliac spine may accompany a hip pointer and should be treated as such.

Anteroinferior Iliac Spine

The anteroinferior iliac spine serves as an attachment for the rectus femoris. As with the anterosuperior iliac spine, apophysitis or a contusion may be treated as a hip pointer (see Treatment for Hip Pointer on p. 375). An avulsion fracture caused by a violent, forceful contraction of the rectus femoris or a violent, forceful passive stretch of the hip into extension should be ruled out by x-ray films. These injuries are seen more often in younger athletes.

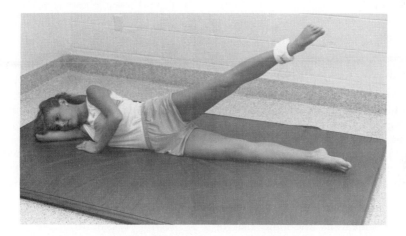

Fig. 22-5. Hip abduction strengthening.

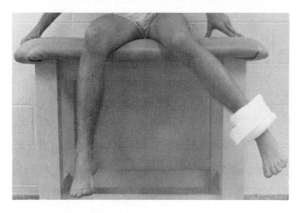

Fig. 22-6. Hip internal rotation strengthening.

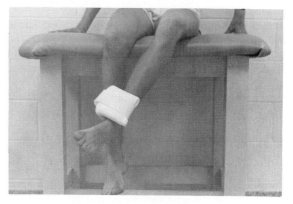

Fig. 22-7. Hip external rotation strengthening.

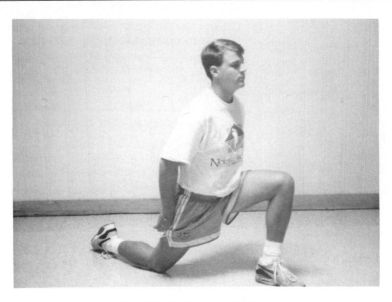

Fig. 22-8. Hip flexor stretching.

Posterosuperior Iliac Spine Contusion

Contusions to the posterosuperior iliac spine must be differentiated from vertebral fractures and more serious internal organ injuries.[1] Depending upon the athlete's pain and range of motion, an x-ray film should be taken to rule out vertebral fractures and vertebral transverse process fractures. Other injuries to this area are not common because of the lack of muscle attachments.[19] Avulsion fractures may not be seen in this area; a fracture of the posterosuperior iliac spine should be ruled out. The injury may be painful but usually does not cause disability.

EVALUATION AND CLINICAL FINDINGS. An athlete with a contusion to the posterosuperior iliac spine may complain of pain on palpation and have swelling that is usually not extensive. The athlete's gait cycle may look normal except in severe cases, when the athlete may take short, choppy steps to avoid the pain associated with landing at heel strike. In severe cases, the athlete's posture may show a slight forward flexion tilt of the trunk. This athlete may show full active range of motion of the trunk, with mild discomfort. In moderate-to-severe cases, up to 3 days of rest may be needed before return to competition.

TREATMENT AND REHABILITATION. Ice massage may be used for the first 3 days, followed by pulsed ultrasound in the less severe cases. The athlete may usually begin hot packs with pain-free stretching ex-

ercises within the first 3 days, as long as the active swelling has been controlled (Figures 22-8 through 22-13). Exercises should include active and passive trunk and hip flexion and extension. A protective doughnut pad should be worn for competition.

Treatment of contusions to the posterosuperior iliac spine

PHASE I: *Days 1-3*
1. Ice (massage).
2. Ultrasound (pulse).
3. Hot packs.
4. Pain-free active and passive range-of-motion exercises of the trunk and hip. Stretches are held for 30 seconds times 5 repetitions daily. Active exercises are performed as 3 sets of 10 repetitions daily.

PIRIFORMIS SYNDROME SCIATICA

The sciatic nerve is a continuation of the sacral plexus as it passes through the greater sciatic notch and descends deeply through the back of the thigh. Hip pain is often diagnosed as sciatic nerve irritation. The sciatic nerve may be irritated by a low back problem, but it is also subject to trauma where the nerve passes underneath or through the piriformis muscle, in which case sciatic nerve irritation is also called *piriformis syndrome.* In approximately 15% of the pop-

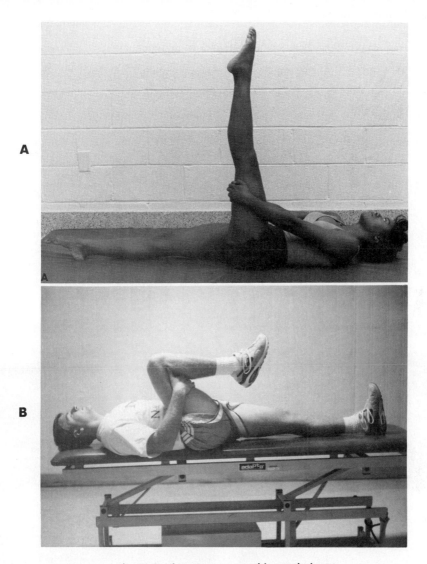

Fig. 22-9. Hip extensor stretching techniques.

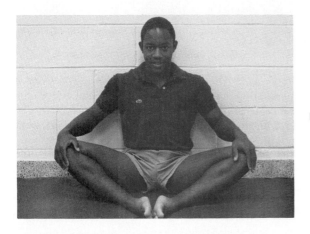

Fig. 22-10. Hip adductor stretching.

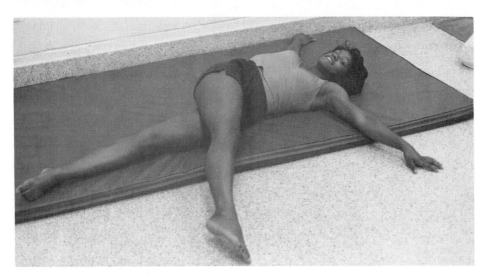

Fig. 22-11. Hip abductor stretching.

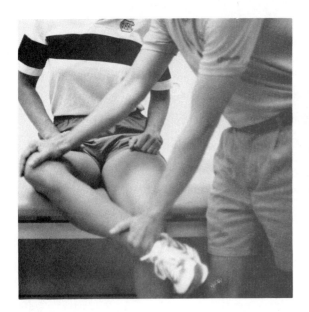

Fig. 22-12. Hip internal rotator stretching.

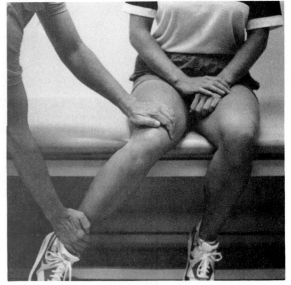

Fig. 22-13. Hip external rotator stretching.

ulation, the sciatic nerve passes through the piriformis muscle, separating it in two. This condition is seen in more women than men, and the cause of piriformis syndrome may be a tight piriformis muscle.[7]

Injury to the hamstring muscles may also cause sciatic nerve irritation as can irritation from ischial bursitis.[7] In a traumatic accident that causes posterior dislocation of the femoral head, the sciatic nerve may be crushed or severed and require surgery.[7]

The most common cause of sciatic nerve irritation in athletics, especially contact sports, is a direct blow to the buttock. Because of the large muscle mass, this injury is not usually disabling when the sciatic nerve is not involved. When the sciatic nerve is involved, however, the athlete may experience pain in the but-

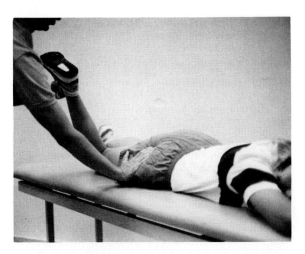

Fig. 22-14. Evaluating tightness of the piriformis.

tock, extending down the back of the thigh, possibly into the lateral calf and foot.[19] Sciatic pain is usually a burning sensation.

With sciatica, the sports therapist must rule out disk disease before starting any exercise rehabilitation program. Stretching exercises that are indicated for sciatica, such as trunk and hip flexion, may be contraindicated for disk disease. To differentiate low back problems (disk disease) from piriformis syndrome as the cause of sciatica, determine if the athlete has low back pain with radiation into the extremity. Back pain is most likely midline, exacerbated by trunk flexion and relieved by rest.[10] Coughing and straining may also increase back pain and possibly the radiation. Muscle weakness and sensory numbness may also be found in an athlete with disk disease.[10] Athletes with piriformis syndrome may have the same symptoms without low back pain.

If, after treatment and rehabilitation, the athlete still maintains neurological deficits, further evaluation should be performed, and disk disease should be ruled out again.

EVALUATION AND CLINICAL FINDINGS. In the case of piriformis syndrome, the athlete may report a deep pain in the buttock without low back pain and possibly radiating pain in the back of the thigh, lateral calf, and foot, also indicating sciatica.[7] The sports therapist's evaluation should include the low back, as well as the hip and thigh. The athlete's gait cycle could include lack of a heel strike, landing in the foot-flat phase, a shortening of the stride, and possible ambulation with a flexed knee. The athlete's posture, in severe cases, shows a flexed knee with the leg ex-

ternally rotated. Palpation in the sciatic notch could also produce pain.

With the athlete lying supine and the hip in a neutral position with the knee in extension, active resistive external rotation and passive internal rotation of the hip may reproduce the pain[7] (Figure 22-14). Straight leg raises performed passively or actively may also cause symptoms. With the athlete in the same position as above and relaxed, a decrease in passive internal rotation of the hip joint as compared to the uninjured side may indicate piriformis tightness.

Severe sciatica caused by piriformis syndrome may put the athlete out of competition for 2 to 3 weeks.

TREATMENT AND REHABILITATION. If the sciatic nerve is irritated and the athlete complains of radiation into the extremity, the first 3 to 5 days should consist of modalities to decrease the pain associated with sciatica. Ice or heat, in contrast form or alone, at the sciatic notch and hamstring areas may decrease symptoms.

After the acute pain has been controlled, the athlete may perform pain-free stretching exercises for the low back, hip, and hamstring muscles, as long as disk disease has been ruled out. The piriformis muscle is stretched by passive internal rotation of the hip (Figure 22-15). Contract-relax techniques (PNF) may aid in lengthening the piriformis muscle. The athlete should also concentrate on hamstring stretching exercises, performed pain-free while maintaining a lordotic curve in the lumbar area while the athlete stretches. Piriformis strengthening may be accomplished through resistive external rotation of the hip (see Figure 22-7).

Reviewing a normal gait cycle may also aid in gaining range of motion if the athlete has been ambulating with a flexed knee. The hamstrings, as well as the sciatic nerve, may have shortened in this case.

The athlete should be capable of performing pain-free activity, such as running and cutting, before being allowed to return to competition. Developing chronic problems poses danger if the athlete participates with radiation into the extremity. The best method of treatment is prevention by instituting a good flexibility exercise program for athletes.

Treatment of piriformis syndrome sciatica
PHASE I: *Days 1-3*
1. Ice.
2. Heat (superficial).
PHASE II: *Days 3-5*
3. Pain-free piriformis stretching exercises in in-

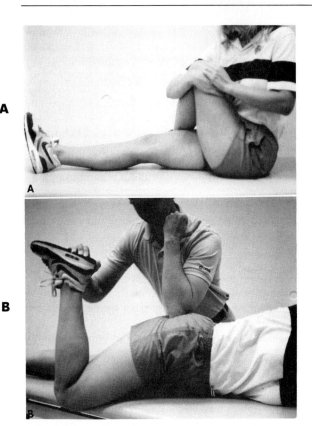

Fig. 22-15. Piriformis stretching techniques.

ternal rotation. Hold stretch for 30 seconds times 5 repetitions twice a day.
4. Pain-free hamstring stretching exercises maintaining lumbar lordotic curve. Hold stretch for 30 seconds times 5 repetitions twice a day.
5. Pain-free low-back stretching exercises knee to chest. Hold stretch for 30 seconds times 5 repetitions twice a day.

PHASE III: *From day 5*
6. Jogging.
7. Sport-specific activities.

BURSITIS OF THE HIP

Bursitis and other disorders of the bursa are often mistaken for other injuries because of the location of numerous other structures around the bursa. The bursa is a structure that normally lies within the area of a joint and produces a fluid that lubricates the two surfaces between which it lies.[11] It has also attached, very loosely, to the joint capsule, tendons, ligaments, and skin. Therefore it is indirectly involved with other close structures.[11] The function of the bursa is to dissipate friction caused by two or more structures moving against one another.

Bursitis is usually caused by direct trauma or overuse stress. Bursitis associated with bleeding into the bursa is the most disabling form. Swelling and pain may limit motion with a hemorrhagic bursitis.[18] The sports therapist must also consider the possibility of an infected bursa. If it is suspected, the athlete should be referred for blood tests.

Trochanteric Bursitis

The most commonly diagnosed hip bursitis is greater trochanteric bursitis. The greater trochanteric bursa lies between the gluteus maximus and the surface of the greater trochanter.[7]

One possible cause for trochanteric bursitis may be irritation caused by the iliotibial band, when the gluteus maximus inserts into it.[7] Repetitive irritation, such as running with one leg slightly adducted (as on the side of a road), may cause trochanteric bursitis on the adducted side.

Trochanteric bursitis caused by overuse is mostly seen in women runners who have an increased Q angle or a possible leg-length discrepancy.[1] Tight adductors may cause a runner's feet to cross over the midline and thus put an exceptional amount of force on the trochanteric bursa.[12]

Lateral heel wear in running shoes may also cause excessive hip adduction, which may indirectly cause trochanteric bursitis. In contact sports, a direct blow may result in a hemorrhagic bursitis, which could be extremely painful to the athlete.[11]

EVALUATION AND CLINICAL FINDINGS. Traumatic trochanteric bursitis is more easily diagnosed than overuse trochanteric bursitis. Palpation produces pain over the lateral hip area and greater trochanter. In both cases the athlete's gait cycle may be slightly abducted on the affected side to relieve pressure on the bursa. An athlete's attempt to remove weight from the affected extremity may cause a shortened weight-bearing phase. The athlete may report an increase in pain on activity, and active resistive hip abduction may also reproduce the pain.

This athlete could miss 3 to 5 days of competition, depending on the severity of the bursitis.

TREATMENT AND REHABILITATION. A complete history must be taken to determine the cause of trochanteric bursitis. The athlete's gait cycle, posture, flexibility, and running shoes should be examined. Oral antiinflammatory medication usually helps decrease pain and inflammation initially. For the first 2 to 3 days, ice in conjunction with compression (especially with hemorrhagic bursitis) should be used. When active swelling has been controlled, ultrasound may be used, with pain-free hip adduction stretching exercises for the iliotibial band. The hip stretching exercises should be performed with the knee extended and with the knee flexed. With all bursa injuries, ice and compression are the keys to decreasing swelling, inflammation, and pain.

An orthotic evaluation should be performed to check for any malalignment that may have caused dysfunction or leg-length discrepancy. Hip abduction progressive resistive strengthening exercises may be performed when the athlete is free of pain. For contact sports, a pad should be worn upon return to competition (see Treatment for Hip Bursitis).

Ischial Bursitis

The ischial bursa lies between the ischial tuberosity and the gluteus maximus. Ischial bursitis is often seen in people who sit for long periods.[7] In athletes, ischial bursitis is more commonly caused by direct trauma, such as falling or a direct hit when the hip is in a flexed position that exposes the ischial area.

EVALUATION AND CLINICAL FINDINGS. The athlete may report trauma to the area. With the hip in a flexed position, palpation over the ischial tuberosity may reproduce the pain. The athlete may experience pain on ambulation when the hip is flexed during the gait cycle. Also, stair climbing and uphill walking and running may reproduce pain. Depending on injury severity, this athlete need not miss competition time.

TREATMENT AND REHABILITATION. Treatment for ischial bursitis consists of positioning the athlete with the hip in a flexed position to expose the ischial area (i.e., lying on the side with hip flexed). Ice is used for 2 to 3 days, followed by heat. Hip and trunk flexion stretching exercises may be performed when the athlete is free of pain. Oral antiinflammatory medication may help decrease the pain and promote range of motion. Avoiding direct trauma to the area usually allows healing within 3 to 5 days. For contact sports, a pad should be worn (see Treatment for Hip Bursitis).

Iliopectineal Bursitis

Rarely seen in athletes, iliopectineal bursitis could potentially be caused by a tight iliopsoas muscle.[7] Osteoarthritis of the hip may also cause iliopectineal bursitis.[7] It may often be mistaken for a strain of the iliopsoas muscle and can be difficult to differentiate.

EVALUATION AND CLINICAL FINDINGS. Resistive hip flexion—sitting with the knee bent or lying supine with the knee extended—may reproduce the pain associated with iliopectineal bursitis. Also, passive hip extension with the knee extended may produce pain. Palpable pain in the inguinal area may also help in evaluating the athlete. In some cases, the nearby femoral nerve may become inflamed and cause radiation into the front of the thigh and knee.[7] Osteoarthritis must be ruled out in evaluating iliopectineal bursitis.

TREATMENT AND REHABILITATION. Oral antiinflammatory medication may be helpful initially. A form of deep heat or ice massage may be used to aid in decreasing inflammation and pain. The iliopsoas tendon must be stretched, and progressive resistive strengthening exercises of the hip flexors may be performed within a pain-free range of motion.

Treatment of hip bursitis

PHASE I: *Days 1-3*
1. Ice.
2. Compression.
3. Pain-free hip stretching exercises to the muscles involved. Hold stretch for 30 seconds times 5 repetitions twice a day.
4. Protective pad.
5. Oral antiinflammatory medication.

PHASE II: *From day 3*
6. Ultrasound.
7. Pain-free hip flexion progressive resistive strengthening exercises: 3 sets of 10 repetitions performed 3 days a week.
8. Sport-specific activities.

PUBIC INJURIES

Pain in the area of the pubic symphysis may be difficult to diagnose. Unless the athlete reports being hit or experiencing some kind of direct trauma, pubic pain may be caused by osteitis pubis, fractures of the inferior ramus (stress fractures and avulsion fractures), and groin strains.

Osteitis Pubis

Because an overuse situation predisposes an athlete to this injury, osteitis pubis is seen mostly in distance running, football, wrestling, and soccer. Repetitive stress on the pubic symphysis, caused by the insertion of muscles to the area, creates a chronic inflammatory condition at the site.[1] Constant movement of the symphysis in sports such as football and soccer produces inflammation and pain. Direct trauma to the symphysis may also cause periostitis. Symptoms develop gradually, may be mistaken for muscle strain, and can be difficult to differentiate. Exercises that aid muscle strains may cause more irritation to the symphysis; thus early active exercises are contraindicated.[12]

Referral to a physician to rule out hernia problems and prostatitis may be helpful in evaluating osteitis pubis.[12] X-ray film changes may take 4 to 6 weeks to show. The athlete should be treated symptomatically in the meantime.

EVALUATION AND CLINICAL FINDINGS. An athlete with osteitis pubis may have pain in the groin area and may complain of an increase in pain with running, sit-ups, and squatting.[1] The athlete may also complain of lower abdominal pain with radiation into the inner thigh. Differentiating osteitis pubis from a muscle strain may be confusing.

Palpation over the pubic symphysis may reproduce pain. In severe cases the athlete may show a waddling gait because of the shear forces at the symphysis.[21] Infection should be ruled out before treatment is begun. In most cases, the athlete may miss 3 to 5 days of competition. In severe cases, from 3 weeks up to 3 months of rest and treatment may be necessary.

TREATMENT AND REHABILITATION. Rest is the main course of treatment. The lower body must be protected from shear forces to the symphysis area. Ice with ultrasound may be used to decrease inflammation and pain. Oral antiinflammatory medication may also help to relieve pain.

Hip adductor stretching exercises may be performed as soon as pain has decreased. Strenthening exercises for the abdominal muscles, low back muscles, hip abductors, hip adductors, hip flexors, and hip extensors may be performed within a pain-free range of motion. Strengthening, in the later phases, helps develop stability at the pubic symphysis.

Treatment of pubic injuries

PHASE I: *Days 1-3*
  1. Rest.
  2. Ice.
  3. Ultrasound.
  4. Oral antiinflammatory medication.

PHASE II: *Days 3-5*
  5. Pain-free hip adductor muscle stretching exercises. Hold the stretch for 30 seconds times 5 repetitions twice a day.

PHASE III: *From day 5*
  6. Pain-free abdominal strengthening exercises, 3 sets of 10 repetitions daily.
  7. Pain-free low back strengthening exercises, 3 sets of 10 repetitions daily.
  8. Pain-free hip abductor strengthening exercises, 3 sets of 10 repetitions daily.
  9. Pain-free hip adductor strengthening exercises, 3 sets of 10 repetitions daily.
  10. Pain-free hip flexor strengthening exercises, 3 sets of 10 repetitions daily.
  11. Pain-free hip extensor strengthening exercises, 3 sets of 10 repetitions daily.
  12. Sport-specific activities.

Fractures of the Inferior Ramus

Stress and avulsion fractures should be ruled out before treating the pubic area for injury. Avulsion fracture of the inferior ramus is usually caused by a violent, forceful contraction of the hip adductor muscles or forceful passive movement into hip abduction, as in a split. The extent of the avulsion must be diagnosed by x-ray film. A palpable mass may be detected under the skin. In some cases, surgical repair should be considered.

Stress fractures may occur from overuse. The patient may report the same symptoms as in osteitis pubis. X-ray films may appear normal until the third or fourth week. Taking a good history may aid in diagnosing a stress fracture. An athlete with a stress fracture may miss 3 to 6 weeks of competition. An avulsion fracture may keep an athlete out of competition for up to 3 months.

TREATMENT AND REHABILITATION. Rest is the key in treating fractures of the inferior ramus. Ice or heat may be used to decrease pain. The timetables presented in Treatment of Pubic Injuries should be lengthened accordingly. Hip stretching and strengthening exercises may be performed within a pain-free range of motion. Return to activity should be gradual, deliberate, and, by all means, free of pain.

Groin Strain

A groin strain may occur to any muscle in the inner hip area. Whether it is to the sartoris, rectus femoris, the adductors, or the iliopsoas, the muscle and degree of injury must be determined and the injury treated accordingly.[3]

A groin strain may develop from overextending and externally rotating the hip or from forcefully contracting the muscles involved, as in running, jumping, twisting, and kicking. Diagnosis and treatment may be difficult because of the number of muscles in the area.

Discomfort may start as mild but develop into moderate-to-severe pain with disability if not treated correctly. A chronic strain may cause bleeding into the groin muscles. Myositis ossificans could form in the groin area (see the section on myositis ossificans); in chronic groin strains, it may be palpated and should be treated accordingly (see the section on thigh injuries). If a groin strain is treated correctly, myositis ossificans can be avoided.

EVALUATION AND CLINICAL FINDINGS

Grade I groin strain. The athlete may complain of mild discomfort with no loss of function and full range of motion and strength. Point tenderness may be minimal, with negative swelling. The gait cycle may be normal. Depending upon the severity of the injury, this athlete need not miss competition time.

Grade II groin strain. Palpation may reproduce pain and a minimal-to-moderate defect. Swelling may also be detected. This athlete may show an abnormal gait cycle. Ambulation may be slow, and the stride length may be shortened on the affected side. The athlete may tend to hike the hip rather than drive the knee through during the swing-through phase. Range of motion may be severely limited, and resistance could cause an increase in pain. This athlete may miss 3 to 14 days of competition, depending on the severity of injury.

Grade III groin strain. This athlete may need crutches to ambulate. A moderate-to-severe defect may be detected in the involved muscle or tendon. Point tenderness may be severe, with noticeable swelling. Range of motion may be severely limited. The athlete may splint the legs together and be apprehensive about allowing movement in abduction. Resistance may not be tolerated. The athlete could potentially miss 3 weeks to 3 months of competition, depending on the severity of the injury.

Differentiating a hip adductor strain from a hip flexor strain is the first step in treating this injury. Resistive adduction while lying supine with the knee in extension may significantly increase pain if the hip adductors are involved. Flexing the hip and knee and resisting hip adduction may also increase pain. If the injury is a pure hip adductor strain, the supine position with the knee extended may reproduce more discomfort than flexing the hip and knee. If resistive adduction with the hip and knee flexed produces more discomfort, the hip flexor may also be involved.

With the athlete lying supine, resistive hip flexion with the knee in extension tests for an iliopsoas strain. Resistive hip flexion with the knee flexed tests for a rectus femoris strain.

After determining the muscle or muscles involved and the degree of the injury, treatment and rehabilitation is the next step.

TREATMENT AND REHABILITATION

Grade I groin strain. Ice and ultrasound should be started immediately, with pain-free hip adductor stretching exercises (see Figure 22-10). Pain-free progressive resistive strengthening exercises may also be performed (see Figures 22-4, 22-6, and 22-7). Care must be taken not to further aggravate the injury.

Treatment of grade I groin strain
PHASE I: *From day 1*
1. Ice.
2. Ultrasosund.
3. Pain-free progressive resistive strengthening exercises, 3 sets of 10 repetitions daily.
4. Pain-free hip stretching exercises. Hold the stretch for 30 seconds times 5 repetitions daily.

Grade II groin strain. Ice should be started immediately, with gentle, pain-free, active range-of-motion exercises of the hip. Electrical muscle stimulation modalities can be very useful in the early stages to decrease inflammation and pain and to promote increases in range of motion.[20] Isometrics should also be performed as soon as they can be managed without pain. A normal gait cycle should be taught to the athlete, even if it involves using crutches for 1 to 3 days. Ater the third day, ultrasound may be used. The athlete may perform pain-free hip adductor stretching exercises and also perform progressive resistive strengthening exercises within a pain-free range of motion, progressing in motion and weight as discomfort decreases. On approximately day 5 the athlete may be able to start biking, swimming, and possibly jogging. Activities should be gradually increased without pain to full activity.

Hip adductor strains usually take longer to treat and rehabilitate than hip flexor strains of the same grade. Treatment and rehabilitation should be modified accordingly.

Treatment of grade II groin strain

PHASE I: *Days 1-3*
1. Ice.
2. Compression.
3. Electrical muscle stimulation modalities.
4. Crutches.
5. Pain-free isometric exercises.
6. Pain-free active range-of-motion exercises.

PHASE II: *Days 3-5*
7. Ultrasound.
8. Pain-free progressive resistive strengthening exercises, 3 sets of 10 repetitions daily.

PHASE III: *From day 5*
9. Biking.
10. Swimming.
11. Jogging.
12. Sport-specific activities.
13. Closed-kinetic chain exercises
    A. Squats: With feet shoulder width apart, descend until hips are equal with or slightly below knee level, keeping knees over feet (Figure 22-16).
    B. Leg Press: With high foot placement and feet shoulder width apart, descend until hips are slightly below knee level, keeping knees over feet.

Grade III groin strain. Grade III groin strains should be iced, compressed, and immobilized, and the athlete should use crutches. Electrical muscle stimulation modalities are useful in the acute stage to decrease inflammation and pain and to promote range of motion.[20] Rest for 1 to 3 days is recommended, with compression at all times.

After surgery has been ruled out, the athlete may perform pain-free isometric exercises between days 3 and 5. Slow, pain-free active range-of-motion exercises may also be performed during days 3 to 5. A normal gait cycle should be emphasized by using crutches. Crutches should not be eliminated until the athlete can ambulate with a normal, pain-free gait cycle.

Heat modalities in the form of ultrasound, hot packs, or diathermy should be used before exercise on approximately day 5.

During days 7 to 10, the athlete may perform pro-

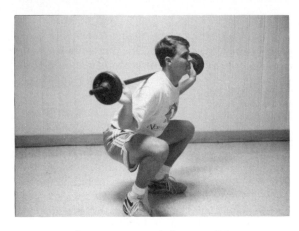

Fig. 22-16. Squats below parallel.

gressive resistive strengthening exercises without pain, progressing in weight and motion. Gentle, pain-free stretching exercises should also be performed. The athlete needs to achieve a good strength level, usually within 10 days after starting progressive resistive strengthening exercises, to perform functional activities such as biking, swimming, and jogging. Treatment and rehabilitation timetables may be modified. The modifications should be based on the degree of injury within the grade presented.

Treatment of grade III groin strain

PHASE I: *Days 1-3*
1. Rest.
2. Ice.
3. Compression.
4. Electrical muscle stimulation modalities.
5. Crutches and immobilization.

PHASE II: *Days 3-5*
6. Pain-free isometric exercises.
7. Pain-free active range-of-motion exercises.
8. Crutches continued if necessary.

PHASE III: *Days 5-14*
9. Heat modalities.
10. Pain-free progressive resistive strengthening exercises, 3 sets of 10 repetitions daily.
11. Pain-free stretching exercises. Hold stretch for 30 seconds times 5 repetitions twice a day.

PHASE IV: *Days 14-21*
12. Biking.
13. Swimming.
14. Jogging.

15. Sport-specific activities.
16. Squats as instructed.
17. Leg press as instructed.
18. Slide board.

HIP DISLOCATION

Dislocation of the hip joint takes a considerable amount of force because of the deep-seated ball-in-socket joint. When dislocation occurs, it is generally a posterior dislocation that takes place with the knee in a flexed position. Fractures may be associated with a dislocation and should always be considered. However, this injury is extremely rare in athletics. If it should occur, it should be treated as a medical emergency. The athlete should be checked for distal pulses and sensation. The sciatic nerve should be examined to see if it has been crushed or severed.[19] Do this by checking sensation and foot and toe movements. If the sciatic nerve is damaged, knee, ankle, and toe weakness may be pronounced.

Hip dislocations may also lead to avascular necrosis, which is a degenerative condition of the head of the femur caused by a disruption of blood supply during dislocation.[1]

EVALUATION AND CLINICAL FINDINGS. The athlete may be totally disabled, in severe pain, and usually unwilling to allow movement of the extremity. The trochanter may appear larger than normal with the extremity in internal rotation, flexed, and adducted.[19] X-ray studies should be performed before anesthetized reduction.

TREATMENT AND REHABILITATION. Two to three weeks of immobilization and bed rest is initially needed. Rehabilitation of the thigh and ankle may also be included at this time. Pain-free hip isometric exercises may be performed. Electrical muscle stimulation modalities may be used initially to promote muscle reeducation and retard muscle atrophy.[20]

At approximately 3 to 6 weeks, pain-free active range-of-motion exercises can be performed. Crutch walking is progressed and performed until the athlete can ambulate with a normal gait cycle and without pain. At approximately 6 weeks, the athlete may perform gentle progressive resistive strengthening exercises with a weight cuff or weight boot. All six movements of the hip should be included in the progressive resistive strengthening exercises (hip flexion, abduction, extension, adduction, internal rotation, and external rotation; see Figures 22-2 through 22-7). Pain-free stretching exercises should not be performed for 8 to 12 weeks. At approximately 12 weeks, the athlete may perform Nautilus hip and low back, abduction and adduction, and possibly leg press exercises. Swimming and biking may also be performed at 12 weeks. At 16 weeks, the athlete may progress to functional activities such as jogging and possibly light squats.

Treatment of hip dislocation

PHASE I: *Weeks 2-3*

1. Immobilization.
2. Bed rest.
3. Thigh and ankle rehabilitation. Quadriceps and hamstring isometrics performed throughout the day, daily. Ankle isometrics and progressive resistive strengthening exercises performed with Theraband (dorsiflexion, plantarflexion, eversion, inversion) daily.
4. Electrical muscle stimulation modalities.
5. Hip isometrics in all six movements (hip flexion, abduction, extension, adduction, and internal and external rotations) throughout the day, daily.

PHASE II: *Weeks 3-6*

6. Pain-free active range-of-motion exercises in all six movements, 3 sets of 10 repetitions daily.
7. Crutch walking, teaching normal gait.

PHASE III: *Weeks 6-12*

8. Pain-free progressive resistive strengthening exercises in all movements, 3 sets of 10 repetitions 3 days per week.
9. Pain-free hip stretching exercises at approximately weeks 8 to 12. Stretching in all six movements, holding the stretch for 30 seconds times 3 to 5 repetitions for each movement daily.

PHASE IV: *Weeks 12-16*

10. Nautilus (hip and low back, abduction and adduction, leg press, 3 sets of 10 repetitions 3 days per week.)
11. Biking.
12. Swimming.

PHASE V: *From week 16*

13. Jogging.
14. Light squats, 4 sets of 6 to 8 repetitions 2 days per week.
15. Sport-specific activities.

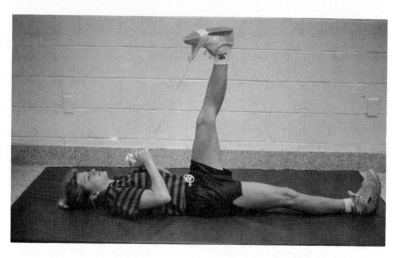

Fig. 22-17. Hamstring stretches maintaining lordotic curve.

HAMSTRING INJURIES
Ischial Tuberosity

The ischial tuberosity is a common site of injury to the hamstring muscle group (the biceps femoris, semitendinosus, and semimembranosus). All three hamstring muscles originate from the ischial tuberosity.

The most common ischial injury, as it relates to the hamstring group, is an avulsion fracture of the tuberosity. This injury usually results from a violent, forceful flexion of the hip, with the knee in extension.[19] A less severe irritation of the hamstring origin at the ischial tuberosity may also develop.

Less Severe Injury

EVALUATION AND CLINICAL FINDINGS. An athlete with the less severe injury or irritation of the hamstring origin at the ischeal tuberosity may complain of discomfort on sitting for extended periods and discomfort on palpation. The athlete may ambulate with a normal gait cycle. This athlete may also complain of pain while walking up stairs or uphill. Also, the athlete may be able to jog normally, but pain may be present with attempts at sprinting. Resistive knee flexion and resistive hip extension with the knee in an extended position may reproduce the pain. Passive hip flexion with the knee in extension may also cause discomfort. This athlete may not miss competition time.

TREATMENT AND REHABILITATION. Ice and ultra-

sound may be started on day 1, with gentle, pain-free hamstring stretching exercises. Also, heat in the form of hot packs may be used before competition while the athlete is stretching. To isolate the hamstring muscles while stretching, the athlete should maintain a lordotic curve in the lumbar back area while flexing at the trunk to stretch the hamstrings (Figure 22-17). Pain-free hamstring muscle progressive resistive strengthening exercises may also be performed on day 1.

Treatment of hamstring injuries
PHASE I: *From day 1*
1. Ice.
2. Ultrasound.
3. Hot packs.
4. Pain-free hamstring stretching exercises. Maintain a lumbar curve, and hold stretch for 30 seconds times 5 repetitions daily.
5. Pain-free hamstring progressive resistive strengthening exercises, 4 sets of 10 repetitions 3 days a week.
6. Pain-free hip extension progressive resistive strengthening exercises, 4 sets of 10 repetitions, 3 days a week.
7. Squats as instructed.
8. Leg press as instructed.

Avulsion Fracture

EVALUATION AND CLINICAL FINDINGS. The more severe ischial tuberosity avulsion fracture presents a

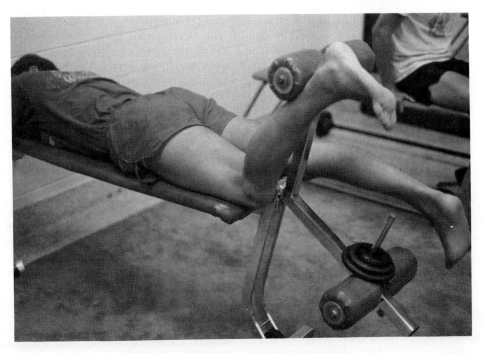

Fig. 22-18. Isotonic hamstring strengthening.

different clinical picture. Palpation may produce moderate-to-severe pain, and the athlete may be in moderate-to-severe pain with a very abnormal gait cycle. The athlete's gait cycle may lack a heel-strike phase and have a very short swing-through phase. The athlete may attempt to keep the injured extremity behind or below the body to avoid hip flexion during the gait cycle. Resistive knee flexion and hip extension with the knee in an extended or flexed position may reproduce the pain. Passive hip flexion with the knee extended and with the knee flexed may cause moderate-to-severe pain at the ischial tuberosity. X-ray films may or may not show the injury.[19]

TREATMENT AND REHABILITATION. Surgery is usually not necessary. Immobilization and limiting physical activity are usually enough to allow healing. Ice and limited physical activity that involves hip flexion and forceful hip extension and knee flexion for the first 3 weeks is usually all that is necessary. Crutches may be needed for the first 3 weeks while normal gait cycle is taught.

During weeks 3 through 6, the athlete may begin heat modalities (hot packs, ultrasound, diathermy, whirlpool), with pain-free active range-of-motion lying prone and sitting. Pain-free hamstring stretching

exercises may also be performed. Regaining full range of motion during the rehabilitation program is very important. Many athletes never regain full hip flexion range of motion after this injury.

Weeks 6 through 12 are a progressive phase for hamstring progressive resistive strengthening exercises (Figure 22-18). Swimming, biking, and jogging may also be performed in this phase, but the athlete should avoid forceful knee and hip flexion and forceful hip extension.

After week 12, the athlete without pain may progress to sport-specific activities.

Further treatment for injuries to the hamstrings
PHASE I: *Weeks 1-3*
1. Ice.
2. Immobilization (avoid hip and knee flexion and active hip extension).
3. Crutch walking.

PHASE II: *Weeks 3-6*
4. Heat modalities.
5. Pain-free hamstring active range-of-motion exercises. Lying prone and sitting, flex the knee through a pain-free range of motion, 3 sets of 10 repetitions daily.

6. Pain-free hamstring stretching exercises maintaining a lumbar lordotic curve. Hold the stretch for 30 seconds times 5 repetitions daily.

PHASE III: *Weeks 6-12*

7. Pain-free hamstring progressive resistive strengthening exercises, 4 sets of 10 repetitions 3 days per week.
8. Swimming.
9. Biking.
10. Jogging.

PHASE IV: *From week 12*

11. Sport-specific activities.
12. Squats as instructed.
13. Leg press as instructed.

Hamstring Strains

Hamstring strains are common, and the causes are numerous. A quick, explosive contraction of the hamstrings while the hip is in flexion with the knee extended bringing the hip into extension and flexing the knee, could lead to a strain of the hamstring muscles. Many theories try to explain the cause of hamstring strains. Imbalance with the quadriceps is one theory, according to which the hamstring muscles should have 60% to 70% of the quadriceps muscles strength. Other possibilities are hamstring muscle fatigue, running posture and gait, leg-length discrepancy, decreased hamstring range of motion, and an imbalance between the medial and lateral hamstring muscles.[1]

EVALUATION AND CLINICAL FINDINGS

Grade I hamstring strain. With a grade I hamstring strain, the athlete may complain of sore hamstring muscles, with pain on palpation and swelling. The athlete's gait cycle may be normal. Hip flexion range of motion is probably normal, with a tight feeling reported at the extreme range of hip flexion. Resistive knee flexion and hip extension with the knee extended is probably free of pain or possibly produces a tight feeling with good strength present.

This athlete may not miss competition but should be watched closely. Rehabilitation and strengthening should begin immediately to avoid further injury.

Grade II hamstring strain. With a grade II hamstring strain, the athlete may report having heard or felt a pop during the activity. The athlete usually ambulates with an abnormal gait cycle. The athlete may lack heel strike and land during the foot-flat phase of the gait cycle. Swing-through phase may be limited because of the athlete's unwillingness to flex the hip and knee. The athlete may tend to ambulate with a flexed knee. After the first or second day, moderate ecchymosis may be observed. Palpation may produce moderate-to-severe pain, and a defect in the muscle belly may be evident, with noticeable swelling. Resistive knee flexion and hip extension with the knee extended may cause moderate-to-severe pain. The athlete may also have a noticeable weakness on resistive knee flexion and hip extension with the knee extended and flexed. Resistive hip extension with the knee flexed also tests the strength of the gluteus maximus muscle.

Passive hip flexion with the knee extended may also produce moderate-to-severe pain. The athlete's range of motion may be moderately to severely limited in hip flexion with the knee extended and moderately limited in hip flexion with the knee flexed.

An athlete with a grade II hamstring strain could miss 5 to 21 days of competition.

Grade III hamstring strain. With a grade III hamstring strain, the athlete may be unable to ambulate without the aid of crutches. The athlete may report having heard or felt a pop during the activity. The sports therapist may detect swelling and severe pain on palpation. A noticeable defect in the muscle belly may be present. After the first through third days, moderate-to-severe ecchymosis may be observed. The athlete may have poor strength and be unable to resist knee flexion and hip extension with the knee extended. The athlete may have fair strength upon resistive hip extension with the knee flexed because of the gluteus maximus muscle. Resisting these motions usually causes pain. Passive hip flexion, knee extended, may not be tolerated because of pain. Passive hip flexion, knee flexed, may be moderately to severely limited.

An athlete with a grade III hamstring strain could miss 3 to 12 weeks of competition.

TREATMENT AND REHABILITATION

Grade I hamstring strain. On the first day, the athlete may begin ice and compression, with gentle, pain-free hamstring stretching exercises while maintaining a lumbar lordotic curve to isolate the hamstring muscles. After the acute stage, heat, in the form of hot packs or whirlpool, may be used before activity with stretching exercises. Pain-free hamstring progressive resistive strengthening exercises may also be performed immediately to prevent further injury to the hamstring muscles during activity.

Ultrasound may be used after ice or hot packs and

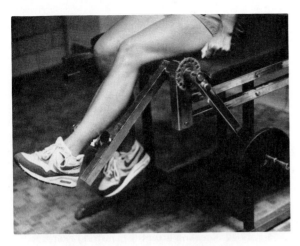

Fig. 22-19. NK table hamstring exercise.

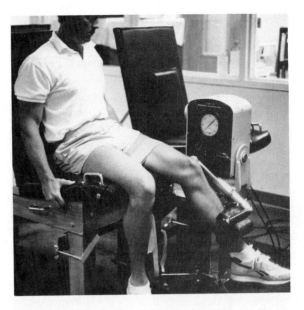

Fig. 22-20. Isokinetic exercise of the hamstrings and quadriceps.

before strengthening exercises. Using an NK table is preferable for hamstring progressive resistive strengthening exercises (Figure 22-19) because the sitting position gives the hamstring muscles a bio-mechanical advantage in working through a full range of motion. By sitting (the hip is flexed) and using an NK table, the hamstrings are stretching at the buttock, and they are allowed to be more efficient during knee flexion exercises, in comparison to lying prone and performing hamstring progressive resistive strength-ening exercises. Isokinetic exercises, in the form of an Orthotron or Cybex, may be used in conjunction with the NK table isotonic exercises (Figure 22-20).

Treatment of grade I hamstring strain

PHASE I: *From day 1*
1. Ice.
2. Compression.
3. After the acute stage, heat (hot packs, whirl-pool, ultrasound).
4. Pain-free hamstring stretching exercises. Hold stretch for 30 seconds times 5 repetitions daily. Always maintain a lumbar lordotic curve while stretching the hamstrings.
5. Pain-free hamstring progressive resistive strengthening exercises. Isotonics performed on the NK table, 4 sets of 10 repetitions 3 days per week.
6. Isokinetics 3 days per week.
7. Prone lying isotonic single leg hamstring curls, 4 sets of 10 repetitions 3 days per week.

Grade II hamstring strain. An athlete with a grade II hamstring strain should be treated conservatively because of the potentially chronic nature of this in-jury.

A pain-free normal gait cycle should be taught as soon as possible, and crutches should be used to ac-complish a normal gait cycle. Ice, compression, and gentle, pain-free hamstring stretching exercises, mak-ing sure the athlete maintains a lumbar lordotic curve to isolate the hamstring muscles, are performed on day 1. Electrical muscle stimulation modalities may be used to promote range of motion and to decrease pain.[20] Active range of motion while lying prone may also be performed between days 1 and 3, if the athlete can do so without pain. Hamstring isometric exer-cises may be taught as soon as possible, again within pain-free limits. Pain-free motion is very important and usually decreases the length of time an athlete misses competition. At approximately day 3, the ath-lete may begin heat in the form of hot packs and whirlpool, combined with pain-free stretching exer-cises, or ultrasound followed by pain-free stretching exercises. Using the NK table, hamstring progressive resistive strengthening exercises may also be per-formed on day 3, if pain free. Isokinetics may be valu-able in conjunction with isotonics (NK table). Swim-ming and biking may be added between days 3 and 6. Jogging and sport-specific activities may be added accordingly, beginning with day 6.

In the later phases of all three grades of hamstring

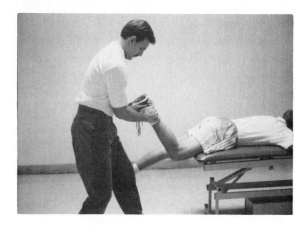

Fig. 22-21. Manual resistance to fatigue hamstrings.

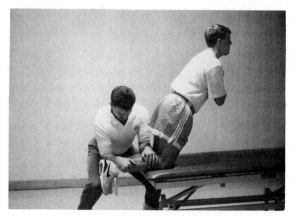

Fig. 22-22. Kneeling eccentric hamstring exercises.

muscle strains, the athlete should be educated in performing full range-of-motion leg press exercises on Nautilus and light-weight squats (see Figure 22-16). These two exercises are very helpful in strengthening the hamstrings in a weight-bearing position.

All activities should be followed by ice treatments to decrease inflammation and discomfort.

Treatment of grade II hamstring strain

PHASE I: *Days 1-3*
1. Ice.
2. Compression.
3. Electrical muscle stimulation modalities.
4. Pain-free hamstring stretching exercises. Hold for 30 seconds times 5 repetitions daily. Maintain lumbar lordotic curve.
5. Pain-free hamstring active range-of-motion exercises lying prone, 3 sets of 10 repetitions daily.
6. Pain-free hamstring isometric exercises.

PHASE II: *Days 3-6*
7. Heat (hot packs, whirlpool, ultrasound).
8. Pain-free hamstring progressive resistive strengthening exercises. Isotonics on the NK table, 4 sets of 10 repetitions 3 days per week.
9. Isokinetics 3 days per week.
10. Swimming 2 days per week.
11. Biking 2 days per week.
12. Prone lying isotonic single leg hamstring curls, 4 sets of 10 repetitions 3 days per week.
13. Manual resistance to fatigue. Athlete lies prone with knee over the edge of treatment table. With the athlete in full knee extension,

resistance is applied to the back of the heels as the athlete contracts concentrically to full knee flexion for a count of 5 seconds. After a 2 second pause at full flexion, resistance is applied into extension for a count of 5 as the athlete contracts the hamstrings eccentrically. This is repeated contracting as fast as possible for 3 sets of 10 to 12 repetitions or until failure, 1 to 2 days per week (Figure 22-21).
14. Kneeling eccentric hamstring lowering exercises. With the athlete kneeling on a treatment table and feet hanging over the end, the sports therapist stabilizes the lower leg as the athlete lowers the body to the prone position, eccentrically contracting the hamstrings. The athlete should maintain a lumbar lordotic curve and stay completely erect, avoiding any hip flexion. The athlete should perform 3 sets of 10 to 12 repetitions or until failure 1 to 2 days per week (Figure 22-22).

PHASE III: *From day 6*
15. Jogging.
16. Sport-specific activities.
17. Leg press exercises, 3 sets of 10 repetitions 2 days per week.
18. Squats, 4 sets of 6 to 8 repetitions 2 days per week.

Grade III hamstring strain. After surgery has been ruled out, an athlete with a grade III hamstring strain may take 3 to 8 weeks to rehabilitate and in more severe cases up to 3 months.

Ice, compression, and crutches should be started immediately. Electrical muscle stimulation modalities may be used in the early stages to decrease inflammation and pain and promote range of motion.[20] The athlete should remain on crutches for 3 to 14 days to rest the injury and learn normal gait cycle. Resting the injury for at least 3 to 5 days is usually necessary to decrease inflammation, pain, and splinting and to prepare the athlete for active range-of-motion exercises.

On approximately day 5, the athlete may perform pain-free, active, range-of-motion exercises lying prone, with gentle, pain-free hamstring stretching exercises. Ice or heat, in the form of hot packs and ultrasound, may be used before or during stretching. Pain-free hamstring isometric exercises may be performed on approximately day 5.

Between days 10 to 14, the athlete may perform pain-free hamstring progressive resistive strengthening exercises by using the NK table and isokinetic machines. The athlete who can do so without pain may swim and bike. This athlete needs to develop good (and preferably excellent) hamstring strength before progressing to jogging and sport-specific activities after 14 days. This conservatism is because of the possibility of reinjury.

The athlete should be educated in performing full range-of-motion leg press exercises on Nautilus and light-weight squats. Especially with this injury, the time parameters presented have to be modified depending on the degree of injury within its grade.

Treatment of grade III hamstring strain

PHASE I: *Days 1-5*
1. Ice.
2. Compression.
3. Electrical muscle stimulation modalities.
4. Crutches.
5. Rest.

PHASE II: *Days 5-10*
6. Pain-free hamstring active range-of-motion exercises lying prone daily.
7. Heat (hot packs, whirlpool, ultrasound).
8. Pain-free hamstring stretching exercises while maintaining a lumbar lordotic curve. Hold stretch for 30 seconds times 5 repetitions daily.
9. Pain-free hamstring isometric exercises daily.

PHASE III: *Days 10-14*
10. Pain-free hamstring progressive-resistive strengthening exercises. Isotonics on NK table, 4 sets of 10 repetitions 3 days per week.
11. Isokinetics 3 days per week.

12. Swimming 2 days per week.
13. Biking 2 days per week.
14. Prone lying isotonic single leg hamstring curls, 4 sets of 10 repetitions 3 days per week.

PHASE IV: *From day 14*
15. Jogging.
16. Sport-specific activities.
17. Leg press exercises, 3 sets of 10 repetitions 2 days per week.
18. Squats, 4 sets of 6 to 8 repetitions 2 days per week.
19. Manual resistance to fatigue.
20. Kneeling eccentric hamstring lowering exercises.

Hamstring Tendon Strains

Another injury that occurs to the hamstring muscles is a strain of the hamstring tendons near their attachments to the tibia and fibula. This injury has also been diagnosed as tendinitis. The athlete may report pain but may not experience disability. An athlete with a hamstring tendon strain or tendinitis may present a history of overuse and chronic pain for a few days.

EVALUATION AND CLINICAL FINDINGS. Palpation helps to isolate which tendon or tendons are involved, and resistive knee flexion, with the tibia in internal and external rotation, aids in the evaluation. The gastrocnemius muscle tendons in the same area must be ruled out. If resistive ankle plantar flexion with the knee in extension does not reproduce symptoms, gastrocnemius involvement may be ruled out.

TREATMENT AND REHABILITATION. An athlete who presents with this condition responds nicely to 1 to 2 days of rest with oral antiinflammatory medication. Ice massage and ultrasound are helpful in decreasing inflammation and pain. Gentle hamstring stretching exercises with the hip in internal and external rotation help to isolate the tendon or tendons involved and should be performed on day 1. Hamstring progressive resistive exercises can be performed on day 1 if they can be done without pain.

Treatment of hamstring tendon strains

PHASE I: *From day 1*
1. Ice.
2. Rest.
3. Ultrasound.
4. Pain-free hamstring stretching exercises with the leg in internal and external rotation held for 30 seconds times 5 repetitions daily.

5. Pain-free hamstring progressive resistive strengthening exercises. Isotonics on the NK table, 4 sets of 10 repetitions 3 days per week.
6. Isokinetics 3 days per week.

FEMORAL FRACTURES

Fractures of the femur may be classified as stress fractures, avulsion fractures, or traumatic fractures.

Stress Fractures

Stress fractures of the femur are rare but may be seen because of repetitive microtrauma.[7] Young athletes are more likely to develop this injury.

EVALUATION AND CLINICAL FINDINGS. The athlete may complain of pinpoint pain that increases during activity. The initial x-ray films are usually negative. Obtaining a good history is very important and should include activities, change in activities, and running gait analysis.[7]

TREATMENT AND REHABILITATION. As with all stress fractures, finding the cause is the first step in treatment and rehabilitation. While the athlete is in the nonweight–bearing phase of rehabilitation, nonweight–bearing activities should be used. Biking, swimming, and upper body ergometers may be used. The athlete may perform pain-free thigh strengthening exercises and progress as shown in the lists outlining treatment of grades II and III hamstring strain (pp. 392-393) and grades II and III quadriceps strain (pp. 397-398).

Avulsion Fractures

Athletes may suffer an isolated avulsion fracture of the femoral trochanters. When the greater trochanter is involved, the cause is usually a violent, forceful contraction of the hip abductor muscles. An avulsion fracture of the lesser trochanter occurs because of a violent, forceful contraction of the iliopsoas muscle.[7]

EVALUATION AND CLINICAL FINDINGS. Palpation may produce pain and possibly a noticeable defect of the greater trochanter. Resistive movements and passive range of motion of the hip may reproduce pain. X-ray films must be taken to confirm the injury.

TREATMENT AND REHABILITATION. Immobilization may be the treatment of choice for an incomplete avulsion fracture. With a complete avulsion fracture, internal fixation is usually required.

The athlete performs isometric hip exercises on the first day of rehabilitation, with isometric quadriceps exercises and ankle strengthening exercises. Crutches are used for at least 6 weeks until a pain-free normal gait cycle can be accomplished. After 6 weeks, the athlete may perform pain-free active range-of-motion exercises and pain-free straight leg raise exercises involving hip flexion, abduction, extension, and adduction. During approximately week 8, the athlete may perform hip progressive resistive straight leg raises in all four movements (flexion, abduction, extension, and adduction).

Biking and swimming are performed when range of motion allows. The athlete is then progressed to jogging and sport-specific activities.

Treatment of avulsion fractures

PHASE I: *Weeks 1-6*
1. Immobilization.
2. Crutches.
3. Isometric exercises daily (hip, thigh, and ankle exercises).

PHASE II: *Weeks 6-8*
4. Pain-free hip active and passive range-of-motion exercises daily (hip flexion, abduction, extension, adduction, and internal and external rotation).

PHASE III: *From week 8*
5. Pain-free hip progressive resistive exercises daily (hip flexion, abduction, extension, adduction, and internal and external rotation).
6. Biking.
7. Swimming.
8. Jogging.
9. Sport-specific activities.

Traumatic Fractures

A femoral neck fracture is associated with osteoporosis and is rarely seen in athletics.[7,11,22] However, a twisting motion combined with a fall may produce this fracture. Because the femoral neck fracture may disrupt the blood supply to the head of the femur, avascular necrosis is often seen later. This injury must receive proper treatment.

TREATMENT AND REHABILITATION. After surgery or during immobilization, isometric hip exercises are started immediately. Athletes, especially younger athletes, are progressed slowly. Within 2 to 3 months, gentle active and passive hip range-of-motion exercises are performed. Muscle strengthening exercises (see Treatment of Avulsion Fractures on p. 395) and a normal gait cycle should be taught to the athlete.

In some cases, exercise has been shown to increase bone density and reverse the rate of osteoporosis.[7,22,23]

QUADRICEPS MUSCLE STRAIN

A strain to the large quadricep muscles in the front of the thigh may be very disabling, especially when the rectus femoris muscle is involved. With no history of direct contact to the quadriceps area, the injury can be treated as a muscle strain.

A quadriceps strain usually occurs because of a sudden violent, forceful contraction of hip and knee flexion, with the knee initially extended. An overstretch of the quadriceps, with the hip in extension and the knee flexed, may also cause a quadriceps strain.

Tight quadriceps, imbalance between quadricep muscles, and leg-length discrepancy may predispose someone to quadriceps strain.[21]

Grade I Quadriceps Strain

EVALUATION AND CLINICAL FINDINGS. With a grade I quadriceps strain, the athlete may complain of tightness in the front of the thigh. The athlete may be ambulating with a normal gait cycle and present with a history of the thigh feeling fatigued and tight. Swelling may not be present, and the athlete usually has negative discomfort on palpation or very mild discomfort when the rectus femoris is involved.

With the athlete sitting over the edge of a table, resistive knee extension may not produce discomfort. If the athlete is lying supine with the knee flexed over the edge of a table, resistive knee extension may produce mild discomfort, if the rectus femoris is involved. With the athlete lying prone, active knee flexion may produce a full pain-free range of motion, with possible tightness at extreme flexion.

An athlete with a grade I quadriceps strain may not miss competition but should be watched closely and started on a rehabilitation and strengthening program immediately.

Grade II Quadriceps Strain

EVALUATION AND CLINICAL FINDINGS. With a grade II quadriceps strain, the athlete may have an abnormal gait cycle. The knee may be splinted in extension. The athlete may present an externally rotated hip to use the adductors to pull the leg through during the swing-through phase, especially when the rectus femoris is involved. In severe cases, it may also be accompanied by hiking the hip during the swing-through phase.

The athlete may have felt a sudden twinge and pain down the length of the rectus femoris during activity.[21] Swelling may be noticeable, and palpation may produce pain. A defect in the muscle may also be evident in a grade II strain. Resistive knee extension, when both sitting and lying supine, may reproduce pain. Lying supine and resisting knee extension may be more painful when the rectus femoris is involved. With the athlete lying prone, active knee flexion range of motion may present a noticeable decrease, in some cases a decrease up to 45 degrees. With a quadriceps strain, any decrease in knee flexion range of motion should classify the injury as a grade II or III strain.

This athlete may miss 7 to 21 days of competition, depending on the amount of active range of motion present. The lack of range of motion and the number of competition days missed are usually directly correlated.

Grade III Quadriceps Strain

EVALUATION AND CLINICAL FINDINGS. An athlete with a grade III quadriceps strain may be unable to ambulate without the aid of crutches and may be in severe pain, with a noticeable defect in the quadriceps muscle. Palpation may not be tolerated, and swelling may be present almost immediately. The athlete may not be able to extend the knee actively and against resistance. An isometric contraction may be painful and may produce a bulge or defect in the quadriceps muscle, especially the rectus femoris. With the athlete lying prone, active knee flexion range of motion may be severely limited and may not be tolerated.

This athlete may miss 3 to 12 weeks of competition. In severe cases, surgery may be a consideration.

Grade I Quadriceps Strain

TREATMENT AND REHABILITATION. Ice, compression, active range of motion, and isometric quadriceps exercises may be performed immediately. Pain-free

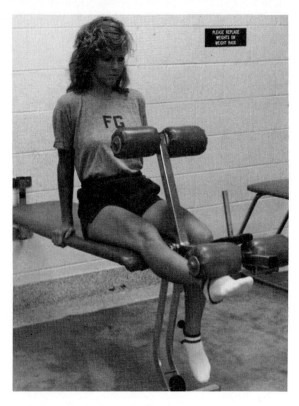

Fig. 22-23. Quadriceps isotonics on universal.

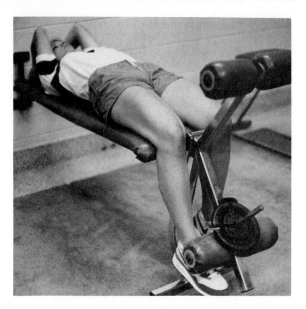

Fig. 22-24. Quadriceps strengthening for rectus femoris.

quadriceps progressive resistive strengthening exercises may be performed within the first 2 days (Figure 22-23). Compression should be used at all times until the athlete is free of pain and no longer complaining of a tight feeling.

Treatment of grade I quadriceps strain

PHASE I: *Days 1-2*
1. Ice.
2. Compression.
3. Quadriceps muscle active range of motion performed lying prone, sitting, and lying supine, 3 sets of 10 repetitions daily.
4. Quadriceps isometric exercises throughout the day, daily.

PHASE II: *From day 2*
5. Pain-free quadriceps progressive resistive strengthening exercises. Isotonic exercises using the NK table, 4 sets of 10 repetitions 3 days a week.
6. Isokinetics 3 days per week.

Grade II Quadriceps Strain

TREATMENT AND REHABILITATION. Ice, compression, and crutches may be used immediately for 3 to 5 days. Electrical muscle stimulation modalities may be used acutely to decrease swelling, inflammation, and pain and promote range of motion.[20] At approximately day 3, the athlete may perform quadriceps isometric exercises and pain-free quadriceps active range-of-motion exercises. These exercises are performed lying prone and sitting and then progressing to the supine position to allow more efficiency to the rectus femoris muscle (Figure 22-24). Ice used in conjunction with active range of motion is very helpful in regaining motion and strengthening the quadricep muscles without pain. Passive stretching exercises to the quadricep muscles are not recommended until later phases of the rehabilitation program. Compression is continued throughout the rehabilitation period. A pain-free normal gait cycle is reviewed and emphasized, with and without crutches.

During approximately days 3 to 7, the athlete may begin heat (hot packs, whirlpool, ultrasound) before exercise. During this phase of rehabilitation, pain-free straight leg raises without weight, progressing to straight leg raises with weight, are performed (Figure 22-25).

Days 7 through 14 are pain-free quadriceps pro-

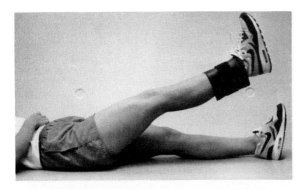

Fig. 22-25. Straight leg raises with weight boot.

gressive resistive strengthening exercise days. The NK table is used because of its ability to change the force on the quadricep muscles by changing the lever arms and torque (Figure 22-26). Isokinetics are also performed in this phase. Pain-free leg press exercises and squats may be performed in the later part of this phase. Training the quadriceps eccentrically and in a weight-bearing position by using leg press exercises and squats is very helpful in the rehabilitation program and in preventing reinjury. Swimming and biking can also be performed as long as the athlete avoids forceful kicking. The bike seat should be adjusted to accommodate a pain-free range of motion. Pain-free quadriceps-stretching exercises are not performed until days 7 to 14. When the athlete has full pain-free range of motion, jogging and sport-specific activities may be added to the rehabilitation program.

Treatment of grade II quadriceps strain
PHASE I: *Days 1-3*
1. Ice.
2. Compression.
3. Crutches.
4. Electrical muscle stimulation modalities.

PHASE II: *Days 3-7*
5. Pain-free quadriceps isometric exercises throughout the day daily with and without ice.
6. Pain-free quadriceps active range-of-motion exercises lying prone, sitting, and lying supine, 3 sets of 10 repetitions daily with and without ice.
7. Heat (hot packs, whirlpool, ultrasound).
8. Straight leg raises daily progressing to weights, 4 sets of 10 repetitions 3 days per week.

PHASE III: *Days 7-14*
9. Pain-free quadriceps progressive resistive

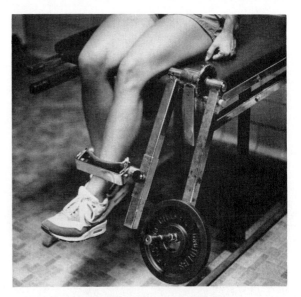

Fig. 22-26. NK table quadriceps exercises.

strengthening exercises. Isotonics using the NK table, 4 sets of 10 repetitions 3 days per week.
10. Isokinetics 3 days per week.
11. Swimming 2 to 3 days per week.
12. Biking 2 to 3 days per week.
13. Begin quadriceps stretching exercises. Hold stretch for 30 seconds times 5 repetitions daily.
14. Leg press exercise, 3 sets of 10 repetitions 2 days per week.
15. Squats, 4 sets of 6 to 8 repetitions 2 days per week.

PHASE IV: *From day 14*
16. Jogging.
17. Sport-specific activities.

Grade III Quadriceps Strain

TREATMENT AND REHABILITATION. An athlete with a grade III quadriceps strain should be on crutches for 7 to 14 days to allow for rest. Compression, ice, and electrical muscle stimulation modalities may be used immediately. Quadriceps stretching exercises are not performed until later phases. Compression is maintained until the athlete has full pain-free range of motion.

On approximately day 7, the athlete may begin

pain-free quadriceps isometric exercises. Gentle, pain-free quadriceps active range-of-motion exercises while the athlete is lying prone may be performed if special attention is paid to avoiding overstretching the quadricep muscles. Ice, in conjunction with active range of motion while sitting over the end of a table, is very useful in regaining range of motion. Heat (hot packs, whirlpool, ultrasound) may be used on approximately days 7 to 10. Pain-free straight leg raises without weight may be performed. Weight may be added after days 10 to 14.

Depending upon active range of motion, pain-free quadriceps active progressive resistive strengthening exercises may be performed after the third week. Isokinetics may also be added to the rehabilitation program along with swimming and biking. The bicycle seat height should be adjusted to accommodate the athlete's available range of motion.

At approximately 4 to 5 weeks, leg press exercises and squats may be performed pain free. Depending on the severity of the injury, the athlete should have full active range of motion by the fourth week. Only when full active range of motion is accomplished should quadriceps stretching exercises be performed. The athlete is then progressed to jogging and sport-specific activities.

Treatment of grade III quadriceps strain

PHASE I: *Week 1*
1. Ice.
2. Compression.
3. Electrical muscle stimulation modalities.
4. Crutches.

PHASE II: *Week 2*
5. Pain-free quadriceps isometric exercises daily.
6. Pain-free quadriceps active range-of-motion exercises daily (see Treatment of Grade I Quadriceps Strain, p. 396).
7. Heat (hot packs, whirlpool, ultrasound).
8. Straight leg raises with no weights daily, 4 sets of 10 repetitions.

PHASE III: *Week 3*
9. Straight leg raises with weights, 4 sets of 10 repetitions 3 days per week.

PHASE IV: *Week 4*
10. Pain-free quadriceps progressive resistive exercises. Isotonics using the NK table, 4 sets of 10 repetitions 3 days per week.
11. Isokinetics 3 days per week.
12. Swimming 2 to 3 days per week.
13. Biking 2 to 3 days per week.

14. Quadriceps stretching exercises. Hold stretch for 30 seconds times 5 repetitions daily.

PHASE V: *Week 5*
15. Leg press exercises, 3 sets of 10 repetitions 2 days per week.
16. Squats, 4 sets of 6 to 8 repetitions 2 days per week.

PHASE VI: *Week 6*
17. Jogging.
18. Sport-specific activities.

QUADRICEPS CONTUSION

Because the quadricep muscle is in the front of the thigh, a direct blow to the area that causes the muscle to compress against the femur can be very disabling.[1] A direct blow to the anterior portion of the muscle is usually more serious and disabling than a direct blow to the lateral quadriceps area because of the differences in muscle mass present in the two areas. Blood vessels that break cause bleeding in the area where muscle tissue has been damaged.[21] If not treated correctly or treated too aggressively, a quadriceps contusion may lead to the formation of myositis ossifans (see p. 401).

At the time of injury, the athlete may develop pain, loss of function to the quadriceps mechanism, and loss of knee flexion range of motion. How relaxed the quadriceps were at the time of injury and how forceful the blow was determine the grade of injury.

Grade I Quadriceps Contusion

EVALUATION AND CLINICAL FINDINGS. With a grade I quadriceps contusion, the athlete may present a normal gait cycle, negative swelling, and only mild discomfort on palpation. The athlete's active knee flexion range of motion while lying prone may be within normal limits. Resistive knee extension while sitting and lying supine may not cause discomfort.

This athlete may not miss competition, but compression and protective padding should be worn during competition until the athlete is symptom free.

Grade II Quadriceps Contusion

EVALUATION AND CLINICAL FINDINGS. Before notifying the trainer, this athlete may attempt to continue to participate while the injury progressively becomes disabling. The athlete's gait cycle may be abnormal.

The knee may be splinted in extension, and the athlete may avoid knee flexion while bearing weight because of the feeling of the knee wanting to give out. This athlete may also externally rotate the extremity to use the hip adductors to pull the leg through during the swing-through phase. This move may be accompanied by hiking the hip at push off.

Swelling may be moderate to severe, with a noticeable defect and pain on palpation. While the athlete is lying prone, active range of motion in the knee may be limited, with possibly 30 to 45 degrees of motion lacking. Resistive knee extension while sitting and lying supine may be painful, and a noticeable weakness in the quadriceps mechanisms may be evident.

This athlete may miss 3 to 21 days of participation, depending upon the severity of injury.

A grade II quadriceps contusion to the lateral thigh area is usually less painful because of the lack of muscle mass involved in the injury. The athlete may experience pain on palpation but may not be disabled. While the athlete is lying prone, knee flexion range of motion may be within normal limits, with possibly a small decrease in range present. Resistive knee extension while the athlete is sitting and lying supine may cause mild discomfort with good strength present.

The athlete with a grade II quadriceps contusion to the lateral thigh area may not miss competition time.

Grade III Quadriceps Contusion

EVALUATION AND CLINICAL FINDINGS. With a grade III quadriceps contusion, the muscle may herniate through the fascia to cause a marked defect, severe bleeding, and disability.

The athlete may not be able to ambulate without crutches. Pain, severe swelling, and a bulge of muscle tissue may be present on palpation. When the athlete is lying prone, knee flexion active range of motion may be severely limited. Active resistive knee extension while the athlete is sitting and lying supine may not be tolerated, and severe weakness may be present.

An athlete with a grade III quadriceps contusion may miss 3 weeks to 3 months of competition time.

Grade I Quadriceps Contusion

TREATMENT AND REHABILITATION. The athlete may begin ice and compression immediately. Compression should be continued until all signs and symptoms are absent.

Gentle, pain-free quadriceps stretching exercises may be performed on the first day. Quadriceps progressive resistive strengthening exercises may also be performed pain free. Isokinetics may be used with isotonic exercises.

The athlete's active range of motion should be carefully monitored. If motion decreases, the injury should be updated to a grade II contusion and treated as such.

Compression and protective padding should be worn at all times during competition.

Treatment of grade I quadriceps contusion

PHASE I: *From day 1*

1. Ice.
2. Compression.
3. Pain-free quadriceps stretching exercises. Hold for 30 seconds times 5 repetitions daily.
4. Pain-free quadriceps progressive resistive strengthening exercises. Isotonics using the NK table, 4 sets of 10 repetitions 3 days per week.
5. Isokinetics 3 days per week.

Grade II Quadriceps Contusion

TREATMENT AND REHABILITATION. This athlete should be treated very conservatively. Crutches should be used until a normal gait can be accomplished free of pain. Ice, compression, and electrical muscle stimulation modalities may be started immediately to decrease swelling, inflammation, and pain and to promote range of motion.[20] Compression should be applied at all times to counteract bleeding into the area.

Pain-free quadriceps isometric exercises may be performed as soon as possible, usually within the first 3 days. Between days 3 and 5, ice is continued with pain-free active range of motion, while the athlete is sitting and lying prone. Passive stretching is not used until the later phases of rehabilitation. Massage and heat modalities are also contraindicated in the early phases because of the possibility of promoting bleeding.

At approximately day 5, the athlete may perform straight leg raises without weights and then progress to weights, pain free. As active range of motion increases to approach 95 to 100 degrees of knee flexion, biking may be performed if the seat height is adjusted to the athlete's available range of motion.

Between days 7 and 10, heat in the form of hot packs, ultrasound, or whirlpool may be used as long as swelling is negative and the athlete is approaching full active range of motion while lying prone. Pain-free quadriceps progressive resistive strengthening exercises may be performed with the NK table. Isokinetics may be performed in conjunction with isotonic exercises. Ice or heat modalities, with active range of motion, may be continued before all exercises.

Swimming and jogging are performed on approximately days 10 to 14. Pain-free quadriceps stretching exercises may be added at approximately the fourteenth day. The athlete may progress to leg press exercises and squats, also after the fourteenth day. Jogging and sport-specific activities may be used in the last phase to prepare the athlete for competition. Compression and protective padding are continued during competition to avoid reinjury.

Treatment of grade II quadriceps contusion
PHASE I: *Days 1-3*
1. Rest.
2. Crutches.
3. Ice.
4. Compression.
5. Electrical muscle stimulation modalities.
6. Quadriceps isometric exercises daily.

PHASE II: *Days 3-5*
7. Pain-free active range-of-motion exercises lying prone and sitting.
8. Straight leg raises without weights daily.

PHASE III: *Days 5-7*
9. Straight leg raises with weights, 4 sets of 10 repetitions 3 days per week.
10. Biking 2 days per week.

PHASE IV: *Days 7-14*
11. Heat (hot packs, ultrasound, whirlpool).
12. Pain-free quadriceps progressive resistive strengthening exercises. Isotonics using the NK table, 4 sets of 10 repetitions 3 days per week.
13. Isokinetics 3 days per week.
14. Swimming 2 days per week.
15. Pain-free quadriceps stretching exercises. Hold for 30 seconds times 5 repetitions daily.

PHASE V: *From day 14*
16. Leg press exercises, 3 sets of 10 repetitions 2 days per week.
17. Squats, 4 sets of 6 to 8 repetitions 2 days per week.

18. Jogging.
19. Sport-specific activities.

Grade III Quadriceps Contusion

TREATMENT AND REHABILITATION. With a grade III quadriceps contusion the athlete should use crutches, rest, ice, compression, and electrical muscle stimulation modalities immediately to decrease pain, bleeding, and swelling and counteract atrophy.[20]

After surgery has been ruled out, the athlete may begin pain-free isometric quadriceps exercises between days 5 and 7. Ice and compression may be continued after day 7, with pain-free active range-of-motion exercises while the athlete is lying prone and sitting. At approximately day 10, the athlete may perform straight leg raises without weights and then progress to weights by day 14. Electrical muscle stimulation modalities may be very helpful in this phase to counteract muscle atrophy and reeducate muscle contraction.

After day 14, the athlete may use heat in the form of hot packs or whirlpool, as long as the swelling has decreased and the athlete has gained active range of motion. At approximately the third week of rehabilitation, pain-free quadriceps progressive resistive strengthening exercises may be performed in conjunction with isokinetics.

Swimming and biking may be added; adjust the bicycle seat height to accommodate the athlete's range of motion. Pain-free quadriceps stretching may also be performed if the athlete is careful not to overstretch the quadricep muscles.

Leg press exercises and squats may be performed after the fourth week, and the athlete can then progress to jogging and sport-specific activities. Compression and protective padding should be worn at all times during competition.

The rehabilitation timetables presented for grade II and III quadriceps contusions may be modified, depending upon the severity of the injury within its given grade.

Treatment of grade III quadriceps contusion
PHASE I: *Days 1-5*
1. Crutches.
2. Rest.
3. Ice.
4. Compression.
5. Electrical muscle stimulation modalities.

PHASE II: *Days 5-7*

6. Pain-free quadriceps isometric exercises daily.

PHASE III: *Days 7-14*

7. Pain-free quadriceps active range-of-motion exercises while lying prone and sitting daily.
8. Straight leg raises first without weights and progressing to weights, 4 sets of 10 repetitions 3 days per week.
9. Electrical muscle stimulation modalities continued.

PHASE IV: *Days 14-21*

10. Heat (hot packs, whirlpool).

PHASE V: *Week 3*

11. Pain-free quadriceps progressive resistive strengthening exercises. Isotonics using the NK table, 4 sets of 10 repetitions 3 days per week.
12. Isokinetics 3 days per week.
13. Pain-free quadriceps stretching exercises. Hold for 30 seconds times 5 repetitions daily.
14. Biking 2 days per week.
15. Swimming 2 days per week.

PHASE VI: *Week 4*

16. Leg press exercises, 3 sets of 10 repetitions 2 days per week.
17. Squats, 4 sets of 6 to 8 repetitions 2 days per week.
18. Jogging.
19. Sport-specific activities.
20. Protective padding upon return to activity.

MYOSITIS OSSIFICANS

With a severe direct blow or repetitive direct blows to the quadricep muscles that cause muscle tissue damage, bleeding, and injury to the periosteum of the femur, ectopic bone production may occur.[1,15] In 3 to 6 weeks, calcium formation may be seen on x-ray films. If the trauma was to the quadricep muscles only and not the femur, a smaller bony mass may be seen on x-ray films.[1]

If quadriceps contusion and strain are properly treated and rehabilitated, myositis ossificans may be prevented. Myositis ossificans can be caused by trying to "play through" a grade II or III quadriceps contusion or strain and by early use of massage, stretching exercises, ultrasound, and other heat modalities for grade II and III quadriceps contusion or strain.[1]

TREATMENT AND REHABILITATION. After 1 year, surgical removal of the bony mass may be helpful. If the bony mass is removed too early, the trauma caused by the surgery may actually enhance the condition.

After diagnosis by x-ray film, treatment and rehabilitation should follow that of a grade II or III quadriceps contusion or quadriceps strain. (See treatments for grade II and III quadriceps contusions and strains.)

The bony mass usually stabilizes after the sixth month.[12] If the mass does not cause disability, the athlete should be closely monitored and follow the rehabilitation programs outlined in Treatment of Grade II Quadriceps Contusion (p. 400) and Treatment of Grade III Quadriceps Contusion (pp. 400-401).

SUMMARY

1. Injuries to the hip and thigh can be extremely disabling and often require a substantial amount of time for rehabilitation.
2. Hip pointers are contusions of the soft tissue in the area of the iliac crest and must be treated aggressively during the first 2 to 4 hours after injury.
3. Piriformis syndrome sciatica should be specifically differentiated from other problems that produce low back or radiating pain in the buttocks and leg. Rehabilitation programs are extremely variable for different conditions and may even be harmful if used inappropriately.
4. Trochanteric bursitis is relatively common in athletes, as is ischial bursitis. Treatment involves efforts directed at protection and reduction of inflammation in the affected area.
5. Strains of the groin musculature, the hamstring, and the quadriceps muscles can require long periods of rehabilitation for the athlete. Early return often exacerbates the problem.
6. Protection is the key to treatment and rehabilitation of quadriceps contusions and accompanying myositis ossificans.

REFERENCES

1 Arnheim DD, Prentice WE: *Principles of athletic training,* St Louis, 1993, Mosby.
2 Coole WG, Gieck JH: An analysis of hamstring strains and their rehabilitation, *J Orthop Sports Phys Ther* 9(2):77-85, 1987.
3 Daniels L, Worthingham C: *Muscle testing, techniques of manual examination,* ed 3, Philadelphia, 1972, WB Saunders.
4 DeLorme TL, Watkins AL: *Progressive resistive exercises: tech-*

I would like to thank Jim Case, M.A., A.T. C., Assistant Athletic Trainer at Cornell University, for his contribution to various portions of this chapter.

nique and medical application, New York, 1952, Appleton-Century-Crofts.

5 DePalma BF, Zelko RR: Knee rehabilitation following anterior cruciate ligament injury or surgery, *Ath Train* 21:3, 1986.

6 Gordon EJ: Diagnosis and treatment of common hip disorders, *Med Tra Tech Q* 28(4):443, 1981.

7 Gould JA III: *Orthopedic and sports physical therapy,* St Louis, 1990, Mosby.

8 Hollinshead WH: *Functional anatomy of the limbs and back,* Philadelphia, 1976, WB Saunders.

9 Hoppenfield S: *Physical examination of the spine and extremities,* New York, 1976, Appleton-Century-Crofts.

10 Harvey J, editor: *Rehabilitation of the injured athlete clinics in sports medicine,* Philadelphia, 1985, WB Saunders.

11 Hunter-Griffen L, editor: *Oversue injuries: clinics in sports medicine,* Philadelphia, 1987, WB Saunders.

12 Kuland DN: *The injured athlete,* Philadelphia, 1982, JB Lippincott.

13 Lewinneck G: The significance and comparison analysis of the epidemiology of hip fractures, *Clin Orthop* 152:35, 1980.

14 Lewis A: *Normal human locomotion,* Hamden, Conn, 1977, Quinnipiac College.

15 Lipscomb AB: Treatment of myositis ossificans traumatica in athletes, *J Sports Med* 4:61, 1976.

16 Magee DJ: *Orthopedic physical assessment,* Philadelphia, 1987, WB Saunders.

17 Moore KL: *Clinical oriented anatomy,* Baltimore, 1985, Williams & Wilkins.

18 Norkin L, LeVange P: *Joint structure and function,* Philadelphia, 1983, FA Davis.

19 O'Donoghue DH: *Treatment of injuries to athletes,* Philadelphia, 1976, WB Saunders.

20 Prentice WE: *Therapeutic modalities in sports medicine,* St Louis, 1990, Mosby.

21 Roy S, Irvin R: *Sports medicine: prevention, evaluation, management, and rehabilitation,* Englewood Cliffs, NJ, 1983, Prentice-Hall.

22 Stevens J: The incidence of osteoporosis in patients with femoral neck fractures, *J Bone Joint Surg* [Fr] 44:520, 1962.

23 Tinker R, editor: *Ramamurti's orthopaedics in primary care,* Baltimore, 1979, Williams & Wilkins.

24 Torg J, Vegso J, Torg P: *Rehabilitation of athletic injuries: a guide to therapeutic exercise,* St Louis, 1987, Mosby.

25 Tortora GJ: *Principles of human anatomy,* New York, 1980, Harper & Row.

Knee Rehabilitation

23

Marc Davis and William E. Prentice

OBJECTIVES

After completion of this chapter, the student should be able to do the following:

- Describe the injury mechanisms of the most common knee injuries.

- Explain the five phases of rehabilitation and how each phase relates to a specific pathology.

- Outline specific rehabilitation protocols for the various knee pathologies.

- Discuss the functional parameters for a safe return of the athlete to activity.

The growth of scientific knowledge has been exponential since the beginning of the twentieth century, and fortunately for the athlete, the treatment of knee injuries has advanced rapidly also. For example, the introduction of arthroscopic techniques has greatly reduced the actual trauma of many reparative and reconstructive procedures, not to mention the accuracy of the diagnosis. Research into biomechanics has furthered the knowledge of knee kinematics, illuminating the functions of the supporting structures of the knee, while computer technology and manufacturing have allowed for the development of a myriad of devices for research, testing, and exercise. Yet all of this equipment and knowledge is of marginal benefit if the people involved do not make optimal use of the information available and if lines of communication between the patient, the surgeon, the sports therapist, the family, and the coach are limited or restricted.

The sports therapist has an obligation to the injured athlete to understand the nature of the injury, the function of the structures damaged, the technique of repair or reconstruction, and the different methods available to safely rehabilitate the athlete. The sports therapist must understand the treatment philosophy of the athlete's physician and be careful in applying different treatment regimens because what may be a safe but outdated technique in the opinion of one physician may be the treatment of choice to another. Communication is crucial to prevent misunderstandings and a subsequent loss of rapport with either the athlete or physician. The successful sports therapist must demonstrate flexibility in their approach to rehabilitation of the injured knee by incorporating techniques that are sound and effective but somewhat variable from patient to patient and physician to physician. Hence the purpose of this chapter is to present different approaches to knee rehabilitation. Clinics may differ in treatment philosophy, equipment, and expertise of staff yet may produce equally gratifying results.

The restoration of normal knee function is the goal of the rehabilitation process and is quantified by a full range of motion, normal strength, stability, no swelling, a relative pain-free state with activity, and normal patterns of sport-specific movements.[13,29] The rehabilitative process should be designed with these parameters in mind and with the realization that attainment of these goals will be affected by the type of injury, treatment option chosen (surgical vs. nonsurgical), length of immobilization, and the availability and quality of therapy.

Under ideal conditions, the physician, the sports therapist, the athlete, and his or her family will communicate freely and function as a team. This group is intimately involved with the rehabilitative process, beginning with patient assessment, treatment selection, and implementation and ending with functional exercises and return to activity. The sports therapist directs the postacute phase of the rehabilitation, and it is crucial that the athlete understand that this part of the recovery is just as crucial as surgical technique to the return of normal joint function and the subsequent return to athletic competition. This is the area of the sports therapist's specialization and where he or she can provide a strong link in the treatment chain.

Two basic principles must be followed to develop a safe and successful rehabilitation program: 1) the effects of immobilization must be minimized and 2) healing tissues must be cautiously and progressively stressed to facilitate return of normal function. Given these two principles, equal and even consideration will allow the sports therapist to develop a safe program, and the athlete will complete the process with as healthy and functional a knee as is currently possible.

GENERAL PRINCIPLES OF REHABILITATION
Range of Motion

After injury to the knee, some loss of motion is likely. This loss may be caused by the effects of the injury, the trauma of surgery, or the effects of immobilization. Waiting for ligaments to heal completely is a luxury that cannot be afforded in an effective rehabilitation program. Ligaments do not heal completely for 18 to 24 months, yet periarticular tissue changes can begin within 4 to 6 weeks of immobilization.[24] This is marked histologically by a decrease in water content in collagen and by an increase in collagen cross linkage.[4,24] The initiation of an early range-of-motion program can minimize these harmful changes. Controlled movement should be initiated early in the recovery process and progress based on healing constraints and patient tolerance toward a normal range of approximately 0 to 130 degrees.

Pitfalls that can slow or prevent regaining normal range of motion include imperfect surgical technique (improper placement of an anterior cruciate replacement), development of joint capsule or ligament contracture, and muscular resistance caused by pain.[20,24,38] The surgeon must address motion lost from technique, but the sports therapist can successfully deal with motion lost from soft tissue contracture or muscular resistance.

To effectively alleviate lost motion, the cause of the limitation must be identified. An experienced sports therapist can detect soft tissue resistance to motion by the quality of the feel of the resistance at the end of the range. Muscular resistance, which restricts normal physiological movement, has a firm end feel and can best be treated by using PNF stretching techniques in combination with appropriate therapeutic modalities (that is, heat, ice, electrical stimulation, etc.).[20] Joint capsule or ligamentous contractures have a leathery end feel and may not respond to conventional simple passive, active–assistive, and active motion exercises.[20] These contractures can limit the accessory motions of the joint, and until the accessory motions are restored, conventional exercises will not produce positive results.

Accessory motions are movements that occur between articulating joint surfaces and are necessary for normal joint function but are not under the active or voluntary control of the patient. Accessory motions in the knee joint must occur between the patella and femur, the femur and tibia, and the tibia and fibula. Restriction in any or all of these accessory motions must be addressed early in the rehabilitation program.

Mobilization of a knee that is restricted by soft tissue constraints may be accomplished by specifically applying graded oscillations to the restricted soft tissue as discussed in Chapter 10. In doing so, the sports therapist is addressing a specific limiting structure rather than assaulting the entire joint with a "crank till you cry" technique. After the release of the soft tissue contracture, accessory motion should improve, and thus so should physiological motion.

THE USE OF CONTINUOUS PASSIVE MOTION. Continuous passive motion (CPM) devices have recently been recommended postsurgically in an attempt to maintain motion, assist in pain control, and decrease inflammation (Figure 23-1).[33] McCarthy et al. reported that the use of CPM after ACL reconstruction reduced the amount of pain medication requested by the patient.[33] Also, they have stated that current research is sparse regarding the effectiveness of CPM and that studies evaluating CPM protocols are needed. The use of CPM after joint replacement is common, while use after ACL reconstruction varies from surgeon to surgeon.

Strengthening

The second goal of rehabilitation is the return of normal strength to the musculature surrounding the knee. Along with the return of muscular strength, it

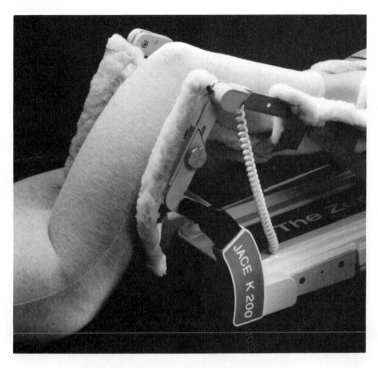

Fig. 23-1. Constant passive motion machine.

is also important to improve muscular endurance and power. These terms are related but not interchangeable. Strength is the force that a muscle can generate, power is the amount of force that can be produced per unit of time, and endurance refers to the ability of the muscle to produce strength and power over a prolonged period of time.[2,20]

It is critically important to understand that strength will be gained only if the muscle is subjected to overload. However, it is also essential to remember that healing tissues may be further damaged by overloading the injured structure too aggressively. Especially during the early phases of rehabilitation, muscular overload needs to be carefully applied to protect the damaged structures. The recovering knee needs protection, and the high-resistance, low-repetition program designed to strengthen a healthy knee may compromise the integrity of the injured knee.[30] The strengthening phase of rehabilitation must be gently progressive and will generally progress from isometric to isotonic to isokinetic to functional exercise.

MUSCLE STRENGTHENING TECHNIQUES. Strengthening exercises in the rehabilitation of the injured knee should use a closed-kinetic chain technique as dis-

cussed in Chapter 7. Closed-kinetic chain exercises may be safely introduced early in the rehabilitation process for virtually all types of knee injury.[12,42,43] For years, open-kinetic chain exercises were the treatment of choice. However, recently closed-kinetic chain exercise has been widely used and recommended. Also, closed-kinetic chain exercises are more functional in nature and may speed return to activity. Closed-kinetic chain activities may involve isometric, isotonic, and even isokinetic techniques.

Isometric exercise occurs when there is a muscle contraction without joint motion or a change in muscle fiber length. Strength is gained within 10 degrees of the position of the joint during the exercise, and the greatest strength gain will occur if a maximal contraction is held for at least 6 seconds.[2] These exercises are used preoperatively and postoperatively as a means of muscle education and form the basis for strength training when only a minimal amount of stress is allowed at the healing tissues. They are also used in the treatment of patellofemoral dysfunction and tibiofemoral arthrosis, both cases where strength is desired but joint irritation needs to be minimized. Recent investigations have looked at the possibility of increasing muscle tension during isometric con-

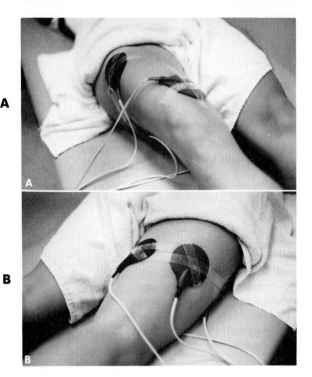

Fig. 23-2. Co-contraction of the quadriceps and hamstrings using a four-pad configuration during electrical stimulation. A, Two pads on quadriceps. **B,** Two pads on hamstrings.

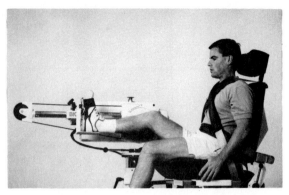

Fig. 23-3. Biodex closed-kinetic chain testing device for the lower extremity.

traction by using electrical stimulation to the muscle (Figure 23-2).[21]

Isotonic exercise occurs when a muscle contracts and shortens/lengthens and joint motion results. These are the classic strengthening exercises popularized by DeLorme and involve raising and lowering a weight against the force of gravity. The major disadvantage for this type of exercise is that the muscle can only be loaded to the maximum of the weakest point within the joint's range of motion. The development of variable resistance devices (for example, Nautilus, Eagle, and Universal) was an attempt to adjust the resistance to accommodate normal strength variations. The current trend in rehabilitation of the knee joint has moved away from the use of the exercise machines that require open-kinetic chain activities. Isotonic closed-kinetic chain activities including mini-squats, stepping exercises, and terminal knee extensions, are both safer and more functional than previously recommended open-chain exercises (see Figures 7-9 and 7-10). They have also been described as an effective means of treating patellar/extensor mechanism dysfunction.[9,24,35]

Isokinetic exercise occurs when there is a muscle contraction and the limb moves at a constant velocity even though the resistance may vary. This type of exercise has become available during the past two decades with development of isokinetic devices (for example, Cybex, Kin Com, Lido, Biodex, Merac, and Areil System). With this type of exercise, it is possible to offer fast-speed, maximum-resistance exercise. Most isokinetic devices operate in an open kinetic chain. However, several companies, including Biodex and Areil, are developing closed-chain isokinetic exercise and testing equipment (Figure 23-3). To reduce joint stresses, isokinetic activity usually starts at higher velocity and gradually progresses to slower speeds.

MUSCLE ENDURANCE. Endurance is another component of muscle function that needs to be addressed early in the rehabilitation program. Endurance exercise needs to be started as early as feasible because immobilization depletes the type 1 (slow twitch, endurance) muscle fibers of the oxydative enzymes needed for prolonged muscle contraction.[29,30]

Any exercises that involve repetitive high-speed contractions, such as cycling, swimming, or rowing, are effective in maintaining local muscular endurance. These activities should be continued throughout the entire rehabilitation period and, as function improves, be augmented by the repetition of sport-specific activities.

Phases of Rehabilitation

It is convenient to break the rehabilitation process into stages, and this has been done by several clinicians.[20,30] Programs for the various knee pathologies can be logically designed using these phases as a guide. By assessing patient response to the exercise progressions, the sports therapist can safely advance the treatment protocol. The patient must be closely watched for pain, effusion, changes in motion, and psychological response and that these changes guide the advancement of the rehabilitation process.

PHASE I - *Maximum protection*
Treat the inflammation, achieve primary tissue healing, maintain function. Use controlled range of motion.

PHASE II - *Moderate protection*
Tissue maturation, strengthening, endurance, protective development. Use crutch walking and low-intensity strengthening exercises.

PHASE III - *Minimum protection*
Determination of time segment needed for tissue maturation/reorientation, light functional activity, skill acquisition. Use moderate strengthening, protected activity, and protected function.

PHASE IV - *Advanced rehabilitation*
Functional program, return to demanding environment, requisition of skill. Use advanced rehabilitation techniques, isokinetic training, intense strengthening.

PHASE V - *Maintenance*[20,30]

Criteria for Return to Activity

Specific criteria for return to full activity after rehabilitation of the injured knee is determined to a large extent by the nature and severity of the specific injury, but it also depends on the philosophy and judgment of both the physician and the sports therapist. Traditionally, return to activity has been dictated through both objective and subjective evaluations. Objective evaluation techniques have made use primarily of isokinetic testing and arthrometry. The advantage of testing with an isokinetic device that indicates levels of strength and an arthrometer that measures joint laxity is that the sports therapist is provided with some hard, quantifiable data relative to the athlete's progress in the rehabilitation program. Recently however, considerable debate has taken place in the sports-medicine community on the functional application of isokinetic testing. The question

has been raised whether the ability to generate torque at a fixed speed is indicative of the athlete's capability of returning to an activity in which success more often depends on the ability to generate force at a high velocity.

For the athlete, it may be more practical to base criteria for return on functional capabilities as indicated by performance on specific functional tests that are more closely related to the demands of a particular sport. Performance on functional tests, such as those described in Chapter 12 (that is, hop test, co-contraction test), should serve as primary determinants of the athlete's capability to return to full activity. Currently data on the majority of these tests are limited. Thus at present they remain as purely subjective evaluations until research data become available to objectively quantify performance on various functional tests. Once results are objectively quantified, these functional tests will be extremely useful and valuable tools for determining readiness to return to full activity.

REHABILITATION CONSIDERATIONS FOR VARIOUS KNEE INJURIES

Injuries to the soft tissues that support the knee occur when these tissues are not able to resist abnormal tension.[24] This abnormal tension develops when the knee is forced through an abnormal motion. The direction of these forces determines which structures within the knee are damaged, and these forces may act in a straight direction (medial, lateral, anterior, or posterior), rotational manner, or in combination.

Anterior Cruciate Ligament

In simple terms, the ACL functions to prevent anterior translation of the tibia on the femur. It works in conjunction with the posterior cruciate ligament to control the gliding and rolling of the tibia on the femur during normal flexion and extension. The twisted configuration of the fibers of the ACL and the shape of the femoral condyles allow for the screw home mechanism of the knee during the final 20 degrees of extension when the tibia externally rotates on the femur. The ligament is under some degree of tension in all positions of knee motion, with lesser tension present from 30 to 90 degrees.[24,25,41]

ACL rehabilitation should be designed to do the following:

1. Enhance the ability of the knee to resist anterior

and rotational displacement. This goal can be addressed by surgical technique and a rehabilitation program that in addition to general muscle strengthening emphasizes retraining the hamstring group to augment ACL function.

2. Avoid the ranges of motion where the ACL is under greatest tension.

Most ACL injuries occur from a twisting motion of the knee with the foot firmly planted. Contact with another athlete is not necessary to cause the injury. Simply the rotational force of the body twisting over the fixed limb can focus a damaging rotational force on the knee. The athlete will usually report either hearing or feeling a "pop" with subsequent swelling within the joint.

In many instances the ACL will be injured after the application of an external force to the knee, and this type of trauma may involve numerous structures in the knee. O'Donohue's unhappy triad (ACL, MCL, and meniscus) is the classic example. Certainly the more structures damaged, the more complicated the assessment, the surgery, and the rehabilitation.

After the diagnosis of injury to the ACL, the athlete, the physician, the sports therapist, and the athlete's family are faced with various treatment options. The conservative approach is to allow the acute phase of the injury to pass and to then implement a vigorous rehabilitation program. If it becomes apparent that normal function cannot be recovered with rehabilitation and if the knee remains unstable even with normal strength and hamstring retraining, then reconstructive surgery is considered. For a sedentary individual, this approach may be acceptable, but most athletes prefer a more aggressive approach. Also some surgeons feel that surgery is necessary to prevent the early onset of degenerative changes within the knee.[25] Wilk and Andrews state that any active individual with a goal of returning to stressful pivoting activities should undergo surgical ACL reconstruction.[45]

In the case of a partially torn ligament, the medical community is split on treatment approach. Some feel that a partially damaged ACL is incompetent, and the knee should be viewed as if the ligament were completely gone. Others prefer a prolonged initial period of immobilization and limited motion, hoping that the ligament will heal and remain functional. This is clearly a case where the athlete may wisely seek several opinions before choosing the treatment course.

Successful surgical repair/reconstruction of the ACL deficient knee is dependent upon patient selec-

tion.[24] The older and more sedentary the individual, the less appropriate a reconstruction. This individual may not have the inclination nor the time for an extensive rehabilitation program and may not be greatly inconvenienced by some degree of knee instability. The ideal patient is a young, motivated, and skilled athlete who is willing to make the personal sacrifices necessary to successfully complete the rehabilitation process.

The surgical approach to ACL pathology is either repair or reconstruction. With a surgical repair, the damaged ligament is sutured if the tear is in the midsubstance of the ligament or the bony fragment is reattached in the case of an avulsion injury. In the case of suturing, the repair may be augmented with an internal splint or an extraarticular reconstruction.

Surgical reconstruction is performed using either an extraarticular or intraarticular technique. An extraarticular reconstruction involves taking a structure that lies outside of the joint capsule and moving it so that it can affect the mechanics of the knee in a manner that mimics normal ACL function. The iliotibial band is the most commonly used structure. This procedure is effective in reducing the pivot shift phenomena that is found in anterolateral rotational instability but cannot match the normal biomechanics of the ACL.[24,30] Isolated extraarticular reconstructions may be effective in patients with mild-to-moderate instability. Also it may be the treatment of choice in patients who cannot afford the commitment of time and resources for an intraarticular reconstruction.[24] The rehabilitation after an extraarticular reconstruction is aggressive and permits an earlier return to functional activities; however as an isolated procedure it is not recommended for high-level athletes.

Intraarticular reconstruction involves placing a structure within the knee that will roughly follow the course of the ACL and will functionally replace the ACL. Patellar tendon grafts are the current state of the art, using human autografts/allografts.[15,24,31,41,46] Problems with autografts include decreased strength at the donor site, resulting in tendinitis and possible failure.[15] Surgical technique is crucial to a successful outcome. The improper placement of the tendon graft by only a few millimeters can prevent the return of normal motion. Patient selection is also important for success, and it is recommended that it be reserved for the following special situations:

- ACL injury in the highly athletic individual
- Active persons with instability and unwillingness to alter their lifestyles

- Instability in normal activities
- Recurrent effusions
- Failure at rehabilitation and instability after 6 months of intensive rehabilitation[24]

Rehabilitation after ACL reconstruction has become more aggressive as a result of the reports of success by Shelbourne and Nitz.[32] An accelerated protocol has been developed emphasizing full knee extension day 1 postoperatively, immediate weight bearing to tolerance, 100 degrees of flexion by week 2, unlimited ADL by week 4, and a return to light sports activities as early as week 8.[32] They believe that this program returns the patient to normal function early, results in fewer patellofemoral problems, and reduces the number of surgeries to obtain extension, all without compromising stability.[32] Closed-chain exercises are emphasized to reduce the stress on the ACL. Other surgeons allow open-chain exercises in the 90 to 45 degree range, but Shelbourne and Nitz do not.[45] They allow return to competitive athletics at 5 to 6 months, while Fu et al. feel that 6 to 9 months is more reasonable.[15,42,43]

The accelerated rehabilitation protocol is not without its detractors. Some clinicians feel that it places too much stress on vulnerable tissues and that there are not sufficient scientific data to justify the protocol.[15,45] It is paramount that the sports therapist understand the surgeon's preference of protocol and realize that different physicians may prefer different approaches.

The accelerated protocol emphasizes the following:
- Immediate motion, including full extension.
- Immediate weight bearing within tolerance.
- Early closed-chain exercise for strengthening and neuromuscular control.
- Return to activity at 2 months and to competition at 5 to 6 months.[42,43]

The traditional protocol emphasizes the following:
- Slow progression to regain flexion and extension.
- Partial or nonweight-bearing postoperatively.
- Closed-chain exercises at 3 to 4 weeks postoperatively.
- Return to activity at 6 to 9 months.[10,15,45]

ACL REHABILITATION PROTOCOL (ACCELERATED PROTOCOL)

POSTOPERATIVE - *0 to 6 days*

Bracing—0 to 90 degrees, locked at 0 degrees for ambulation.

ROM—CPM 0 to 90 degrees, patellar mobilization.

Crutches—weight bearing as tolerated, full weight bearing (FWB) acceptable.

Exercise—ankle pumps, electrical stimulation with co-contraction, ice, and elevation.

PHASE I - *7 days to 5 weeks*

Bracing—set 0 to 110 degrees.

ROM—emphasis on gaining and maintaining full extension, move toward full flexion.

Crutches—FWB without crutches by 2 weeks, still in brace.

Exercise—wall slides, prone hangs, hamstring curls, bilateral closed-chain exercise for terminal knee extension (TKE) (quarter squats, leg press 0 to 60 degrees, stair climber), bicycle, swimming with 90 degrees of flexion. Some surgeons allow open-chain extension with light weights within the limits of 90 to 45 degrees.

PHASE II - *5 weeks to 10 weeks*

Bracing—FWB without brace and crutches by week 6.

ROM—130 degrees approaching full range.

Exercise—continue phase I, begin unilateral closed-chain exercises, increase weight-room activities, begin rotational exercises for heel slides, begin lateral motions.

PHASE III - *10 weeks to 20 weeks*

Bracing—measure for derotational brace for activity.

ROM—full, work to maintain.

Exercise—advance weight-room activities, begin running program, isokinetic testing (Shelbourne[43] at week 6, Andrews[45] at week 12).

PHASE IV - *return to activity 5 to 6 months*

If isokinetic, stability, and functional testing are satisfactory, competition may be resumed.

PHASE V - *Maintenance*—Minimum of twice per week.[12,42,43]

ACL REHABILITATION PROTOCOL (TRADITIONAL PROTOCOL)

POSTOPERATIVE - *0 to 6 days*

Bracing—15 to 75 degrees.

ROM—CPM 15 to 75 degrees, patellar mobilization.

Crutches—touch down weight bearing, brace locked at 15 degrees.

Exercise—Straight leg raises (SLR) with 30 degrees of flexion, quadriceps sets at 30 degrees flexion, ankle pumps, electric stimulation for co-contraction.

PHASE I - *7 days to week 4*

Bracing—10 degrees extension to full motion by week 4.

ROM—move to full by week 4, slowly to full extension, patellar mobilizations.

Crutches—move to FWB in brace locked at 10 degrees, discontinue crutches by week 4.

Exercise—SLR, quadriceps sets, ankle pumps, TKE against towel and tubing, hamstring curls, bicycling.

PHASE II - *4 weeks - 8 weeks*

Bracing—out at home and while sleeping at 6 weeks, out completely at 8 weeks.

ROM—full, work to maintain.

Exercise—continue phase I, bilateral closed- or open-chain exercises may be done safely from 90 to 45 degrees at 8 weeks, swimming.

PHASE III - *8 weeks to 24 weeks*

Bracing—measure for derotational brace.

ROM—full, work to maintain.

Exercise—increase weight-room activities, begin unilateral closed chain, (leg press 0-60 degrees, step-ups), begin straight ahead jogging and running program at week 20.

PHASE IV - *return to activity 6 to 9 months*

Increase strength, endurance, balance with isokinetic test at 24 weeks, return to full competitive activity at 9 to 12 months.*

PHASE V - *Maintenance*

ACL DEFICIENT KNEE REHABILITATION PROTOCOL

This protocol may be accelerated as symptoms allow emphasis on hamstring function.

PHASE I - *0- 3 weeks*

Bracing—initially locked between 15 to 90 degrees and advancing toward 90 to 0 degrees by week 3.

ROM—as allowed by brace.

Exercise—done in brace: heel slides, quadriceps sets, co-contractions, ankle ROM, hip flexion, extension, patellar mobilizations, progressive resistive exercises—90 to 45 degrees extension at week 2, standing hamstring curls at week 2, electrical stimulation as needed.

Crutches—PWB to FWB

PHASE II - *3 weeks to 6 weeks*

Bracing—90 to 0 degrees at fifth week.

ROM—active out of brace.

Exercise—quadriceps sets, co-contractions, SLR,

progress PRE 90 to 45 degrees, begin hamstring PRE, stationary cycling, swimming, hip strengthening (all planes), electrical stimulation as needed, PNF emphasizing hamstring function, closed-chain exercises bilateral.

Crutches—discontinued.

PHASE III - *6 weeks to 9 weeks*

Bracing—discontinue except for stressful activities; should be fitted for derotational brace for activity.

ROM—flexion as tolerated, terminal extension without weight.

Exercise—quadriceps PRE—90 to 45 degrees, hamstring PRE—advance rapidly as patient tolerates, TKE closed-kinetic chain—unilateral, rotational exercises—PNF, using tubing, cycling, swimming, isokinetic exercises 90 to 45 degrees using antishear device.

PHASE IV - *9 weeks plus*

Bracing—wear derotational brace for activity.

ROM—assisted as needed.

Exercise—progress to phase III, begin jogging program, progressing to running, sprinting, cutting, cross overs, and return to sport-specific activity, backward running for hamstring function.

PHASE V - *Maintenance*—minimum twice per week.*

Posterior Cruciate Ligament

The posterior cruciate ligament (PCL) functions with the ACL to control the rolling and gliding of the tibiofemoral joint and has been called the primary stabilizer of the knee. More specifically the PCL prevents the posterior translation of the tibia on the femur. This is evident in the PCL deficient knee when upon descending an incline, the force of gravity works to increase the anterior glide of the femur on the tibia, and without the PCL the femur will sublux on the tibia from mid-stance to toe-off where the quadriceps are less effective in controlling the anterior motion of the femur on the tibia.[9,30] In athletics, the most common mechanism of injury to the PCL is with the knee in a position of forced hyperflexion with the foot plantar flexed. The PCL may also be injured when the tibia is forced posteriorly on the fixed femur or the femur is forced anteriorly on the fixed tibia.[25,30]

Surgery to reconstruct a PCL deficient knee may

*References 7, 10, 13, 15, 30, 37, 38, 44, 45.

*References 7, 10, 13, 24, 30, 37, 41, 44.

involve a reconstructive procedure that used the semitendinous tendon, the tendinous part of the medial gastrocnemius, or the patellar tendon to replace the lost PCL. Both autografts and allografts have been used. Some surgeons prefer nonoperative treatment for isolated PCL tears. Panlie and Bergfield reported over 80% success with nonoperative treatment, while Clancey reported a high incidence of femoral condylar articular injury in patients 4 years after PCL injury.[32] Rehabilitation should emphasize protection of the patella, protection of the lateral stabilizers, evaluation of joint articulating surfaces, bracing for athletic activities, and achieving a high degree of strength, power, and endurance. Pusey reported that patients treated successfully nonoperatively had quadriceps strength greater than 100% of the uninvolved side.[31] After surgical reconstruction of the PCL, it is important to limit hamstring function to reduce the posterior translational forces.[31]

Medial Collateral Ligament

The medial collateral ligament (MCL) is divided into two parts, the stronger superficial portion and the thinner and weaker "deep" medial ligament or capsular ligament, with its accompanying attachment to the medial meniscus. The MCL functions as the primary static stablizer against valgus stress. In the normal knee, valgus loading is greatest during the push-off phase of gait when the foot is planted and the tibia externally rotated relative to the femur. The MCL is taut at full extension and begins to relax between 20 to 30 degrees of flexion and comes under tension again at 60 to 70 degrees of flexion, although a portion of the ligament is taut through the range of motion.[25,46]

The most common mechanism of injury to the MCL is a valgus force upon the slightly flexed knee while the foot is planted.[11,25,30] The treatment of MCL injuries is largely non-surgical with immobilization in the case of all isolated grade I and II tears and in the majority of isolated grade III tears.[30,46] However, grade III injuries that display gross instability or the involvement of other stabilizing structures will require surgery. Three conditions must be met for healing to occur at the MCL: 1) the ligament fibers must remain in continuity or within a well-vascularized soft-tissue bed, 2) there must be enough stress to stimulate and direct the healing process, and 3) there must be protection from harmful stresses.[46] The emphasis for MCL rehabilitation is to protect the knee from valgus stress while the joint heals. Controlling functional stress at the knee is accomplished by the use of cast bracing, splints, functional bracing, or crutch walking. Full range of motion is regained as quickly as patient tolerance allows. External rotation of the tibia on the femur and hip adduction exercises are avoided early in the rehabilitation process. At approximately 12 months after injury, maximal maturation occurs with the ligament regaining 70% to 75% of its original strength.[46]

Lateral Collateral Ligament

The lateral collateral ligament (LCL) functions with the illiotibial band, the popliteus tendon, the arcuate ligament complex, and the biceps tendons to support the lateral aspect of the knee. The LCL is under constant tensile loading, and the thick, firm configuration of the ligament is well designed to withstand this constant stress.[11,25] The incidence of injury to the LCL is much less than either to the ACL or the MCL, and the mechanism is usually a varus stress. A complete disruption of the LCL usually involves one or both cruciate ligaments.[25,30] Severe injury to the LCL is rare in athletics since most athletic injuries result from a stress placed on the lateral aspect of the knee.[25,30]

Fortunately, the lateral aspect of the knee is well supported by secondary stabilizers, which can also provide support for an injured LCL. Except in extreme cases, injuries respond quite well to conservative treatment. The ligament should be protected from varus stress during the recovery phase, and general range of motion and strengthening exercises can be initiated as soon as symptoms permit.

CAPSULAR REPAIR—MCL, LCL, CAPSULAR DAMAGE REHABILITATION PROTOCOLS

(The time frame may be accelerated for grade I injuries and extended for more involved injuries.)

PHASE I - *0 - 7 days*

Bracing—hinged brace set for patient comfort, avoid full extension.

ROM—as allowed by the brace.

Exercise—in the brace: quadriceps sets, co-contractions, electrical stimulation for quadriceps, ankle ROM, hip flexion, extension, patellar mobilizations, SLR.

Crutches—weight bearing to patient tolerance.

PHASE II - *7 days - 2 weeks*

Bracing—set to comfort.

ROM—push to full extension and flexion, bicycle.

Exercise—out of brace: quadriceps sets, co-contractions, quadriceps PRE—90 to 45 degrees (submaximal), hamstring PRE (submaximal), bicycle if ROM sufficient, for MCL—hip adductor exercises, tibial internal rotation, closed-chain bilateral exercises.

Crutches—FWB in brace, discontinue crutches.

PHASE III - *2 weeks - 4 weeks*
Bracing—discontinue.
ROM—normal, work to maintain.
Exercise—quadriceps sets, co-contractions, SLR (4 planes), quadriceps PRE progress to TKE, hamstring PRE progress to gastrocnemius strengthening, cycling, swimming, unilateral closed-chain exercises, begin running program.

Crutches—FWB.

PHASE IV - *4 weeks - 6 weeks*
Bracing—functional brace for activity if needed.
ROM—normal.
Exercise—begin eccentric quadriceps and hamstring exercises, begin isokinetic quadriceps and hamstrings, progress functional activity.

PHASE V - *Maintenance*[9,21,22,33,35]

Progress through this rehabilitation protocol should be as quick as patient tolerance will allow. Any increase in pain, swelling, or loss of motion indicates that the progression is too rapid and stressful, and it should be slowed.

Meniscal Injury

Injuries to the menisci may be isolated or occur in conjunction with injuries to other structures. The injury is caused by either a traction or compression force and usually occurs when the knee is flexed and rotated. Noncontact injuries are common.

The menisci function to aid in joint lubrication, to increase joint congruency, which aids stability, to act as a shock absorber, and to distribute weight-bearing forces.[8,11,20,29] Traditional surgical treatment required the total removal of the damaged meniscus with the concomitant loss of these functions. With the advent of arthroscopic surgery, the need for total meniscectomy has been virtually eliminated. Maximum preservation of the undamaged meniscus is attempted and, if possible, meniscal repair undertaken.

Three choices are possible for the athlete with a damaged meniscus: total meniscectomy, partial menisecomy, and meniscal repair. The outer third of the cartilage is highly vascular, and if the damage occurs in this region, repair and healing are possible. If the

tear is in the inner two thirds of the cartilage, then removal of the damaged portion can be accomplished leaving viable meniscal tissue behind to continue the above-mentioned functions. If the damage is extensive, then total meniscectomy may be required.

The repair of a damaged meniscus involves the use of absorbable sutures, vascular access channels drilled from vascular to nonvascular areas, and the insertion of a fibrin clot.[8] Rehabilitation after meniscal repair requires that joint motion be limited. The menisci move during knee motion, approximately 12 millimeters anterior to posterior with the tibia during flexion and extension, and during rotation they follow the femur.[8,30] Hence motion must be restricted to prevent stress at the repair site. Rehabilitation after repair is more prolonged than following partial or total meniscectomy where motion does not need to be restricted. Recommendations for immobilization after repair range from immediate weight bearing as tolerated to 3 to 4 weeks nonweight-bearing (NWB). Obviously, it is important to understand the surgeon's protocol for such cases.[8]

Rehabilitation after arthroscopic surgery for partial or total meniscectomy with no associated capsular damage is rapid, and the likelihood of complications is minimal. Immediate postoperative care consists of wound care for the portal sites, compression to control edema, and a rapid progression of range-of-motion and strengthening exercises.

PARTIAL OR COMPLETE MENISCECTOMY REHABILITATION PROTOCOL

PHASE I - *generally not required*
PHASE II - *0 - 10 days*
Bracing—compressive brace for control of swelling.
ROM—as tolerated.
Exercise—quadriceps sets, SLR (4 planes), co-contractions, cycling to tolerance, add weights to SLR in later stage
Crutches—PWB to FWB quickly.

PHASE III - *10 days - 3 weeks*
Bracing—compressive as needed.
ROM—normal.
Exercise—as above, quadriceps PRE—90 to 30 degrees, advance to 0 degrees, hamstrings PRE, isokinetic exercise at 3 weeks, swimming when wound healing complete.

PHASE IV - *progress phase 3*

MENISCAL REPAIR REHABILITATION PROTOCOL

PHASE I - *0 - 3 weeks*

Bracing—80 to 30 degrees.

ROM—passive in brace.

Exercise—in brace: quadriceps sets, co-contractions, SLR (3 planes—avoid adduction with medial meniscectomy, abduction with lateral), electrical stimulation as needed, all exercise in this phase must be submaximal.

Crutches—NWB.

PHASE II - *3 - 10 weeks*

Bracing—increase 10 degrees in flexion and extension each week.

ROM—follows bracing toward 0 to 120 degrees at 8 weeks.

Exercise - quadriceps sets, SLR with weight, quadriceps PRE—90 to 30 degrees, hamstrings PRE at week 6 with limited extension, cycling, swimming.

Crutches—PWB at onset progressing to FWB at end phase.

PHASE III and IV - *As in meniscal removal*

REHABILITATION OF THE PATELLOFEMORAL JOINT

Complaints of patellofemoral pain are exceedingly common among the athletic population. Until recently, almost every athlete who walked into a sports-medicine center complaining of anterior knee pain was diagnosed as having condromalacia patella. However, there can be many other causes of anterior knee pain, and the treatment and rehabilitation of patients complaining of anterior knee pain can be very frustrating for the sports therapist. The more conservative approach to treatment of patellofemoral pain described below should be used initially. If this approach fails, surgical intervention may be required.

Common Signs and Symptoms

Athletes presenting with patellofemoral pain typically exhibit relatively common symptoms. They complain of nonspecific pain in the anterior portion of the knee. It is difficult to place one finger on a specific spot and be certain that the pain is there. Pain seems to be increased when either ascending or descending stairs or when moving from a squatting to a standing position. Athletes also complain of pain when sitting for long periods of time. This has occasionally been referred to as the *movie goer's sign*. Reports of the knee

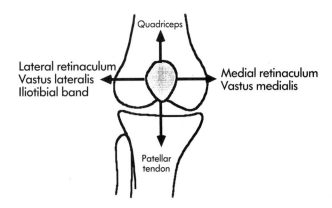

Fig. 23-4. Static and dynamic patellar stabilizers.

"giving away" are likely, although typically no instability is associated with this problem.

Assessment of Patellofemoral Mechanics

When evaluating the mechanics of the patellofemoral joint, the sports therapist must assess static alignment, dynamic alignment, and patellar orientation.

STATIC ALIGNMENT. Static stabilizers of the patellofemoral joint act to maintain the appropriate alignment of the patella when no motion is occurring (Figure 23-4). The superior static stabilizers are the quadriceps muscles (vastus lateralis, vastus intermedius, vastus medialis, rectus femoris). Laterally, static stabilizers include the lateral retinaculum, vastus lateralis, and iliotibial band. Medially, the medial retinaculum and the vastus medialis are the static stabilizers. Inferiorly, the patellar tendon stabilizes the patella.

DYNAMIC ALIGNMENT. Dynamic alignment of the patella must be assessed during functional activities. It is critical to look at the tracking of the patella from an anterior view during normal gait. Muscle control should be observed while the athlete engages in other functional activities including stepping, bilateral squats, or one-legged squats.

There are a number of different anatomical factors that can affect dynamic alignment. It is essential to understand that both static and dynamic structures must create a balance of forces about the knee. Any change in this balance may produce improper tracking of the patella and patellofemoral pain.

Increased Q-angle. The Q-angle (Figure 23-5) is

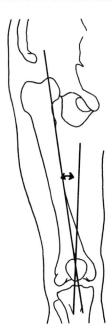

Fig. 23-5. Measuring the Q-angle.

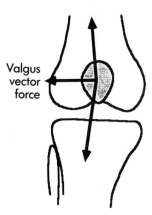

Fig. 23-6. A lateral valgus vector force created when the quadriceps is contracted.

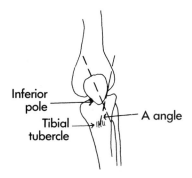

Fig. 23-7. Measurement of the A-angle.

formed by drawing a line from the anterosuperior iliac spine to the center of the patella. A second line drawn from the tibial tubercle to the center of the patella that intersects the first line forms the Q-angle. A normal Q-angle falls between 10 to 12 degrees in the male and 15 to 17 degrees in the female. Q-angle may be increased by lateral displacement of the tibial tubercle, external tibial torsion, or femoral neck anteversion. The Q-angle is a static measurement that may have no direct correlation with patellofemoral pain.[17] However, dynamically this increased Q-angle may increase the lateral valgus vector force, thus encouraging lateral tracking, resulting in patellofemoral pain (Figure 23-6).

A-angle. The A-angle (Figure 23-7) measures the patellar orientation to the tibial tubercle. It is created by the intersection of lines drawn bisecting the patella longitudinally and from the tibial tubercle to the apex of the inferior pole of the patella. An angle of 35 degrees or greater has been correlated with patellofemoral pathomechanics, which results in patellofemoral pain.[1]

Iliotibial band. The distal portion of the iliotibial band interdigitates with both the deep transverse retinaculum and the superficial oblique retinaculum. As the knee moves into flexion, the iliotibial band moves posteriorly, causing the patella to tilt and track laterally.[17]

Vastus medialis oblique insufficiency. The vastus medialis oblique (VMO) functions as an active and dynamic stabilizer of the patella. Anatomically it arises from the tendon of the adductor magnus.[6] Normally, the VMO is tonically active electromyographically throughout the range of motion. In individuals with patellofemoral pain, it is phasically active, and it tends to lose fatigue resistant capabilities.[40] The VMO is innervated by a separate branch of the femoral nerve; therefore it can be activated as a single motor unit.[2] In normal individuals the VMO to vastus lateralis (VL) ratio has been shown to be 1:1.[39] However in individuals who complain of patellofemoral pain the VMO:VL ratio is less than 1:1.

Vastus lateralis. The vastus lateralis interdigitates

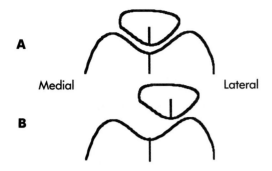

Fig. 23-8. Positive lateral glide. A, Normal positioning.
B, Positive lateral glide component.

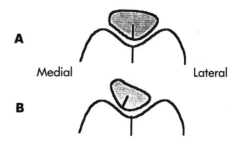

Fig. 23-9. Positive lateral tilt. A, Normal positioning.
B, Positive lateral tilt component.

with fibers of the superficial lateral retinaculum. Again, if this retinaculum is tight or if a muscle imbalance exists between the vastus lateralis and the vastus medialis with the lateralis being more active, lateral tilt or tracking of the patella may occur dynamically.[16]

Excessive pronation. Excessive pronation may result from existing structural deformities in the foot. With overpronation there is excessive subtalar eversion and adduction with an obligatory internal rotation of the tibia, increased internal rotation of the femur, and thus an increased lateral valgus vector force at the knee that encourages lateral tracking.[20] Various structural deformities in the feet that may cause knee pain should be corrected biomechanically according to techniques recommended in Chapter 26.

Tight hamstring muscles. Tight hamstring muscles cause an increase in knee flexion. When the heel strikes the ground, there must be increased dorsiflexion at the talocrural joint. Excessive subtalar joint motion may occur to allow for necessary dorsiflexion. As stated previously, this produces excessive pronation with concomitant increased internal tibial rotation and a resultant increase in the lateral valgus vector force.

Tight gastrocnemius muscle. A tight gastrocnemius muscle will not allow for the 10 degrees of dorsiflexion necessary for normal gait. Once again this produces excessive subtalar motion, increased internal tibial rotation, and increased lateral valgus vector force.[20]

Patella alta. In patella alta, the ratio of patellar tendon length to the height of the patella is greater than the normal 1:1 ratio. In patella alta the length of the patellar tendon is 20% greater than the height of the patella. This creates a situation where greater flexion is necessary before the patella assumes a stable position within the trochlear groove, and thus there is an increased tendency toward lateral subluxation.[23]

PATELLAR ORIENTATION. Patellar orientation refers to the positioning of the patella relative to the tibia. Assessment should be done with the athlete in supine position. Four components should be assessed when looking at patellar orientation: the glide component, the tilt component, the rotation component, and the anteroposterior tilt component.

Glide component. This component assesses the lateral or medial deviation of the patella relative to the trochlear groove of the femur. Glide should be assessed both statically and dynamically. Figure 23-8 provides an example of a positive lateral glide.

Tilt component. Tilt is determined by comparing the height of the medial patellar border with the lateral patellar border. Figure 23-9 shows an example of a positive lateral tilt.

Rotational component. Rotation is identified by assessing the deviation of the longitudinal axis (line drawn from superior pole to inferior pole) of the patella relative to the femur. The point of reference is the inferior pole. Thus if the inferior pole is more lateral than the superior pole a positive external rotation exists (Figure 23-10).

Anteroposterior tilt component. This must be assessed laterally to determine if a line drawn from the inferior patellar pole to the superior patellar pole is parallel to the long axis of the femur. If the inferior pole is posterior to the superior pole the athlete has a positive anteroposterior tilt component (Figure 23-11).

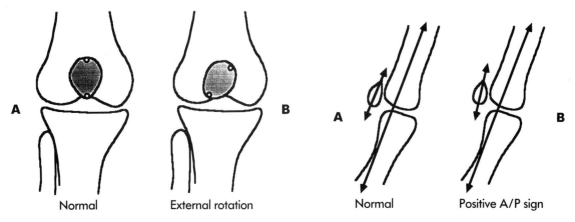

Fig. 23-10. Positive external rotation. A, Normal positioning. **B,** Positive external rotation component.

Fig. 23-11. Positive inferior anteroposterior tilt. A, Normal positioning. **B,** Positive inferior anteroposterior tilt component.

Rehabilitation Techniques

Traditionally, rehabilitation techniques for athletes complaining of patellofemoral pain tended to concentrate on avoiding those activities that exacerbated pain (for example, squatting or stair climbing), occasional immobilization, and strengthening of the quadriceps group using open-kinetic chain exercises. The current treatment approach has a new direction and focus that includes strengthening of the quadriceps through closed-kinetic chain exercise, regaining optimal patellar positioning and tracking, and regaining neuromuscular control to improve lower limb mechanics.

STRENGTHENING EXERCISES. Earlier in this chapter, closed-kinetic chain exercises were recommended for strengthening in the rehabilitation of ligamentous knee injuries. These same exercises are also useful in the rehabilitation of patellofemoral pain not because anterior shear is reduced but because of how they affect patellofemoral joint reaction force (PFJRF).

More traditional rehabilitation techniques focused on reducing the compressive forces of the patella against the femur and reducing PFJRF. PFJRF increases when the angle between the patellar tendon and the quadriceps tendon decreases (Figure 23-12). PFJRF also increases when the quadriceps tension increases to resist the flexion moment created by the lever arms. However PFJRF can be minimized by maximizing the area of surface contact of the patella on the femur. As the knee moves into greater degrees of

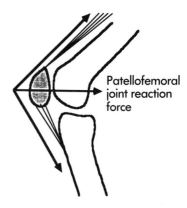

Fig. 23-12. Patellofemoral joint reaction forces (PFJRF).

flexion, the area of surface contact increases, distributing the forces associated with increased compression over a larger area (Figure 23-13). Therefore the compressive forces per unit area are minimized.[19]

Rehabilitation techniques involving closed-kinetic chain exercises try to maximize the area of surface contact. With closed-kinetic chain exercises, as the angle of knee flexion decreases, the flexion moment acting on the knee increases. This requires greater quadriceps and patellar tendon tension to counteract the effects of the increased flexion moment arm, resulting in an increase in PFJRF as flexion increases. However the force is distributed over a larger patellofemoral contact area, thus minimizing the increase

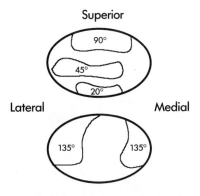

Fig. 23-13. Compression force and contact stress. Even though compression forces increase with increasing knee flexion, the amount of contact stress per unit area decreases.

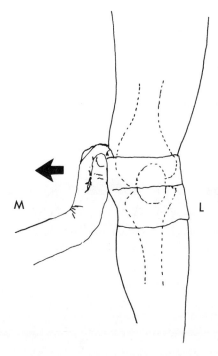

Fig. 23-14. Application of base tape.

in contact stress per unit area. Therefore it appears that closed-kinetic chain exercises may be better tolerated by the patellofemoral joint than open-kinetic chain exercises.

Closed-kinetic chain exercises were discussed in detail in Chapter 7. In the case of patellofemoral rehabilitation, mini-squats from 0 to 40 degrees, leg press from 0 to 60 degrees, lateral step-ups using an 8 inch step and stepping machine, and a stationary bike are all examples of closed-kinetic chain strengthening exercises that may be used in patellofemoral rehabilitation.

REGAINING OPTIMAL PATELLAR POSITIONING AND TRACKING. This second goal in our current treatment approach is based on the work of an Australian physiotherapist, Jenny McConnell.[18,34] This goal may be accomplished by stretching the tight lateral structures, correcting patellar orientation, and improving the timing and force of the VMO contraction.

Stretching. Successfully stretching the tight lateral structures involves a combination of both active and passive stretching techniques. Active stretching techniques include mobilization techniques as discussed in Chapter 10. Specific techniques should involve medial patellar glides and medial patellar tilts along the longitudinal axis of the patella.

Passive stretch is accomplished through a long duration stretch created by the use of very specific taping techniques to alter patellar alignment and orientation.

Correcting patellar orientation. After a thorough assessment of patellofemoral mechanics as described earlier, the sports therapist should have the athlete perform an activity that produces patellofemoral pain such as step-ups or double or single leg squats to establish a baseline for comparison.

From the beginning of this discussion it should be stressed that not all individuals who complain of patellofemoral pain exhibit some positive patellar orientation component. In those athletes who do, patellofemoral orientation may be corrected to some degree by using tape. Correction of patellar positioning and tracking is accomplished by using passive taping of the patella in a more biomechanically correct position. In addition to correcting the orientation of the patella, the tape provides a prolonged stretch to the soft tissue structures that affect patellar movement.

Taping should be done using two separate types of highly adhesive tape available from several different manufacturers. A base layer using white tape is applied directly to the skin from the lateral femoral condyle to just posterior to the medial femoral condyle, making certain that the patella is completely covered by the base layer (Figure 23-14). This tape is used as a base to which the other tape is adhered to correct patellar alignment. The glide component

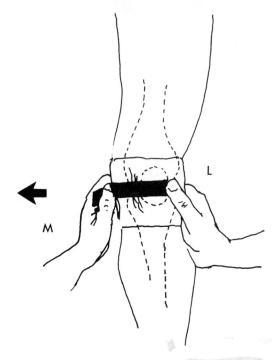

Fig. 23-15. Taping to correct positive lateral glide.

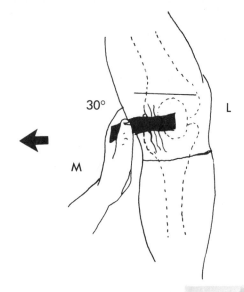

Fig. 23-16. Taping to correct positive lateral tilt.

should always be corrected first, followed by the component found to be the most excessive. If no positive glide exists, begin with the most pronounced component found.

The glide component should always be corrected with the knee in full extension. To correct a positive lateral glide, attach the tape one thumb's breadth from the lateral patellar border, push the patella medially, gather the soft tissue over the medial condyle, push toward the condyle, and adhere to the medial condyle (Figure 23-15).

The tilt component should be corrected with the knee flexed 30 to 45 degrees. To correct a positive lateral tilt, from the middle of the patella pull medially to lift the lateral border. Again, gather the skin underneath, and adhere to the medial condyle (Figure 23-16).

The rotational component is corrected in 30 to 40 degrees of flexion. To correct a positive external rotation, from the middle of the inferior border pull upward and medially while rotating the superior pole externally (Figure 23-17).

To correct a positive anteroposterior inferior tilt, place the knee in full extension. Adhere a 6-inch strip

of tape over the upper half of the patella, and press directly posterior, adhereing with equal pressure on both sides (Figure 23-18).

One piece of tape may be used to correct two components simultaneously. For example, when correcting a lateral glide along with an anteroposterior inferior tilt, follow the same taping procedure for the glide component except that the tape should be applied to the upper half of the patella.

After this taping procedure, the sports therapist should reassess the activity that caused the athlete's pain. In many cases the athlete will indicate improvement almost immediately. If not, the order of the taping or the way the patella is taped may have to be changed considerably. The tape should be worn 24 hours a day initially, and the sports therapist should instruct the athlete how to adjust and tighten the tape as necessary.

It is important to understand that taping changes the forces acting on the patella and thus the kinematics of the knee joint. Taping essentially attempts to decrease the lateral pull on the patella. This, when combined with an increase in the force and timing of the VMO contraction, will result in alteration of the balance of forces on the patella. Interestingly, a study by Bockrath et al. demonstrated that patellar taping reduced pain in patients with anterior knee pain, but radiographic studies before and after taping revealed no change in patellofemoral congruency or

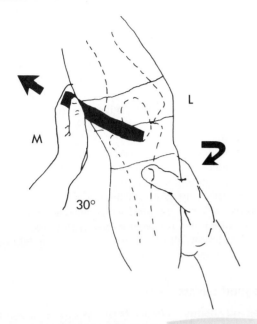

Fig. 23-17. Taping to correct positive external rotation.

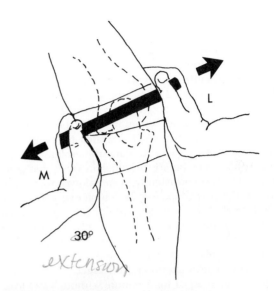

Fig. 23-18. Taping to correct positive inferior anteroposterior tilt.

patellar rotational angles. Hence the reduction in pain was not associated with positional change of the patella.[5]

ESTABLISHING NEUROMUSCULAR CONTROL. Establishing neuromuscular control involves improving the timing and force of VMO contraction. It is perhaps most important for the sports therapist to emphasize the quality rather than the quantity of the contraction. This means that training the VMO should concentrate more on motor skill acquisition rather than on strengthening activities. Strengthening should occur concomitantly with improvement in motor skill.

As mentioned previously the VMO:VL strength ratio should be 1:1. In athletes who have a VMO:VL ratio of less than 1:1 with patellofemoral pain, training efforts should focus on selectively strengthening the VMO. Isolating and training the VMO selectively requires concentration on the part of the athlete. Techniques of facilitation, such as manually stroking or taping the VMO or the use of biofeedback, are recommended. The use of a dual channel biofeedback unit capable of monitoring both VMO and VL electromyographic activity can help the athlete gain neuromuscular control over both the force of contraction and timing for the firing of the VMO.

Since the VMO is a tonic muscle that acts to sta-

bilize the patella both statically and dynamically, it should be active throughout the range of motion. Training goals should be directed toward increasing the force of the VMO contraction both concentrically and eccentrically throughout the range of motion. Since the VMO arises from the adductor magnus tendon, adduction exercises may be used to facilitate VMO contraction. The VMO should be trained to respond to a new length-tension relationship between the agonist (VMO) and the antagonist (VL).

Several sources have indicated that the VMO has a separate nerve supply from the rest of the quadriceps, although this is in our opinion somewhat debatable.[2,6,14] Nevertheless, assuming this is the case, then the athlete should be taught to fire the VMO before the VL. Neuromuscular control of the VMO firing should help the athlete maintain appropriate patellar alignment.

VMO exercises should concentrate on controlling the firing of the VMO. Exercises should be performed slowly and with concentration to selectively activate muscles. The sports therapist should address concentric and eccentric control in a variety of functional tasks and positions. Mini-squats, step-ups or step-downs, and leg presses are good exercises for establishing concentric and eccentric control. Training on a BAPS board or KAT system is useful for proprioceptive training. It is extremely important to concentrate on VMO control during gait training activities.

TAPING AND VMO TRAINING. Taping should continue throughout the VMO training period. Again, tape should initially be worn 24 hours/day. The athlete may be weaned from tape progressively when he or she demonstrates VMO control. Examples of functional criteria for weaning would be when the athlete can keep the VMO activated for 5 minutes during a walking gait and when the athlete can fire the VMO either before or simultaneously with the vastus lateralis consistently in step-downs for 1 minute. At this point, tape may be left off every third day for 1 week, then every second day for 1 week, then worn only during activity, and finally worn only if pain is present. Taping may be eliminated altogether when the athlete can perform step-downs for 5 minutes with appropriate timing and when they can sustain a ¼ to ½ squat for 1 minute without VMO loss.

Jumper's Knee

Jumper's knee occurs when chronic inflammation develops in the patellar tendon, especially at the distal pole. It usually develops in athletes involved in activities that require repetitive jumping; hence the name. Point tenderness on the posterior aspect of the inferior pole of the patellar is the hallmark of this condition. This condition is felt to be related to the shock absorbing function that the quadriceps provides upon landing from a jump, an eccentric contraction.

Besides the conventional treatment previously mentioned for patellofemoral disorders, success has been reported using eccentric strengthening exercises for the quadriceps and the ankle dorsiflexors.[9,26,35] Curwin and Stanish have theorized that a graded program of eccentric stress will stimulate the tendon to heal.[9] They feel that rest does not stimulate healing, while low-to-moderate level eccentric exercise will. Their program consists of five parts: warm-up, stretching, eccentric squatting, stretching, and ice.[9] The eccentric squats, called *drop squats,* are performed with the patient moving slowly from standing to a squat position and return. To increase stress, the speed of the drop is increased until a mild level of pain is experienced. The goal is to perform 3 sets of 10 repetitions at a speed that causes mild pain during the last set. The presence of mild pain is

indicative of the mild stress. Jensen and DiFabio have suggested treating patellar tendinitis with a program of isokinetic eccentric quadriceps training.[26] The program begins with 6 sets of 5 repetitions at 30 degrees per second 3 times per week progressing over an 8-week period to 4 sets of 5 repetitions each at 30/50/70 degrees per second.[26] Vigorous quadriceps and hamstring stretching precede and follow each workout.

Transverse friction massage has also been recommended as a treatment for jumper's knee. This technique attempts to facilitate the healing process by exacerbating acute inflammation. The technique involves a 5 to 7 minute friction massage performed every other day for approximately 1 week. During this treatment, all other medicative or modality efforts to reduce inflammation should be eliminated.

Osgood Schlatter's Disease

Osgood Shlatter's disease (OSD) is characterized by pain and swelling over the tibial tuberosity that increases with activity and decreases with rest. Traditionally OSD was described as either a partial avulsion of the tibial tubercle or an avascular necrosis of the same. Current thinking views it more as an apophysitis or inflammation of a portion of the extensor mechanism, and is treated as such. OSD occurs mostly in adolescents, and most sufferers have related extensor mechanism deficiencies that need to be addressed in the treatment program. Especially prominent are quadriceps atrophy and hamstring tightness.[11,35] Treatment is symptomatic with emphasis placed on icing, quadriceps strengthening, hamstring stretching, and activity modification. Only in extreme cases is immobilization necessary.

SUMMARY

1. To be effective in a knee rehabilitation program, the sports therapist must have a good understanding of the nature of the injury, the function of the structures damaged, and the technique of repair or reconstruction.
2. Range of motion may be restricted by lack of either physiological motion, which may be corrected by stretching, or by lack of accessory motions, which may be corrected by mobilization techniques. Constant passive motion may be used postoperatively to assist the athlete in regaining range of motion.

3. Techniques of strengthening involving closed-ki-netic chain isometric, isotonic, and isokinetic exercises are recommended after injury to the knee because of their safety and because they are more functional than open-chain exercises.

4. The current surgical procedure of choice for ACL reconstruction uses an extraarticular patellar tendon graft.

5. Recent trends in rehabilitation after ACL reconstruction are toward an aggressive, accelerated program that emphasizes immediate motion, immediate weight bearing, early closed-chain strengthening exercises, and early return to activity.

6. PCL, MCL, and LCL injuries are generally treated nonoperatively, and the athlete is progressed back into activity rapidly within their limitations.

7. The current trend in treating meniscal tears is to surgically repair the defect if possible or perform a partial meniscectomy arthroscopically. Repaired menisci should be immobilized NWB for 3 to 4 weeks.

8. It is critical to assess the mechanics of the patellofemoral joint in terms of static alignment, dynamic alignment, and patellar orientation to determine what specifically is causing pain.

9. Rehabilitation of patellofemoral pain concentrates on strengthening of the quadriceps through closed-kinetic chain exercises, regaining optimal patellar positioning and tracking, and regaining neuromuscular control to improve lower limb mechanics.

REFERENCES

1 Arno S: The A-angle: a quantitative measurement of patellar alignment and realignment, *JOSPT* 12[C]:237-242, 1990.

2 Basmajian J, DeLuca C: *Muscles alive, their functions revealed by electromyography,* Baltimore, 1985, Williams & Wilkins.

3 Bennet J, Stauber W: Evaluation and treatment of anterior knee pain using eccentric exercise, *Med Sci Sports Exerc* 18(5), 1986.

4 Bernhardt D, editor: *Sports physical therapy,* New York, 1986, Churchill Livingstone.

5 Bockrath K: *Effect of patellar taping on patellar position and perceived pain,* Poster Presentation, 1993, APTA Combined Sections, San Antonio, Texas.

6 Bose K, Kanagasuntheram R, Osman M: Vastus medialis oblique: an anatomic and physiologic study, *Orthopaedics,* 3:880-883, 1980.

7 Brewster C, Moynes D, Jobe F: Rehabilitation for the anterior cruciate reconstruction, *JOSPT* 5:121-126, 1983.

8 Cavenaugh J: *Rehabilitation following meniscal surgery.* In Engle R, editor: *Knee ligament rehabilitation,* New York, 1991, Churchill Livingstone.

9 Curwin S, Stanish WD: *Tendinitis: its etiology and treatment,* New York, 1984, Collamore Press.

10 DePalma B, Zelko R: Knee rehabilitation following anterior cruciate injury or surgery, *JNATA* 21(3):200-206, 1986.

11 Ellison A, chairman: *Athletic training and sports medicine,* American Academy of Orthopaedic Surgery Annual Meeting, 1984.

12 Engle R, Giesen D: *ACL reconstruction rehabilitation.* In Engle R, editor: *Knee ligament rehabilitation,* New York, 1991, Churchill Livingstone.

13 Ferguson D: Return to functional activities, *Sports Medicine Update* 3(3):6-9, 1988.

14 Ficat P, Hungerford D: *Disorders of the patellofemoral joint,* Baltimore, 1977, Williams & Wilkins.

15 Fu F, Woo S, Irrgang J, et al: Current concepts for rehabilitation following ACL reconstruction, *JOSPT* 15(6):270-278, 1992.

16 Fulkerson J: Evaluation of peripatellar soft tissues and retinaculum in patients with patellofemoral pain, *Clin Sports Med* 8(2):197-202, 1989.

17 Fulkerson J, Hungerford D: *Disorders of the patellofemoral joint,* Baltimore, 1990, Williams & Wilkins.

18 Gerrard B: The patellofemoral pain syndrome: a clinical trial of the McConnell program, *Aust J Physiother* 35(2):71-80, 1989.

19 Goodfellow J, Hungerford D, Woods C: Patellofemoral mechanics and pathology. II. Chondromalacia patella, *J Bone Joint Surg* 58[B]:287, 1976.

20 Gould J, Davies G: *Orthopaedic and sports physical therapy,* St Louis, 1990, Mosby.

21 Hartsell H: Electrical muscle stimulation and isometric exercise effects on selected quadriceps parameters, *JOSPT* 8(4):211, 1986.

22 Hughston J, Walsh W, Puddu G: *Patellar subluxation and dislocation,* Philadelphia, 1984, WB Saunders.

23 Insall J: Chondromalacia patella: patellar malalignment syndromes, *Orthop Clin North Am* (10):117-125, 1979.

24 Jackson D, Drez D: *The anterior cruciate deficient knee,* St Louis, 1987, Mosby.

25 Jenkins D: *Ligament injuries and their treatment,* Rockville, Maryland, 1985, Aspen Publications.

26 Jensen J, DiFabio R: Evaluation of eccentric exercise in the treatment of patellar tendinitis, *Phys Ther* 69(3):211-216, 1989.

27 Johnson D: Controlling anterior shear during isokinetic knee exercise, *JOSPT* 4(1):27, 1982.

28 Kramer P: Patellar malalignment syndrome: rationale to reduce lateral pressure, *JOSPT* 8(6):301, 1983.

29 Kuland D: *The injured athlete,* ed 2, Philadelphia, 1988, JB Lippincott.

30 Mangine R: *Physical therapy of the knee,* New York, 1988, Churchill Livingstone.

31 Mangine R, Eifert-Mangine M: *Postoperative PCL reconstruction rehabilitation.* In Engle R, editor: *Knee ligament rehabilitation,* New York, 1991, Churchill Livingstone.

32 Mansmann K: *PCL reconstruction.* In Engle R, editor: *Knee ligament rehabilitation,* New York, 1991, Churchill Livingstone.

33 McCarthy M, Yates C, Anderson J, et al: The effects of immediate CPM on pain during the inflammatory phase of soft tissue healing following ACL reconstruction, *JOSPT* 17(2):96-101, 1993.

34 McConnell J: The management of chondromalacia patella: a long-term solution, *Aust J Physiother* 32(4):215-223, 1986.

35 Mellion M, editor: *Office management of sports injury and athletic problems,* Philadelphia, 1987, Hanley and Belfus.

36 Paulos L, Noyes F, Grood E: Knee rehabilitation after anterior cruciate ligament reconstruction and repair, *Am J Sports Med* 9:140-149, 1981.

37 Prentice W: A manual resistance technique for strengthening tibial rotation, *JNATA* 23(3):230-233, 1988.

38 Quillen W, Gieck J: Manual therapy: mobilization of the motion restricted knee, *JNATA* 23(2):123-130, 1988.

39 Reynold L, Levin T, Medoiros J, et al.: EMG activity of the vastus medialis oblique and the vastus lateralis and their role in patellar alignment, *Am J Phys Med* 62(2):61-71, 1983.

40 Richardson C: *The role of the knee musculature in high speed oscillating movements of the knee,* MTAA 4th Biennial Conference Proceedings, Brisbane, Australia, 1985.

41 Saal J, editor: *Physical medicine and rehabilitation: rehabilitation of sports injuries,* Philadelphia, 1987, Hanley and Belfus.

42 Shelbourne K, Klootwyk T, DeCarlo M, et al.: Update of accelerated rehabilitation after ACL reconstruction, *JOSPT* 15(6):303-308, 1992.

43 Shelbourne K, Nitz P: Accelerated rehabilitation after ACL reconstruction, *JOSPT* 15(6):256-264, 1992.

44 Torg J, Vesgo J, Torg E: *Rehabilitation of athletic injuries: an atlas of therapeutic exercise,* St Louis, 1987, Mosby.

45 Wilk K, Andrews J: Current concepts in treatment of ACL disruption, *JOSPT* 15(6):279-293, 1992.

46 Wilk K, Clancey W: *Medial collateral ligament injuries: diagnosis, treatment, and rehabilitation.* in Engle R, editor: *Knee ligament rehabilitation,* New York, 1991, Churchill Livingstone.

Rehabilitation of Lower Leg Injuries

24

Rich Riehl

OBJECTIVES

After completion of this chapter, the student should be able to do the following:

- Differentiate between anterior and posterior shin splints.

- Explain the concept of eccentric overload as it relates to overuse syndromes.

- Explain why the Achilles tendon is susceptible to overuse conditions.

- Design and apply an eccentric strengthening program for Achilles tendinitis rehabilitation.

- Define the four compartments of the lower leg, and differentiate between acute and chronic compartment syndromes.

- Discuss the bone remodeling theory as it pertains to stress fractures.

- Design and implement an effective rehabilitation program for any lower leg pathology.

Injuries to the lower leg are common. Brody[3] has reported that approximately 30% of all running injuries involve the lower leg. The appropriate recognition, treatment, and rehabilitation of these injuries are important if the incidence of injuries is to be prevented from rising.

The purpose of this chapter is to present various approaches to rehabilitation that are designed to return the athlete to activity as quickly as possible. Many times sports therapists end up using the same old treatments day in and day out. Although nothing is wrong with that approach, the intent of this chapter is to present different ideas that can add a little diversity to the rehabilitation of injuries without compromising the objectives.

RECONDITIONING EXERCISES FOR THE LOWER LEG
Range of Motion

Range-of-motion exercises should be started as early as possible in the rehabilitation process. Both active and passive movements should be included. The therapist should monitor the athlete for any increase in inflammatory signs and symptoms after the onset of range-of-motion exercises. Range-of-motion exercises serve many purposes[23]:

- Prevent muscle atrophy (active only)
- Help align collagen fibers along areas of stress
- Restore normal joint motion
- Decrease edema and pain
- Retard loss of connective tissue tensile strength

Range-of-motion exercises for lower leg pathology should include both the ankle and knee joints. It is important to maintain normal range of motion of the joints above and below the injured area. This will help to maintain a normal kinetic chain and decrease the potential of abnormal mechanics on the injured area. The gastrocnemius muscle is of prime importance. This muscle, being the only muscle to span both the knee and ankle joints, as well as being a powerful plantarflexor, must be adequately stretched. Appropriate stretching of the gastrocnemius requires simultaneous dorsiflexion of the ankle and extension of the knee.

Passive motion exercises should be done initially

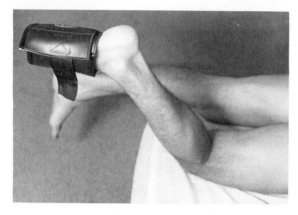

Fig. 24-1. Bent-leg position for plantarflexion strengthening exercises using ankle weights.

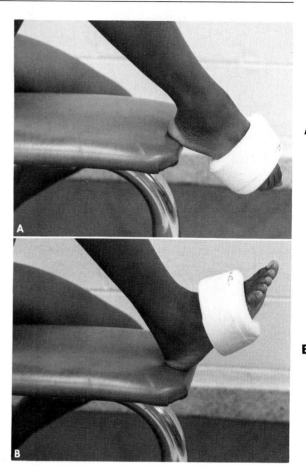

Fig. 24-2. Dorsiflexion strengthening exercises. **A,** Starting position. **B,** Terminal position.

with the help of the sports therapist, who should perform and instruct the athlete in the proper stretching technique. A towel can be used to help with the passive movements once the athlete has been shown how to do the exercises properly. Plantarflexion and dorsiflexion, along with inversion and eversion, are the desired movements. The stretching should be done for 30 to 45 seconds and repeated 3 to 4 times for each direction. A good approach, initially, would be the application of ice massage followed by the stretching exercises, both active and passive movements, and then another ice application.

Strengthening Exercises

Isometric exercise is quite useful when an injury is immobilized for a prolonged period of time. The lower leg pathology that falls into this category would be post Achilles tendon repair of immobilization after a fracture. When using an isometric program, the athlete should be instructed to contract the desired muscle for approximately 5 to 10 seconds and then relax. This should be repeated 10 to 15 times several times throughout the day. One drawback to isometric work is that strength gains are only found at the angle at which the exercise is being performed. Thus the athlete should also be instructed to perform isometric work every 20 to 30 degrees through a complete range of motion. This will help to prevent isolation of strength gains.

Isotonic exercises, by far the most common, can be divided into two types: concentric and eccentric muscular contractions. Concentric muscle contrac-

tions cause a shortening of the muscle; eccentric contractions are a lengthening of the muscle. Eccentric muscle contractions are used for antigravity or deceleration types of actions. An example is the contraction of the posterior tibial muscle in a person who hyperpronates.

A comprehensive rehabilitation plan should include both types of isotonic exercises, however, the concept of eccentric work is especially important when rehabilitating lower leg injuries. The etiology of injuries to the tendons and muscles of the lower leg is often a repeated eccentric muscle contraction. Proper rehabilitation of these injuries must include eccentric strength training as part of the total rehabilitation program.

One of the most frequently used isotonic methods

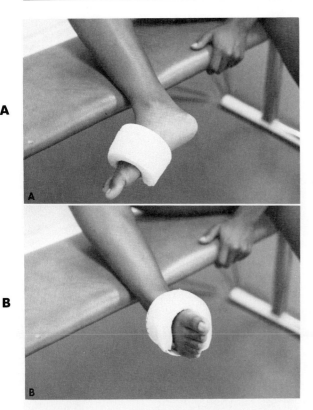

Fig. 24-3. Inversion strengthening exercises. A, Starting position. **B,** Terminal position.

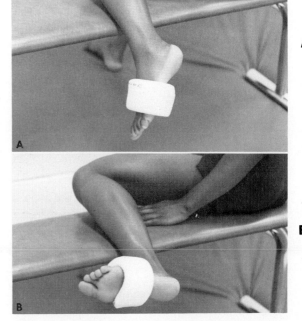

Fig. 24-4. Eversion strengthening exercises. A, Starting position. **B,** Terminal position.

of acquiring lower leg strength is through the use of ankle weights. This method allows motion in all four ranges (Figures 24-1 to 24-4).

A typical program involves 3 sets of 15 repetitions with a 30 to 45 second rest between sets. The resistance should be determined by athlete discomfort. Muscular fatigue during the third set of exercises is appropriate and indicates that the muscles are being properly overloaded. If during the third set of activity the athlete does not experience any local muscular fatigue, then the weight should be increased to properly overload the muscle. If the athlete completes the third set of work with little or no muscular fatigue, then the weight should be adjusted up. A good starting point is usually 5 pounds.

A similar resistance program can be done with surgical tubing. The tubing is fixed around something sturdy, such as a table or chair. All four motions (plantarflexion, dorsiflexion, inversion, and eversion) should be worked. The same guidelines outlined for

the ankle weights should be followed (Figures 24-5 to 24-8).

Toe raises also provide an effective method for strength gains. This type of exercise will primarily work the plantarflexors, both eccentrically and concentrically. Curwin and Stanish[6] and Fyfe and Stanish[11] have outlined an eccentric conditioning program using heel drops. The program has three main variables:

1. **Length of the muscle tendon unit—** Stretching the muscle tendon unit will decrease the strain placed on the structures. Thus establishing proper length is a vital component of the program.
2. **Proper load application during the exercise—** The body must be properly overloaded to achieve strength gains. Thus establishing the proper load is equally important and is a criteria for progression through the program.
3. **Speed of contraction—** With an eccentric

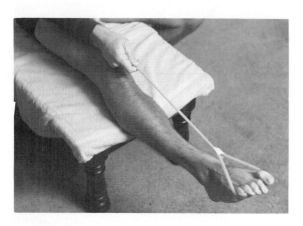

Fig. 24-5. Plantarflexion strengthening exercises using rubber tubing.

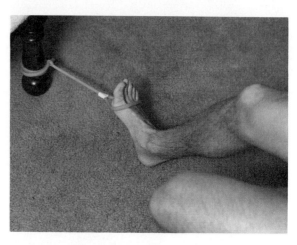

Fig. 24-6. Dorsiflexion strengthening exercises using rubber tubing.

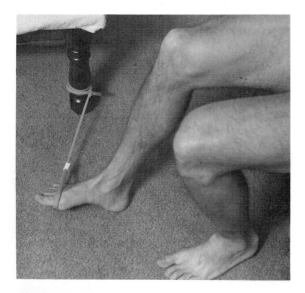

Fig. 24-7. Inversion strengthening exercises using rubber tubing.

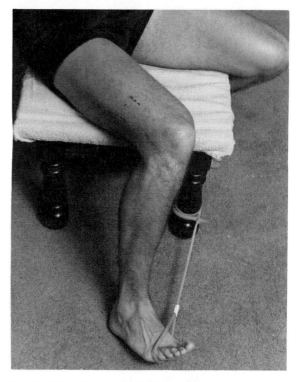

Fig. 24-8. Eversion strengthening exercises using rubber tubing.

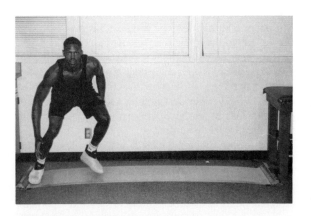

Fig. 24-9. Slide board use for lower leg strengthening and cardiovascular training.

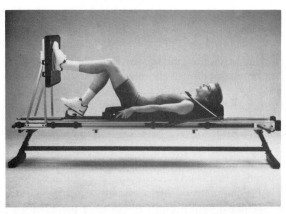

Fig. 24-10. Double legged closed-chain exercises using the Shuttle 2000.

muscle contraction, the greater the speed of contraction, the greater the force that is being generated within the muscle. Thus by increasing the speed of contraction a greater load is being applied to the muscle tendon unit; thus greater strength gains should be experienced.

The program consists of having the athlete stand on a step with the ankle in neutral and then lower the heel until a stretch is felt. This exercise should be done initially with both feet at the same time and at a slow speed. Three sets of 10 repetitions are performed. The final 10 repetitions should cause mild discomfort, which indicates if the level is adequate or if the athlete should progress. Their exercise program is based on a 7-day progression with speed of contraction and load being the two main variables. The progression would go as follows:

1. Weight is supported equally on both feet.
2. Increase shifting of weight to the symptomatic leg.
3. Weight is only on the symptomatic leg.
4. Gradually increase the speed of dropping.
5. Add weight to the shoulders (10% of the body weight at the start).

Wherever the athlete is along the progression of proper load, they should also be adjusting the speed of contraction. This variable is also based on a 7-day progression. The criteria for advancement is the athlete's perception of pain.

Days 1-2   Slow contractions
Days 3-4   Moderate contractions
Days 6-7   Fast contractions

For a much more detailed description of the above program, the reader should refer to the works cited.

Another variation of strengthening is grasping small objects with the toes and moving them from one place to another. The object can be anything from marbles to rocks to scraps of tape. The heel should remain stationary during this exercise. Start by making three different piles of the objects, pick up one object and move it to another pile, and continue rotating the objects among the different piles. Two sets of 50 are a desired workout.

The use of a slide board has become very popular in rehabilitating lower leg injuries (Figure 24-9). Incorporating both strengthening and proprioceptive training, the slide board will allow the athlete to train in a very functional manner. Another positive aspect of this type of training is that the stress the athlete is subjected to is controlled.

A general guideline for exercise protocols would be to have the athlete perform work-rest intervals of 30 seconds. The athlete should be monitored to ensure that technique is not compromised for speed of movement.

Another fairly new rehabilitation device is called the Plyometronic (Figure 24-10). This device is a horizontal resistance exerciser that allows the athlete to perform closed-chain activities while reducing the effects of gravity. It is very beneficial when attempting to place eccentric loads on the body in a closed-chain situation. This is a very nice transitional tool when attempting to progress the athlete back to a functional type of training. Numerous types of closed-chain strengthening programs can be applied using this machine.

Isokinetic programs are extremely useful in improving strength gains because maximal resistance can be attained throughout the entire range of motion. Specific protocols for rehabilitation are quite varied. The speed of contraction should be changed during the workout to provide both muscular endurance and power. Three speeds commonly used are 180, 270, and 300 degrees per second. Plantarflexion and dorsiflexion are the most frequently used exercises. Inversion and eversion should also be done if the equipment has the capability. In a study currently being reviewed for publication from the Department of Sports Medicine at Pepperdine University, the investigators found that excessive rear-foot motion could be significantly reduced after a concentric and eccentric isokinetic strength training program involving inversion and eversion of the lower leg muscles.[8]

Isokinetic machines do have their disadvantages: they are inconvenient for exercising more than one joint; the set-up is often time-consuming; eccentric contractions are not possible, except in the most sophisticated equipment; and, finally, the equipment is usually quite expensive. If isokinetic equipment is available under the proper supervision, however, then it should be used because the benefits far outweigh the drawbacks.

Cardiovascular Fitness

The athlete's cardiovascular fitness must be maintained while the lower leg is rehabilitated. Athletes are often concerned that they will lose their fitness level during the rehabilitation period. The sports therapist is often challenged to supply cardiovascular workouts that stimulate the athlete both physically and psychologically without compromising the healing process. Several ideas that have gained widespread acceptance are stationary bicycling and swimming.

Stationary bicycles are a very effective means of cardiovascular fitness. A variety of workouts can be done, including interval training, sprints, or slow/long distance. This exercise is usually well received by the athlete because it often mimics their normal workouts. A good guideline to follow when establishing the proper duration of the workout is a 3 to 1 ratio, using running distances as the baseline. Thus for every mile the athlete was supposed to run, he or she should ride 3 miles.

One important variable when stationary cycling is the proper adjustment of the seat height. The seat should be adjusted so that when the pedal is at the bottom of the stroke, the knee should be in a slightly flexed position. When the pedal is at 3 o'clock and 9 o'clock, the knee should be directly over the center of the crank. Proper seat height will help reduce improper stroke mechanics, which might be an extrinsic factor leading to an injury.

Swimming also provides an excellent workout. Swimming will benefit most athletes who are attempting to build a cardiovascular base. A recommendation would be to be very cautious when having athletes, such as baseball pitchers or tennis players, use swimming as a cardiovascular training tool. Shoulder impingement with these types of athletes is a serious concern; we as sports therapists should not put that group in a situation that might put further stress on the shoulder.

A good guideline when establishing swimming workouts is to use a 4 to 1 ratio with running distances. Every quarter-mile swum is the equivalent of 1 mile run.[11] While training in the pool, the athlete can either just use their arms, their legs, or a combination. Vary the workouts, and structure them so that the athlete will receive maximum benefits.

The use of a pool need not be limited to swimming. One type of exercise that is gaining popularity is running in water, either running in the shallow end or using a flotation device to keep the athlete above the waterline while in the deep end. The athlete can simulate sport-specific running patterns without placing the extremities in a weight-bearing position.

Another type of exercise that is extremely beneficial for athletes with lower leg dysfunction is the use of an upper body ergometer (UBE). This machine is designed specifically for the athlete who cannot or should not use their legs for any type of activity. Athletes with limited range of motion or those who are immobilized can benefit from this tremendously. One suggestion for those sports therapists who don't have a machine designed specifically for upper body ergometry is to rotate a stationary bicycle on its handlebars and then have the athlete hold onto the pedals (Figure 24-11).

Whereas general cardiovascular conditioning is quite important and should not be neglected, sport-specific training should be emphasized whenever possible. In the early stages of rehabilitation, cardiovascular fitness should be maintained however possible. As the athlete progresses through the initial stages of rehabilitation, a much more sport-specific program

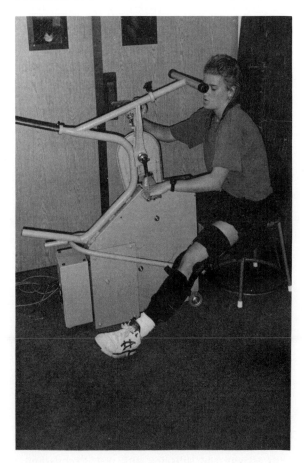

Fig. 24-11. Upper body ergometry using a stationary bicycle.

should be designed. For example, there is very little functional crossover between swimming and playing competitive basketball. A baseline of cardiovascular fitness is very important, but to return an athlete to a functional, competitive situation, the athlete must be trained with specificity in mind.

The importance of maintaining an athlete's cardiovascular fitness cannot be overstated. Deterioration of the athlete's fitness level delays return to full activity and may put the athlete at risk for reinjury.

Restoration of Smooth, Coordinated Movement

Restoration of smooth coordination is a vital part of any rehabilitation program. An athlete must be able to perform sports-related functional activities before returning to competition. Proprioception and sport

specific—skill testing are the two primary objectives during this phase.

Proprioception—the body's awareness of where the extremities are in space at any moment in time— is often disrupted after injury. Proper joint proprioception can be restored with a teeter board. Many variations and foot placements can be done. Plantar-flexion-dorsiflexion, inversion-eversion, single leg, and both legs should be worked. The number of combinations is limited only by the sports therapist's imagination. A good progression is as follows:

1. Two-footed, front to back.
2. Two-footed, side to side.
3. Two-footed, front to back with legs staggered.
4. One-footed, front to back.
5. One-footed, toe in.
6. One-footed, toe out.

The athlete need not master each level before proceeding to the next. This progression lists the easiest progressions first and then proceeds to the more difficult ones. Athletes should challenge themselves to see how long they can maintain their balance. A way to add difficulty to this progression would be to have the athletes close their eyes while performing the exercises. This will eliminate the visual cues that are used to aid in balance and make the athletes rely solely on intrinsic ability and proprioception.

Included in coordinated movement is training the athlete functionally. Sport-specific skills should be performed before the athlete's return to activity. These skills involve running, jumping, cutting, kicking, and throwing. The importance of training the athlete functionally cannot be overstated. We are not providing a complete rehabilitation program for our athletes if we release them before assessing their functional level and potentially assisting them in restoration of a coordinated functional movement. This chapter does not detail a progression for each skill. Common sense should dictate the progression. A conservative approach is better than an aggressive approach.

Maintenance

The rehabilitation program should not be stopped once the athlete has returned to competition. A proper maintenance program includes stretching and strengthening the affected body parts. Most lower leg injuries need a continuing flexibility program for the Achilles tendon because of the increased workloads placed on the posterior musculature.

Strengthening programs also should be continued.

Muscles will gain strength with the exercise demands placed on them, but a light maintenance program will complement the athlete's return to activity. The athlete should concentrate on invertors and evertors, both eccentrically and concentrically.

INJURIES TO THE LOWER EXTREMITY

A common misconception is that all lower leg pain should be termed *shin splints*. The AMA defines shin splints as pain and discomfort in the leg from running on hard surfaces or forcible excessive use of the foot flexors; the diagnosis should be limited to musculotendinous inflammation, excluding a fatigue fracture or ischemic disorder.[1] This definition might be accurate for one type of lower leg injury, but it by no means includes all forms of lower leg pathology. All lower leg pain is not produced by shin splints. This chapter provides enough information to differentiate between various lower leg pathologies and then explains proper rehabilitation methods.

Achilles Tendinitis

Achilles tendinitis is a common disorder of the lower extremity. James, Bates, and Osternig[13] have documented that 11% of all running injuries can be attributed to Achilles tendinitis. Achilles tendinitis is an overuse type of injury. A typical runner who jogs 1 mile encounters 1500 heel strikes.[26] With such a high demand placed on the posterior musculature and Achilles tendon, how an overuse condition can develop should be apparent.

The Achilles tendon is the common tendon of the gastrocnemius and soleus muscles. The primary action is plantarflexion. These muscles account for 95% of the muscular activity during plantarflexion.[14] A unique characteristic of the tendon is its rotatory component. The tendon has lateral rotation as it descends toward its insertion on the calcaneus. This region, 2 to 5 centimeters proximal to the calcaneus, is also the area of poorest blood supply.[15] This combination of factors has led researchers to believe that this region is the most frequently injured.

Several researchers have documented that the pain associated with Achilles tendinitis is located in this area.[5,16] The Achilles tendon, similar to most tendons, has a very low metabolical rate,[22] which may be significant during the recovery phase of injury. The decreased metabolism delays the healing rate and could account for the prolonged rehabilitation often

needed with Achilles tendon injuries. These various anatomical factors are important considerations when examining the etiologies of Achilles tendinitis. The underlying mechanism is that the tensile strength of the tendon is inadequate to enable it to meet the demands.[6]

Several etiologies have been associated with the microtrauma produced by eccentric loading of fatigued muscles and the inflexibility of the gastrocnemius-soleus muscle group.[21,26] Clement, Taunton, and Smart[5] have identified training errors in 75% of all patients who suffered from Achilles tendinitis. These errors include hill training, a sudden increase in mileage, improper warm-up, training on uneven ground, and an increase in intensity. Hyperpronation is mentioned in 56% of all cases.[5] The rotatory component of the Achilles tendon, as mentioned previously, is accentuated by a foot that hyperpronates and creates snapping action of the tendon that may produce microtears and an inflammatory response.

Poor flexibility and strength of the calf muscles increase the demand placed on the Achilles tendon. If this increased demand is for a prolonged time, it could lead to an inflammatory condition. Achilles tendinitis is likely when any of these factors are present in combination with excessive use of the calf muscles.

EVALUATION AND CLINICAL FINDINGS. An athlete who is experiencing Achilles tendinitis usually complains of pain in a region 2 to 5 centimeters proximal to the insertion on the calcaneus. The pain increases with activity and subsides with rest. Crepitation is usually present along the Achilles tendon and increases with activity. Poor flexibility and palpable tightness of the gastrocnemius-soleus complex are usually apparent.

TREATMENT AND REHABILITATION. The initial concern in treating Achilles tendinitis is to identify which of these factors is causing the problem. Specific changes should be made to prevent further aggravation once the cause is established.

The pain and inflammation of Achilles tendinitis can best be controlled through a modified activity program, cryotherapy, and NSAIDs. Severe pain responds best to several days of complete rest. The use of NSAIDs is beneficial during the early stages of injury. Steroid injections directly into the tendon, however, should be avoided. Several authors have attributed Achilles tendon rupture to steroid injections.[12,27]

Gentle, passive stretching should be begun as soon as the pain allows. An important range-of-motion exercise involves the posterior musculature, specifically

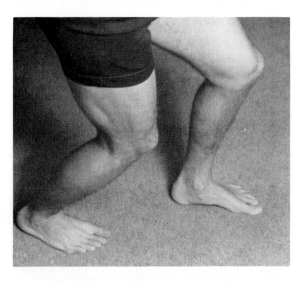

Fig. 24-12. Bent-knee stretch for soleus.

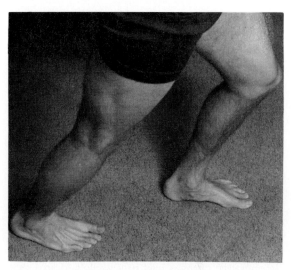

Fig. 24-13. Straight knee stretch for gastrocnemius.

the Achilles tendon. The Achilles tendon and gastrocnemius should be stretched in two distinct ways, with the leg straight and then bent at approximately 45 degrees (Figures 24-12 and 24-13). The bent-knee method is used to isolate the soleus muscle and allow it to be stretched to a greater degree by putting the gastrocnemius in a relaxed condition. This stretching can also be accomplished with the help of an incline board. This exercise should be done for 30 to 45 seconds and repeated several times. This protocol should be done three times a day. Again, both straight- and bent-leg methods should be used. Ice massage, before and after any stretching program, helps to decrease the pain, thus increasing the capability to stretch. Quarter-inch to half-inch heel lifts should be placed in both shoes to help take the stress off the Achilles tendon.[16] Orthotics can be used to correct any biomechanical flaw, which is especially important in a person who hyperpronates. Strengthening the gastrocnemius and soleus muscles, which is of prime importance, is best accomplished by using an eccentric program, as previously outlined in the chapter. This exercise increases the strength of the Achilles tendon to the point of returning the athlete to activity.

A stretching program should be continued as well. Ice massage followed by ultrasound can be used quite effectively before any exercise. Immediately after exercise the Achilles tendon should be iced for about 20 minutes.

A modified activity program should be continued until the athlete is completely pain free and has good strength and flexibility. Before returning to full activity the athlete should be placed in a progressive running program. This is the most appropriate guideline for returning to activity. If pain is felt during the course of the program, the program should be modified to decrease the intensity or duration. Emphasis must be placed on running on flat, soft surfaces. Jumping activities during this time period should be carefully structured. Achilles tendon stretching after the return to activity must be continued. The athlete who has progressed to the point of returning to activity should be monitored very judiciously during activity.

Achilles tendinitis treatment

PHASE I
1. Identify etiological factors; biomechanical correction.
2. Ice.
3. Rest.
4. NSAIDs.
5. Nonweight–bearing cardiovascular conditioning.

PHASE II
1. Cryotherapy.
2. Gentle, passive stretching (both straight and bent leg).
3. Ultrasound.
4. Heel lifts.

5. Progressive cardiovascular fitness (limited toe push-off).
6. Eccentric strengthening program.

PHASE III

1. Progressive running program.
2. Stretching and strengthening programs.
3. Cryotherapy after activity.
4. Gradual progression to full activity.

Achilles Tendon Rupture

Complete rupture of the Achilles tendon is a relatively uncommon injury in a young, athletic population. The injury is much more frequent with older men who are recreational athletes. Williams[32] has suggested that Achilles tendon ruptures are associated with a previous pathological condition of the tendon. These degenerative changes lead to a weakened area that, if placed under stress, might rupture. The most common site for ruptures is 2 to 6 centimeters proximal to the calcaneus. This area is the same that is associated with Achilles tendinitis, perhaps because of the poor blood supply in that area.[15]

EVALUATION AND CLINICAL FINDINGS. The two distinct mechanisms for Achilles tendon rupture are a violent dorsiflexion of the foot and a direct blow while the muscle is contracted. After a complete rupture, the athlete experiences a sudden pain and often an audible snap. The pain often quickly diminishes. This disorder is usually associated with a weakness during push-off. On examination the sports therapist can note a palpable defect of the Achilles tendon where it has ruptured and an area of marked discoloration that might be distal to the actual site of rupture because of gravitational effects. A positive Thompson test also helps in evaluating this condition (Figure 24-14).

TREATMENT AND REHABILITATION. The primary objective of treatment is to restore the Achilles tendon to its preinjury strength and flexibility. Immediately after injury, treatment should include ice, compression, elevation, and immobilization. A suspected Achilles tendon rupture should be referred to a physician for accurate diagnosis and care.

A conservative nonsurgical approach involves prolonged immobilization. Two months generally provides adequate time for proper healing. A very gradual stretching and strengthening program should follow immobilization. This process is slow and should be undertaken very gradually. Heel lifts should be placed in both shoes to diminish the stress placed on the Achilles tendon.

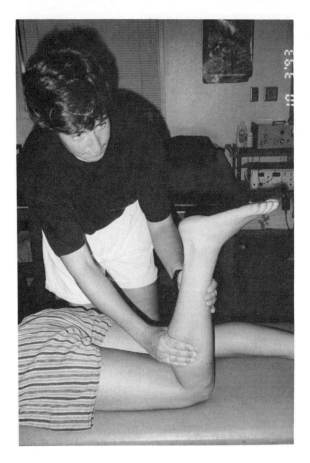

Fig. 24-14. Thompson test for assessment of Achilles tendon rupture.

The athlete may return to activity when full range of motion and strength have been restored. Rehabilitation should be done in a progressive manner with careful monitoring of the athlete's pain and type of activities. In the early stages of return, ballistic types of movements should be avoided to decrease the chance of rerupture. A conservative approach has several drawbacks. First, the chance of rerupture is quite high, between 22%[12] and 35%.[23] Moreover, the athlete must understand that the rehabilitation process is extremely long. If surgery is elected, the postsurgical rehabilitation program follows a course similar to the nonsurgical program. After immobilization, usually 6 to 8 weeks, range-of-motion exercises should be initiated. The range of motion, specifically dorsiflexion, should be much easier to attain after surgery than after conservative treatment. A gradual resistive exercise program should be initiated when range of motion is back to normal. The athlete's activity should be monitored after return to sports activity to decrease the chance for rerupture.

Achilles tendon rupture treatment

PHASE I
1. Ice.
2. Compression.
3. Elevation.
4. Immobilization.

PHASE II
1. Conservative: immobilization for 2 to 3 months.
2. Surgical: surgical repair.

PHASE III
1. Heel lifts.
2. Passive and active range-of-motion exercises.
3. Progressive resistance exercises.
4. Ice after workout.

Tennis Leg

The term **tennis leg** is synonymous with a partial tear of the medial head of the gastrocnemius. This injury usually occurs in sports where a ballistic, side-to-side movement is common. The cause is a sudden overload of the muscle. Abrupt dorsiflexion of the ankle while extending the knee often produces enough force to cause this overload. The weakest point of the gastrocnemius-soleus complex is the insertion of the medial head of the gastrocnemius into the soleus fascia.[33] This area accounts for the majority of cases of tennis leg.[20]

EVALUATION AND CLINICAL FINDINGS. An athlete who experiences a tear of the medial head of the gastrocnemius is usually unable to continue activity. On examination the area around the medial head is point tender, discolored, and swollen. A palpable defect is usually present, and pain is present with dorsiflexion.

TREATMENT AND REHABILITATION. Immediate treatment for this injury consists of rest, ice, compression, and elevation. The athlete should use crutches to avoid putting weight on the injured leg if the injury is severe enough to alter gait. The use of NSAIDs is beneficial during the first several days after the injury,[4] and heel lifts should be used to relieve stress on the gastrocnemius.

A program of passive and active stretching should be initiated as early as the pain allows. This program should progress to a form of resistive exercise to strengthen the posterior musculature. During this phase, heat treatments can replace cold. Ultrasound may provide a very effective treatment.

Return to activity, as with any injury to the lower leg, should be based on bilateral flexibility and strength measurements. A progressive activity program should be used. Any type of ballistic activity may lead to reinjury and should be monitored. A maintenance program of stretching and strengthening should be adhered to after return to activity.

Tennis leg treatment

PHASE I
1. Rest.
2. Ice.
3. Compression.
4. Elevation.
5. Nonweight-bearing.
6. NSAIDs.

PHASE II
1. Passive range-of-motion stretching.
2. Active range-of-motion stretching.
3. Progressive resistance exercises.
4. Heel lifts.
5. Thermotherapy.

PHASE III
1. Progressive running program.
2. Gradual return to activity.
3. Maintenance stretching and strengthening.

Shin Splint Syndromes

Shin splints are a musculotendinous overuse condition. They generally occur to athletes who are unconditioned and initiate a training program too vigorously. Two distinct shin splint conditions, anterior and posterior, can be differentiated by the location of pain.

Many factors contribute to shin splint syndromes. The three common etiologies of shin splints are abnormal biomechanical function, poor conditioning, and improper training methods. They may be present individually or in combination. A proper assessment of these contributing factors not only can help to differentiate between anterior and posterior shin splints but also can help to direct the rehabilitation. If the athlete is allowed to return to competition before the underlying cause of the injury is determined, then the chance of reinjury is significant.

ANTERIOR SHIN SPLINTS

Anterior shin splints usually elicit pain and tenderness lateral to the tibia and over the anterior compartment. The muscles that are the most involved are the anterior tibial, the long extensor of toes, and the long extensor of great toe. The muscles associated with anterior shin splints are active during toe-off, heel-strike, and the entire swing phase.[29]

Anterior shin pain is often a result of hard heel strike during the landing phase of running. A forceful eccentric contraction of the dorsiflexors, primarily the anterior tibial, follows a hard heel strike. This action assists in decelerating the forefoot and cushioning the impact of the body.

As is the basic premise of any overuse type of injury, the muscles are unable to handle the stresses placed upon them. Thus weak foot dorsiflexor muscles contribute to this condition. Biomechanical factors also play a role. A person with forefoot varus requires an increase in anterior tibial activity to help prevent foot slap.[2]

POSTERIOR SHIN SPLINTS

Posterior shin splints usually cause pain along the posterior medial border of the lower third of the tibia.[25] This pain is often associated with inflammation of the posterior tibial, long flexor of toe, and long flexor of great toe muscles. These muscles are active during the first 80% of stance phase.[10] The subtalar joint normally goes from a supinated position at heel strike to a pronated position during midstance, and then during toe off it returns into supination. A foot that hyperpronates during midstance places a tremendous amount of stress on these muscles.[31] The posterior muscles contract eccentrically to combat this hypermobility. This condition may eventually lead to an inflammatory response of the involved muscles.[19] Training errors, a tight Achilles tendon, and improper footwear in conjunction with a hyperpronating foot can contribute to this type of condition.

Evaluation and clinical findings. A detailed history should help to differentiate between anterior and posterior shin splints, but the location of the pain is the best indicator. Anterior shin splints elicit pain lateral to the tibia along the anterior compartment. Posterior shin splints usually manifest pain along the medial border of the lower third of the tibia. This pain is often described as a dull ache that often increases with the intensity of work. The onset of pain is often associated with constant exercise. Depending on the severity of the condition, pain might be felt only during activity or, in more progressed cases, during inactive times. The injury is generally quite tender to palpation. In the early stages, tenderness is quite lo-

calized, which makes evaluation much easier. A muscle weakness can usually be determined in the affected muscles.

Treatment and rehabilitation. A thorough history to determine the underlying cause of the condition should be the first step in treatment. More often than not, a biomechanical abnormality or training error will be the contributing factor.

Clinical treatment for shin splints is basically the same whether the condition is anterior or posterior. As with any overuse condition, the affected muscles must be allowed to rest. Depending on the severity of the pain, this rest period can range from 1 day to many weeks. Ice and NSAIDs are indicated during this time, and any biomechanical abnormality should be corrected.

Biomechanical correction for these two types of lower leg problems is often accomplished through the use of orthotics. The reader should refer to Chapter 26. When the pain has decreased to a level where the athlete is able to exercise with minimal soreness, resistance exercises, including any of the previously mentioned strengthening programs, should be started. Athletes with anterior shin splints should emphasize the anterior muscle groups. Athletes with posterior shin pain should work on inversion-eversion exercises done both eccentrically and concentrically.

Therapeutic modalities can be used during this phase. Heat and cold are both effective methods of treatment. Smith, Winn, and Parette[28] have shown that ultrasound, ice, and phonophoresis are equally effective in terms of treating the pain associated with shin splints.

Modified activity is important. Stationary bicycling (being careful not to push off with the toes) and running in water are excellent alternatives. A progressive running program should be used to return the athlete to activity gradually.

Before allowing the athlete to return to competition the biomechanical and training errors must be corrected. This point cannot be overemphasized. Without the proper corrections, the chance of reinjury is quite high.

Shin splint treatment

PHASE 1
1. Rest.
2. Ice massage.
3. NSAIDs.
4. Nonweight–bearing cardiovascular training.
5. Biomechanical corrections.

6. Upper body strengthening.

PHASE II

1. Ice.
2. Stretching (both anterior and posterior muscles).
3. Progressive resistance exercises.
4. Heat (ultrasound).

PHASE III

1. Progressive running program.
2. Continued stretching and strengthening.
3. Gradual return to activity.
4. Ice after activity.

Retrocalcaneobursitis

Retrocalcaneobursitis is an inflammatory overuse condition involving the retrocalcaneal bursa. It is located just anterior to the Achilles tendon insertion on the calcaneus. Often it is misdiagnosed as Achilles tendinitis. The two can be differentiated by a careful examination.

EVALUATION AND CLINICAL FINDINGS. An athlete who is experiencing retrocalcaneobursitis feels pain and tenderness between the talus and the Achilles tendon. This sensation can help the examiner differentiate between the two structures. Pain associated with retrocalcaneobursitis is not directly on the Achilles, as with tendinitis. Pain increases with activity and is often accompanied by mild swelling. This condition is usually brought on by an irritation of the shoe heel counter.

TREATMENT AND REHABILITATION. Early treatment measures should be aimed at correcting the irritation caused by the shoe. Raising the heel with lifts and softening the heel counter both relieve irritation. Exercise should be modified to decrease the irritation to the bursa. Ice, phonophoresis with hydrocortisone, and NSAIDs are all effective treatments. Upon return to activity, a well-fitting shoe should be worn to decrease the friction on the bursa.

In extreme cases, surgical intervention might be indicated. An 8-week immobilization period is usually indicated. After removal of the cast, range-of-motion exercises and a strengthening program should be initiated and continued until strength and flexibility are bilaterally equal.

Retrocalcaneobursitis treatment

PHASE I

1. Ice.
2. NSAIDs.

3. Shoe modification.
4. Correcting any errors in training.

PHASE II

1. Ice.
2. Phonophoresis with hydrocortisone cream.

PHASE III

1. Progressive return to competition.

Compartment Syndromes

Compartment syndromes of the lower leg are a result of an increased compartmental pressure. Among the many factors that can contribute to them are direct trauma, fracture, or muscle hypertrophy. Compartment syndromes can be acute or chronic. The pathology is basically the same, an increase in compartmental pressure, for both acute and chronic syndromes. A chronic compartment syndrome gets better with rest; an acute compartment syndrome gets worse with time.

The lower leg can be divided into four distinct compartments: the anterior, lateral, superficial, and deep posterior. The following structures are contained in each compartment:

- *Anterior:* anterior tibial muscle, deep peroneal nerve, anterior tibial artery and vein, extensor muscles of the foot and toes
- *Lateral:* superficial peroneal nerve, short and long peroneal muscle
- *Superficial posterior:* soleus muscle, plantaris and gastrocnemius tendons
- *Deep posterior:* posterior tibial muscle, long flexor muscle of toe, long flexor muscle of great toe, peroneal artery and vein, tibial nerve, posterior tibial artery and vein

ACUTE COMPARTMENT SYNDROME

Acute compartment syndrome is caused by a sudden trauma that causes swelling within the compartment. The increase in tissue volume within the compartment produces an increase in compartmental pressure that may occlude the blood vessels and produce an ischemic condition. This increased pressure may also produce excessive pressure on the nerves within the compartment that may lead to a neurological deficit. An acute compartment syndrome is considered a medical emergency.

Irreversible damage occurs to the structures within the compartment if it is left untreated. Loss of motion is dependent on the severity and length of the condition and can range from complete drop foot to a partial limitation of the toe and ankle extensors.

Evaluation and clinical findings. An athlete who is experiencing an acute compartment syndrome complains of severe pain in the affected muscles. In the case of a traumatic acute compartment syndrome, such as a contusion to the lower leg, pain progresses from a dull aching sensation to a very sharp pain.

Passively stretching the affected compartment's muscle group produces an increase in pain. Local temperature increases, and the area is swollen and feels tense. Paresthesia is often present in the space between the first and second toes with an anterior compartment involvement. Only in extreme cases are distal pulses lost.

Treatment and rehabilitation. The only effective treatment of acute compartment syndrome is an immediate surgical fasciotomy of the involved compartment. This procedure releases the pressure that has been affecting the tissues within the compartment. Any attempt to treat this condition conservatively only increases the chances for permanent damage to the muscles within the compartment.

Immediately after surgery, the athlete is advised to limit activities and keep the affected leg elevated. Gentle active and passive stretching can be initiated. Ice bags should be applied to the surgical area three to four times a day. Walking can be done as tolerated after the first 2 days.

A more aggressive rehabilitation program should be initiated once the athlete has a full, pain-free range of motion. This program should include Achilles tendon stretching and a manual resistance exercise program. Strengthening programs should not be too aggressive in this phase of rehabilitation. Muscular hypertrophy is contraindicated after fasciotomy. Walking for a longer duration and stationary bicycling should be started and continued in conjunction with a stretching program. A progressive running program should be used as the guideline for returning the athlete to competition.

CHRONIC COMPARTMENT SYNDROMES

Chronic compartment syndrome (CCS) has also been called *exertional compartment syndrome*. Symptoms of CCS often are produced by exercise or by muscle exertion. Not all individuals who exercise, however, experience CCS. Individual differences in the size of the lower leg musculature and compartmental dimensions justify why some people experience problems and others do not. Detmer[7] has concluded that muscle mass increases by 20% during heavy exercise. The increase in muscle mass may produce an increase in compartmental pressure and in some people may lead to CCS. The increase in pressure may produce a local ischemic condition in the muscle. The ischemic response may produce pain that persists until the compartmental pressure diminishes and normal circulation is sufficient to meet the demands of the working muscles. The pain eventually subsides completely with rest.

Athletes may experience bilateral compartment syndromes. Reneman[24] found that 58 out of 61 athletes examined experienced bilateral symptoms. However, the dominant leg usually had more severe symptoms.

Evaluation and clinical findings. A thorough history helps to determine if a chronic compartment syndrome is occurring. The athlete is usually able to tell an exact time, intensity level, or distance during the workout when the symptoms present. The patient often complains of transient pain with exercise that is described as a deep, cramping feeling. It is often a bilateral condition. The athlete also complains of muscle weakness in the affected muscles. If a chronic compartment syndrome is suspected, then diagnosis should be confirmed by comparing compartmental pressure measurements during exercise and rest.

Treatment and rehabilitation. Conservative treatment of CCS generally does not help alleviate the problem. Rest, ice, stretching, and NSAIDs all have been used with limited success. Remember that pain is a symptom of a pathological condition and not one itself. For athletes who wish to continue at a competitive activity level, fasciotomy may be the treatment of choice. Rehabilitation after surgical fasciotomy should be the same as was previously described.

Compartment syndromes treatment (postfasciotomy)

PHASE I
1. Rest.
2. Elevation.
3. Ice 3 to 4 times per day.

PHASE II: *2 to 3 days after surgery*
1. Walking as tolerated.
2. Passive range-of-motion exercises.
3. Active range-of-motion exercises.
4. Ice.

PHASE III
1. Passive or active range-of-motion exercises.
2. Manual resistance (begin with very light work).
3. Bike riding, walking.
4. Ice.

PHASE IV

1. Progressive running program.
2. Stretching.
3. Gradual return to activity.
3. Ice after activity.

Stress Fractures

A **stress fracture** in the lower leg can be defined as a fracture of the tibia or fibula caused by the bones being unable to withstand repeated stress. They are quite common in athletics. McBryde[17] found that 10% of all athletic injuries were stress fractures. Lower leg stress fractures are the most common types. The tibia is the body's primary weight bearer in the lower extremity, and 49% of all stress fractures involve the tibia. The fibula, which plays a lesser role in weight bearing, is only involved in 7% to 10% of the cases.[18]

Stress fractures are very different than acute fractures. Generally no one specific episode of training produces a stress fracture. Frankel[9] has identified four etiological factors associated with stress fractures:

1. Overload placed on bone by continuous muscle contractions.
2. Stress distribution in the bone altered by continued activity in the presence of muscle fatigue.
3. Change in running surface.
4. High repetition of stress, even if the intensity is low.

These four factors all place stress on the body, specifically the lower leg. The body's normal response is to adapt to this increased demand. Bone is in a constant state of remodeling that involves removal of old bone and then a replacement with new bone. The sites for this remodeling are based on increased blood flow and specific stress sites. During this remodeling, problems can arise if the stress placed on the body exceeds the recovery time and the body does not have enough time to form new bone. Eventually a weakened area develops that is highly susceptible to a stress fracture. These overloads are often a result of improper training. Taunton, Clement, and Webber[30] have identified the following training errors:

27%	A rapid increase in training
10%	A single severe session
8%	A rapid increase in mileage
6%	A sudden increase in hill training
5%	Faulty footwear
44%	Combination of faulty footwear and training errors

These factors are indicative of all types of stress fractures, not just lower leg. However, a good parallel can be drawn because 52% of the cases examined involved either the tibia or the fibula.

EVALUATION AND CLINICAL FINDINGS. Obtaining a careful history is important. Noting type and location of pain and when it occurs can help to differentiate between soft tissue and bony involvement. An athlete with a suspected stress fracture complains of a well-localized pain. Initially this pain occurs only after activity. As the condition progresses, the pain starts earlier, during activity. The intensity of pain is also much greater and lasts for a longer period of time.

On examination some swelling might be present from a local periosteal reaction. Percussion distal to the area of suspected fracture often elicits pain. Suspected stress fractures should be followed up with a bone scan to provide an accurate diagnosis. X-ray films at an early stage are often not conclusive.

TREATMENT AND REHABILITATION. The most effective rehabilitation program revolves around a modified activity program. Stress fractures are an overuse syndrome, and the only way they can heal is through rest. In extreme cases, immobilization of the lower leg might be needed. However, a complete abstention from all activity can be very difficult to enforce. Thus alternative cardiovascular training and a very gradual progression of pain-free activity must be implemented.

Relief from the symptoms can be accomplished by rest, ice, and NSAIDs. However, these measures should not mask any pain that the athlete is experiencing because adequate feedback is necessary when the athlete returns to activity.

Strength should be developed in the ankle dorsi and plantarflexors to decrease the stresses placed on the body when the athlete returns to activity. Any biomechanical abnormalities that exist should be corrected with orthotics. Before allowing the athlete to return to preinjury activity levels, a progressive running program should be started. The athlete should also be counseled and monitored about training errors.

Stress fracture treatment

PHASE I
1. Rest.
2. Biomechanical correction.
3. Alternative cardiovascular training.
4. Bone scan diagnosis.
5. Strengthening of lower leg musculature.
6. Stretching of Achilles tendon.

PHASE II: *When fracture is healed*
1. Progressive running/activity program.
2. Ice after workout.

PHASE III
1. Gradual return to activity.

SUMMARY

1. Not all lower leg pain is shin splints.
2. Pain is not a pathological condition in itself.
3. Cardiovascular fitness should be maintained throughout the entire rehabilitation process.
4. Eccentric overloading is a common mechanism with overuse injuries to the lower leg.
5. Biomechanical malalignment should be corrected before allowing the athlete to return to activity.
6. A progressive return to competition should be followed.
7. Upon return to activity, the athlete should continue to work actively on building strength and flexibility.

REFERENCES

1. AMA Subcommittee on the Classification of Sports Injuries: *Standard nomenclature of athletic injuries,* Chicago, 1966, American Medical Association.
2. Andrews JR: Overuse syndromes of the lower extremity, *Clin Sports Med* 2:137, 1983.
3. Brody DM: *Running injuries.* In Nicholas JA, Hershmann EB, editors: *The lower extremity and spine in sports medicine,* St Louis, 1986, Mosby.
4. Calabese LH, Rooney TW: The use of non-steroidal antiinflammatory drugs in sports, *Phys Sports Med* 14:89-97, 1986.
5. Clement DB, Taunton JE, Smart GW: Achilles tendinitis and peritendinitis: etiology and treatment, *Am J Sports Med* 12(3):179-184, 1984.
6. Curwin S, Stanish WD: *Tendinitis: its etiology and treatment,* Lexington, Mass, 1984, Collamore Press.
7. Detmer DE: Chronic leg pain, *Am J Sports Med* 8:141-144, 1980.
8. Feltner ME, MacRae HS, MacRae PG, et al.: Strength training effects on rearfoot motion in running, *Med Sci Sports Exerc* submitted for publication.
9. Frankel VH: Editorial comment, *Am J Sports Med* 6:396, 1978.
10. Friedman MA: *Injuries to the leg in athletics.* In Nicholas JA, Hershmann EB, editors: *The lower extremity and spine in sports medicine,* St Louis, 1986, Mosby.
11. Fyfe I, Stanish WD: The use of eccentric training and stretching in the treatment and prevention of tendon injuries, *Clin Sports Med* 11(3):601-624, 1992.
12. Jacobs D, Martens M, VanAudekercke R, et al.: Comparison of conservative and operative treatments of Achilles tendon rupture, *Am J Sports Med* 6:107, 1978.
13. James SL, Bates BT, Osternig LR: Injuries to runners, *Am J Sports Med* 6:40-50, 1978.
14. Jesse J: *Hidden causes of injury, prevention and correction for running athletes and joggers,* Pasadena, Calif, 1977, The Athletic Press.
15. Lagergren C, Lindholm A: Vascular distribution: the Achilles tendon, *Acta Chir Scand* 116:491, 1958.
16. Leach RE, James S, Wasilewski S: Achilles tendinitis, *Am J Sports Med* 9:93-98, 1981.
17. McBryde AM: Stress fractures in athletics, *Am J Sports Med* 3:212-217, 1975.
18. Matheson GO, Clement D, McKenzie D, et al.: Stress fractures in athletics: a study of 320 cases, *Am J Sports Med* 15:46-57, 1987.
19. Michael RH, Holder LE: The soleus syndrome: a cause of medial tibial stress (shin splints), *Am J Sports Med* 13:87-94, 1985.
20. Millar AP: Strains of the posterior calf musculature (tennis leg), *Clin Sports Med* 2:175, 1983.
21. O'Connor P, Kersey RD: Achilles peritendinitis, *Ath Train* 15:159-166, 1980.
22. Peacock EE: A study of the circulation in normal tendons and healing grafts, *Ann Surg* 149:415, 1959.
23. Persson S, Wredmark T: The treatment of total rupture of the Achilles tendon by plaster immobilization, *Int Orthop* 3:149-152, 1979.
24. Reneman RS: The anterior and lateral compartment syndrome of the leg due to intense use of muscles, *Clin Orthop* 113:69, 1975.
25. Scheuch PA: Tibialis posterior shin splints: diagnosis and treatment, *Ath Train* 19:271-274, 1984.
26. Shields CL: Achilles tendon injuries and disabling conditions, *Phys Sports Med* 10:77-84, 1982.
27. Skeoch DU: Spontaneous partial subcutaneous rupture of the tendon Achilles: review of the literature and evaluation of 16 involved tendons, *Am J Sports Med* 9:20, 1981.
28. Smith W, Winn F, Parette R: Comparative study using four modalities in shin splint treatments, *J Orthop Sports Phys Ther* 8:77-80, 1986.
29. Subotonick SI: *Podiatric sports medicine,* Mt Kisco, NY, 1975, Futura Publishing.
30. Taunton JE, Clement DB, Webber D: Lower extremity stress fractures in athletics, *Phys Sports Med* 9:77-86, 1981.
31. Viitasalo JT, Kvist M: Some biomechanical aspects of the foot and ankle in athletics with and without shin splints, *Am J Sports Med* 11:125-130, 1983.
32. Williams JGP: Achilles tendon lesions in sport, *Sports Med* 3:114-135, 1986.
33. Zarins B, Ciullo JV: Acute muscle and tendon injuries in athletics, *Clin Sports Med* 2:175, 1983.

Rehabilitation of Ankle Injuries

25

Skip Hunter

OBJECTIVES

After completion of this chapter, the student should be able to do the following:

- Identify types of ankle sprains and the mechanisms of injury.

- Identify the stages of rehabilitation for the ankle.

- Discuss the various treatment options available for each of the stages of rehabilitation.

- Discuss criteria for return to activity after ankle injury.

The most frequently injured part of the musculo-skeletal system is the lateral ankle.[3,9] The turned ankle is the second greatest cause of days lost from work.[8] Management of these injuries ranges from no treatment to surgical repair and reconstruction. Rehabilitation techniques are varied, and the equipment used may be as simple as a $1 piece of tubing or as sophisticated as a $50,000 isokinetic device.

MECHANISMS OF INJURY

Injuries to the ligaments of the ankle may be graded so that grade I is mild, grade II is a greater ligamentous disruption, and grade III is a complete tear.[9] Chapter 1 contains a detailed description of the most commonly used system of grading ankle sprains.

Injuries to the ligaments of the ankle may also be classified according to the site of occurrence. The lateral ankle sprain is by far the most common. The anterior talofibular ligament is the weakest of the three lateral ligaments. Its major function is to stop forward subluxation of the talus. It is injured in an inverted, plantarflexed, and internally rotated position.[23,41] The calcaneofibular and posterior talofibular ligaments are commonly involved in lateral sprains as the force of the injury is increased and the mechanism is slightly altered. Increased inversion force is

needed to tear the calcaneofibular ligament. Because the posterior talofibular ligament prevents posterior subluxation of the talus, its injuries are severe such as complete dislocations.[4]

The medial ankle sprain is less common than the lateral ankle sprain. More often it may involve an avulsion fracture of the tibia before the deltoid ligament tears.[6] Although eversion sprains are uncommon, their severity is such that this category of sprain may take longer to heal than the simple lateral sprain.[33]

The tibiofibular ligaments are stronger and less prone to injury than the other ligaments of the ankle.[45] These ligaments extend between the tibia and fibula up the leg as the interosseous ligament. These ligaments are torn with increased rotational force and are often torn in conjunction with a severe sprain of the medial and lateral ligament complexes. Initial rupture of this ligament occurs distally at the tibiofibular ligament above the ankle mortise. As the force of disruption is increased, the interosseous ligament is torn more proximally. Sprains of the tibiofibular and interosseous ligaments are extremely hard to treat and often take months to heal. Treatments for this problem are essentially the same as for medial or lateral sprains, with the difference being an extended period of immobilization. Functional activities and

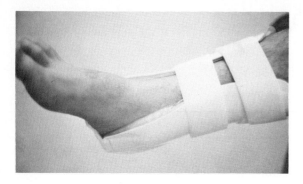

Fig. 25-1. Commerically available aircast ankle stirrup.

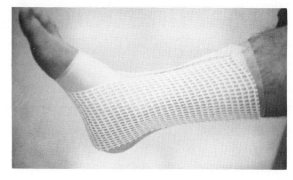

Fig. 25-2. Molded Hexalite ankle stirrup.

return to sport may be delayed for a longer period of time than for the more common sprains.

TREATMENT AND REHABILITATION OF ANKLE SPRAINS
Phase I (Early Phase)

During the initial phase of ankle rehabilitation, the major goals are reduction of postinjury swelling, bleeding, and pain and protection of the already healing ligament. All initial treatment should be directed toward limiting the amount of swelling. Initial management includes protection, rest, ice, compression, and elevation.

PROTECTION. The injured ligament must be maintained in a stable position so that healing can occur. In the past, this objective was accomplished by casting until the acute effects of the sprain were over. Recent literature suggests that limited stress on the ankle may promote faster and stronger healing.[4,34] These studies found that protected motion facilitated proper collagen reorientation and thus increased the strength of the healing ligament.

Several appliances are available to accomplish this early protected motion. Quillen[35] recommends the ankle stirrup, which allows motion in the sagittal plane while limiting movement of the frontal plane and thus avoids stressing the ligaments through inversion and eversion (Figure 25-1). Several commercially available braces accomplish this goal and also apply cushioned pressure to help with edema.[40] When a commercially available product is not feasible, a similar protective device may be fashioned from thermoplastic materials such as Hexalite or Orthoplast (Figure 25-2).

The open Gibney taping technique also accom-

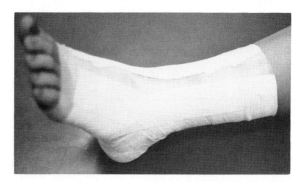

Fig. 25-3. Correctly done open Gibney tape.

plishes this early medial and lateral protection while allowing plantarflexion and dorsiflexion. It also is an excellent edema control mechanism (Figure 25-3).

Gross, Lapp, and Davis compared the effectiveness of a number of commercial ankle orthoses and taping in restricting eversion and inversion. All of these support systems significantly reduced inversion and eversion immediately after application and after exercise when compared to preapplication measures. Of the orthoses tested, taping provided the least support after exercise.[18] Early application of these devices allows early ambulation. Partial weight bearing with crutches helps control several complications to healing. Muscle atrophy, proprioceptive loss, and circulatory stasis are all reduced when even limited weight bearing is allowed. Weight bearing also inhibits contracture of the tendons, which may lead to tendinitis. For these reasons, early ambulation, even if only touchdown weight bearing, is essential.

REST. In the early phase of rehabilitation, vigorous exercise is discouraged. The studies cited previously

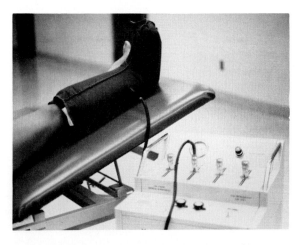

Fig. 25-4. Jobst intermittent air compression device.

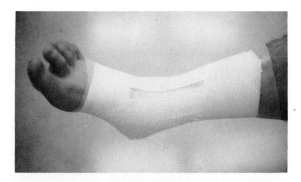

Fig. 25-5. Do not close the open Gibney tape.

show that a healing ligament needs a certain amount of stress to heal properly.

Contralateral exercises may be performed to obtain cross-transfer effects on the muscles of the injured side.[25] Isometric exercises may be performed very early in dorsiflexion, plantarflexion, inversion, and eversion. The athlete should hold these for a 6 to 8 count in all of the major ankle movements. These types of exercises may be performed to prevent atrophy without fear of further injury to the ligament. Active plantarflexion and dorsiflexion may be initiated early because they also do not endanger the healing ligament as long as they are done pain free. An excellent method is two sets of 40 of active plantarflexion and dorsiflexion while the athlete is iced and elevated. Inversion and eversion are to be avoided, since they might initiate bleeding and further traumatize ligaments.

ICE. The use of ice on acute injuries has been well documented in the literature. Ice has received attention not only as an aid in acute situations but also for continued use in chronic conditions. The initial use of ice has its basis in constricting superficial blood vessels to prevent hemorrhage. Long-term benefits may be from reduction of pain and spasticity.[2] Garrick suggests the use of ice for a minimum of 20 minutes once every 4 waking hours.[15] Ice should not be used longer than 30 minutes, especially over superficial nerves such as the peroneal and ulnar nerves. Prolonged use of ice in such areas may produce transient nerve palsy.[10]

One of the most frequently asked questions in sports medicine is "When do I use ice, and when do I use heat?" Current literature suggests that ice can be used during all phases of rehabilitation.[26] The sooner it is started, the more effective it is.[20] Ice can certainly do no harm if used properly, but heat, if applied too soon after injury, may lead to increased swelling.

Ice should be used as a rehabilitative tool until the process plateaus. At that point the sports therapist may elect to change to heat in an effort to progress the rehabilitative process. Often the switch from ice to heat cannot be made for weeks or months.

COMPRESSION. Ice alone is apparently not as effective as ice used in conjunction with compression.[39] Many devices are available that apply external compression to the ankle to reduce swelling. Most of these use either air or cold water within an enclosed bag to provide pressure to reduce swelling. The most commonly used device of this type is the intermittent air compression device (Figure 25-4).

Several methods may be used to control edema when the patient is away from the treatment area. An Ace wrap can prevent or control swelling. It should be applied evenly, wrapping distal to proximal with enough force so that it does not fall. Uneven pressure or uncovered areas over any part of the extremity may allow the swelling to accumulate.

Open Gibney tape may be applied under an Ace wrap to provide additional support. Care should be taken not to compartmentalize this treatment by placing tape across the top and bottom of the open area of the open Gibney (Figure 25-5). In cases of severe swelling, tissue may be forced through this compartmental window and cause damage to the skin. As swelling begins to reduce, a bulky dressing may be taped closed with several layers of prewrap or gauze

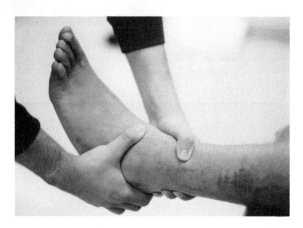

Fig. 25-6. Manual joint mobilization techniques.

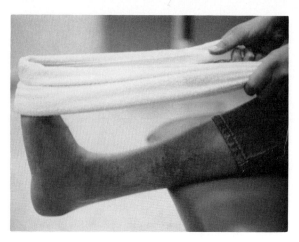

Fig. 25-7. Towel stretch for plantarflexion.

with tape lightly applied over the top. To add more compression, a horseshoe-shaped felt pad may be inserted under the wrap over the area of maximum swelling.

Electrical stimulation has been used to help control edema. Michlovitz, Smith, and Watkins[30] used high-voltage pulsed galvanic stimulation at varying pulse rates in conjunction with ice. Although descriptive data indicated some pain relief, the addition of electrical stimulation to the treatment protocol made no significant difference in the amount of acute edema in the first 3 days.

ELEVATION. Elevation is an essential part of edema control. Pressure in any vessel below the level of the heart is increased, which may lead to increased edema.[7] Several publications have stated that any treatment done in the dependent position allows edema to increase.[30,38] Elevation allows gravity to work with the lymphatic system rather than against it and decreases hydrostatic pressure to decrease fluid loss and also assist venous and lymphatic return through gravity.[7]

An attempt should be made to treat in the elevated position rather than the gravity dependent position. Patients should be asked to maintain an elevated position as often as possible during the early phase of rehabilitation.

OTHER TREATMENT. Cardiorespiratory conditioning should be maintained during the entire rehabilitation process. Pedaling a stationary bike such as an Airdyne or UBE with the hands provides excellent cardiovascular exercise without placing stress on the ankle. Swimming can also be beneficial if it is pain free.

Summary of treatments for phase I

1. *Protection:* Air or gel casts, open Gibney taping, self-made Hexalite splints.
2. *Rest:* Crutches with partial weight bearing, isometric exercises progressing to isometric inversion-eversion exercises with active plantarflexion and dorsiflexion.
3. *Ice:* Ice throughout the entire rehabilitation process, although heat may be substituted when progress is not noted with ice.
4. *Compression:* Intermittent compression devices in conjunction with ice and electrical stimulation. An Ace wrap, open Gibney taping, or closed taping using a bulky dressing can reduce edema.
5. *Elevation*

Phase II (Rehabilitation Phase)

The end of the early protective phase and beginning of the rehabilitation phase is marked by two events: (1) swelling stops increasing and (2) pain lessens, indicating that the ligaments have reached that point in the healing process at which they are not in danger from minimal stress.

This phase of rehabilitation increases motion and strength. This increased activity should aid circulation and help eliminate residual inflammatory agents.

RANGE OF MOTION. In the early stages of the rehabilitation phase, inversion and eversion should be minimized. Light joint mobilization concentrating on dorsiflexion and plantarflexion should be started first. It can be accomplished by manual joint mobilization

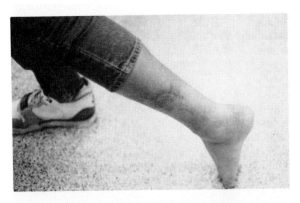

Fig. 25-8. Toe stretch for dorsiflexion.

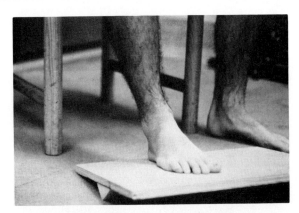

Fig. 25-9. Seated wedge board.

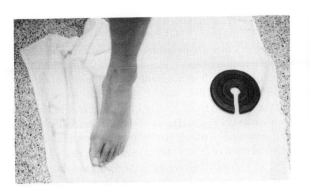

Fig. 25-10. Towel pull with weight added.

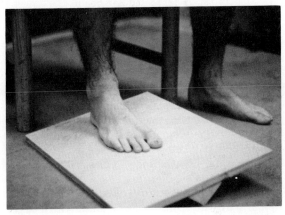

Fig. 25-11. Seated wedge board for inversion and eversion.

in the anteriorposterior direction (Figure 25-6) or through exercises such as dorsiflexion stretches with a towel (Figure 25-7) and standing toe stretches for plantarflexion (Figure 25-8). Both exercises may be done while ice is being applied. Athletes are encouraged to do these exercises slowly, without pain, and to use high repetitions (two sets of 40). A wedge board may be beneficial for range of motion, as well as a beginning exercise for proprioception. These exercises should at first be done seated (Figure 25-9).

As tenderness over the ligament decreases, inversion-eversion exercises may be initiated in conjunction with plantarflexion and dorsiflexion exercises. Early exercises include pulling a towel from one side to the other by alternatively inverting and everting the foot (Figure 25-10) and alphabet drawing in an ice bath, which should be done in capital letters to ensure that full range is used. A wedge board may be turned so that inversion-eversion is the primary movement (Figure 25-11). These exercises may be supplemented with a seated biomechanical ankle platform (BAP) board technique by rotating the foot through its entire range both clockwise and counterclockwise for two sets of 20 repetitions (Figure 25-12).

A wedge-BAP board exercise should follow a progression. Initially the athlete should start in the seated position with a wedge board in the plantarflexion-dorsiflexion direction. As pain decreases and ligament healing progresses, the board may be turned in the inversion-eversion direction. As the athlete performs these movements easily, a seated BAP board may be used for full range-of-motion exercises. When seated exercises are performed with ease, standing balance

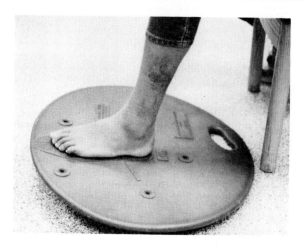

Fig. 25-12. Seated BAP board.

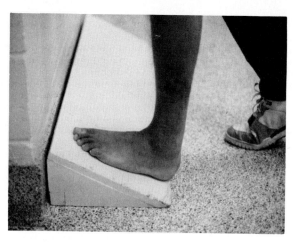

Fig. 25-13. Heelcord stretching using an incline board.

exercises should be initiated. They may be started on one leg standing without a board. The athlete then supports weight with the hands and maintains balance on a wedge board in either plantarflexion-dorsiflexion or inversion-eversion. Next, hand support may be eliminated while the athlete balances on the wedge board. The same sequence is then used on the BAP board. The BAP board is initially used with assistance from the hands. Then balance is practiced on the BAP board unassisted.

Each time a BAP board is used, the progression should start with a small ball and finish with a larger ball before moving to the next step.

Vigorous heelcord stretching should be initiated as soon as possible (Figure 25-13). McCluskey, Blackburn, and Lewis[27] found that the heelcord acts as a bowstring when tight and may increase the chance of ankle sprains.

The author advocates that athletes have available something on which the foot can rest to stretch the heelcords, perhaps at a location where they stand during the day, such as by the phone, in front of a mirror, or in front of the sink, to ensure that they stretch at least a few minutes each day.

STRENGTHENING. Isometrics may be done in the four major ankle motion planes, frontal and sagittal. They may be accompanied early in the rehabilitative phase by plantarflexion and dorsiflexion isotonic exercises, which do not endanger the ligaments. They may be done with a device as simple as an ankle weight or as sophisticated as an isokinetic device. As the ligaments heal further and range of motion in-

creases, strengthening exercises may be begun in all planes of motion (Figure 25-14). Pain should be the basic guideline for deciding when to start inversion-eversion isotonic exercises. Light resistance with high repetitions has fewer detrimental effects on the ligaments (two to four sets of 10 repetitions).

Tubing exercises and ankle weights around the foot are excellent methods of strengthening inversion and eversion. Tubing has advantages in that it may be used both eccentrically and concentrically (Figure 25-15). Isokinetics have advantages in that more functional speeds may be obtained (Figure 25-16). Care must be taken when exercising the ankle in inversion and eversion to avoid tibial rotation as a substitute movement. Have the athlete palpate the tibial tubercle to ensure that the proper movement is occurring.

PROPRIOCEPTION. The role of proprioception in repeated ankle trauma has been questioned.[5,12,14,32] The literature suggests that proprioception is certainly a factor in recurrent ankle sprains. Rebman[36] reported that 83% of his patients experienced a reduction in chronic ankle sprains after a program of proprioceptive exercises. Glencross and Thornton[17] found that the greater the ligamentous disruption, the greater the proprioceptive loss. Early weight bearing has previously been mentioned as a method of reducing proprioceptive loss. During the rehabilitation phase, standing on both feet with closed eyes with progression to standing on one leg is an exercise to recoup proprioception. This exercise may be followed by standing and balancing on a BAP board, which should be done initially with support from the hands. As a

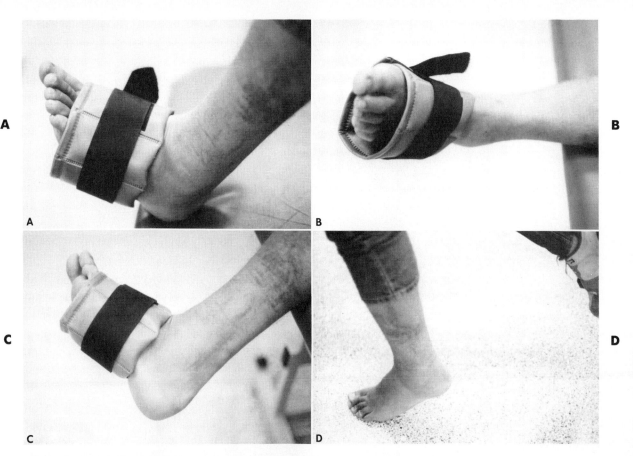

Fig. 25-14. Isotonic stengthening. A, Dorsiflexion using ankle weight. **B,** Inversion using ankle weight. **C,** Eversion using ankle weight. **D,** Plantar flexion using toe raises.

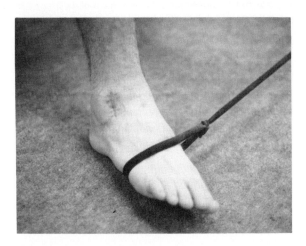

Fig. 25-15. Ankle strengthening technique using rubber tubing.

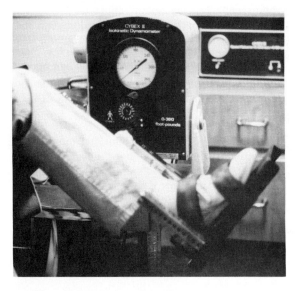

Fig. 25-16. Isokinetic strengthening using an isokinetic device.

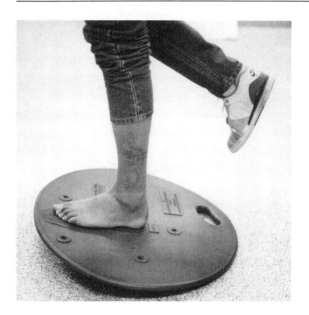

Fig. 25-17. Strengthening while free standing on a BAP board.

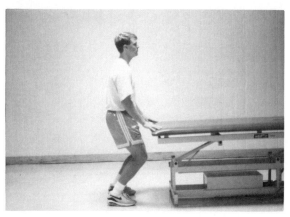

Fig. 25-18. Mini-squats. Mini-squats and other closed-chain exercises may be used to help establish neuromuscular control on the involved side.

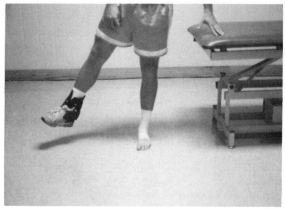

Fig. 25-19. Hip movement. Hip movement of the uninvolved side while weight bearing on the involved side may encourage neuromuscular control.

final-stage exercise, the athlete can progress to free standing and controlling the board through all ranges (Figure 25-17).

Other closed-kinetic chain exercises may be beneficial. Leg press and mini-squats on the involved leg will encourage weight bearing and increase proprioceptive return (Figure 25-18). Hip abduction, adduction, extension, and flexion of the uninvolved side while weight bearing on the affected side will increase both strength and proprioception. This may be accomplished either free standing (Figure 25-19) or on a machine.

OTHER TREATMENT. As noted in Chapter 26 the foot and ankle function together very close. As the foot pronates or supinates, the ankle also rotates with the leg.[10,31] Orthotic therapy after an ankle sprain has proved very helpful in lessening pain.[42] The author feels that this is particularly helpful after interosseous and medial sprains.

Summary of treatments for phase II

1. Range-of-motion exercises beginning with plantarflexion and dorsiflexion may be initiated early. As swelling and pain decrease, inversion and eversion may be started with manual mobilization, active exercises, or devices such as a BAP board.

2. Strengthening may be begun with isometrics with a progression to isotonic or isokinetics as pain decreases.
3. Proprioceptive exercises may be begun early in phase II to limit proprioceptive loss.
4. Orthotic therapy may be of benefit for certain sprains.

Phase III (Return to Activity)

Estimates are that 30% to 40% of all inversion injuries result in reinjury.[12,21,22,29,37] In the past, athletes were simply returned to sports once the pain was low enough to tolerate the activity. Thanks to pioneers such as Donley, this procedure has been replaced by a gradual return to practice through a functional progression.[24] The actual process of return to activity is started the first day after the injury with conditioning exercises and continued strength training on the unaffected joints. This practice not only keeps the athlete physically ready for return but also fosters a healthy mental attitude. Stationary bicycling is a good way to maintain fitness. For lower extremity injuries that may cause pain with regular bicycling, an upper extremity ergometer is recommended. If nothing else is available, place a stationary bike on a table, and have the athlete pedal it with the hands rather than the legs. Running in a pool, using a float vest, or swimming are also good cardiovascular exercises. As the athlete begins to progress functionally so that stress on the ankle is tolerated, several measures may be taken to further protect the ankle. Although taping does not appear to interfere with motor performance,[13,27] it does have a stabilizing effect on unstable ankles.[16,43] McCluskey and others[27] suggest taping the ankle and also taping the shoe onto the foot to make the shoe and ankle function as one unit. High-topped footwear may further stabilize the ankle.[19] If cleated shoes are worn, cleats should be outset along the periphery of the shoe to provide stability.[27]

The athlete should have complete range of motion and 80% to 90% of preinjury strength before considering a return to the sport. This return should include a gradual progression of functional activities that slowly increase the stress on the ligament. The specific demands of each individual sport dictate the individual drills of this progression. Functional progressions may be as complex or simple as needed. The more severe the injury, the more the need for a detailed functional progression. The typical progression begins early in the rehabilitation process as the athlete becomes partially weight bearing. Full weight bearing should be started when ambulation is performed without a limp. Running may be begun as soon as ambulation is pain free. Pain-free hopping on the affected side may also be a guideline to determine when running is appropriate. A method that allows early running is pool running. The athlete is placed in the pool in a swim vest that supports the body in water. The athlete then runs in place without touching the bottom of the pool. Proper running form should be stressed. Eventually the athlete is moved into shallow water so that more weight is placed on

the ankle while running is performed. Progression is then to running on a smooth, flat surface, ideally a track. Initially the athlete should jog the straights and walk the curves and then progress to jogging the entire track. Speed may be increased to a sprint in a straight line.

The cutting sequence should begin with circles of diminishing diameter. Cones may be set up for the athlete to run figure eights as the next cutting progression. The predetermined crossover or sidestep is next.[1] The athlete sprints to a predesignated spot and cuts or sidesteps abruptly. When this progression is accomplished, the cut should be done without warning on the command of another person.

The exercise progression begins with plantarflexion-dorsiflexion exercises and gradually involves inversion-eversion also. The BAP board exercises progress from sitting to standing. Jumping and hopping exercises should be started on both legs simultaneously and gradually reduced to only the injured side.

The athlete may perform on different levels for each of these functional sequences. One functional sequence may be done at half speed while another is done at full speed. An example of this is the athlete who is running full speed on straights of the track while doing figure eights at only half speed. Once the upper levels of all the sequences are reached, the athlete may return to limited practice, which may include early teaching and fundamental drills. Finally, if full practice is tolerated without insult to the injured part, the athlete may return to competition.

Summary of treatments for phase III
1. Exercises to maintain fitness are continued in this phase.
2. Functional exercises are performed that are specific toward returning the athlete to the individual sport.

SUMMARY

1. Ankle sprains are very common. Lateral sprains are more common than medial sprains. Medial and interosseous sprains are usually more severe than lateral sprains.
2. Inversion sprains usually involve the lateral ligaments of the ankle, and eversion sprains frequently involve the medial ligaments of the ankle. Rotational injuries often involve the tibiofibular and interosseous ligaments and may be very severe.

3. Treatment of ankle sprains may be divided into an early phase, a rehabilitation phase, and a return to activity phase.

4. The early phase of treatment uses PRICE. *Protection* and *Rest* include a gradual increase in stress on the healing ligament through protected weight bearing. *Ice* should be used until progress reaches a plateau. At that time heat may be initiated to see if progress resumes. *Compression* and *Elevation* are essential components in reducing and preventing swelling.

5. The rehabilitative phase begins as swelling and pain lessen. The purpose of this phase is to increase strength and range of motion. Joint mobilization, towel exercises, wedge boards, BAP boards, tubing, and isokinetic devices may be used to accomplish this purpose. Proprioceptive exercises should be started during this phase.

6. The return to activity phase begins immediately after the injury. Conditioning exercises that do not involve the injured extremity are started as soon as possible. Before returning to the sport, the athlete should be taken through a gradual functional progression, including drills that involve cutting and mimic the sport.

REFERENCES

1 Andrews JR, McClod W, Ward T, et al.: The cutting mechanism, *Am J Sports Med* 5:111-121, 1977.

2 Arnheim D, Prentice W: *Principles of athletic training,* St Louis, 1993, Mosby.

3 Bosien WR, Staples OS, Russell SW: Residual disability following acute ankle sprains, *J Bone Joint Surg* 37[A]:1237, 1955.

4 Bostrum L: Treatment and prognosis in recent ligament ruptures, *Acta Chir Scand* 132:537-550, 1966.

5 Burgess PR, Wei J: Signalling of kinesthetic information by peripheral sensory receptors, *Ann Rev Neurosci* 5:171-187, 1982.

6 Calliet R: *Foot and ankle pain,* Philadelphia, 1968, FA Davis.

7 Canoy WF: *Review of medical physiology,* ed 7, Los Altos, Calif, 1975, Lange Medical Publications.

8 Choi J: Acute conditions: incidence and associated disability, *Vital Health Statistics* 120:10, 1978.

9 Cutler JM: *Lateral ligamentous injuries of the ankle.* In Hamilton WC, editor: *Lateral ligamentous injuries of the ankle,* New York, 1984, Springer-Verlag.

10 Donatelli R: Normal biomechanics of the foot and ankle, *J Orthop Sports Phys Ther* 7:91-95, 1985

11 Drez D, Faust D, Evans P: Cryotherapy and nerve palsy, *Am J Sports Med* 9:256-257, 1981.

12 Freeman M, Dean M, Hanhan I: The etiology and prevention of functional instability at the foot, *J Bone Joint Surg* 47[Br]:678-685, 1965.

13 Fumich RM, Ellison A, Guerin G, et al.: The measured effect of taping on combined foot and ankle motion before and after exercise, *Am J Sports Med* 9:165-169, 1981.

14 Garn SN, Newton RA: Kinesthetic awareness in subjects with multiple ankle sprains, *J Am Phys Ther Assoc* 68:1667-1671, 1988.

15 Garrick JG: When can I...? A practical approach to rehabilitation illustrated by treatment of an ankle injury, *Am J Sports Med* 9:67-68, 1981.

16 Garrick JG, Requa RK: Role of external supports in the prevention of ankle sprains, *Med Sci Sports Exerc* 5:200, 1977.

17 Glencross D, Thornton E: Position sense following joint injury, *J Sport Med Phys Fitness* 21:23-27, 1981

18 Gross M, Lapp A, Davis M: Comparison of Swed-O-Universal ankle support and Aircast Sport Stirrup orthoses and ankle tape in restricting eversion-inversion before and after exercise, *J Orthop Sports Phys Ther* 13(1):11-19, 1991.

19 Hirata I: Proper playing conditions, *J Sports Med* 4:228-234, 1974.

20 Hocutt JE, Jaffe R, Rylander C, et al.: Cryotherapy in ankle sprains, *Am J Sports Med* 10:316-319, 1982.

21 Isakov E, Mizrahi J, Solzi P, et al.: Response of the peroneal muscles to sudden inversion of the ankle during standing, *Int J Sports Biomech* 2:100-109, 1986.

22 Itay S: Clinical and functional status following lateral ankle sprains: followup of 90 young adults treated conservatively, *Orthop Rev* 11:73-76, 1982.

23 Kelikian H, Kelikian AS: *Disorders of the ankle,* Philadelphia, 1985, WB Saunders.

24 Kergerris S: The construction and implementation of functional progressions as a component of athletic rehabilitation, *J Orthop Sports Phys Ther* 5:14-19, 1983.

25 Klein KK: A study of cross transfer of muscular strength and endurance resulting from progressive resistive exercises following surgery, *J Assoc Phys Mental Rehab* 9:5, 1955.

26 Kowal MA: Review of physiologic effects of cryotherapy, *J Orthop Sports Phys Ther* 5:66-73, 1983.

27 McCluskey GM, Blackburn TA, Lewis T: Prevention of ankle sprains, *Am J Sports Med* 4:151-157, 1976.

28 Mandelbaum BR, Finerman G, Grant T, et al.: Collegiate football players with recurrent ankle sprains, *Phys Sports Med* 15(11):57-61, 1987.

29 Mayhew JL, Riner WF: Effects of ankle wrapping on motor performance, *Ath Train* 3:128-130, 1974.

30 Michlovitz S, Smith W, Watkins M: Ice and high voltage pulsed stimulation in treatment of acute lateral ankle sprains, *J Orthop Sports Phys Ther* 9:301-304, 1988.

31 Morris JM: Biomechanics of the foot and ankle, *Clin Orthop* 122:10-17, 1977.

32 Nawoczenski DA, Owen M, Ecker M, et al.: Objective evaluation of peroneal response to sudden inversion stress, *J Orthop Sports Phys Ther* 7:107-119, 1985.

33 Nicholas JA, Hershman EB: *The lower extremity and spine in sports medicine,* St Louis, 1990, Mosby.

34 Noyes FR: Functional properties of knee ligaments and alterations induced by immobilization: a correlative biomechanical and histological study in primates, *Clin Orthop* 123:210-243, 1977.

35 Quillen S: Alternative management protocol for lateral ankle sprains, *J Orthop Sports Phys Ther* 12:187-190, 1980.

36 Rebman LW: Ankle injuries: clinical observations, *J Orthop Sports Phys Ther* 8:153-156, 1986.

37 Sammarco JG: Biomechanics of foot and ankle injuries, *Ath Train* 10:96, 1975.

38 Sims D: Effects of positioning on ankle edema, *J Orthop Sports Phys Ther* 8:30-33, 1986.

39 Sloan JP, Guddings P, Hain R: Effects of cold and compression on edema, *Phys Sports Med* 16:116-120, 1988.

40 Stover CN, York JM: Air stirrup management of ankle injuries in the athlete, *Am J Sports Med* 8:360-365, 1980.

41 Tippett SR: A case study: the need for evaluation and reevaluation of acute ankle sprains, *J Orthop Sports Phys Ther* 4:44, 1982.

42 Tropp H, Askling C, Gillquist J: Prevention of ankle sprains, *Am J Sports Med* 13:259-266, 1985.

43 Vaes P, DeBoeck H, Handleberg F, et al.: Comparative radiologic study of the influence of ankle joint bandages on ankle stability, *Am J Sports Med* 13:46-49, 1985.

44 Yablon IG, Segal D, Leach RE: *Ankle injuries,* New York, 1983, Churchill Livingstone.

Rehabilitation of Foot Injuries

26

Skip Hunter

OBJECTIVES

After completion of this chapter, the student should be able to do the following:

- Discuss the actions of the subtalar and midtarsal joints.

- Define **pronation** and **supination.**

- Discuss the effect the position of the midtarsal joint may have on the forefoot.

- List the causes of pronation.

- Discuss the effect of forefoot varus and valgus on the foot and lower extremity.

- Describe the biomechanical examination of the foot.

- Discuss the methods by which a pronator may be recognized.

- Describe the three types of orthotics.

- Describe an orthotic fabrication.

- Discuss shoe selection in terms of pronation and supination.

- Identify problems associated with the foot and the treatment options for each.

Rehabilitation of injuries to the foot requires not only a proper knowledge of therapeutic modalities and exercises but also an understanding of foot biomechanics. Biomechanical understanding leads to a treatment that addresses not only the symptoms of an injury but also the underlying cause.

The foot must possess many functional components to function properly. It must be rigid enough to provide a lever upon which the body propels itself. Conversely, it must be adaptive enough to accommodate uneven surfaces and absorb shock during gait. To accomplish both of these tasks, the foot stays in a constant state of change during gait. At heel strike, the foot is in a supinated position, followed by a short period of pronation, then resupinated for toe off. It is important to understand from the very beginning that supination and pronation are normal motions during a gait cycle. Pronation and supination become abnormal when they occur at the wrong time or when they become excessive.[30]

The two major joints that determine the functional stability of the foot are the subtalar joint and the midtarsal joint.

THE SUBTALAR JOINT

The subtalar joint consists of three articulations between the talus and the calcaneus.[28] Supination and pronation are the normal movements of the subtalar joint through which it acts as a torque convertor to translate leg rotation into the foot as pronation-supination.[32,36] These movements are triplanar movements, that is, movements in all three planes that occur simultaneously.[10,21,24] In weight bearing, supination consists of the talus abducting and dorsiflexing on the calcaneus while the calcaneus inverts on the talus. Without weight bearing, supination consists of the calcaneus inverting as the talus adducts and plantarflexes. The foot moves into adduction, plantarflexion, and inversion in supination.[10] These movements are exactly the opposite in pronation. The foot everts, abducts, and dorsiflexes. In weight bearing, the talus adducts and plantarflexes while the calcaneus everts on the talus. Without weight bearing, the calcaneus everts as the talus abducts and dorsiflexes.[10,21]

THE MIDTARSAL JOINT

An old axiom in rehabilitation is that for distal mobility, proximal stability is necessary. The function of the midtarsal joint is a prime example. The midtarsal joint consists of two distinct joints: the calcaneocuboid and the talonavicular joint. The midtarsal joint depends mainly on ligamentous and muscular tension to maintain position and integrity. Midtarsal joint stability is directly related to the position of the subtalar joint. As the midtarsal joint becomes more or less mobile, it affects the distal portion of the foot because of the articulations at the tarsal-metatarsal joint.

Effects of Midtarsal Joint Position During Pronation

During pronation, the talus adducts and plantarflexes and makes the joint articulations of the midtarsal joint more congruous. The long axes of the talonavicular and calcaneocuboid joints are more parallel and thus allow more motion. The resulting foot is often referred to as a "loose bag of bones."[10,28]

As more motion is allowed at the midtarsal joint, the lesser tarsal bones, particularly the first metatarsal and first cuneiform, become more mobile. These bones comprise a functional unit known as the **first ray.** With pronation of the midtarsal joint, the first ray is more mobile because of its articulations with that joint. One of the original descriptions was Morton's paper describing the now classic Morton's toe.[23] The first ray is also stabilized by the attachment of the long peroneal tendon, which attaches to the base of the first metatarsal. The long peroneal tendon passes laterally around the base of the lateral malleolus and then through a notch in the cuboid to cross the foot to the first metatarsal. The cuboid functions

as a pulley to increase the mechanical advantage of the peroneal tendon. Stability of the cuboid is essential in this process. In the pronated position, the cuboid loses much of its mechanical advantage as a pulley; therefore the peroneal tendon no longer stabilizes the first ray effectively. This condition creates hypermobility of the first ray and increased pressure on the other metatarsals.

Calluses under the metatarsal heads of the second and third toes are common in individuals with excessive pronation for this reason. Many pronators have bunions. As the hypermobility of the first ray occurs, the metatarsal heads splay apart, and the tendons attached to the toe continue to pull in a straight line. This process is one method by which a bunion is formed.

Effects of Midtarsal Joint Position During Supination

During supination, the talus abducts and dorsiflexes, which raises the level of the talonavicular joint superior to that of the calcaneocuboid joint and allows lesser surface areas of both joint articulations to become congruous.[27] Also the long axes of the joints become more oblique. Both allow less motion to occur at this joint, making the foot very rigid and tight. Since less movement occurs at the calcaneocuboid joint, the cuboid becomes hypomobile. The long peroneal tendon has a greater amount of tension since the cuboid has less mobility and thus will not allow hypermobility of the first ray. In this case the majority of the weight is borne by the first and fifth metatarsals.

CAUSES OF PRONATION

Most of these pronatory motions occur as compensatory mechanisms for abnormal osseous relationships in the foot. Many of these deformities are the result of faulty rotation of the limb during embryology.[21] Root and others list six congenital defects of the foot that may cause pronation: (1) forefoot varus, (2) plantarflexed fifth ray, (3) forefoot valgus, (4) lateral instability during propulsion caused by a plantarflexed fifth ray, (5) rearfoot varus, and (6) ankle joint equinus.[28]

Forefoot Varus and Valgus

Forefoot varus has been identified by Subotnick as the leading cause of pronation.[31] Its effect on the prox-

TALUS ADDUCTS/PLANTAR FLEXES
↓
FOOT MUSCLES FIRE OUT OF SYNC
↓
LOWER EXTREMITY INTERNALLY ROTATES
↓
MIDTARSAL JOINT HYPERMOBILE
↓
CUBOID PULLEY IS LESS EFFICIENT
↓
PERONEAL TENDON LESS FUNCTIONAL
↓
FIRST RAY HYPERMOBILE
↓
2ND & 3RD METATARSALS BEAR TOO MUCH WEIGHT
↓
METATARSALS SPLAY APART
↓
BUNIONS, FRACTURES, CALLOUSES

Fig. 26-1. Diagram illustrating the effects of a forefoot varus.

Talus abducts/dorsiflexes
↓
Lower extremity externally rotates
↓
Midtarsal joint hypomobile
↓
Cuboid pulley is less mobile
↓
Peroneal tendon held more rigid
↓
First ray hypomobile
↓
1st & 5th metatarsals bear most weight

Fig. 26-2. Diagram illustrating the effects of a forefoot valgus.

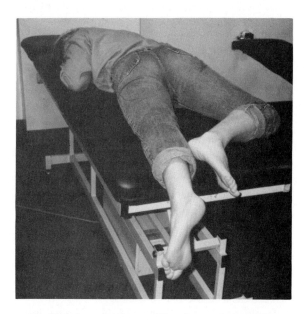

Fig. 26-3. Examination position for neutral position.

imal foot and extremity is shown in Figure 26-1. Forefoot valgus causes the foot to become rigid as the midtarsal joint becomes more oblique (Figure 26-2). This foot is a poor shock absorber and may also contribute to an increased incidence of lateral ankle sprains as the foot rolls out.[32] Forefoot varus and valgus are discussed further in the examination section of this chapter.

EXAMINATION
Neutral subtalar position. The athlete should be prone with the distal third of the leg hanging off the end of the table (Figure 26-3). A line should be drawn bisecting the leg from the start of the musculotendinous junction of the gastrocnemius to the distal portion of the calcaneus[33] (Figure 26-4). With the athlete still prone, the sports therapist palpates the talus while the forefoot is inverted and everted. One finger should palpate the talus at the anterior aspect of the fibula and another finger at the anterior portion of the medial malleolus (Figure 26-5). The position at which the talus is equally prominent on both sides is considered neutral subtalar position.[16] Root, Orien, and Weed [28] describe this as the position of the subtalar joint where it is neither pronated or supinated. It is the standard position in which the foot should be placed to examine deformities.[24] In this position,

the lines on the lower leg and calcaneus should form a straight line. Any variance is considered to be a rearfoot valgus or varus deformity. The most common deformity of the foot is a rearfoot varus deformity.[22] A deviation of 2 to 3 degrees is normal.[35]

Another method of determining subtalar neutral position involves the lines that were drawn previously on the leg and back of the heel. With the athlete prone, the heel is swung into full eversion and inversion, with measurements taken at each position. Angles of the two lines are taken at each extreme. Neutral position is considered two-thirds away from

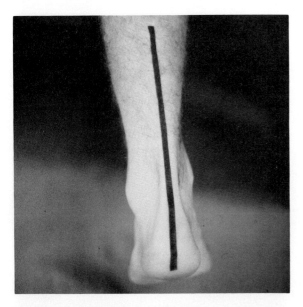

Fig. 26-4. Line bisecting the gastrocnemius and posterior calcaneus.

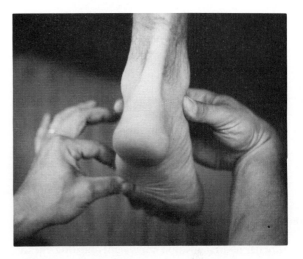

Fig. 26-5. Palpation of the talus to determine neutral position.

maximum inversion or one-third away from maximum eversion. The normal foot pronates 6 to 8 degrees from neutral.[28] For example, from neutral position a foot inverts 27 degrees and everts 3 degrees. The position at which this foot is neither pronated nor supinated is that point at which the calcaneus is inverted 7 degrees.

Forefoot-rearfoot relationship. Once the subtalar joint is placed in neutral position, mild dorsiflexion should be initiated while observing the metatarsal heads in relation to the plantar surface of the calcaneus. Forefoot varus is an osseous deformity in which the medial metatarsal heads are inverted in relation to the plane of the calcaneus (Figure 26-6). Forefoot varus is the most common cause of excessive pronation, according to Subotnick.[31] Forefoot valgus is a position in which the lateral metatarsals are everted in relation to the rearfoot (Figure 26-7). These forefoot deformities are benign in a nonweight–bearing position, but in stance the foot or metatarsal heads must somehow get to the floor to bear weight. This movement is accomplished by the talus rolling down and in and the calcaneus everting for a forefoot varus. For the forefoot valgus, the calcaneus inverts and the talus abducts and dorsiflexes. McPoil, Knecht, and Schmit[22] report that forefoot valgus is the most common forefoot deformity in their sample group.

In a rearfoot varus deformity, when the foot is in

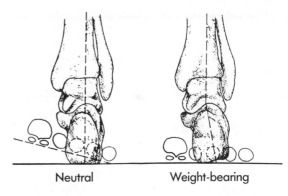

Neutral   Weight-bearing

Fig. 26-6. Forefoot varus. Comparing neutral and weight-bearing positions.

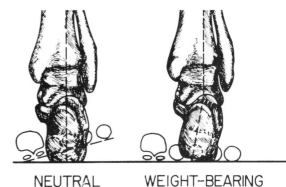

NEUTRAL   WEIGHT–BEARING

Fig. 26-7. Forefoot valgus. Comparing neutral and weight-bearing positions.

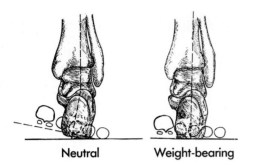

Neutral   Weight-bearing

Fig. 26-8. Rearfoot varus. Comparing neutral and weight-bearing positions.

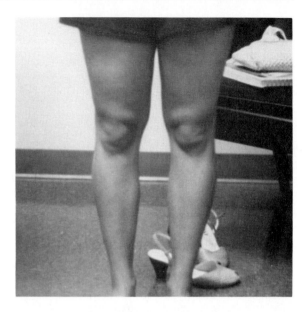

Fig. 26-9. Bowleg deformity.

subtalar neutral position nonweight−bearing, the medial metatarsal heads are inverted as in a forefoot varus, and the calcaneous is also in an inverted position. To get to footflat in weightbearing, the subtalar joint must pronate (Figure 26-8).

Minimal osseous deformities of the forefoot have little effect on the function of the foot. When either forefoot varus or valgus is too large, the foot compensates through abnormal movements to bear weight.

Extrinsic Factors

Several structural deformities originating outside the foot also require compensation by the foot for a proper weight-bearing position to be attained. Tibial varum is the common bowleg deformity.[21] The distal tibia is medial to the proximal tibia[11] (Figure 26-9). This measurement is taken weight bearing with the foot in neutral position.[35] The angle of deviation of the distal tibia from a perpendicular line from the calcaneal midline is considered tibial varum.[12]

Tibial varum increases pronation to allow proper foot function.[5] At heel strike the calcaneus must evert to attain a perpendicular position.[32]

Ankle joint equinus is another extrinsic deformity that may require abnormal compensation. It may be considered an extrinsic or intrinsic problem.

During normal gait, the tibia must move anterior to the talar dome.[21] Approximately 10 degrees of dorsiflexion is required for this movement[32] (Figure 26-10). Lack of dorsiflexion may cause compensatory pronation of the foot with resultant foot and lower extremity pain. Often this lack of dorsiflexion results from tightness of the posterior leg muscles. Other

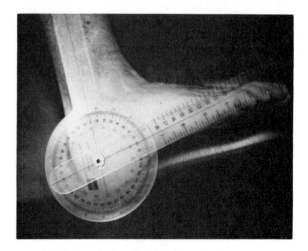

Fig. 26-10. Ten degrees of dorsiflexion.

causes include forefoot equinus, in which the plane of the forefoot is below the plane of the rearfoot.[32] It occurs in many high-arched feet. This deformity requires more ankle dorsiflexion. When enough dorsiflexion is not available at the ankle, the additional movement is required at other sites, such as dorsiflexion of the midtarsal joint and rotation of the leg.

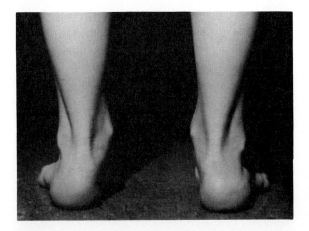

Fig. 26-11. Eversion of the calcaneus indicating pronation.

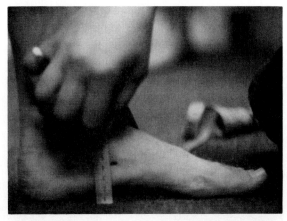

Fig. 26-12. Measurement of the navicular differential.

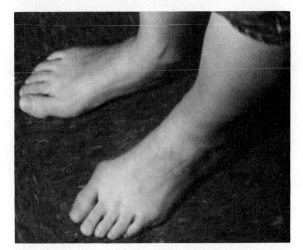

Fig. 26-13. Medial bulge of the talar head indicating pronation.

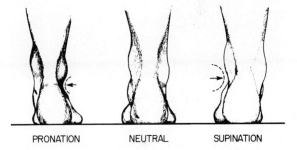

PRONATION   NEUTRAL   SUPINATION

Fig. 26-14. Concavity below the lateral malleolus indicating pronation.

IDENTIFICATION OF ATHLETES WITH EXCESSIVE PRONATION

An accurate biomechanical analysis of the foot and lower extremity should identify those deformities that require abnormal compensatory movements. Several extrinsic keys may be observed that indicate pronation.[28] Excessive eversion of the calcaneus during the stance phase indicates pronation (Figure 26-11). Excessive or prolonged internal rotation of the tibia is another sign of pronation. This internal rota-

tion may cause increased symptoms in the shin or knee, especially in repetitive sports such as running. A lowering of the medial arch accompanies pronation. It may be measured as the navicular differential,[9] the difference between the height of the navicular tuberosity from the floor in a nonweight–bearing position vs. a weight-bearing position (Figure 26-12). As previously discussed, the talus plantarflexes and adducts with pronation. It may be seen as a medial bulging of the talar head (Figure 26-13). This same talar adduction causes increased concavity below the lateral malleolus in a posterior view while the calcaneus everts[21] (Figure 26-14).

ORTHOTICS

Almost any problem of the lower extremity appears at one time to have been treated by orthotic therapy.

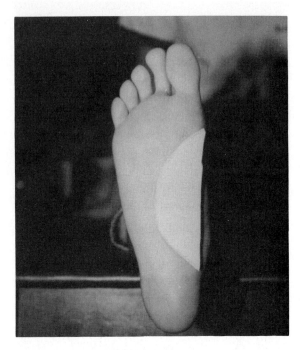

Fig. 26-15. Felt pads.

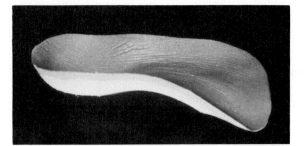

Fig. 26-16. Semirigid orthotics.

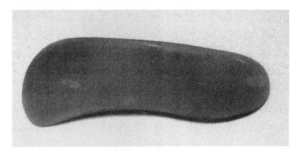

Fig. 26-17. Hard orthotic.

The use of orthotics in control of foot deformities has been argued for many years.* The normal foot functions most efficiently when no deformities are present that predispose it to injury or exacerbate existing injuries. Orthotics are used to control abnormal compensatory movements of the foot by "bringing the floor to the foot."

The foot functions most efficiently in neutral position. By providing support so that the foot does not have to move abnormally, an orthotic should help prevent compensatory problems. For problems that have already occurred, the orthotic provides a platform of support so that soft tissues can heal properly without undue stress.

Basically there are three types of orthotics:[18,32]

1. Pads and soft flexible felt supports (Figure 26-15). These soft inserts are readily fabricated and are advocated for mild overuse syndromes. Pads are particularly useful in shoes, such as spikes and ski boots, that are too narrow to hold orthotics.

2. Semirigid orthotics made of flexible thermoplastics, rubber, or leather (Figure 26-16). These orthotics are prescribed for athletes who have increased symptoms. These orthotics are molded from a neutral cast. They are well tolerated by athletes whose sports require speed or jumping.

3. Functional or rigid orthotics are made from hard plastic and also require neutral casting (Figure 26-17). These orthotics allow control for most overuse symptoms.

Despite arguments in the literature, the author has found orthotic therapy to be of tremendous value in the treatment of many lower extremity problems. This view is supported in the literature by several clinical studies. Donatelli et al.[10] found that 96% of their patients reported pain relief from orthotics and that 52% would not leave home without the devices in their shoes. McPoil, Adrian, and Pidcoe found that orthotics were an important treatment for valgus forefoot deformities only.[20] Riegler reported that 80% of his patients experienced at least a 50% improvement with orthotics.[26] This same study reported improvements in sports performance with orthotics. Hunt

*References 3, 7, 8, 13, 16, 27, 31, 32, 36.

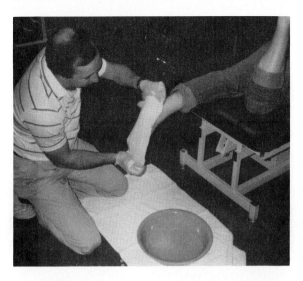

Fig. 26-18. Three layers of plaster form neutral mold.

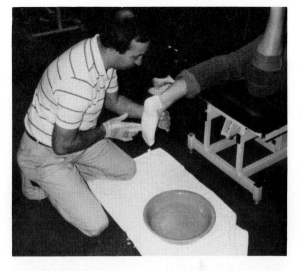

Fig. 26-19. Mild pressure over the fifth metatarsal to lock the midtarsal joint.

reported decreased muscular activity with orthotics.[15]

Orthotic Fabrication

Many sports therapists make a neutral mold, put it in a box, mail it to an orthotic laboratory, and several weeks later receive an orthotic back in the mail. Others like to complete the entire orthotic from start to finish, which requires a much more skilled technician than the mail-in method, as well as approximately $1000 in equipment and supplies. The obvious advantage is cost if many orthotics are to be made.

No matter which method is chosen, the first step is the fabrication of the neutral mold, done with the patient in the same position used to determine subtalar neutral position. Once subtalar neutral is found, three layers of plaster splints are applied to the plantar surface and sides of the foot (Figure 26-18). Subtalar neutral position is maintained as pressure is applied on the fifth metatarsal area in a dorsiflexion direction until the midtarsal joint is locked (Figure 26-19). This position is held until the plaster dries. At this point the plaster cast may be sent out to have the orthotic made or it may be finished (Figure 26-20). If it is mailed out, the appropriate measurements of forefoot and rearfoot positions should be sent, along with any extrinsic measurements.

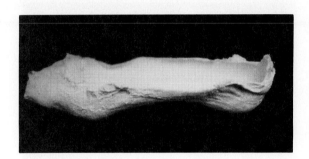

Fig. 26-20. Neutral mold.

If the orthotic is to be fabricated in-house, the plaster cast should be liberally lined interiorly with talc or powder. Plaster of paris should then be poured into the cast to form a positive mold of the foot (Figure 26-21).

Many different materials may be used to fabricate an orthotic from the positive mold. The author uses ⅛ inch Aliplast (Alimed Inc., Boston) covering with a ¼ inch Plastazote underneath. A rectangular piece of each material large enough to completely encompass the lower third of the mold is cut. These two pieces are placed in a convection oven (Figure 26-22) at approximately 275° F. At this temperature the two materials bond together and become moldable in about 5 to 7 minutes. At this time the orthotic

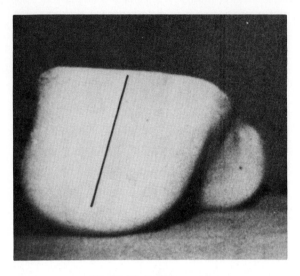

Fig. 26-21. Positive mold.

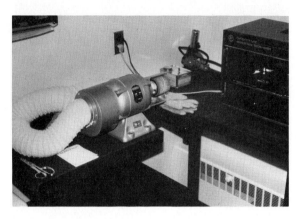

Fig. 26-22. Convection oven and grinder.

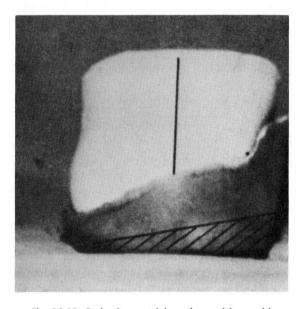

Fig. 26-23. Orthotic material on the positive mold.

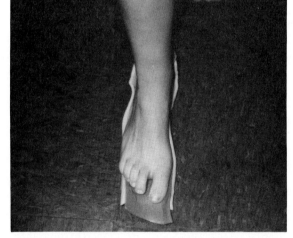

Fig. 26-24. Orthotic mold under the foot with patient sitting.

materials are removed from the oven and placed on the positive mold (Figure 26-23). Ideally a form or vacuum press should be used to form the orthotic to the mold.

Once cooled, the uncut orthotic is placed under the foot while the athlete sits in a chair (Figure 26-24). Excess material is then trimmed from the sides of the orthotic with scissors. Any material that can

be seen protruding from either side of the foot should be trimmed (Figure 26-25) to provide the proper width of the orthotic. The length should be trimmed so that the end of the orthotic bisects the metatarsal heads (Figure 26-26). This style is slightly longer than most orthotics are made, but the author has found that this length provides better comfort.

Next a third layer of medial Plastazote may be

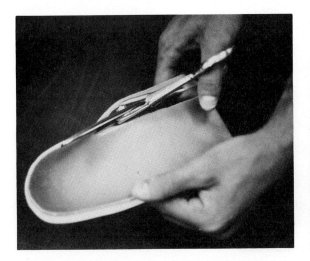

Fig. 26-25. Trim excess material from orthotic.

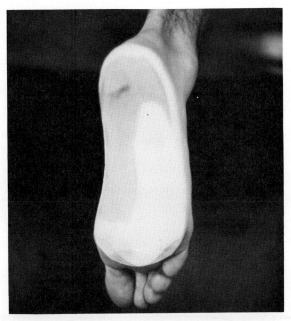

Fig. 26-26. The length of the orthotic should bisect the metatarsal heads.

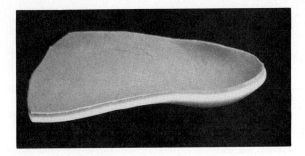

Fig. 26-27. Sides of the orthotic should be leveled inward.

glued to the arch to fill that area to the floor. Grinding begins with the sides of the orthotic, which should be ground so that the sides are slightly beveled inward (Figure 26-27) to allow better shoe fit. The bottom of the orthotic is leveled so that the surface is perpendicular to the bisection of the calcaneus. Grinding is continued until very little Plastazote remains under the Aliplast at the heel. The forefoot is posted by selectively grinding Plastazote just proximal to the metatarsal heads. Forefoot varus is posted by grinding more laterally than medially. Forefoot valgus requires grinding more medially than laterally. The final step is to grind the distal portion of the orthotic so that only a very thin piece of Aliplast is under the area where the orthotic ends. This prevents discomfort under the forefoot where the orthotic stops. If the athlete feels that this area is a problem, a full insole of Spenco or other material may be used to cover the orthotic to the end of the shoe to eliminate the drop off sometimes felt as the orthotic ends. Time must be allowed for proper break-in. The athlete should wear the orthotic for 3 to 4 hours the first day, 6 to 8 hours the next day, and then all day on the third day. Sports activities should be started with the orthotic only after it has been worn all day for several days.

SHOE SELECTION

The shoe is one of the biggest considerations in treating a foot problem. Even a properly made orthotic is less effective if placed in a poorly constructed shoe.

As noted, pronation is a problem of hypermobility. Pronated feet need stability and firmness to reduce this excess movement. Research indicates that shoe compression may actually increase pronation vs. a barefoot condition.[2] The ideal shoe for a pronated foot is less flexible and has good rearfoot control.

Conversely, supinated feet are usually very rigid. Increased cushion and flexibility benefit this type of foot. Several construction factors may influence the firmness and stability of a shoe. The basic form upon which a shoe is built is called the *last*.[2] The upper is fitted onto a last in several ways. Each method has its own flexibility and control characteristics. A slip-

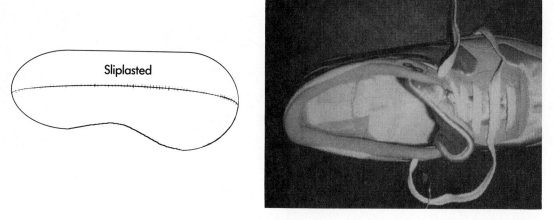

Fig. 26-28. Slip-lasted shoe.

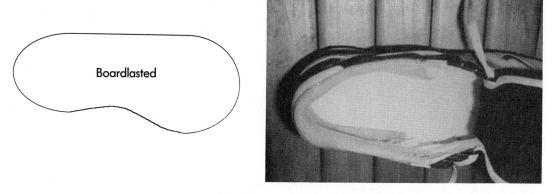

Fig. 26-29. Board-lasted shoe.

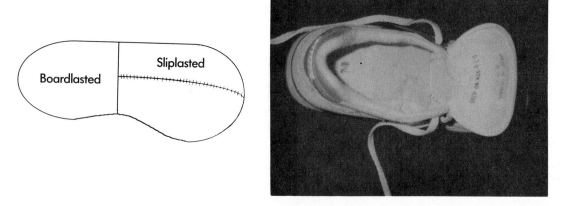

Fig. 26-30. Combination-lasted shoe.

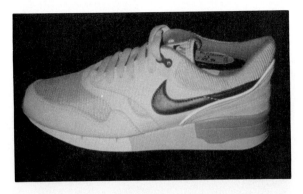

Fig. 26-31. EVA in a midsole.

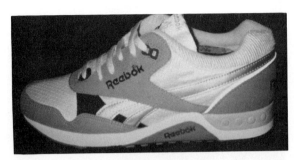

Fig. 26-32. External heel counter.

lasted shoe is sewn together like a moccasin (Figure 26-28) and is very flexible. Board-lasting provides a piece of fiberboard upon which the upper is attached (Figure 26-29), which provides a very firm, inflexible base for the shoe. A combination-lasted shoe is boarded in the back half of the shoe and slip-lasted in the front (Figure 26-30), which provides rearfoot stability with forefoot mobility. The shape of the last may also be used in shoe selection. Most athletes with excessive pronation perform better in a straight-lasted shoe,[2] that is, a shoe in which the forefoot does not curve inward in relation to the rearfoot. Midsole design also affects the stability of a shoe. The midsole separates the upper from the outsole.[6] Ethylene vinyl acetate (EVA) is one of the most commonly used materials in the midsole.[25] Often denser EVA, which is colored differently to show that it is denser, is placed under the medial aspect of the foot to control pronation (Figure 26-31).

In an effort to control rearfoot movement, many shoe manufacturers have reinforced the heel counter both internally and externally, often in the form of extra plastic along the outside of the heel counter[19] (Figure 26-32).

Other factors that may affect the performance of a shoe are the outsole contour and composition, lacing systems, and forefoot wedges.

Shoe Wear Patterns

Athletes with excessive pronation often wear out the front of the running shoe under the second metatarsal (Figure 26-33). Shoe wear patterns are commonly misinterpreted by athletes who think they must be

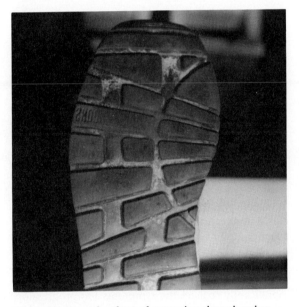

Fig. 26-33. Front forefoot of a running shoe showing the typical wear pattern of a pronator.

pronators because they wear out the back outside edges of their heels. Actually, most people wear out the back outside edges of their shoes. Just before heelstrike, the anterior tibial muscle fires to prevent the foot from slapping forward. The anterior tibial muscle not only dorsiflexes the foot but also slightly inverts it, hence the wear pattern on the back edge of the shoe. The key to inspection of wear patterns on shoes is observation of the heel counter and the forefoot.

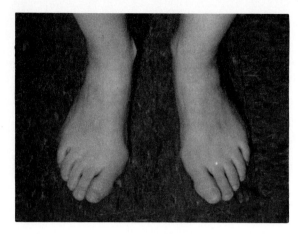

Fig. 26-34. Bunion.

PATHOLOGIES OF THE FOOT

Many of the problems of the foot are biomechanically related. The symptoms of these biomechanical problems may appear in the foot or lower extremity. Even trauma-induced injuries to the foot may be treated by orthotic therapy, as well as modalities and exercises.

Bunions

A bunion is a deformity of the head of the first metatarsal in which the large toe takes a valgus position[1] (Figure 26-34). Many bunions are the result of a biomechanical fault that causes a hypermobility of the first ray segment. Often a neutral orthotic that increases the weight-bearing properties of the first ray significantly reduces the symptoms and progressions of a bunion.[32] Shoe selection may also play an important role in the treatment of bunions. Shoes of the proper width cause less irritation to the bunion area, especially if exostosis is involved from a chronic bunion. Local therapy, including moist heat, soaks, and ultrasound, may alleviate some of the acute symptoms of a bunion. Protective devices such as wedges, pads, and tape can also be used.[1]

Neuroma

A neuroma is a neuromatous mass occurring about the nerve sheath of the common plantar nerve while it divides into the two digital branches to adjacent

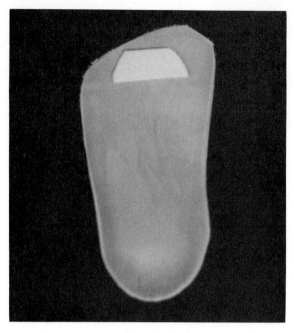

Fig. 26-35. Metatarsal bar.

toes. It occurs most commonly between the metatarsal heads and is the most common nerve problem of the lower extremity. A neuroma may occur in any metatarsal space, but the most common site is the third interspace.[32] Orthotic therapy is essential to reduce the shearing movements of the metatarsal heads. To increase this effect, often a bar is placed just proximal to the metatarsal heads in an attempt to have these splay apart with weight bearing (Figure 26-35). It may decrease pressure on the affected area. The author has used phonophoresis with hydrocortisone with some success in symptom reduction. Shoe selection also plays an important role in treatment of neuromas. Narrow shoes, particularly women's shoes that are pointed in the toe area and certain men's boots, may squeeze the metatarsal heads together and exacerbate the problem. A shoe that is wide in the toe box area should be selected. A straight-laced shoe often provides increased space in the toe box.[29]

Turf Toe

Turf toe is a hyperextension injury of the great toe, either from repetitive overuse or trauma.[34] Many of these injuries occur on unyielding synthetic turf, al-

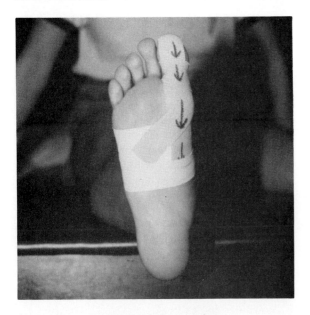

Fig. 26-36. Turf toe taping.

though it can occur on grass also. The author believes that many of these injuries occur because artificial turf shoes often are more flexible and allow more dorsiflexion of the great toe. Some shoe companies have addressed this problem by adding steel or other materials to the forefoot of their turf shoes to stiffen them. Flat insoles that have thin sheets of steel under the forefoot are also available. When commercially made products are not available, a thin, flat piece of Orthoplast may be placed under the shoe insole or may be molded to the foot.[34] Taping the toe to prevent dorsiflexion may be done separately or with one of the shoe stiffening suggestions (Figure 26-36).

Modalities of choice include ice and ultrasound. One of the major ingredients in any treatment for turf toe is rest. The athlete should be discouraged from returning to activity until the toe is pain free.

Plantar Fasciitis

Heel pain is a very common problem in the athletic and nonathletic population. This phenomenon has been blamed on several etiologies, including heel spurs, plantar fascia irritation, and bursitis. Plantar fasciitis is a catch-all term that is commonly used to describe pain in the proximal arch and heel.

The complaints are similar: early pain in the medial arch and medial distal heel that moves to a more central or lateral distribution in the late course of the problem. This pain is particularly troublesome upon arising in the morning or upon bearing weight after sitting for a long period. Orthotic therapy is very useful in the treatment of this problem. The author has found that soft orthotics in combination with exercises can significantly reduce the pain level of these patients.

A soft orthotic works better than a hard orthotic. An extra-deep heel cup should be built into the orthotic. The orthotic should be worn at all times, especially upon arising from bed in the morning. Always have the athlete step into the orthotic rather than ambulating barefooted. When soft orthotics are not feasible, taping may reduce the symptoms. A simple arch taping or alternative taping often allows pain-free ambulation.[38]

Vigorous heelcord stretching should be used, along with an exercise to stretch the plantar fascia in the arch. The old-fashioned exercise of rolling the arch over a rolling pin accomplishes this. The athlete should be cautioned not to roll over the heel area, which usually exacerbates the problem. Another stretch is the use of the "windless" mechanism by controlled dorsiflexion of the talocrural joint and extension of the metatarsophylangeal (MP) joints. Exercises that increase dorsiflexion of the great toe also may be of benefit to this problem.

Cuboid Subluxation

Another problem that often mimics plantar fasciitis is cuboid subluxation. Pronation and trauma have been reported to be prominent causes of this syndrome.[37] This displacement of the cuboid causes pain along the fourth and fifth metatarsals, as well as over the cuboid. This problem often refers pain to the heel area as well. Many times this pain is increased upon arising after a prolonged nonweight–bearing period. Dramatic treatment results may be obtained by manipulating to restore the cuboid to its natural position. The manipulation is done with the athlete prone (Figure 26-37). The plantar aspect of the forefoot is grasped by the thumbs with the fingers supporting the dorsum of the foot. The thumbs should be over the cuboid. The manipulation should be a thrust downward to move the cuboid into its more dorsal position. Often a pop is felt as the cuboid moves back into place. Once the cuboid is manipulated, an orthotic often helps to support it in its proper position.

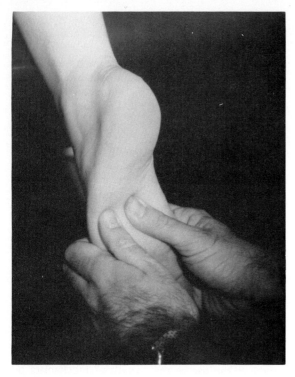

Fig. 26-37. Prone position for cuboid manipulation.

Tarsal Tunnel Syndrome

The tarsal tunnel is a loosely defined area about the medial malleolus that is bordered by the retinaculum, which binds the tibial nerve.[13] Pronation, overuse problems such as tendinitis, and trauma may cause neurovascular problems in the ankle and foot. Symptoms may vary, with pain, numbness, and paresthesia reported along the medial ankle and into the sole of the foot.[4] Tenderness may be present over the tibial nerve area behind the medial malleolus. Neutral foot control may alleviate symptoms in less involved cases. Surgery is often performed if symptoms do not respond to conservative treatment or if weakness occurs in the flexors of the toes.[4]

SUMMARY

1. The foot changes gait to provide for forward movement, adapt to uneven terrain, and absorb shock.
2. The subtalar and midtarsal joints contribute significantly to the stability of the foot. Dysfunction at either joint may have a profound effect on the foot and lower extremity.
3. Certain intrinsic and extrinsic deformities may cause dysfunction at the subtalar and midtarsal joints.
4. Examination of the foot should focus on intrinsic and extrinsic deformities of the foot.
5. Individuals with excessive pronation may be identified by several extrinsic keys.
6. Orthotics may be of great benefit in the treatment of biomechanical problems of the foot and leg. Neutral casting is essential for the production of an orthotic, whether it is to be produced in-house or by someone else.
7. Shoe selection is an important parameter in the treatment of foot problems. Various shoe components may dictate the type of foot that a shoe best suits.
8. Of the many possible pathologies in the foot, many may be treated by orthotic therapy, as well as by modalities and exercise.

REFERENCES

1 Arnheim D, Prentice W: *Principles of athletic training,* St Louis, 1993, Mosby.
2 Baer T: Designing for the long run, *Mech Eng,* pp 67-75, Sept 1984.
3 Bates BT, Osternig L, Mason B, et al.: Foot orthotic devices to modify selected aspects of lower extremity mechanics, *Am J Sports Med* 7:338, 1979.
4 Birnham JS: *The musculoskeletal manual,* 1982, Academic Press.
5 Brody DM: Techniques in the evaluation and treatment of the injured runner, *Orthop Clin North Am* 13:541, 1982.
6 Brunwich T, Wischnia B: Battle of the midsoles, *Runners World,* p 47, April 1987.
7 Cavanaugh PR: *An evaluation of the effects of orthotics force distribution and rearfoot movement during running.* Paper presented at a meeting of the American Orthopedic Society for Sports Medicine, Lake Placid, NY, 1978.
8 Collona P: Fabrication of a custom molded orthotic using an intrinsic posting technique for a forefoot varus deformity, *Phys Ther Forum* 8(5):3, 1989.
9 Delacerda FG: A study of anatomical factors involved in shin-splints, *J Orthop Sports Phys Ther* 2:55-59, 1980.
10 Donatelli R: Normal biomechanics of the foot and ankle, *J Orthop Sports Phys Ther* 7:91-95, 1985.
11 Donatelli R, Hurlbert C, Conaway D, et al.: Biomechanical foot orthotics: a retrospective study, *J Orthop Sports Phys Ther* 10:205-212, 1988.
12 Giallonardo LM: Clinical evaluation of foot and ankle dysfunction, *Phys Ther* 68:1850-1856, 1988.
13 Gill E: Orthotics, *Runners World,* pp 55-57, Feb 1985.
14 Hoppenfield S: *Physical examination of the spine and extremities,* New York, 1976, Appleton-Century-Crofts.

15 Hunt G: *Examination of lower extremity dysfunction.* In Gould J, Davies G, editors: *Orthopedic and sports physical therapy,* vol 2, St Louis, 1985, Mosby.

16 James SL: *Chondromalacia of the patella in the adolescent.* In Kennedy SC, editor: *The injured adolescent,* Baltimore, 1979, Williams & Wilkins.

17 James SL, Bates BT, Osternig LR: Injuries to runners, *Am J Sports Med* 6:43, 1978.

18 Lockard MA: Foot orthoses, *Phys Ther* 68:1866-1873, 1988.

19 McPoil TG: Footwear, *Phys Ther* 68:1857-1865, 1988.

20 McPoil TG, Adrian M, Pidcoe P: Effects of foot orthoses on center of pressure patterns in women, *Phys Ther* 69:149-154, 1989.

21 McPoil TG, Brocato RS: *The foot and ankle: biomechanical evaluation and treatment.* In Gould J, Davies G, editors: *Orthopedic and sports physical therapy,* St Louis, 1985, Mosby.

22 McPoil TG, Knecht HG, Schmit D: A survey of foot types in normal females between the ages of 18 and 30 years, *J Orthop Sports Phys Ther* 9:406-409, 1988.

23 Morton DJ: Foot disorders in general practice, *JAMA* 109:1112-1119, 1937.

24 Oatis CA: Biomechanics of the foot and ankle under static conditions, *Phys Ther* 68:1815-1821, 1988.

25 Pagliano JN: Athletic footwear, *Sports Med Digest* 10:1-2, 1988.

26 Riegler HF: Orthotic devices for the foot, *Orthop Rev* 16:293-303, 1987.

27 Rogers MM, LeVeau BF: Effectiveness of foot orthotic devices used to modify pronation in runners, *J Orthop Sports Phys Ther* 4:86-90, 1982.

28 Root ML, Orien WP, Weed JH: *Normal and abnormal functions of the foot,* Los Angeles, 1977, Clinical Biomechanics.

29 Sims DS, Cavanaugh PR, Ulbrecht JS: Risk factors in the diabetic foot, *Phys Ther* 68:1887-1901, 1988.

30 Subotnick SI: *The running foot doctor,* Mt Vias, Calif, 1977, World Publications.

31 Subotnick SI: The flat foot, *Phys Sports Med* 9:85-91, 1981.

32 Subotnick SI, Newell SG: *Podiatric sports medicine,* Mt Kisko, NY, 1975, Futura Publishing.

33 Tiberio D: Pathomechanics of structural foot deformities, *Phys Ther* 68:1840-1849, 1988.

34 Visnich AL: A playing orthoses for "turf toe," *Ath Train* 22:215, 1987.

35 Vogelbach WD, Combs LC: A biomechanical approach to the management of chronic lower extremity pathologies as they relate to excessive pronation, *Ath Train* 22:6-16, 1987.

36 Williams JGP: The foot and chondromalacia—a case of biomechanical uncertainty, *J Orthop Sports Phys Ther* 2:50-51, 1980.

37 Woods A, Smith W: Cuboid syndrome and the techniques used for treatment, *Ath Train* 18:64-65, 1983.

38 Zylks DR: Alternative taping for plantar fasciitis, *Ath Train* 22:317, 1987.

Index